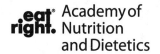

Academy of
Nutrition
and Dietetics

P9-DEA-392

Research
Successful Approaches

Third Edition

Elaine R. Monsen, PhD, RD, and
Linda Van Horn, PhD, RD, Editors

10 9 8 7 6 5

Library of Congress Cataloging-in-Publication Data

Research: successful approaches / Elaine R. Monsen and Linda Van Horn, editors.— 3rd ed.
   p. ; cm.
Includes bibliographical references and index.
   ISBN 978-0-88091-415-4
   1. Nutrition—Research. 2. Dietetics—Research. I. Monsen, Elaine R. II. Van Horn, Linda.
III. American Dietetic Association.
   [DNLM: 1. Nutrition Physiology. 2. Research Design. 3. Data Collection. 4. Dietetics—methods.
5. Epidemiologic Methods. QU 145 R432 2008]

   TX367.R46 2008
   613.2072—dc22
                                                                              2007026887

Contributors

Editors

Elaine R. Monsen, PhD, RD
Editor Emeritus, *Journal of the American Dietetic Association*
Professor Emeritus, Nutrition and Medicine, University of Washington
Seattle, WA

Linda Van Horn, PhD, RD
Professor, Preventive Medicine and Associate Dean for Faculty Development, Northwestern University Feinberg School of Medicine
Editor-in-Chief, *Journal of the American Dietetic Association*
Chicago, IL

Authors

Cheryl L. Achterberg, PhD
Dean, College of Human Sciences, Iowa State University
Ames, IA

Sujata Archer, PhD, RD
Research Assistant Professor, Northwestern University Feinberg School of Medicine
Chicago, IL

Susan I. Barr, PhD, RD
Professor of Nutrition, University of British Columbia
Vancouver, BC, Canada

Judith Beto, PhD, RD
Department Chairperson and Professor, Nutrition Sciences Director, Didactic Program in Dietetics, Dominican University
River Forest, IL

Karil Bialostosky, MS
Deputy Director, Cleveland Department of Public Health
Cleveland, OH

Susan T. Borra, RD
President, International Food Information Council Foundation
Washington, DC

Carol J. Boushey, PhD, MPH, RD
Associate Professor, Department of Foods and Nutrition, Purdue University
West Lafayette, IN

Maureen Brady Moran, MPH
Assistant Professor of Preventive Medicine, Northwestern University Feinberg School of Medicine
Chicago, IL

Ronette R. Briefel, DrPH, RD
Senior Fellow, Mathematica Policy Research
Washington, DC

Suzanne Brodney Folse, PhD, RD
Manager, Research and Outcomes, Health and
    Wellness Institute
Providence, RI

Barbara Bruemmer, PhD, RD
Senior Lecturer, Department of Epidemiology, Nutritional
    Sciences Program Director, Didactic Program in
    Dietetics School of Public Health and Community
    Medicine, University of Washington
Seattle, WA

Laura Byham-Gray, PhD, RD
Associate Professor, Department of Nutritional Sciences,
    University of Medicine and Dentistry of New Jersey
Stratford, NJ

Alicia L. Carriquiry, PhD
Professor of Statistics, Iowa State University
Ames, IA

Mary Cluskey, PhD, RD
Associate Professor, Dietetic Program Director, Department
    of Nutrition and Exercise Sciences, Oregon State University
Corvallis, OR

Beverly Cowart, PhD
Member, Monell Chemical Senses Center
Scientific Director, Monell-Jefferson Taste and Smell Clinic
Philadelphia, PA

Judy A Driskell, PhD, RD
Professor of Nutrition and Health Sciences, University of
    Nebraska
Lincoln, NE

Bonnie L. Gerald, PhD, DTR
Associate Professor of Nutrition and Food Systems,
    University of Southern Mississippi
Hattiesburg, MS

Judith A. Gilbride, PhD, RD, FADA
Department of Nutrition, Food Studies and Public Health,
    New York University
New York, NY

Shelley Goldberg, MPH, RD
Director, Nutrition Communications, International Food
    Information Council
Washington, DC

Geoffery W. Greene, PhD, RD
Professor, Director Dietetic Internship, Department of
    Nutrition and Food Sciences, University of
    Rhode Island
Kingston, RI

Mary B. Gregoire, PhD, RD, FADA
Director, Food and Nutrition Services, Rush University
    Medical Center
Professor and Interim Chair, Clinical Nutrition, Professor,
    Health Systems Management, Rush University
Chicago, IL

Amy E. Griel, PhD
Dietetic intern, Pennsylvania State University
University Park, PA

Jean H. Hankin, DrPH, RD
Researcher, Professor Emeritus
Cancer Research Center, University of Hawaii
Honolulu, HI

Jeffrey E. Harris, DrPH, MPH, RD
Associate Professor and Dietetics Program Director,
    Department of Health, West Chester University
West Chester, PA

James Hollis, PhD
Lecturer in Predictive Nutrition, Institute of Agri-food
    and Land Use
School of Biological Sciences, Queen's University Belfast
Belfast, Northern Ireland

Rachel K. Johnson, PhD, MPH, RD
Dean, College of Agriculture, and Life Sciences Professor
    of Nutrition, University of Vermont
Burlington, VT

Penny M. Kris-Etherton, PhD, RD
Distinguished Professor of Nutrition, Department of
    Nutritional Sciences, Penn State University
University Park, PA

Johanna W. Lampe, PhD, RD
Full Member and Associate Division Director, Cancer
    Prevention Program, Division of Public Health Sciences,
    Fred Hutchinson Cancer Research Center
Seattle, WA

Richard D. Mattes, PhD, RD
Professor of Foods and Nutrition, Department of Foods and
Nutrition, Purdue University
West Lafayette, IN

Shortie McKinney, PhD, RD, FADA
Dean, College of Health Professions, Marshall University
Huntington, WV

Barbara E. Millen, DPH, RD, FADA
Professor of Family Medicine, Department of Family
Medicine Chair, Graduate Programs in Medical Nutrition
Sciences, Boston University School of Medicine
Boston, MA

Elaine R. Monsen, PhD, RD
Editor Emeritus, *Journal of the American Dietetic
Association*
Professor Emeritus, Nutrition and Medicine, University
of Washington
Seattle, WA

Suzanne Murphy, PhD, RD
Nutrition Researcher, Cancer Research Center of Hawaii,
University of Hawaii
Honolulu, HI

Esther F. Myers, PhD, RD, FADA
Director, Scientific Affairs and Research
American Dietetic Association
Chicago, IL

Dianne Neumark-Sztainer, MPH, PhD, RD
Professor, Division of Epidemiology and Community
Health, University of Minnesota
Minneapolis, MN

Ruth E. Patterson, PhD
Director Medical Writing, Amylin Pharmaceuticals, Inc.
San Diego, CA

Jean A.T. Pennington, PhD, RD
National Institutes of Health
Bethesda, MD

Tricia L. Psota, BS
Research Assistant, Pennsylvania State University
University Park, PA

Colleen A. Redding, PhD
Research Professor, Cancer Prevention Research Center,
University of Rhode Island
Kingston, RI

Cheryl L. Rock, PhD, RD, FADA
Professor, Department of Family and Preventive Medicine,
School of Medicine, University of California, San Diego
La Jolla, CA

Leila Saldanha, PhD, RD
President/Managing Member, NutrIQ LLC
Alexandria, VA

Madeleine Sigman-Grant, PhD, RD
Professor and Area Extension Specialist, University of
Nevada Cooperative Extension
Las Vegas, NV

Patricia L. Splett, PhD, RD, FADA
Evaluation Consultant, Splett and Associates, LLC
Adjunct Associate Professor, Nutrition Graduate Program,
University of Minnesota
St. Paul, MN

Cynthia A. Thomson, PhD, RD, FADA
Associate Professor, College of Agriculture and Life
Sciences, University of Arizona
Tucson, AZ

Michele Tuttle, MPH, RD
Nutrition Communications Consultant, Tuttle
Communications
Columbia, MD

Linda Van Horn, PhD, RD
Professor, Preventive Medicine and Associate Dean for
Faculty Development
Northwestern University, Feinberg School of Medicine
Editor-in-Chief, *Journal of the American Dietetic
Association*
Chicago, IL

Jacqueline A. Vernarelli, MS
Research Assistant, Alzheimer's Disease Clinical and
Research Program, Boston University School of
Medicine
Boston, MA

Susan Wohlsdorf-Arendt, PhD, RD
Assistant Professor, Apparel, Educational Studies and
    Hospitality Management, Iowa State University
Ames, IA

Monica E. Yamamoto, DrPH, RD, FADA
Assistant Professor, Department of Epidemiology, School
    of Public Health, University of Pittsburgh
Pittsburgh, PA

Bethany A. Yon, MS
Public Health Nutritionist, Vermont Department of Health
Rutland, VT

Reviewers

Jamie Benedict, PhD, RD
Associate Professor, Nutrition Department, University of
    Nevada, Reno
Reno, NV

LuAnn Soliah, PhD, RD
Professor and Director of Nutrition Sciences
Baylor University, Waco, TX

Second Edition Contributing Authors

Cheryl L. Achterberg, PhD
Sujata Archer, PhD, RD
Karil Bialostosky, MS
Alma J. Blake, PhD, RD
Carol J. Boushey, PhD, MPH, RD
Ronette R. Briefel, DrPH, RD
Lisa Brown, MPH, DSc

Jean C. Burge, PhD, RD
Carrie L. Cheney†, PhD, RD
Ronni Chernoff, PhD, RD, FADA
Anne Dattilo, PhD, RD, CDE
Barbara H. Dennis, PhD, RD
Judith A. Ernst, DMSc, RD
Judith A. Gilbride, PhD, RD, FADA
Geoffery W. Greene, PhD, RD
Mary B. Gregoire, PhD, RD, FADA
Jean H. Hankin, DrPH, RD
Rachel K. Johnson, PhD, MPH, RD
Mark Kestin, PhD, MPH
P.M. Kris-Etherton, PhD, RD
Johanna W. Lampe, PhD, RD
Richard D. Mattes, MPH, PhD, RD
Esther F. Myers, PhD, RD, FADA
Sara C. Parks, PhD, RD
Ruth E. Patterson, PhD, RD
Jean A.T. Pennington, PhD, RD
Judy E. Perkin, DrPH, RD
Cheryl L. Rock, PhD, RD, FADA
M. Rosita Schiller, PhD, RD, FADA
Sandra K. Shepherd, PhD, RD
Bettylou Sherry, PhD, RD
Margaret D. Simko†, PhD, RD, FADA
Jeannie Sneed, PhD, RD
Patricia L. Splett, PhD, RD, FADA
Linda Van Horn, PhD, RD
Carol West Suitor, DSc, RD
Monica E. Yamamoto, DrPH, RD, FADA

†Deceased

Acknowledgments

It was with great pleasure that I asked Linda Van Horn, PhD, RD, and current Editor-in-Chief of the *Journal of the American Dietetic Association* to join me as co-editor of the current edition of *Research: Successful Approaches.* Linda has great clarity of mind and is highly knowledgeable of the diverse areas of dietetics and nutrition research. Her contributions are greatly appreciated.

We both want to recognize the strong support and excellent management that Pamela Woolf, development editor for the American Dietetic Association, has provided over many months. Pamela is professionally focused. She combines steady steering with confirming encouragement, thus ensuring a quality and completed project. Also, Elizabeth Nishiura, ADA's production manager, and David Greenstein, administrative assistant, made valuable contributions. We thank each of you.

Above all, we as editors, and you as readers, are indebted to the excellent authors who contributed so much to the chapters of this book. These authors are experts in their respective fields, and we are grateful to each of them for sharing their expertise with us. It is our hope that you, the readers, will find great value in the multiple components of this text and apply the principles regularly to your own work in nutrition. Research provides the evidence that validates the field of nutrition, thereby supplying the rationale for a career in dietetics. Research is the future.

Elaine R. Monsen, PhD, RD
Editor Emeritus, Journal of the American
Dietetic Association

Contents

Foreword

Since the first edition of *Research: Successful Approaches* was published in 1992, research has played an increasingly prominent role in the American Dietetic Association (ADA). The current ADA philosophy is that "research is the foundation of the profession, providing the basis for practice, education, and policy." More specifically, the Standards of Professional Practice state that each dietetics professional needs to effectively apply, participate in, or generate research to enhance practice. This new edition of *Research: Successful Approaches* is an invaluable resource to meet this standard.

Of the 29 ADA dietetic practice groups, only one, the Research Dietetic Practice Group, has the mission of leading the future of dietetics by promoting the conduct and application of research related to food, nutrition, and dietetics. Our members are the most valued source for conducting, interpreting, and applying research related to food, nutrition, and dietetics. As a profession, we are uniquely positioned for translational research, especially the dissemination of nutrition interventions for improving the health and quality of life of the American population. Consequently, we enthusiastically support the use of this third edition by all professionals engaged in nutrition research.

Dr. Elaine R. Monsen and Dr. Linda Van Horn both have distinguished careers in research and have worked tirelessly to make the *Journal of the American Dietetic Association* the premier journal that it is today. These editors have compiled an august group of researchers for this third edition. The continuum of the research process is addressed from asking the question to writing up the results. Timely and tactical, new chapters include ones on multidisciplinary research (Chapter 5); appetite assessment (Chapter 19); and dietary supplements and complementary and alternative medicine (Chapter 23).

Research drives the profession—for nutrition students, practitioners, and researchers. We believe that the third edition of *Research: Successful Approaches* will advance, promote, and further accelerate nutrition research. Accordingly, we encourage members to use this book and get involved in research. The rewards will be life-long, not only for you as an individual, but also for the populations you serve and the profession at large. Happy reading, researching, and writing!

David H. Holben, PhD, RD
Chair, Research Dietetic Practice Group 2006–2007

Debra A. Krummel, PhD, RD
Chair, Research Dietetic Practice Group 2007–2008

PART 1

An Introduction to Discovery Through Research in Nutrition and Dietetics

1

—ᴍ—

Steering Through the Research Continuum

Linda Van Horn, PhD, RD, and Elaine R. Monsen, PhD, RD

Through well-designed, well-conducted, and carefully analyzed research, our profession advances. Initially, one needs to clearly identify the problem to be studied and select an appropriate research design (eg, observational or experimental). The research site and the selection of participants are important in setting up the parameters of data collection and ensuring that the outcomes support answers to the questions being asked. Once data are available, they need to be analyzed, interpreted, and presented. Through the evidence of the research, decisions can be made that will affect dietetics practice. Future research is generally born from current research; thus, the continuum continues. Steer carefully, and keep your eyes on the road—it is an exciting process.

FORCES FOR RESEARCH

As described by Monsen (1), there are at least four driving forces for research that continue to influence ongoing studies of nutrition. These include recognizing the unexpected, extending existing information, point-counterpoint, and responding to socioeconomic and political environment.

Recognizing the Unexpected

An exciting by-product of a study may lead to the identification of new areas for research. This is more commonly known as the "Aha" moment. The discovery

of the first vitamin is a clear example of recognizing the unexpected. In the 18th century, a British naval surgeon, James Lind, gave a great deal of thought to the prevalence of scurvy among English sailors. The disease was particularly rampant on long voyages. In 1747, Lind completed the first controlled dietary study, in which he proved that citrus fruits cured scurvy. Six years later, he published his treatise (2), and in 1796, 43 years after his publication, the British navy officially introduced lemon juice as a prophylactic against scurvy. More than a century later, in 1906, the concept of accessory food factors was introduced. In 1932, 185 years after Lind's first controlled study, crystalline vitamin C was prepared from lemon juice.

We cannot plan for the breakthrough, but we need to be unceasingly alert for the unexpected. For example, recent findings from the Women's Health Initiative indicate that use of progestin-containing hormone therapy is associated with increased risk of postmenopausal breast cancer (3–5).

Extending Existing Information

Going beyond what is known to better understand what is not known remains a compelling force for research. A classic example is the discovery of the second vitamin. After the idea of accessory food factors was introduced to the scientific community, there was a great deal of research devoted to ascertaining whether other food factors existed, where these food factors were, and what effects they had. From 1913 to 1916, research teams led by McCullum, Osborn, and Mendel (6,7) observed and isolated components from foods that they termed "Fat Soluble A" and "Water Soluble B." Shortly, Fat Soluble A was partitioned into vitamins A, D, E, and K, and Water Soluble B developed into the long series of B vitamins (8). This search for accessory food factors was a highly productive extension of the earlier discovery of vitamin C.

A more current example is the study of glycemic index and glycemic load. Whether these two factors will prove to be vitally related to the development of insulin resistance and/or type 2 diabetes remains to be seen, but awareness that these factors affect postprandial glucose/insulin response offers a new and compelling area for nutrition research (9–11).

Point-Counterpoint

The point-counterpoint concept involves actions and reactions. A current example is the explosion of "functional foods" that have been developed by the food industry, presumably to conveniently meet the nutrient needs of busy people without imposing on them the hassle of buying and preparing raw ingredients. Whether these foods are indeed helpful because of their nutrient contributions—or perhaps are harmful because they introduce extra calories, sugar, salt or other factors—remains to be documented. However, the presence of these products continues to have a growing influence on the modern American diet (12).

Responding to the Socioeconomic and Political Environment

The Special Supplemental Food Program for Women, Infants and Children (WIC) is an outstanding response to the socioeconomic and political environment. Dietetics and nutrition have soared as important influences in WIC. Evaluation and documentation of the WIC program and kindred research are among the prime reasons that the program has been so successful and aided so many citizens. Another example of research undertaken in response to socioeconomic conditions is the Obesity Guidelines produced by the National Heart, Lung, and Blood Institute in response to awareness of the growing obesity epidemic in the United States (13). Ongoing concerns regarding homelessness raise issues related to economic opportunity, needed support of physical and mental health,

and adequate nutrition. Applied research on these topics has the promise of ameliorating such difficult problems.

Public interest in quality nutrition care has been underscored during recent discussions on health care reform. Nutrition has been recognized as a major component in health promotion and disease prevention. Economically, it is logical to include adequate nutrition and access to quality nutrition care in any basic health care benefit package. At least two desirable results will occur if health can be improved through better nutrition: higher quality of life and lower health care costs.

RESEARCH IN THE MODERN ERA

Nutrition research has never been more exciting or more challenging. The forces for research continue to influence new studies and their findings. Registered dietitians (RDs) have the opportunity to take an active role by designing both basic science and clinical studies that will position nutrition as a tool for prevention and treatment of disease in new and evidence-based ways. This is the era for "translational" research intended to take results from bench to bedside and even to curbside, offering timely community health benefits from well-executed experimental and clinical designs. This book offers a wealth of tools and techniques to apply in designing nutrition research studies of your own. This chapter simply introduces a few basic considerations, but the rest of the book offers detailed guidance on nutrition research endeavors.

RDs play an important role in research, both as leaders and as collaborators. By targeting their own areas of expertise, RDs can drive each area of dietetics to its highest level. Training and education in the field are guided and updated by these unique research findings, and, through these efforts, practice guidelines will continue to advance.

Researchers must follow ethical procedures in all aspects of the design and conduct of their research (14,15). Everything from the choice of topics to the samples selected, the interventions designed, and the data collected must adhere to ethical guidelines (see Chapter 3). Data analysis and reporting of data are likewise subject to scrutiny.

Investigators should choose an issue important to their own practice. You may want to consider ideas to improve patient health, increase effectiveness of services and products, test concepts in published literature, or initiate basic research in new areas of advanced study. Chapters 21 through 26 cover key aspects of research in food, nutrition, and dietetics.

DESCRIPTIVE RESEARCH

Descriptive research is an effective way to obtain information used in devising hypotheses and proposing associations. Descriptive research cannot test or verify; analytic research is required to evaluate hypotheses or ascertain cause and effect. Important examples of descriptive investigations are descriptive epidemiologic research and qualitative research studies.

Descriptive research often illustrates a relevant but nonquantified topic involving a well-focused research question. Once the research topic is identified, the research design is determined, the protocol is carefully developed, and a pilot study is undertaken. A trial or pilot study is essential in most National Institutes of Health studies and can greatly improve the proposed study design and methodology. Testing instruments and making adjustments before instigating a major study helps to ensure that data collection is efficient and successful. All data collection should be justified. Data and experience gained from the pilot study can make or break support and funding for the proposed project. See Chapters 4 and 9.

Descriptive Epidemiologic Research

Epidemiologic research is descriptive when data detailing person, place, and time are collected. Descriptive epidemiologic research encompasses correlational studies, case reports, case series, surveys, surveillance systems, demographics, and vital statistics. Epidemiologic research is discussed in detail in Chapters 6 and 8.

Qualitative Research

Qualitative research generates narrative data—that is, data described in words instead of numbers (Chapter 7). A variety of techniques are suitable for securing qualitative data. Observation, in-depth individual interviews, focus-group interviews, nominal group process, the Delphi technique, free elicitation, concept maps, cognitive response tasks, and content analysis are some of the approaches. Such data may produce graphic and dramatic responses to research questions. Impressive applications of descriptive research may be seen in program planning, identification of population needs, and development of educational materials. Methods—some of them computer-based—for analyzing, unitizing, coding, and comparing qualitative data are currently used to interpret qualitative data. Future research will explore strategies for appraising the "confirmability" of qualitative data (akin to evaluating the reliability of quantitative data) and further enhancing the usefulness of qualitative research in nutrition and dietetics.

A qualitative study often precedes other research designs. Its primary purpose is to explore the phenomenon of interest as a prelude to theory development (16). The design is necessarily flexible so the researcher can discover ideas, gain insight, and ultimately formulate a problem for further investigation. Qualitative research is often the means to the end, rather than the end itself. For example, grounded theory research involves collecting and analyzing data "grounded" in real-life observations for the purpose of developing theoretical propositions. Similarly, focus groups or case studies can be useful in formulating hypotheses. Data are usually subjective in nature, but with careful definitions and pre-established boundaries they can provide useful and practical information. Such studies are not usually publishable in major scientific journals, but they can offer valuable guidance for future studies. Chapters 7 and 8 provide more thorough discussion of this type of research.

OBSERVATIONAL AND EXPERIMENTAL RESEARCH

Analytic research techniques, through observational or experimental designs, allow the evaluation of hypotheses and the determination of causal relationships. Observational analytic research encompasses case-control and cohort (follow-up) studies. Observational research designs generate measures of association (relative risk and odds ratios) and measures of effect (attributable risk). Relative risk is calculated from cohort studies, and odds ratios are from case-control studies. Attributable risk indicates a public health impact or an effect on the population.

Experimental analytic research, including clinical trials, involves investigator-controlled interventions and allows cause and effect to be examined. Clinical trials are designed to evaluate clearly defined treatment groups in which the investigator manipulates the variables of interest and compares resulting data from the study groups with the data from a control group. Chapter 9 discusses issues important in designing clinical trials to ensure that the statistical power is sufficient to detect differences among the study groups and that the data generated are generalizable.

Experimental design is a powerful analytic research method. Regardless of whether the subjects are human beings, experimental animals, or inanimate objects, criteria for subject selection need to be established, the appropriate sample size needs to be estimated (Chapter 27), the treatment(s) must be clearly defined, and end points must be established. Randomized controlled clinical trials (RCTs) are the epitome of excellence in research design. Cohort studies and case control studies are likewise examples of scientifically rigorous designs that are intended to yield meaningful, accurate and valid results. Chapters 8, 9,10, 29, and 30 are especially focused on these issues.

INTEGRATIVE AND TRANSLATIONAL RESEARCH

Integrative research is intended to encompass research that brings together multiple research studies or extends prior research, as in meta-analysis (Chapter 11) or the evaluation of existing large databases (Chapter 13). As such, integrative research extends available data through careful and constructive assimilation. Chapter 11 describes the steps of meta-analysis: constructing selection inclusion criteria, making a comprehensive search of existing studies that meet the criteria, and combining and assessing the data from the qualifying studies. Meta-analysis allows data from many empirical studies that meet the specified inclusion criteria of the researchers to be united into a larger unit that may yield more objective conclusions. The uses of well-designed meta-analyses are many, including the formation of public policy and the development of recommendations for evidence-based practice (Chapter 12).

Translational research is a promising type of research whose goal is to translate new science to patient care. Upon this base rests evidence-based practice. Medical nutrition therapy evolves from thoughtful evaluation of the beneficial effects of controlled laboratory studies and clinical investigations. Translational research, as exemplified in evidence-based practice, is a strong link between research and practice.

PRESENTATION OF RESEARCH

Original research can be presented in may ways: as technical reports (interim, summary, and evaluation reports), abstracts (to introduce a report, summarize projects, and submit a report for presentation consideration), posters at technical and scientific meetings, oral presentations, videotape and film presentations, and manuscripts prepared for publication in professional and research journals. The specific format should fit the purpose, the type of presentation, and, of course, the audience. All presentations are enhanced by thoughtful, clear organization.

Chapter 31 examines research publications from the point of view of the writer, the reviewer, and the reader. The writer's goal is to communicate logically, clearly, accurately, and ethically. The reviewer plays a prominent role in maintaining the quality of scientific literature. Peer review is a serious business and a professional responsibility. Peer reviewers must respect the work of their colleagues and maintain its confidentiality. Thoughtful, conscientious review gives clear, constructive direction to authors. The third critical corner of the presentation triangle is the readers. Guidance is provided to aid them in developing skills to evaluate the scientific literature critically. Understanding basic statistics (see Chapter 28) speeds the interpretation of scientific articles. To enhance efficiency in reading the vast scientific literature, it is helpful to look at the title and the list of authors; determine the article's intent; and read the abstract, methods, results, discussion, and recommendations. The skilled reader avoids overgeneralizing the findings by assessing the research design, sample selection, and data collected. A study's findings may be generalized to a population other than the specific study sample only if the study controls well the many variables of the research.

CONCLUSION

Opportunities for research continue to expand as our knowledge base sharpens and broadens in such diverse areas as human genetics, changes in behavior, complementary medicine, foodservice, marketing, and economic analyses of outcomes and effectiveness of care. All these areas are vital in dietetics education and its research component.

Research is exciting. It is based on discovery of new information and can change entire paradigms when the study results are conclusive. Nutrition research offers endless opportunities to investigate ways to improve health and patient care through better choices in diet, nutrition, and lifestyle. The following chapters provide detailed instructions and evidence-based approaches for moving the profession forward. Dietetics professionals have many ways to enhance and lead the profession in useful and exciting directions.

REFERENCES

1. Monsen E. Forces for research. *J Am Diet Assoc.* 1993;93:981–985.
2. Lind J. *A Treatise of the Scurvy. In Three Parts. Containing an Inquiry into the Nature, Causes, and*

Cure, of That Disease. Together with a Critical and Chronological View of What Has Been Published on the Subject. Edinburgh, Scotland: Sands, Murray, and Cochran; 1753.

3. Modugno F, Kip KE, Cochrane B, Kuller L, Klug TL, Rohan TE, Chlebowski RT, Lasser N, Stefanick ML. Obesity, hormone therapy, estrogen metabolism and risk of postmenopausal breast cancer. *Int J Cancer.* 2006;118:1292–1301.

4. Collaborative Group on Hormonal Factors in Breast Cancer. Breast cancer and hormone replacement therapy: collaborative reanalysis of data from 51 epidemiological studies of 52,705 women with breast cancer and 108,411 women without breast cancer. *Lancet.* 1997;350:1047–1059.

5. Chlebowski RT, Hendrix SL, Langer RD, Stefanick ML, Gass M, Lane D, Rodabough RJ, Gilligan MA, Cyr MG, Thomson CA, Khandekar J, Petrovitch H, et al. Influence of estrogen plus progestin on breast cancer and mammography in healthy postmenopausal women: the Women's Health Initiative randomized trial. *JAMA.* 2003;289:3243–3253.

6. Osborne T, Mendell L. *Feeding Experiments with Isolated Food Substances.* Washington DC: Carnegie Institute;1911:156.

7. Osborne T, Mendell L. Amino acids in nutrition and growth. *J Biol Chem.* 1914;17:325–349.

8. Stipanuk M. The vitamins. In: *Biochemical, Physiological Molecular Aspects of Human Nutrition.* 2nd ed. St. Louis, Mo: Saunders; 2006:661–663.

9. Wolever TM, Jenkins DJ, Jenkins AL, Josse RG. The glycemic index: methodology and clinical implications. *Am J Clin Nutr.* 1991;54:846–854.

10. Campfield LA, Smith FJ, Rosenbaum M, Hirsch J. Human eating: evidence for a physiological basis using a modified paradigm. *Neurosci Biobehav Rev.* 1996;20:133–137.

11. Ludwig DS, Majzoub JA, Al-Zahrani A, Dallal GE, Blanco I, Roberts SB. High glycemic index foods, overeating, and obesity. *Pediatrics.* 1999; 103:e26.

12. Kris-Etherton PM, Hecker KD, Bonanome A, Coval SM, Binkoski AE, Hilpert KF, Griel AE, Etherton TD. Bioactive compounds in foods: their role in the prevention of cardiovascular disease and cancer. *Am J Med.* 2002;113(suppl 9B): 71S–88S.

13. National Heart, Lung, and Blood Institute Obesity Education Initiative. *Clinical Guidelines on the Identification, Evaluation, and Treatment of Overweight and Obesity in Adults: The Evidence Report.* Bethesda, Md: National Institutes of Health; 1998.

14. Code of ethics for the profession of dietetics. *J Am Diet Assoc.* 1999;99:109–113.

15. *Honor in Science.* 2nd ed. New Haven, Conn: Sigma Xi, the Scientific Research Society; 1986.

16. Kerlinger FN, Lee HB. *Foundations of Behavioral Research.* 4th ed. New York, NY: Harcourt College Publishers; 2000.

2

Building the Research Foundation: The Research Question and Study Design

Carol J. Boushey, PhD, MPH, RD, Jeffrey Harris, DrPH, MPH, RD, Barbara Bruemmer, PhD, RD, and Sujata L. Archer, PhD, RD

Research is the backbone of nutrition and dietetics. It supports practice, innovation, and progress. Research allows objective measurement of complex environments and rigorous evaluation of the outcomes of procedures and treatments. Through research, associations can be observed, hypotheses tested, programs compared, and protocols evaluated. Research procedures can be used to document practice, to monitor activities, to ensure quality, and to assess cost-effectiveness. The strength of any discipline is associated closely with its research base. Strong research supports a strong profession.

Research may be broadly classified according to its purpose as either descriptive or analytic. Descriptive studies include qualitative research, case series (including case reports), and surveys. Descriptive studies are designed to describe the state of nature at a specific point in time. They are useful for generating hypotheses regarding the determinants of a condition, disease, or characteristic of interest. Descriptive studies provide baseline data and can monitor change over time, as is being done to monitor achievement of the Healthy People 2010 goals and objectives (1). The intent of analytic research is to test a hypothesis concerning causal relationships—perhaps a hypothesis generated from an earlier descriptive study. Experimental design is often considered the gold standard of analytic research: important factors are held constant except those factors manipulated by the investigator. Some observational designs, such as prospective cohort (follow-up) studies and case-control studies, are analytic but not experimental.

DESIGNING A RESEARCH STUDY

Research begins with identifying a relevant important topic and developing a well-considered research question and hypothesis. After the research design has been determined, the research protocol is prepared and, if necessary, a pilot study is undertaken. Throughout each phase, researchers must consider the ethical implications of their actions. This chapter focuses on the development of the research question and study design. Other chapters in this monograph cover research protocols and ethical considerations.

Selecting the Research Topic

Research is a problem-solving, decision-making process involving a series of interrelated decisions. When the researcher focuses on one decision at a time, the research process becomes manageable. Each option can be considered, and the most appropriate option can be selected.

Research projects should be meaningful; they should expand current knowledge and enhance the practice of the profession. Registered dietitians (RDs) can choose issues important to their practices and thereby important to the field of dietetics. Research questions can evolve from many sources, including ideas to improve patient health, suggestions to increase the effectiveness of services and products, untested concepts in published literature, the application of business research methods (2,3), and uncharted boundaries in basic research in all areas of advanced study. An RD can observe and thoughtfully consider the needs of his or her practice. The researcher then divides the overall topic into smaller component parts, and singles out a component that is feasible to study in the given setting. Start with a simple question. Data generated in response to the initial question will lead to many other questions that subsequent studies can address.

Preparing for the Research Project

A good first step in pursuing a research plan is to review the published research literature related to the topic. A thorough review will emphasize current scientific literature, seminal articles, and early published papers on the topic. A computerized literature search can speed and facilitate the review. The National Library of Medicine houses MEDLINE, which is the premier bibliographic database covering the fields of medicine, the health care system, nutrition and dietetics, and the preclinical sciences (4). MEDLINE contains bibliographic citations and author abstracts from more than 4,800 biomedical journals published in the United States and 70 other countries. To search this rich database, PubMed is available as a text-based search and retrieval system. Although many commercial Web-based search engines are available, PubMed is tailored to the biomedical literature.

Multiple papers already published on the topic should not discourage forward progress. A critical review of previous work in the field can be the base upon which to build solid new research projects. Shortcomings in study design or measurements can be improved and suggested new areas developed. Contact experts in the field. Discuss the problem with them by telephone or by e-mail. Actively seek out information that may be useful to you from colleagues in related fields.

Once the topic is solidified and the issue to address is identified, assess available resources and personnel, such as patient populations, laboratory and library facilities, foodservice equipment, nutrient databases, data-processing capabilities, computer facilities, personnel resources, statistical consultants, other consultants, and collaborative opportunities. Team efforts are invaluable; they facilitate quality research that provides major benefits to the profession. Practicing RDs can demonstrate leadership in research by directing team efforts. The direct and indirect costs of performing the research need to be estimated. If a study is well designed and carefully developed, it may be implemented with existing personnel and facilities. If it is necessary to obtain funds, consider a variety of funding sources, such as government agencies and foundations. Guidelines for obtaining funding are highlighted in Chapter 4.

Clearly Stating the Research Question

Preparation for a research project involves both formulating the research question and evaluating its feasibility (5). A concise, simple, straightforward statement of the research question focuses the research design process. Clearly define the question, and strive to keep it uncomplicated. Use objective, measurable, operational terms, such as *identify, compare, differentiate, assess,* and *describe.*

Components of the research question include the following:

- **Who (which)?** The subjects or units being assessed should be defined in broad terms (eg, *patients with diabetes, dietetics students, food items, tray lines,* or *foodservice costs*).
- **What?** The factor of interest should be stated specifically (eg, *body weight, knowledge about dietary recommendations, iron intake, tray error,* or *labor costs*).
- **How assessed?** The outcome to be assessed should be stated specifically (eg, *disease incidence, change in knowledge, alterations in food selection, tray errors per meal,* or *labor costs per patient day*).

A well-developed and focused research question leads directly to a hypothesis. A hypothesis has six essential characteristics: it is measurable; it specifies the population being studied; it identifies a time frame; it specifies the type of relationship being examined; it defines the variables being studied; and it states the level of statistical significance (5,6). Descriptive studies often use a research objective rather than a hypothesis as these studies define distributions of diseases and health-related characteristics in the sample population.

The difference between use of a research objective and use of a hypothesis can be clearly outlined by comparing a descriptive study and an analytic study that each examined the same health problem of overweight and obesity. Ogden et al (7) published the results from a descriptive study outlining the trends in overweight and obesity in the United States. Rather than a hypothesis, these investigators used a research objective. Their objective was "to provide current estimates of the prevalence and trends of overweight in children and adolescents and obesity in adults" using data from the National Health and Nutrition Examination Survey (NHANES) collected in 1999 to 2004. Many of the essential components of a hypothesis are present in their research objective, including being measurable (estimates of prevalence), specifying the population (children, adolescents, and adults from NHANES), identifying a timeframe (1999–2004), and defining variables (overweight or obese status). However, a relationship is not specified nor is a level of statistical significance stated. In other words, no a priori statements about prevalence rates of overweight or obesity or expected differences between groups were suggested by the research objective, which is consistent with a descriptive study.

In contrast, an analytic study will propose an expected difference between groups. Bacon et al (8) hypothesized that among obese, female chronic dieters, aged 30 to 45 years, those randomized to a "health at every size" treatment would statistically significantly improve ($P \le .05$) blood pressure, blood lipid levels, energy expenditure, eating behaviors, and self-esteem compared with those randomized to a traditional weight loss treatment after a 6-month intervention and 2-year follow-up. Note that all six essential components of a hypothesis are present. These two studies, one a descriptive study directed by a research objective (7), the other an analytic study driven by a hypothesis (8), each provided a valuable contribution to the knowledge base in the field.

Designing the Research Project

A clear statement of the research question, along with its accompanying research objective or hypothesis, make the design of the research project easier. Consider several research designs to determine which design is best suited to the research question and the setting. Among items to consider are the dependent and independent variables, which are characteristics or attributes of the persons or objects that vary within the study population (examples could be serum cholesterol and fiber intake). The dependent variable is the outcome variable of interest (eg, serum cholesterol). The independent variable or the exposure (the presumed causal factor) is the factor that is thought to influence the dependent variable and that is manipulated in the experimental design (eg, dietary fiber intake).

Other study design characteristics relate to time and direction of data collection. These characteristics differentiate (a) the cross-sectional study (a study based on data collected from a group of subjects at a single point in time); (b) the longitudinal study (a study based on data collected

at more than one point in time); (c) the prospective study (a study that begins with examination of a presumed cause or exposure, such as fiber intake, and goes forward in time to an observed presumed effect or outcome, such as cardiovascular disease); and (d) the retrospective study (a study that begins with manifestations of an outcome, such as cardiovascular disease, and goes back in time to uncover relationships with a presumed cause, such as fiber intake).

DESCRIPTIVE RESEARCH DESIGNS

Qualitative Research

A qualitative study often precedes other research designs (9). Its primary purpose is to explore the phenomenon of interest as a prelude to theory development (10). The design is necessarily flexible so the researcher can discover ideas, gain insight, and ultimately formulate a problem for further investigation. Qualitative studies are considered formulative or exploratory studies, characterized by a receptive, seeking attitude of the investigator and an intense study of the participants (11). One approach is grounded theory research, where data "grounded" in real-life observations are collected and analyzed with the purpose of developing theoretical propositions (12).

In grounded theory research, study volunteers or participants are selected according to their experience with the phenomenon being explored. Thus, they have special characteristics and are not considered to be typical or representative of the population. Data are collected by such methods as observation, interviews, and questionnaires. The interview format may range from structured (restricting the range of responses) to less structured or unstructured (permitting an unlimited range of responses). The latter type of interview may focus on a particular topic or experience (a focused interview) or may have minimal direction (a nondirective interview) (12,13). A more in-depth discussion of qualitative research can be found in Chapter 7.

A focus group involves a group of respondents assembled to answer questions on a specific topic. Focus groups can be used to examine attitudes toward issues in consumer groups or other target populations (14,15).

EXAMPLE. The factors that influence the consumption of calcium-rich foods among adolescents were examined using focus groups. Using a structured interview, group facilitators conducted focus groups among 200 boys and girls in two age groups

(11–12 years old and 16–17 years old) and representing three ethnic groups (Asian, Hispanic, or non-Hispanic white). The sessions were audiotaped and transcribed. Researchers coded the comments following the principles of grounded research theory. The results of the content analysis procedures highlighted the importance of family influence, stressing the benefits of calcium-rich foods to girls, and focusing on the breakfast meal. Results were also used to develop a quantitative questionnaire for use in larger, more representative population samples (15).

Surveys

A survey is research designed to describe and quantify characteristics of a defined population. A survey usually employs a research objective rather than a hypothesis. The purpose of a survey is to obtain a descriptive profile of the population (7,16). For example, the study by Ogden et al (7) described earlier in this chapter provided a statistical profile of overweight and obesity in the United States. A survey may be designed to assess the nutrient content of the food supply. A survey is an example of the cross-sectional study design: individuals are measured at only one point in time (see Figure 2.1).

Uses of Surveys

A survey may be useful for establishing associations among variables or factors, and often provides clues to direct further study (see Figure 2.2). Surveys can also provide baseline data about the prevalence of a condition or

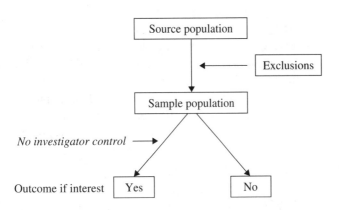

FIGURE 2.1   Basic cross-sectional study design (or survey) for determination of prevalence rates of a health outcome (eg, hypercholesterolemia) or a behavioral outcome (eg, consumption of fruits and vegetables).

factor of interest in the population. A major use of the survey method is for planning health and dietary services. However, a survey does not allow conclusions about causal relationships.

EXAMPLE.   In one hospital, randomly selected patients were questioned with regard to their satisfaction with tray presentation to assist in quality improvement in the hospital's dietary services. Assessments of cold food, hot food, time of delivery, and tray appearance were included. The random survey was repeated periodically so that tray service could be monitored, trends could be observed, and actions could be taken to improve service.

Survey Participant Selection

It is usually not feasible to measure an entire population in a survey. Therefore, a sample is selected based on a probability design, which means that all individuals have an equal chance of being selected. The individuals who consent to participate in the sample are then questioned or examined for the disease or characteristic of interest and other relevant variables.

EXAMPLE.   A survey was conducted to describe the food intake and food sources of macronutrients in the diets of older Hispanic adults in the northeastern United States, as well as to explore relationships between acculturation, years in the United States, and macronutrient intake. The 779 participants in the Massachusetts Hispanic Elders Study sample were selected using a two-stage random cluster sampling technique that ensured a sample that was representative of the older Hispanic adult population in the state of Massachusetts (17).

EXAMPLE.   Foodservice managers in health care and educational institutions were sent a pretested questionnaire covering uses of technology. The sample comprised 2,064 persons randomly selected from the membership listings of several professional organizations related to foodservice management (18).

Results of a survey can be generalized to the entire population of interest with confidence only if the sample is

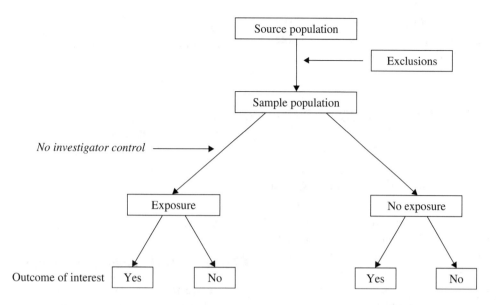

FIGURE 2.2   Basic cross-sectional study design (or survey) for the examination of a relationship between exposure and outcome.

representative of the target population. Thus, the target population must be defined and enumerated, and the sample must be drawn at random from the target population. In a simple random sample, each individual in the target population has the same known chance of being included in the sample; that is, the chances of being selected are specified in the sampling scheme. A sampling method allows the sampling errors to be calculated and increases the likelihood that the study is representative of the target population. A high rate of participation (high response rate) increases the chances that the results are representative, as it is never certain that responders and nonresponders are similar.

Possible sampling schemes range from the simple random method to complex methods using varying selection probabilities among subgroups (strata) of the population. Elwood (19) discusses the rationale for probability sampling in nutrition research, and Moore and McCabe (20) provide details on methodology.

The appropriate sample size for a survey depends upon many factors, including how precisely the sample should estimate the population parameters. Methods for calculating sample size requirements are given by Cohen (21) and are covered in Chapter 27.

A survey based on an accidental or convenience sampling scheme is of limited value, because its results cannot be generalized. The reference population is undefined or is defined by the conscious or unconscious selection biases of the investigator. Further, the selection itself may be influenced by the condition or factor under study.

Survey Data Collection

Data in surveys are most frequently collected by questionnaires or interviews. They also may be generated by physical examination (eg, anthropometric measurement; laboratory evaluation of specimens, such as blood analysis for hemoglobin levels; or direct observation, such as employee productivity).

One of the most difficult aspects of survey methodology is designing a questionnaire (16,22). Depending on the research objectives, standard or tested instruments may be available. If questions must be developed, they must be unambiguous, yet concise and tactful. The length of the questionnaire, its format, and how it is to be administered are also important considerations. Guidelines and suggestions for questionnaire development are provided in the literature (16,22) and are discussed in Chapter 13.

EXAMPLE.   A study conducted to assess the nutritional status of adolescent girls living in Hawaii involved participants aged 9 to 14 years. Anthropometric measurements of height, weight, and skin folds were collected during a clinic visit. Following the visit, the girls completed 3 days of food records and physical activity records. Nutrient and food intakes were compared against recommended intakes as were body mass index and skin fold thicknesses (23).

Surveys or cross-sectional studies are a valuable study design used extensively in nutrition research. Chapter 6 offers more information about descriptive research.

EXPERIMENTAL STUDY DESIGNS (RANDOMIZED TRIALS)

Experimental design is a powerful analytic research method, regardless of whether the participants are human beings, experimental animals, or inanimate objects. In each case, criteria for participation in the study, the appropriate sample size, the treatment or treatments, and end points must be established. After a preliminary study has been conducted and the experiment has been designed, data must be collected and analyzed suitably to permit appropriate interpretation and application.

Randomized Controlled Trials

Uses of the Randomized Controlled Trial

The experimental design in medical research, referred to as a randomized trial, is the most powerful design for evaluating practices and medical treatments. It is used to demonstrate the feasibility and safety of a treatment. After safety has been established, a randomized controlled trial may be designed to determine the optimal treatment regimen to obtain the desired effect. Most commonly, a randomized trial is employed to compare the efficacy of two or more treatments or practices.

EXAMPLE.   Using a randomized controlled trial, the Women's Health Initiative (WHI) examined the effect of following a diet of 20% energy from fat, ≥ 5 servings/day of fruits and vegetables, and ≥ 6 servings/day of grains on the incidence of breast cancer. Eligible women were randomized to the intervention of low-fat dietary pattern or the control group of the usual diet pattern. Randomization was done using a permuted block design. Effects were measured by monitoring incident cases of invasive breast cancer over a 12-year period (24).

Features of the Randomized Controlled Trial

There are three general features of the randomized controlled trial. First, prospective study volunteers are informed about the study purposes and risks and are asked to participate. Second, people consenting to participate are assigned randomly to one of two or more treatment or intervention groups. The individuals randomized to receive the standard treatment constitute the control group. The individuals randomized to receive the experimental treatment constitute the intervention, experimental, or treatment group. The key feature is random assignment; that is, chance determines treatment assignment. Third, participants are observed for the occurrence of particular outcomes or end points following or concurrent with intervention or treatment (see Figure 2.3).

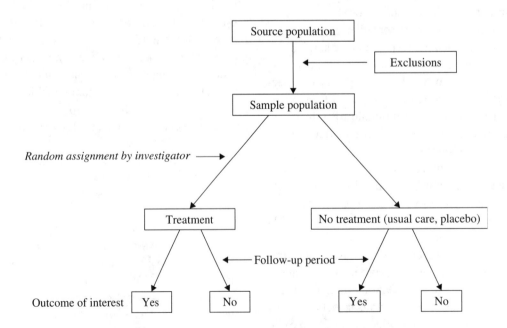

FIGURE 2.3   Basic randomized controlled trial study design.

EXAMPLE.   The effectiveness of death education lessons was assessed by randomly assigning dietetics students to a group that received lessons in death education or to a group who did not. The evaluation instrument measured students' change in knowledge of the grief process, personality traits of empathy and dogmatism, fear of death, fear of interacting with the dying, and attitudes toward working with terminally ill clients. Clinical performance of empathic counseling was assessed by direct observation (25).

Selection of Participants

In a randomized controlled trial, the degree to which a study group is representative of a reference population determines whether the results can be generalized. This issue must be reconciled with the equally important requirement of a high degree of probability that the treatment effect be large enough that it can be measured. For example, in the study of an intervention directed toward lowering dietary fat intakes, if the recruited subjects are already consuming a low-fat diet, additional lowering of dietary fat may not change the outcome enough to be detectable. On the other hand, if the recruited subjects are consuming a high-fat diet, the probability of detecting a change in some biological outcome is higher. In general, the researcher should select participants who are relatively homogeneous in major characteristics (eg, diagnosis and nutritional status) so that extraneous sources of variation are eliminated. When selecting participants, other factors to consider are subject compliance, ease of follow-up, and cost of enrolling and monitoring the subjects (26).

Compliance with the study protocol may be enhanced by offering appropriate incentives to all participants, such as special information or health care. Assessment of compliance prior to the start of the study may also be helpful; this can be done by including a pre-study requirement for all potential participants. Repeated 24-hour urine collections or several days of dietary intake records are useful requirements for judging compliance. Participants who are unable to complete the pre-study tasks are less likely to comply with study demands and should be excluded from the study before it begins. The resulting sample is necessarily biased, composed as it is of persons selected for their compliant behavior.

The ease of follow-up is related, in part, to the study setting. Follow-up is facilitated by highly restrictive settings or in settings in which the participant can be readily observed, such as in hospital settings. Unless the research question is relevant in such restricted settings, however, imposing severe restrictions on participants can impair the study's ability to correspond to a natural setting and can decrease its usefulness.

The cost of enrolling, monitoring, and retaining participants influences the number of subjects in the study. In many cases, investigators can lower the cost per enrollee by employing facilities and resources that are already available and by using information that is collected routinely. Retention of participants for the duration of study is important to maintain the validity of the final results.

Choice of Intervention or Treatment

As with participant selection, the intervention in a randomized controlled trial is chosen to maximize the likelihood that a statistically significant effect can be measured. The more the treatment of the intervention group differs from the treatment of the control group, within the range of safe or acceptable levels, the more likely that measurable differences will be seen. Whenever possible, the control treatment should have a reasonable expectation of benefit at least equal to that of the experimental treatment (26). An untreated group is valid as a control only if there is no recognized treatment. Otherwise, the control group should receive the standard treatment or an accepted treatment for the disease or condition of interest.

If there is no recognized treatment and it is thought that a psychological effect or observer bias is likely, a placebo is recommended as the control treatment. In these cases, a blind (masked) study is conducted, in which the subjects are unaware of the treatment assignment. The placebo, or sham treatment, must be inert and identical to the experimental treatment in appearance and mode of administration. The efficacy of blinding should be evaluated before and during the trial to ensure that blinding is maintained (27). If both subjects and investigators are unaware of the treatment assignment, the trial is a double-blind controlled trial—a powerful design because it eliminates expectation bias on the part of both the study participants and the investigative staff. The effect of expectation cannot be underestimated, as illustrated in the following classic example.

EXAMPLE.   The National Institutes of Health conducted a double-blind randomized controlled trial (a trial in which neither subject nor investigator was informed as to which treatment group the subject was assigned) of the effectiveness of ascorbic acid on reducing the frequency and severity of the common cold. A lactose-capsule placebo that could be easily distinguished from a vitamin C tablet by taste was used. The investigators gave little thought to the possibility that their subjects might actually bite into the capsules. Early in the study, the investigators learned that many of their curious volunteers had bitten into the capsules; as a result, a significant number of subjects knew which medication they were receiving. Although the study was no longer a double-blind study, it did illustrate an association between severity and duration of symptoms and knowledge of the medication taken. Among those subjects who tasted their capsules, those receiving vitamin C had shorter, milder colds, whereas the converse was true for the placebo group. Among those subjects who remained blind to their treatment, no effect of vitamin C was seen (28).

Assignment to Treatment Groups

A random method of treatment assignment is essential in a randomized controlled trial. Researchers are advised to avoid any treatment assignment method that is not random, such as allocation procedures based on characteristics

associated with patients (eg, birth dates or Social Security numbers) or odd-even or other systematic schemes (29). The random method eliminates the selection bias that can occur if the participant or the investigator selects the treatment. It also mitigates unintentional bias, or the chance formation of groups that are not comparable because of differences in factors that affect the response to treatment, such as age or gender. The random method does not guarantee comparable groups, however, and a chance imbalance between groups is possible, especially if the sample size is less than 200. Restricted randomization is a method of randomization that ensures that groups are equal or similar in numbers of subjects with certain characteristics, such as age and gender (29).

A crossover design uses an individual as his or her own control rather than using a separate control group of matched individuals. This design requires fewer participants, because the within-subject variation is less than the between-subject variation. A concept that is important for sample size calculations (see Chapter 27) is useful when the study involves conditions that are chronic and the treatment effects, if present, are not long lasting. In a crossover design, the subjects are randomly assigned to two groups differing in the sequence of treatments (see Figure 2.4). This assignment method ensures that an effect

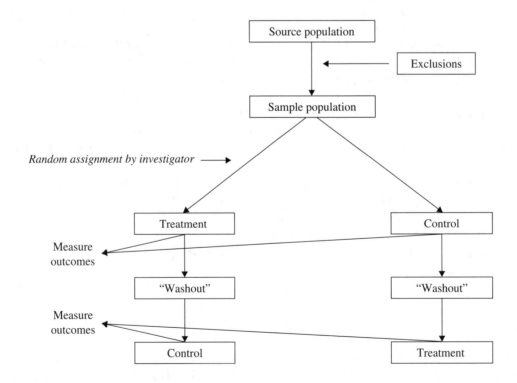

FIGURE 2.4 Basic study design for the crossover randomized controlled trial in which the same individuals participate in both treatment and control (placebo) groups.

due to order of treatment is eliminated from the observed treatment effect (30).

EXAMPLE.   To investigate how consumption of nuts may reduce cardiovascular risk factors, volunteers were randomly assigned to consume peanuts (500 kcal) daily over an 8-week ad libitum diet period or to consume a substitute energy equivalent food item. After a washout period of at least 4 weeks, subjects switched treatments (31).

Although seemingly simple and appealing, the crossover design is difficult to justify in many circumstances because the validity of the comparison rests upon the assumption that the participant enters each time period—treatment and control—in an identical state. This experimental design assumes that there are no carryover effects of the treatment and no appreciable change in the participant's condition. The crossover design is not appropriate when the treatment acts systemically or when the physical condition of the participant is unstable over the time period of the trial. The relevant issues are discussed by Hills and Armitage (30).

Instead of randomizing patients to a control group, it is often tempting to use a historical control group composed of subjects—usually patients—who were treated in some manner recognized as standard in the past. Unfortunately, it is difficult to establish the validity of historical controls. The biases present in such a series of patients are rarely completely identifiable and may irretrievably weight the outcome of the comparison in favor of the new treatment (32). It is not possible to ensure comparability between current and previous patients, or between the treatments used. A suggested alternative is to use both historical and concurrent randomized controls, but only when certain conditions are met, as outlined by Pocock (33).

Some clinical questions cannot be addressed by a randomized controlled trial because a comparison group of internal controls cannot be formed for ethical or logistic reasons. Other comparison groups—external controls—are necessary in such cases. If the external controls are well chosen, the studies can make valuable contributions. General advice on the proper use and interpretation of studies using external controls is offered by Bailar et al (34).

Sample Size

The ability of a clinical trial to detect a difference in outcomes between treatment and control groups depends, in part, on the sample size. Procedures for determining the

sample size yield an estimate only and are based on several assumptions and judgments about circumstances of the study (35). The procedures for estimating the size of a study are detailed by Browner et al (36). The six steps of the procedures for determining sample size are outlined in Chapter 27, which covers details of the calculations and provides examples of approaches to sample size and power estimation.

If the estimated sample size is larger than is reasonable with available resources, the researcher should ask, given the sample size feasible with available resources, what is the chance that a meaningful difference can be detected (ie, what is the power of an attainable study)? The answer can be calculated by the same methods used to estimate the sample size, but by solving for power instead of sample size. A study may not be worth doing if there is a low probability of detecting a relevant difference. If the final analysis shows that sufficient resources cannot be obtained, the project should be redesigned to require fewer assets. The WHI's large sample size of 48,835 turned out to be deceiving (24). Despite the large number of subjects, the level of compliance with the diet was lower than expected, as was the number of incident cases of breast cancer. Thus, the lack of statistically significant results for the main outcomes may have been due to the unexpected reduction in study power.

End Points and Data Collection

The end point of a study is the measurement by which the treatments are compared. The choice of a meaningful end point is often clear from the nature of the research question. However, the preferred end point for some research questions is not measurable; reasons for this may include the length of time required for the end point to occur or the sophisticated equipment necessary to measure the end point. In such cases, a surrogate for the end point is chosen, often an antecedent to the end point. The surrogate or antecedent condition must be highly predictive of the end point for it to serve as a valid answer to the study question (26). Collecting more than a single surrogate may be advisable to help corroborate findings.

As Weiss cautions, whenever a surrogate is used rather than direct measure of an end point, the possibility exists that the treatment affects only the surrogate and not the end point of interest (26). In choosing the surrogate, consider all available information to reduce the risk that the measured value does not reflect the desired outcome.

Measured end points may be "hard" (objective) or "soft" (subjective) evidence or data. Serum cholesterol concentration and body weight are hard data; degree of headache pain and severity of flu symptoms are soft data. Hard variables are preferred because they are more objective, more reliable, and easier to measure. Relevant soft variables should not be dismissed, however, because they are frequently the most interesting and important outcomes and can be useful in interpreting hard data. A useful approach is to combine a few carefully chosen hard and soft variables.

EXAMPLE.   A randomized intervention trial was designed to evaluate the effect of a farmer's market nutrition program, with or without coupons, on fruit and vegetable consumption behavior. Participants were randomized to either education alone or education with farmer's market coupons. A self-administered questionnaire measured attitudes toward fruit and vegetable consumption and intake of fruits and vegetables before and after intervention. Records from the US Department of Agriculture's Special Nutrition Program for Women, Infants, and Children (WIC) were used to document redemption of coupons (37).

Statistical Analysis and Interpretation

Several excellent references describe statistical procedures for testing hypotheses in experiments (6,29,38,39). Among the major problems frequently encountered in analyzing and interpreting results of clinical trials are noncompliance and loss of subjects.

Even with the best efforts to maintain strict adherence to the treatment protocol, noncompliance often occurs. Adherence to treatment should be monitored to learn practical aspects of the treatment. All participants should be followed to the same extent, regardless of their compliance with treatment. At the time of analysis, retain subjects in their originally assigned treatment group whether or not they actually received the treatment (29). This comparison, called the *intent-to-treat comparison,* reflects how the treatments perform in practice (6). A selection bias is introduced if the subjects are excluded or analyzed in groups other than the group to which they were randomly assigned. A secondary analysis could evaluate the outcomes of the treatments actually received, but that analysis should not be given more weight or relevance than the primary intent-to-treat analysis (24).

Withdrawal of subjects presents another opportunity for selection bias to occur. Subjects who are withdrawn

from the study should be followed in the same manner as all other study subjects, if possible (6). As in the problem of noncompliance, these subjects should be analyzed as part of their original treatment group. Report reasons for withdrawal, and compare them among groups. One treatment may favor withdrawal because it is less acceptable or has unexpected adverse effects.

Reporting adverse effects aids in evaluating the practicality of the treatment and in planning future studies. If follow-up is not possible and the outcome is not known, compare the known characteristics of the withdrawn subjects with the characteristics of the subjects who complete the study. This comparison may help determine the nature of the bias introduced into the results by the subjects' withdrawal. As an additional step in estimating the effect of removing the subjects, a secondary analysis could be done assuming an unfavorable outcome for those subjects. Compare this worst-outcome result with the result obtained using only known end points.

Factorial Design

The study designs previously described in this chapter consider only one study question and investigate only one factor. Their simplicity makes them preferred designs in most settings. If the resources allow, however, it may be useful and efficient to study more than one factor in a single study. This is done using a factorial design. A factorial design includes study groups for all combinations of levels of each factor under study. For example, a two-factor factorial design with two levels per factor would have four treatment groups (see Figure 2.5).

The comparison of levels of factor A is achieved by comparing groups with factor A (cells 1 and 3) with groups without factor A (cells 2 and 4); the comparison of levels of factor B is achieved by comparing groups with factor B (cells 1 and 2) with groups without factor B (cells 3 and 4). These comparisons are made using two-way analysis of variance. This design also allows a synergistic effect (interaction) to be detected. Hulley and coauthors (6) provide details of the design and analysis of factorial experiments.

Partially Controlled or Quasi Experimental Designs

All research involves balancing the ideal with the feasible. In certain situations randomized treatment assignment or assembly of an appropriate control group is impossible.

FACTOR A

		YES	NO	
FACTOR B	YES	Cell 1 Yes–Yes	Cell 2 Yes–No	1 + 2
	NO	Cell 3 No–Yes	Cell 4 No–No	3 + 4
		1 + 3	2 + 4	A × B

FIGURE 2.5   An example of a 2p factorial design in which two factors are at two levels each. The effects of factor A (cells 1 and 3 vs cells 2 and 4), factor B (cells 1 and 2 vs cells 3 and 4) and the interaction of A × B may be calculated using two-way analysis of variance.

Other study design options are available, although each has limitations, and none is as convincing as the randomized controlled trial. Experiments that compare groups that have not been randomized, or that lack a control group, are sometimes termed *quasi experiments.*

Although these studies do involve the manipulation of a treatment or intervention, they are weak in supporting causal inferences. This drawback exists because these studies are far less satisfactory than the randomized controlled trial in controlling for the influence of confounding or distorting variables. Of particular concern is the problem of unmeasured confounding variables, such as lifestyle (6). Other research options to consider are the observational analytic study designs (ie, cohort and case-control studies).

PROSPECTIVE (COHORT, FOLLOW-UP) STUDIES

Prospective (also known as cohort or follow-up) studies are observational analytic studies that are designed to mimic the randomized controlled trial. A prospective study does not involve investigator manipulation and thus is not categorized as experimental. It does test a hypothesis of a possible chronological or temporal sequence in the causal pathway, and thus is analytic in approach.

A cohort is a group of persons followed over time and having a common characteristic or factor of interest. A cohort is assembled on the basis of factors thought to

relate to the development of the end point under study. This organization allows the investigation of a hypothesis concerning the etiology of the outcome of interest. The study involves following the cohort forward in time to observe its experience. The outcome studied is most commonly a disease; for convenience, the following discussion refers to the studied outcome as a disease. This design is by no means limited to the study of diseases, however. Many other conditions, such as overweight (40), can be studied in the same manner. The possible causal factors under investigation, referred to as *exposures,* may cover a wide range of environmental and lifestyle characteristics (see Figure 2.6).

Uses of Prospective Studies

A cohort design is useful for determining the frequency of a newly diagnosed disease or a health-related event and for assessing an exposure-disease relationship. In the cohort design, exposure to a suspected risk factor is identified when individuals are free of detectable disease; that is, the cohort is identified on the basis of exposure to certain factors thought to affect risk but without the presence of disease. Exposure to the factor of interest clearly precedes the detection of disease. Because it helps establish the temporal sequence of risk factor and end point, the cohort design is appealing for the study of causes of disease. A drawback is that sufficient time must elapse between assessing the exposure and detecting the outcome. For example, the

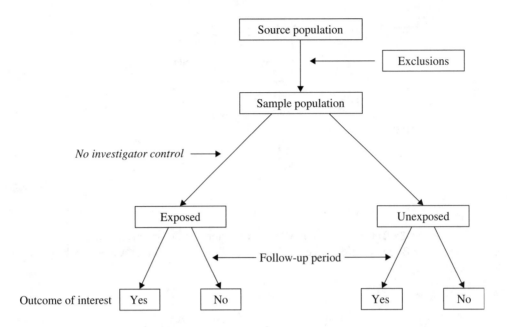

FIGURE 2.6   Basic prospective cohort study design.

latency period of many cancers is 10 years or more; thus, the cohort study would need to span, at a minimum, this same time period. Cohort studies are most useful when the time between exposure and detection of the end point is thought to be relatively short.

EXAMPLE.   Investigators used a prospective cohort design to assess the association between changes in nutritional status in hospitalized patients and the occurrence of infections, the occurrence of complications, length of stay in the hospital, and hospital charges. In patients admitted to the hospital inpatient service for a stay of longer than 7 days, nutritional status at the time of admission and discharge was measured, and change in nutritional status during hospitalization was assessed. Outcome measures included length of stay, complications, infections, and hospital charges (41).

Unless the disease studied is extremely common in the population to be studied, most individuals in a cohort will not develop it. Therefore, a large number of participants is required to allow comparison of incidence between exposure groups. This design is more feasible for conditions that are relatively common in the population studied.

EXAMPLE.   A prospective cohort study design was used to examine demographic and psychosocial factors that predict healthful dietary change. Participants were recruited by random-digit dialing and were followed up with assessments 2 years later. At baseline, participants were interviewed to obtain demographic characteristics, attitudes and behaviors related to cancer risk, and psychosocial factors related to diet. Dietary fat intake was measured at baseline and follow-up by the use of a validated 12-item questionnaire that asked about fat-related dietary habits over the previous 3 months. At the same time, fruit and vegetable intakes were assessed using a validated 6-item questionnaire. Baseline characteristics were examined for their ability to predict changes in dietary fat-related behaviors and fruit and vegetable intakes (42).

Features of Prospective Cohort Studies

The members in a cohort are apparently free of the disease under study at the time of selection, and are selected on the basis of the presence or absence of a factor of interest, or exposure. Subjects are then followed forward in time to determine the occurrence of the disease or of a specific end point serving as an indicator of the disease. The direction of the study is always prospective, because the exposure is identified before the disease is detected. However, the follow-up period may be concurrent (prospective) or nonconcurrent (retrospective). Follow-up may proceed at the same time as the study is conducted (concurrent follow-up); in these cases, current records generate data on disease occurrence. Alternatively, follow-up may have occurred earlier (nonconcurrent follow-up); existing records yield data on disease occurrence. Clearly, the latter scheme alleviates the need to wait for the cohort to go through time.

EXAMPLE.   A nonconcurrent (retrospective) cohort design was used to determine whether stature is a useful prognostic factor in cystic fibrosis survival. The cohort was assembled from the national registry maintained by the Cystic Fibrosis Foundation in the United States. The registry maintains records on numerous variables related to patient morbidity and mortality. Individuals were included in the cohort if they were born between 1980 and 1989, had a minimum of four records each, were alive at age 7 years, and had a recorded height measurement at age 7 to 8 years. Vital status, along with the date of death if it had occurred, was obtained from the registry (43).

Selection of Participants in Cohort Studies

The subjects who make up a cohort must be at risk for developing the disease or outcome of interest but free of the disease at the start of the study. The subjects may be members of a single cohort and classified according to their exposure to the factor of interest, or the subjects may be members of different cohorts, selected from different exposure groups so that the exposed cohort can be compared with the unexposed cohort. The validity of the comparison between cohorts depends upon the assumption that the cohorts are comparable in all relevant factors other than the exposure.

Assessing Exposure Status

Exposure to the factor of interest is observed or measured for each subject at the start of a cohort study. A standardized assessment is used to improve reliability. Information relating to exposure and other important characteristics can be collected from direct measurement, existing records, personal interviews, or questionnaires.

Analytic epidemiology studies are discussed in Chapter 8.

Assessing dietary intake poses special problems. Dietary intake methodology is the subject of continuing investigation; no single method has been shown to be reliable and valid for all types of research. When selecting the method for collecting dietary data, the researcher should review three issues thoroughly. These issues are discussed in Chapter 14.

A difficulty inherent in cohort studies is that a change in exposure status may occur during the follow-up period. A change in exposure status may dilute the study's ability to detect a difference in risk between exposed and unexposed groups. Repeated measurement of the factor during the follow-up period reduces the likelihood of this error.

Assessing Outcomes (Diseases)

The disease or health outcome in a cohort study should be defined in detail. The method and type of follow-up should be identical for all subjects, regardless of exposure status. Achievement of this goal is facilitated by making the evaluators unaware of the subjects' exposure status (ie, blind assessment). Blinding ensures that the efforts for follow-up and the assessment methods used will be applied equally and will not be biased by the investigators' expectations.

The outcome events are counted as they occur during the follow-up period. However, outcomes occurring immediately after assessment of the exposure status cannot be counted when it is not clear that the exposure preceded the end point. This decision depends on what is known or believed to be true about the length of the induction or latent period for the disease or primary end point in question.

Complete follow-up on all members of the cohort is vitally important. Loss of subjects can seriously distort the study's results. Make vigorous efforts to assess the outcome of each subject at the end of the follow-up period.

The length of follow-up depends on the hypothesis and related knowledge of the latency period or the mechanisms of action of the risk factor. The longer the follow-up period, the more difficult the follow-up becomes due to changes of residence, death from other causes, changes in exposure status, and the added staffing expenses for monitoring subjects and collecting data. Those considerations must be balanced with the need to allow sufficient time for the proposed effect to become manifest.

Statistical Analysis and Interpretation

Baseline characteristics of the cohort are described using distributions and frequencies. The usual inferential comparative analysis of prospective studies involves determining the incidence of disease and estimating the incidence ratio for exposed vs unexposed subjects. The incidence ratio is known as the relative risk and measures the strength of the association between the exposure factor and the disease or outcome of interest (39). Thus, the result is a statement that those with the exposure are more likely (or less likely) to develop the disease compared with those without the exposure.

The weakness in this observational study design is that a relationship is not clearly causal. All factors are not held constant, as they are in an experiment. These limitations need to be considered in the interpretation of the final results. The criteria for determining causation based on the collective results from observational and experimental studies are reviewed in Chapter 8.

CASE-CONTROL STUDIES

Case-control studies involve observational analytic designs that investigate hypotheses of causal relationships. These designs support retrospective, historically oriented studies, also known as *case-referent studies* or *case-comparison studies*. Because case-control designs do not involve intervention by the investigators, they are not experimental but do adhere to as many principles of experimental design as possible.

Uses of Case-Control Studies

A case-control design is used to explore etiology by comparing the prevalence of the exposure to factors of interest in persons who have a disease with that of a group without the disease. The design is useful in studies of rare diseases or end points. In general, case-control studies are less expensive to conduct and require less time than cohort studies. An entire issue of the *Journal of Chronic Diseases* is devoted to the use and methods of the case-control design and is a classic reference (44).

Features of Case-Control Studies

The case-control study design assesses exposure status after disease status is known and thus is retrospective. The comparison groups are formed on the basis of disease or outcome status, either with disease diagnosis (cases) or without disease diagnosis (controls). Subjects are then investigated for the current presence of, or previous exposure to, a factor or factors of interest. The prevalence of the factor or factors is compared between cases and controls (see Figure 2.7).

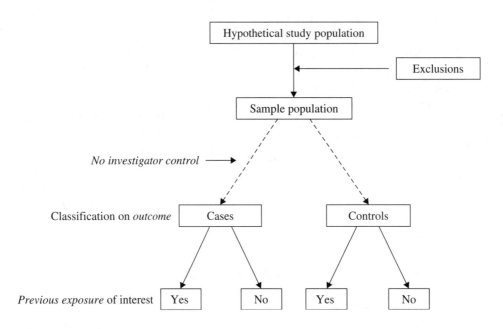

FIGURE 2.7   Basic case-control study design involves ascertainment of cases after onset of disease and assessment of exposure as recall prior to onset of disease.

EXAMPLE.   Inadequate antioxidant defenses against free-radical toxicity have been implicated in the etiology of amyotrophic lateral sclerosis (ALS). A case-control study was designed to assess diet as a predisposing factor for the development of ALS. Over a 4-year study period, 180 patients newly diagnosed with ALS met study criteria. Controls were identified by random-digit dialing of households in the same residential areas (counties) as the cases. An in-person structured interview and a self-administered food frequency questionnaire were used to obtain information on lifestyle and diet exposures (45).

Selection of Cases

In a case-control study, the goal in selection of cases is to obtain a sample that is representative of cases arising from a defined target population. This goal is difficult or impossible to attain in most circumstances. The ideal compromise is to select all incident (newly developed or detected) cases arising in a defined population over some specified period. Selecting incident cases rather than existing (prevalent) cases is preferred because factors related to survival, and thus to selection for the study, may differ from causal factors but cannot be distinguished from one another in a case-control study when prevalent cases are used. The definition of a case should be specific and objective to minimize the bias of personal judgment.

EXAMPLE.   To investigate the hypothesis that a high intake of fruits and vegetables, and nutrients involved in antioxidant activities contributes to the risk of developing non-Hodgkin's lymphoma (NHL), a case-control study was planned using the Surveillance, Epidemiology, and End Results cancer registry (SEER). During a 3-year period, 1,321 of 2,248 potentially eligible incident case subjects between 20 and 74 years old with NHL were enrolled as cases. The control group members younger than 65 years were identified by random dialing, and those age 65 and older were randomly identified from Medicare files. Controls were frequency matched to cases by age (within 5 years), geographic location, race, and gender. Subjects were mailed a self-administered quantitative food frequency questionnaire to assess usual intake of foods including fruits and vegetables 1 year prior to disease for cases and the same time period for

controls. The reported fruit and vegetable intakes (both quantity and type) were compared between cases and controls (46).

Selection of Controls

Selection of an appropriate comparison group in a case-control study depends largely upon the hypothesis. The goal in selecting the control subjects is that controls should be representative of the population from which the cases arose. A random probability sample is ideal and is feasible if information is available on the sampling units (or community). A random probability sample is also feasible if the population is a closed one, such as participants in a prepaid health plan or inpatients in an institution. Samples of convenience are often used, but the validity of the study rests upon the assumption that the subjects are similar to the reference or target population with regard to the factors of interest; this assumption may or may not be reasonable.

Considerations in choosing a control group include cost, response rate, and interview setting. Compromises may have to be made to reduce the cost of accessing a control subject while maximizing the response rate. Insofar as possible, the interview setting should be comparable to the setting for cases. Much of the information is elicited by recall and self-report, and factors bearing on those methods should be as identical as possible between the groups.

A selection bias in controls is undesirable but possible. Minimize bias by planning a structured selection system with established criteria for selecting control subjects. The criteria should be applied without the investigators' knowledge of the individuals' exposure status. Other sources of bias, such as differences in age, gender, or socioeconomic status, may be eliminated by matching in the selection or by stratification in the analysis. How to select appropriate controls is not always clear; several authors review problems and give suggestions (47,48).

EXAMPLE.   Studies have suggested that tea may be protective against cancers of the urinary tract. Using a case-control design, investigators examined the association between usual adult tea consumption and risk of bladder and kidney cancers in a population-based study. Newly diagnosed cases of bladder and kidney cancer were identified through the Iowa Cancer Registry. Controls younger than 65 years old were selected from

Iowa drivers' license records, and controls aged 65 years and older were selected from US Health Care Financing Administration records. Cases were frequency matched to controls by gender and 5-year age group. Usual tea intake, as well as intakes of coffee and other beverages, was assessed by self-report using a mailed questionnaire. Subjects who were reluctant to complete the detailed questionnaire (5.8%) were offered a 15-minute abbreviated telephone interview. Tea use was categorized into four levels of intake, and distribution of tea use was compared between cases and controls using odds ratios, adjusted for potential confounding factors (49).

Assessing Exposure to the Factor of Interest

In case-control studies, historical information, including the exposure to the factor of interest, may be obtained from existing records, examinations, direct measurements, or personal interviews or questionnaires. The starting point for developing any data-gathering tool is a list of all pertinent variables, including the extent of detail needed. The methods for assessing past diet in case-control studies have been studied in a variety of settings (50,51). Issues involved with selecting a dietary assessment method are covered in Chapter 14.

EXAMPLE. A population-based case-control study was conducted to examine the association between selected nutrients, foods, and diet behaviors and bladder cancer. Bladder cancer cases diagnosed within a 4-year period were identified from the SEER cancer registry for Western Washington State. Controls were identified through random dialing for the same residential area. A food frequency questionnaire was used to estimate usual food intake. Subjects were asked to estimate this intake for the year that was the midpoint of the 10-year reference period (that is, 7 years prior to diagnosis for cases and a similar reference period for controls) (52).

Regardless of the instrument used, the procedure for gathering information should be the same for cases and controls. The comparability of the procedure is increased if the interviewer or evaluator does not know whether the subject is a case or a control. This goal may not be possible in a personal interview but may be feasible for a person gathering other objective data.

Statistical Analysis and Interpretation

In a case-control study, the frequencies of the exposure of interest are presented for cases and controls. The association between the exposure and the disease is expressed by estimating the odds ratio, a statistical comparison of the prevalence of exposure between cases and controls (39). Thus, the results are expressed as the statement that those with the disease are more likely (or less likely) to have had the exposure compared with those without the disease.

The observational methodology and retrospective nature of the case-control study present limitations that should be kept in mind in the interpretation of the results. There are always alternatives to a causal explanation for an association. Chief among the alternatives are the following:

- In a case-control study, it may be unclear whether the factor preceded the disease or resulted from it.
- The self-report is influenced by the presence of the disease, especially if the subject is aware of the hypothesis being tested. This recall bias is likely to cause the observed association to overestimate the actual association.
- The comparability of cases and controls may be questionable. The choice of control group is crucial to a valid study.

CONCLUSION

Nutrition and dietetics offer many opportunities to pursue a compelling research question. To examine a proposed research question, an investigator needs to first summarize the literature on the topic complemented with observations from the working environment. This step will aid in the refinement of the hypothesis or research objective. Qualitative, descriptive, or analytic study approaches are options available to address a variety of research questions. Selecting the best study design will allow valid conclusions to be inferred from the data collected. The strengths and weaknesses of the different study designs need to be considered within the framework of available resources. Throughout the research process, the investigator uses brainstorming, attention to the detail of data collection, and teamwork.

REFERENCES

1. US Department of Health and Human Services. Healthy People 2010. January 30, 2001. Available at: http://www.healthypeople.gov. Accessed July 27, 2006.

2. Bryman A, Bell E. *Business Research Methods.* New York, NY: Oxford University Press; 2003.

3. Blank SC. *Practical Business Research Methods.* Westport, Conn: AVI Publishing; 1984.

4. National Library of Medicine. National Institutes of Health. NLM Web site. Available at: http://www.nlm.nih.gov. Accessed June 26, 2006.

5. Boushey C, Harris J, Bruemmer B, Archer SL, Van Horn L. Publishing nutrition research: a review of study design, statistical analyses, and other key elements of manuscript preparation, Part 1. *J Am Diet Assoc.* 2006;106:89–96.

6. Hulley SB, Cummings SR, Browner WS, Grady D, Hearst N, Newman TB. *Designing Clinical Research: An Epidemiological Approach.* 2nd ed. Philadelphia, Pa: Lippincott Williams & Wilkins; 2001.

7. Ogden CL, Carroll MD, Curtin LR, McDowell MA, Tabak CJ, Flegal KM. Prevalence of overweight and obesity in the United States, 1999–2004. *JAMA.* 2006;295:1549–1555.

8 Bacon L, Stern JS, Van Loan MD, Keim NL. Size acceptance and intuitive eating improve health for obese, female chronic dieters. *J Am Diet Assoc.* 2005;105:929–936.

9. Borra S, Kelly L, Tuttle M, Neville K. Developing actionable dietary guidance messages: dietary fat as a case study. *J Am Diet Assoc.* 2001;101:678–684.

10. Kerlinger FN, Lee HB. *Foundations of Behavioral Research.* 4th ed. New York, NY: Harcourt College Publishers; 2000.

11. Hoyle RH, Judd CM, Harris MJ. *Research Methods in Social Relations.* 7th ed. New York, NY: Wadsworth Publishing Co; 2002.

12. Patton MQ. *Qualitative Evaluation and Research Methods.* 2nd ed. London, UK: Sage; 1990

13. Sobal J. Sample extensiveness in qualitative nutrition education research. *J Nutr Educ.* 2001;33: 184–192.

14. Dahlke R, Wolf KN, Wilson SL, Brodnik M. Focus groups as predictors of dietitians' roles on interdisciplinary teams. *J Am Diet Assoc.* 2000;100:455–457.

15. Auld G, Boushey CJ, Bock MA, Bruhn C, Gabel K, Gustafson D, Holmes B, Misner S, Novotny R, Peck L, Pelican S, Pond-Smith D, Read M. Perspectives on intake of calcium rich foods among Asian, Hispanic, and white preadolescent and adolescent females. *J Nutr Educ.* 2002;34:242–251.

16. McColl E, Jacoby A, Thomas L, Soutter J, Bamford C, Steen N, Thomas R, Harvey E, Garratt A, Bond J. Design and use of questionnaires: a review of best

practice applicable to surveys of health service staff and patients. *Health Technol Assess.* 2001;5: 204–244.

17. Bermúdez OI, Falcón LM, Tucker KL. Intake and food sources of macronutrients among older Hispanic adults: association with ethnicity, acculturation, and length of residence in the United States. *J Am Diet Assoc.* 2000;100:665–673.

18. McCool AC, Garand MM. Computer technology in institutional foodservice. *J Am Diet Assoc.* 1986;86: 48–56.

19. Elwood PC. Epidemiology for nutritionists: 2. sampling. *Hum Nutr Appl Nutr.* 1983;37:265–269.

20. Moore DS, McCabe GP. Producing data. In: Moore DS, McCabe GP, eds. *Introduction to the Practice of Statistics.* New York, NY: WH Freeman; 2006: 191–250.

21. Cohen J. *Analysis for the Behavioral Sciences.* 2nd ed. Matwah, NJ: Lawrence Erlbaum; 1988.

22. Dillman DA. *Mail and Internet Surveys: The Tailored Design Method.* 2nd ed. New York, NY: Wiley; 1999.

23. Daida Y, Novotny R, Grove JS, Acharya S, Vogt TM. Ethnicity and nutrition of adolescent girls in Hawaii. *J Am Diet Assoc.* 2006;106:221–226.

24. Prentice RL, Caan B, Chlebowski RT, Patterson R, Kuller LH, Ockene JK, Margolis KL, Limacher MC, Manson JE, Parker LM, Paskett E, Phillips L, Robbins J, Rossouw JE, Sarto GE, Shikany JM, Stefanick ML, Thomson CA, Van Horn L, Vitolins MZ, Wactawski-Wende J, Wallace RB, Wassertheil-Smoller S, Whitlock E, Yano K, Adams-Campbell L, Anderson GL, Assaf AR, Beresford SAA, Black HR, Brunner RL, Brzyski RG, Ford L, Gass M, Hays J, Heber D, Heiss G, Hendrix SL, Hsia J, Hubbell A, Jackson RD, Johnson KC, Kotchen JM, LaCroix AZ, Lane DS, Langer RD, Lasser NL, Henderson MM. Low-fat dietary pattern and risk of invasive breast cancer. *JAMA.* 2006;295:629–642.

25. Oakland MJ. The effectiveness of a short curriculum unit in death education for dietetic students. *J Am Diet Assoc.* 1988;88:26–28.

26. Weiss NS. *Clinical Epidemiology: The Study of the Outcome of Illness.* 3rd ed. New York, NY: Oxford University Press; 2006.

27. Farr BM, Gwaltney JM Jr. The problems of taste in placebo matching: an evaluation of zinc gluconate for the common cold. *J Chronic Dis.* 1987;40:875–879.

28. Karlowski TR, Chalmers TC, Frenkel LD, Kapidian AZ, Lewis TL, Lynch JM. Ascorbic acid for

the common cold. A prophylactic and therapeutic trial. *JAMA.* 1975;231:1038–1042.

29. Meinert CL. *Clinical Trials: Design, Conduct, and Analysis.* New York, NY: Oxford University Press; 1986.

30. Hills M, Armitage P. The two-period cross-over clinical trial. *Br J Clin Pharmacol.* 1979;8:7–20.

31. Alper CM, Mattes RD. Peanut consumption improves indices of cardiovascular disease risk in healthy adults. *J Am Coll Nutr.* 2003;22:133–141.

32. Sacks H, Chalmers TC, Smith H. Randomized versus historical controls for clinical trials. *Am J Med.* 1982;72:233–240.

33. Pocock SJ. The combination of randomized and historical controls in clinical trials. *J Chronic Dis.* 1976;29:175–188.

34. Bailar JC, Louis TA, Lavori PW, Polansky M. Studies without internal controls. *N Engl J Med.* 1984;311: 156–162.

35. Browner WS, Newman TB, Hearst N, Hulley SB. Getting ready to estimate sample size: hypotheses and underlying principles. In: Hulley SB, Cummings SR, Browner WS, Grady D, Hearst N, Newman TB. *Designing Clinical Research: An Epidemiological Approach.* 2nd ed. Philadelphia, Pa: Lippincott Williams & Wilkins; 2001:51–63.

36. Browner WS, Newman TB, Cummings SR, Hulley SB. Estimating sample size and power: the nitty-gritty. In: Hulley SB, Cummings SR, Browner WS, Grady D, Hearst N, Newman TB. *Designing Clinical Research: An Epidemiological Approach.* 2nd ed. Philadelphia, Pa: Lippincott Williams & Wilkins; 2001:65–91.

37. Anderson JV, Bybee DI, Brown RM, McClean DF, Garcia EM, Breer ML, Schillo BA. 5 a day fruit and vegetable intervention improves consumption in a low income population. *J Am Diet Assoc.* 2001;101: 195–202.

38. Moore DS, McCabe GP. *Introduction to the Practice of Statistics.* 5th ed. New York, NY: WH Freeman; 2006.

39. Rosner B. *Fundamentals of Biostatistics.* 6th ed. Belmont, Calif: Duxbury/Thomson Brooks/Cole; 2006.

40. Berkey CS, Rockett HRH, Field AE, Gillman MW, Colditz GA. Sugar-added beverages and adolescent weight change. *Obes Res.* 2004;12:778–788.

41. Braunschweig C, Gomez S, Sheean PM. Impact of declines in nutritional status on outcomes in adult patients. *J Am Diet Assoc.* 2000;100:1316–1322.

42. Kristal AR, Hedderson MM, Patterson RE, Neuhouser ML. Predictors of self-initiated, healthful dietary change. *J Am Diet Assoc.* 2001;101:762–766.

43. Beker LT, Russek-Cohen E, Fink RJ. Stature as a prognostic factor in cystic fibrosis survival. *J Am Diet Assoc.* 2001;101:438–442.

44. The case-control study: consensus and controversy. *J Chronic Dis.* 1979;32:1–144.

45. Nelson LM, Markin C, Longstreth WT, McGuire V. Population-based case-control study of amyotrophic lateral sclerosis in western Washington State. II. Diet. *Am J Epidemiol.* 2000;151:164–173.

46. Kelemen LE, Cerhan JR, Lim U, Davis S, Cozen W, Schenk M, Colt J, Hartge P, Ward MH. Vegetables, fruit, and antioxidant-related nutrients and risk of non-Hodgkin's lymphoma: a National Cancer Institute-Surveillance, Epidemiology, and End Results population-based case-control study. *Am J Clin Nutr.* 2006;83:1401–1410.

47. Newman TB, Browner WS, Cummings SR, Hulley SB. Designing an observational study: cross-sectional and case-control studies. In: Hulley SB, Cummings SR, Browner WS, Grady D, Hearst N, Newman TB. *Designing Clinical Research: An Epidemiological Approach.* 2nd ed. Philadelphia, Pa: Lippincott Williams & Wilkins; 2001:107–124.

48. Breslow NE, Day NE, Davis W. *Statistical Methods in Cancer Research: The Analysis of Case-Control Studies.* New York, NY: Oxford University Press; 1993.

49. Bianchi GD, Cerhan JR, Parker AS, Putnam SD, See WA, Lynch CF, Cantor KP. Tea consumption and risk of bladder and kidney cancers in a population-based case-control study. *Am J Epidemiol.* 2000;151: 377–383.

50. Thompson FE, Subar AF. Dietary assessment methodology. In: Coulston AM, Rock CL, Monsen ER, eds. *Nutrition in the Prevention and Treatment of Disease.* San Diego, Calif: Academic Press; 2001:3–30.

51. Boushey CJ. Nutritional epidemiology: dietary assessment methods. In: Weaver CM, Heaney RP, eds. *Calcium in Human Health.* Totowa, NJ: Humana Press; 2006:39–64.

52. Bruemmer B, White E, Vaughan TL, Cheney CL. Nutrient intake in relation to bladder cancer among middle-aged men and women. *Am J Epidemiol.* 1996;144:485–495.

PART 2

—ᴡ—

Establishing and Maintaining a Research Environment

3

—ɯ—

Conducting and Presenting Research Ethically

Elaine R. Monsen, PhD, RD

Ethics encompasses the rules and principles that govern right conduct, and the values and guidelines that should govern decisions in science and medicine. Thus, ethical behavior and decisions are of critical import in conducting and presenting research.

The American Dietetic Association (ADA) has adopted a code of ethics, as have other responsible professional groups. The current version of the code, which became effective in 1999, delineates 19 principles to guide dietetics professionals in their conduct, commitments, and obligations to "self, client, society, and the profession" (1). According to the code of conduct, practitioners act with objectivity and respect for the unique needs and values of individuals; avoid discrimination; maintain confidentiality; base practices on scientific principles and current information; conduct professional affairs with honesty, integrity, and fairness; and remain free of conflicts of interest.

In addition to being grounded in ethical judgments, many evaluations and decisions are based on considerations of practicality, aesthetics, or professional values (2,3). Ethical judgments frequently reflect divergent opinions. Cases can be evaluated on an individual basis; indeed, case analysis is a pillar of moral reasoning (4). Despite these differences, people of all cultures and eras have been found to agree on which actions are basically constructive—or destructive—to human interaction. Ethical conduct emphasizes behavior that supports positive relationships between persons and facilitates scientific progress.

At each step of research, ethical issues arise. Designing, conducting, reporting, and interpreting research, as well as planning future research, all involve decisions in which professional ethics is pivotal (5).

RESEARCH ERROR, HUMAN ERROR, AND FRAUD

Scientific errors can seriously impede scientific progress, whether they are the consequences of flawed design, improper conduct of research, unintentional mistakes, or intentional misrepresentation. The repercussions of such errors may be manifold. Time and finances can be wasted in pursuing blind alleys, misapplication of research can be damaging to society, scientific careers can be threatened, and the education of prospective professionals in the field can be compromised. Poor supervision is not acceptable in scientific enterprises. It is critical that researchers assume responsibility and facilitate investigation if misconduct is charged in any research project in which they have participated.

Researchers are obligated to, and generally can, prevent research errors—those of design, execution, analysis, or presentation (6). Research errors may be categorized into six types:

- Sampling errors
- Noncoverage errors
- Nonresponse errors
- Measurement errors
- Errors of data distortion and overgeneralization
- Errors of misrepresentation to human subjects, in authorship, and in conflicts of interest

29

Quality research demands that research errors be minimized; moreover, allowing such errors may cause major ethical dilemmas in the future. Depending on the conduct of the researcher, an error may or may not represent an ethical breach of conduct.

Human errors are generally more obscure and less readily detectable than research errors. Human error is an unfortunate—and, it is hoped, an uncommon—element of research. Three sources of human error need to be differentiated:

- Inadvertent errors
- Negligence
- Intentional deception

Because scientists are fallible, inadvertent errors occur. An honest mistake is acceptable to the scientific community and the public if it is promptly and properly handled once uncovered. However, preventable mistakes attributable to carelessness or negligence are not tolerated by either science or society; sloppy science is a form of intentional error. It is critical, therefore, that researchers be vigilant and maintain a strong leadership role throughout the research process.

Fraud, or intentional deception, destroys science by eroding trust and integrity. Fraud comes in various forms, including concealing data not supportive of a particular hypothesis and presenting only supportive data ("selective" reporting or data "cooking"), revising observed data to conform to a chosen hypothesis (data "trimming"), and blatantly fabricating data. Every deception is intentional, although the extent of misconduct varies dramatically. Researchers rarely falsify or fabricate data, but when they do, it has a calamitous impact that can shut down laboratories and cripple participating institutions. Plagiarism, where one puts forth the work or words of others as one's own, is another category of intentional fraud. The original authors and subjects experience the damaging effects of plagiarism keenly, and the perpetrators can face severe castigation by both the scientific community and the public.

ETHICS IN RESEARCH INVOLVING HUMANS

Nuremberg Code and Declaration of Helsinki

Guidelines and regulations regarding human experimentation have been evolving since the middle of the 20th century, in reaction to public and scientific outcry over a few unrelated cases of gross human injustice. One of the first such incidents to receive public scrutiny was the heinous behavior of physicians toward the inmates of Nazi concentration camps in Germany during World War II. Following the war, 20 of these doctors were tried in Nuremberg before an international tribunal for war crimes and crimes against humanity. The resulting Nuremberg Code of 1947 established 10 principles that must be followed in human experimentation to satisfy moral, ethical, and legal standards (7). These principles first established that the informed voluntary consent of human subjects was essential.

The second major international code of ethics was the Declaration of Helsinki, adopted by the World Medical Association in 1964, with the proviso that the text be reviewed periodically. The basic principles in the Declaration of Helsinki were extended by the 29th World Medical Assembly in Tokyo in 1975, and were further revised in 1983 (8). The 12 basic principles delineate the process of submitting experimental protocols to an independent committee for consideration, comment, and guidance. This concept was the genesis of the institutional review board, which has become a major force in protecting the rights of human subjects. The Helsinki Declaration also counseled researchers to exercise caution in conducting research that could affect the environment and to respect the welfare of animals used for research.

Belmont Report

Another important document supporting the rights of human subjects is the 1978 Belmont Report, issued by the National Commission for the Protection of Human Subjects of Biomedical and Behavioral Research (9). This president's commission was formed in 1974, in a rapid response to the disclosure of two scandalous research studies of the 1930s (10). The first study, which concerned the immune response, involved the injection of live, malignant cells into several elderly patients in a chronic disease hospital without the patients' prior consent. The second study involved long-term observation of the "natural" course of syphilis in men who were recruited into the study without their informed consent. The men were observed for several decades but did not receive penicillin, even though its effectiveness in the treatment of syphilis had been established several years after the initiation of the study.

Respect for persons, beneficence, and justice are the three basic principles upheld in the Belmont Report. The report argues that "respect for persons" incorporates at least two basic ethical convictions (or assurances): that individuals be treated as autonomous agents and that individuals in need of protection because of diminished autonomy are entitled to protection. Beneficence is understood to encompass acts of kindness and charity that go beyond strict obligation. Beneficent actions extend from doing no harm to maximizing possible benefits and minimizing possible harms. Justice demands that each person be treated fairly. It requires that burdens and benefits be shared equally, and that those in a position to reap the benefits of the research are also those who should shoulder the risk. Collectively, these ethical convictions serve as the foundation of effective team-based research that benefits human beings.

The reports issued by the National Commission for the Protection of Human Subjects of Biomedical and Behavioral Research established recommendations for the protection of special categories of human subjects, including human fetuses, children, prisoners, and people institutionalized as mentally infirm. To protect the rights of subjects, institutional review boards were empowered through federal regulations.

In all aspects of human experimentation, it is critical that researchers avoid misrepresentation to human participants. The primary strategy for avoiding this type of research error relies on the three ethical principles of respect, beneficence, and justice. These principles support full and comprehensible disclosure to subjects; noncoerced consent; confidentiality (11); protection of privacy; equity in subject selection; autonomous right of free choice, including the right of the subject to terminate participation without penalty; and the termination of the research project at any point if the data warrant such action. For example, if a study is scheduled to last 7 years, but benefits from the treatment protocol become apparent sooner, the research must be terminated so that control subjects or subjects receiving ineffective treatments may benefit from the effective treatment protocol.

ETHICS IN DESIGNING, CONDUCTING, AND ANALYZING RESEARCH

Confidentiality of medical and personal information is a pillar of scientific ethics. Participants agree, through the informed consent process, to have specific clinical, psychological, or physiological data collected. Researchers must manage the data in a manner that maintains subject confidentiality. Once the data have been collected, the "contract" of informed consent is concluded, and further testing or analysis of samples is prohibited. After a specified period of time for final data analysis, samples should be destroyed. Only when additional consent has been obtained may further analysis be done. Any records indicating the identities of subjects must be maintained securely, with restricted access.

The use of "banked samples" (eg, blood samples taken at the time of an ongoing experiment and carefully stored for subsequent analysis at a time researchers deem appropriate but that is undetermined when the samples are taken) is ethically questionable. The new analysis may be of scientific interest, but there can be no presumption of consent. Another unethical practice is "blanket consent," the assumption of consent to tests and analyses not included in the original agreement. For example, subsequent analyses not governed by the consent agreement could shed light on medical conditions and have a major impact on subjects' lives by influencing insurance coverage, as well as medical and employment decisions.

The scientific method is the basis for research design (6). First, the existing body of scientific knowledge is carefully assessed. Questions important to science and society are formulated, and in response to the research questions a rigorous research design is crafted. Ethical scientific conduct includes accurate recording of data in such a way that they are readily available and understandable to current and future colleagues. To ensure appropriate accessibility, the data need to be recorded at the time they are generated both accurately and in sufficient detail to allow for ready comprehension. Original records need to be carefully secured and maintained, and they must be made available if requested. Subject confidentiality must be maintained as well.

Throughout the process, researchers must carefully attend to details of subject selection, method choice, and execution (12). When critical details are disregarded and sloppy science is allowed, ethical predicaments usually develop.

Dillman (13), who is recognized for his research on survey methodology, outlined four research errors that invalidate a study: sampling error (eg, study sample does not represent actual sample); noncoverage error (eg, a sample that excludes some individuals); nonresponse error (eg, a low response rate or a loss of subjects to follow-up); and measurement error (eg, use of slanted questions and/or use of instruments that lack reliability and validity). The impact of these errors extends beyond survey design to other descriptive research techniques and to analytic research as well. By minimizing and, if possible, eliminating these errors, researchers can make their work substantially more useful. It is unethical in science to be aware of such errors and proceed as though they are of no consequence.

Sampling Errors

Errors of sampling result from differences between the study sample and the population (12,13). For a true probability sample, each individual in the study population must have an equal chance of being selected as a subject. Sampling errors may be random; that is, they may occur by chance as samples from the same population are drawn. Ensuring that each individual within the study population has the same likelihood of participating will minimize random sampling errors.

Another key to minimizing sampling error is ensuring that the sample size is appropriate for the goals of the research (see Chapter 26). The incidence of random sampling errors generally decreases as the sample size increases. A useful guideline is that quadrupling the sample size reduces the rate of random sampling error by half (13).

Noncoverage Errors

Noncoverage errors result from a sampling format that excludes some individuals within the study population as a result of the way subjects are selected. Noncoverage errors, in general, are systematic and difficult to eliminate (13). They are caused by bias in specifying or selecting the study sample (12). For example, subjects may be selected from outdated lists, which would exclude recent additions; from published telephone listings, which would exclude people with unlisted numbers; or from a group of people who are able to attend lectures in the evening, which would exclude people who work at that time. Bias generally occurs when samples of convenience are selected (eg, members of a specific group, volunteers responding to advertisements, or people from different health care institutions in whom a specific disease is diagnosed). Such biases affect the degree to which the data generated represent the population at large.

When bias cannot be eliminated, it is particularly important to recognize it and acknowledge it to the people who are considering the results of the study.

Nonresponse Errors

The third category of error is that of nonresponse. In surveys, the response rate is the percentage of people who actually answer the survey queries (13). A low response rate raises serious questions as to whether the observed data accurately represent the study population—whether the nonresponders differ significantly from the responders. In many studies, researchers strive to improve the response rate by devising various strategies to motivate, remind, and cajole subjects to respond.

Unfortunately, researchers may pay little attention to a modest response rate unless there is a marked disparity between projected and actual observations. One way to lessen concern over a low response rate is to evaluate demographic and other available data related to both nonresponders and responders to ascertain whether important differences exist between the two groups. Another dilemma results when responders provide incomplete data sets—for example, omitting responses or supplying partial responses to some questions in a survey. Researchers can limit inadequate response to survey questions by evaluating and pilot testing the survey carefully, ensuring clarity and ease of response.

A corollary of nonresponse in clinical trials is error resulting from the loss of subjects to follow-up. To minimize such loss, researchers make concerted efforts to complete the data sets. For example, to secure 25 years of follow-up data, some researchers have commissioned private detectives to investigate the whereabouts and life vs death status of individuals in cohorts. Other sources of nonresponse error are missing laboratory values or anthropometric measurements and incomplete food intake records. In each case, the complete and incomplete data sets must be evaluated to ascertain whether the missing data skew the results.

Unless the researcher can be confident that the inclusion of incomplete data is not misleading, the complete and incomplete data sets should be handled separately, rather than as a single, blended group of data. To do otherwise is to present the research results in an unethical manner.

Measurement Errors

Measurement error is the fourth type of research error. Whereas the first three types of error result from nonobservation, measurement error is an error of observation (13). Errors in conducting or executing the research are a source of measurement error. For example, if a question is worded in such a way that it cannot be answered accurately or if a questionnaire is structured so that extra emphasis is placed on certain questions, measurement error will result. It is critical to recognize that slanted questions and selective organization produce biased answers. Subject characteristics may also produce measurement error. An all-too-common measurement error arises from instruments that lack reliability and validity.

Therefore, instruments used in research need to be evaluated and validated prior to use.

Other Sources of Bias

Other biases (12) in executing research projects also need to be recognized and avoided. A common error results when the experimental group and control group are treated differently in ways beyond what is designated by the specified intervention, such as giving additional attention or care to the experimental group. When the control group does not receive care and attention equal to what the experimental group receives, differences in outcome may be inaccurately attributed to the intervention. A masked study design in which subjects and researchers are blinded to treatment and control group assignments can help prevent treatment bias. However, it is difficult to maintain a masked design if certain end points (eg, body weight and blood pressure) are monitored during the study as a component of usual patient care.

Another type of research bias occurs when issues of efficacy become confounded with those of compliance, which may occur when the experimental design requires patients to adhere to specified therapies. For example, some subjects may have a low rate of attendance at the education sessions for a program being evaluated. As suggested in the discussion of nonresponse error, the researcher should compare the complete data sets with the incomplete data sets to determine whether the data can be merged. Similarly, subjects who either withdraw or are withdrawn from an experiment may differ systematically from those who remain, resulting in withdrawal bias. Furthermore, preconception bias is likely to occur unless the experimental design is masked, or blinded, with methods established to allow the investigation to proceed and data to be collected without influence or bias from either subject or investigator.

Well-Crafted Design

The well-crafted research design minimizes research errors. All people in the population that the investigator wishes to observe have an equal probability of being subjects, so that noncoverage error is avoided. Individual subjects within that population are randomly selected, and the number selected is sufficiently large to provide the desired precision, so that sampling error is minimized. Subject sampling criteria are guided by official research policies; for example, children as a category are defined by set standards. Every subject selected responds and no subject is lost

to follow-up, so that response error is not a factor. The techniques for estimating response are precise, accurate, reproducible, and equally valid for each subject; each subject complies fully with the assigned regimen, thus limiting measurement error; and all data are truthfully and fully recorded.

Thoughtful and adequate supervision is essential in all research projects to ensure that the data are properly collected. Each person in a research team must assume responsibility for all aspects of the research in his or her domain and maintain awareness of the project in its entirety. The team includes graduate students, research assistants, intradisciplinary and interdisciplinary professionals, and faculty. Although the chief supervisor must assume ultimate accountability, responsibility for ethical conduct falls on everyone's shoulders.

ETHICAL PRESENTATION AND INTERPRETATION OF RESEARCH

Honesty, truthfulness, and full disclosure are necessary in the presentation of research. It is the researcher's obligation to publish valid data, to analyze the data objectively and dispassionately, and to present a fair and unbiased interpretation to readers (14,15). Inferences must be supported by the data. Authors must recognize the power of inference and avoid misleading the reader.

For their part, readers are obligated to use data ethically, without distortion (16). The Council of Biology Editors (now the Council of Scientific Editors) contends that equal degrees of care must be exercised by researchers and authors in preparing the message they send and by readers in interpreting the message they receive and use (15).

Presentation of the Whole Truth, and Nothing but the Truth

The ethical investigator truthfully reports and fully discloses research data and the methods whereby the data were generated. At all times, scientific proof must be rigorous and without bias (17). Limitations of the study design—for example, subject bias—should be clearly stated. The ethical investigator objectively evaluates the data and provides a fair interpretation. To do otherwise is ethically insupportable.

Several data handling practices are considered unethical and may constitute data distortion: data dredging, selective reporting of findings, fragmentation of reports, redundant publication, and inappropriate statistical tests (15). Data dredging is the process of combing through a large pool of data to pick out "significant findings" from research that was not designed to produce those results. Data dredging is particularly damaging when only "positive" results are reported and "negative" results are ignored, making the former appear to be important rather than significant merely by chance. Because the accepted level of statistical significance is .05 or less, the chance that a relationship would be considered significant is 1 in 20. Thus, if the number of comparisons were large, which could be the case if data collected from 10 laboratory values and the dietary intake of 10 nutrients were compared, the potential comparisons would undoubtedly yield several "significant relationships" (perhaps 5 out of 100 in the present example), most of which would occur by chance and would thus lack relevance.

The relationships that are appropriate for evaluation are those specified in the original research design, driven by the research question and hypothesis. Chance observations may encourage further research, and if the new research question results in data that replicate the earlier "positive" results, publication of the findings is justified.

Selective reporting of research findings is a form of intentional fraud, often motivated by the desire to support a chosen hypothesis when the data do not provide adequate support. Such actions as concealing data, presenting solely favorable data, or otherwise shaping or trimming data to accommodate the hypothesis amount to a disregard for scientific and ethical principles. Such conscious acts are ignoble, premeditated efforts to distort data and mislead colleagues and the public.

Research findings that are fragmented and published in multiple, small units are a disservice to readers. The whole picture is not visible, and interrelationships are lost. Scientific editors discourage the submission of "least publishable units," commonly called LPUs, and refer to such fragmentation as "salami science." A similar wasteful practice is duplicate or redundant publication, the presentation of essentially the same study in more than one place with little, if any, modification. Copyright laws prohibit such actions.

Statistics in Data Interpretation

Statistics is the art and science of interpreting quantitative data. It includes framing questions that are answerable, designing the study, exercising quality control of the data to limit researcher-initiated variance and bias, drawing inferences from data, and generalizing results to other situations (12,15,17).

Fienberg (18) suggests that the following eight points be addressed in a statistical review of a submitted manuscript. The points are of equal usefulness in designing, conducting, and reporting research.

- What do the original data consist of? How have they been transformed for use in the statistical analyses?
- Is information given on uncertainty and measurement error?
- How were the statistical analyses done, and are they accurately described in the paper?
- Are the statistical methods that were used appropriate for the data?
- Have the data or analyses been "selected," and does such selection distort the "facts"?
- What population do the data represent? Does the design for data collection allow for the inferences and generalizations made?
- Are additional analyses possible that would be enlightening?
- Are the conclusions sensitive to the methodological and substantive assumptions? If so, is this fact acknowledged? Do reported measures of uncertainty reflect this sensitivity?

The core of the scientific method, and hence of science, is inference: learning about unobserved phenomena by studying and interpreting relevant data on observed phenomena (12,15,17). Inference must be protected, not abused through such distorting actions as selective reporting and data dredging. Data need to be honest and honestly presented.

ETHICS IN PUBLICATION

It is your responsibility to submit manuscripts that are appropriate for publication consideration and peer review; in other words, the data need to be accurate, responsibly analyzed, and responsibly interpreted. The research design and the materials and methods used need to be clearly and fully presented. All relevant sources require full and accurate citation. It is unethical and deceptive to present data selectively, to withhold contradictory data, or to revise data for the purpose of impact.

Questions often arise as to the amount of data that should be presented in a manuscript. The goal should be to proffer the optimal publishable unit, not to disperse the data in a number of LPUs. With tenure evaluations focusing more on quality per unit published and less on number of units published, LPUs will be viewed as a negative factor in a researcher's list of publications. If a researcher is allowed to offer five original publications for tenure consideration, the advantage will go to a well-crafted and reasoned article rather than a single fragment of a research project.

Peer review is the primary instrument that science uses to monitor itself. The scientist accepts the dual professional responsibility of submitting research for peer review and serving as an objective, ethical reviewer for the work of peers. Reviewers assume the responsibility of ensuring the scientific integrity of published literature, and their confidentiality is a critical component of ethical behavior toward an author. Should legitimate conflicts of interest become apparent to peer reviewers, they should decline the review rather than jeopardize a sound review process. It is obviously unethical to take advantage of authors by invading the confidentiality of the peer review process or by using their work before its official publication.

In the interpretation and application of data, it is tempting to overpresent the data to the media and the public (19). The desire to make a point or to support a bias or preconception must not override the accurate use of scientific data. For example, a research study showing lower serum cholesterol concentrations in men who consumed a diet low in saturated fat cannot be generalized to the population at large (all other men), let alone to infants, children, adolescents, women, or the elderly. To overgeneralize erodes the credibility both of the researcher and of science in general (20). It is particularly disturbing when data are overgeneralized in an effort to perpetrate prejudice or patronage. Honest differences of opinion exist, and they should be stated clearly, with recognition given to opposing views. However, inappropriately representing one's own data or the data of others is scientifically reprehensible, because it misleads others.

ETHICAL ISSUES RELATED TO AUTHORSHIP

Authorship implies a substantial contribution to a published article and conveys responsibility for the content. Collaboration in research allows input from the vantage point of each participant and can improve research design, conduct, presentation, and dissemination. Also, effective collaboration sets the stage for further joint research endeavors (20).

The Uniform Requirements for Manuscripts Submitted to Biomedical Journals delineate three criteria to determine whether someone has contributed sufficiently to be designated as an author. The criteria, all of which

must be satisfied, include substantial contributions to (a) design or analysis and interpretation of the data, (b) drafting or revision of the article critically for important intellectual content, and (c) final approval of the version to be published (21).

Authorship cannot be justified for a person whose participation is limited to the acquisition of funding, administration of the department or unit, or the collection of the data. General, as opposed to specific, supervision of the research group is also considered inadequate to warrant authorship. Each section critical to the main conclusions of the article must be the product of one or more of the designated authors. For an article consisting of contributions of researchers from diverse fields, only the key people responsible for the article should be specified as authors; other contributors should be recognized and thanked in an acknowledgment.

An author must make major contributions to the genesis and presentation of the research data. In addition, an author not only is responsible for the published data but also must be prepared to defend the data and the interpretation of the data. Discussion continues on how extensive an individual's contribution must be to qualify as an author, and how accountable to both peers and the public an author must be for the paper in its entirety. One obvious dilemma is the extent of accountability an author assumes when collaborating with scientists and professionals in diverse fields. At minimum, individual authors are responsible for all aspects of work that are within and proximate to their fields of expertise.

The primary or lead author has a special position that results from having made the major intellectual input to the article. The primary author also should have made outstanding, positive, and creative contributions; provided the major intellectual input; participated actively in the work, data tabulation, and interpretation; and provided key scientific leadership throughout the research design, conduct, analysis, and presentation (15). It is customary to reward the individual who is the primary author of the manuscript with the first author position.

CONFLICTS OF INTEREST

Conflicts of interest occur whenever financial or other personal considerations compromise, or appear to compromise, an investigator's professional actions in designing, conducting, or reporting research. Conflicts of interest may also bias other aspects of an investigator's research activities, such as the choice of methods, the length of time subjects are studied, purchases of materials, hiring of support staff, or the choice of statistical analyses. Other scholarly activities are also affected by conflicts of interest; for example, in the preparation of review articles, financial and personal interests may interfere with professional objectivity.

It is customary for investigators to disclose any possible conflicts. The editors of professional journals expect acknowledgment of each author's funding sources and institutional and corporate affiliations to appear on the title page of articles submitted for publication. In addition, consultancies, stock ownership, or other equity interests or patent licensing issues should be disclosed to the journal editor in a cover letter at the time articles are submitted (15,22). It is important for full disclosure to be made, because the appearance of conflict may be as professionally damaging as proven conflict (23). Many reputable scientists are subject to one or several actual or perceived conflicts of interest. Their disclosure provides a platform for unbiased, open evaluation.

Concerns over conflicts of interest should not deter an investigator from seeking ethical financial and corporate relations. Problems develop when financial interests are not disclosed. It is ethically irresponsible for a scientist, because of a personal conflict of interest and thus a possible desirable or undesirable financial impact, to repress negative data, to expose only selected findings, or to distort the presentation of data in any other way. Financial interest should neither interfere with professional objectivity nor drive professional activities.

CONCLUSION

The three principles of respect for persons, beneficence, and justice are excellent guides, not only in considerations concerning human subjects, but also in interactions with close colleagues, professional peers, clients, the public, and the media. Conflicts of interest require full disclosure to ensure that others are not misled. In such an ethical climate, research accomplishments will grow and survive.

The application of ethics in scientific research can be encapsulated in the statement that one needs to act responsibly in every aspect of research, from design to presentation.

REFERENCES

1. American Dietetic Association. Code of Ethics for the profession of dietetics. *J Am Diet Assoc.* 1999;99:103–113.

2. Fieber LK. Practice points: ethical considerations in dietetics practice. *J Am Diet Assoc.* 2000;100:454.

3. Woteki CE. Conflicts of interest in presentations and publications and dietetics research. *J Am Diet Assoc.* 2006;106:27–31.

4. Jonsen AR, Toulmin S. *The Abuse of Casuistry: A History of Moral Reasoning.* Berkeley: University of California Press; 1988.

5. Monsen ER, Vanderpool HY, Halsted CH, McNutt KW, Sandstead HH. Ethics: responsible scientific conduct. *Am J Clin Nutr.* 1991;54:1–6.

6. Committee on the Conduct of Science, National Academy of Sciences. *On Being a Scientist.* Washington, DC: National Academies Press; 1995.

7. *Trials of War Criminals Before the Nuremberg Military Tribunal Under Control Council Law No. 10.* Vol 2. Washington, DC: US Government Printing Office; 1949.

8. 18th World Medical Assembly. The Helsinki Declaration of 1964. In: Reich WT, ed. *Encyclopedia of Bioethics.* Vol 4. New York, NY: Free Press; 1978:1770–1771.

9. National Commission for the Protection of Human Subjects of Biomedical and Behavioral Research. *The Belmont Report: Ethical Principles and Guidelines for the Protection of Human Subjects of Research.* Washington, DC: US Government Printing Office; 1978. DHEW publication (OS) 78–0012; Appendix I, DHEW publication (OS) 78–0013; Appendix II; DHEW publication (OS) 78–0014.

10. Levine RI. *Ethics and Regulation of Clinical Research.* 2nd ed. New Haven, Conn: Yale University Press; 1988.

11. Botkin JR. Protecting the privacy of family members in survey and pedigree research. *JAMA.* 2001;258:207–211.

12. Riegelman RK. *Studying a Study and Testing a Test.* 4th ed. Philadelphia, Pa: Lippincott Williams & Wilkins; 2000.

13. Dillman DA. *Mail and Internet Surveys: The Tailored Design Method.* 2nd ed. New York, NY: John Wiley and Sons; 1999.

14. Block BH. Ethical and legal issues in medical writing. *J Am Podiatr Med Assoc.* 1998;88:45–46.

15. Council of Biology Editors. *Ethics and Policy in Scientific Publication.* Bethesda, Md: Council of Biology Editors; 1990.

16. Kagarise MJ, Sheldon GF. Translational ethics: a perspective for the new millennium. *Arch Surg.* 2000;135:39–45.

17. Huth EJ. *Writing and Publishing in Medicine.* 3rd ed. Baltimore, Md: Williams & Wilkins; 1999.

18. Fienberg SE. Statistical reporting in scientific journals. In: *Ethics and Policy in Scientific Publications.* Bethesda, Md: Council of Biology Editors; 1990.

19. Fahmy S. *Research Integrity and the Media. CBE Views.* Vol 22. Bethesda, Md: Council of Biology Editors; 1999:151.

20. Gardner JK, Rall, LC, Peterson, CA. Lack of multidisciplinary collaboration is a barrier to outcomes research. *J Am Diet Assoc.* 2002;122:65–71.

21. International Committee of Medical Journal Editors. Uniform requirements for manuscripts submitted to biomedical journals. *Ann Intern Med.* 1988;108:258–265.

22. Krinsky S, Rothenberg LS. Financial interest and its disclosure in scientific publications. *JAMA.* 1998;280:225–226.

23. Inbody T. *Conflicts of Interest in Relation to Articles. CBE Views.* Vol 22. Bethesda, Md: Council of Biology Editors; 1999:188.

4

How to Write Proposals and Obtain Funding

Dianne Neumark-Sztainer, PhD, MPH, RD

The primary reason for writing grant proposals is to obtain funding to implement a research idea. The grant proposal is a venue for selling our ideas to potential funders (1). Thus, our ideas need to be conveyed in a manner that will invoke enthusiasm amongst the reviewers and funding agency, and convince them that the proposed research questions are worthy of exploration, the research team is qualified to implement the study, and the methods being proposed are feasible, well-planned, and appropriate for the research questions being addressed.

GRANT PROPOSALS

A grant proposal is a detailed blueprint of a research plan. Writing a proposal helps researchers clarify why the proposed study is important and guides the development of a polished, well-thought-out plan for addressing the research questions of interest. Thus, even though the primary reason for writing a grant proposal is to obtain funding, an additional benefit is that the process of writing the proposal helps in developing a well-thought-out research plan and guiding its implementation.

Writing grant proposals can also offer individuals benefits in terms of career development and independence on the job. Individuals who are able to write successful grant proposals will be more attractive employees to hire and may be more likely to progress up the career ladder. Furthermore, individuals who can bring in money to fund their research ideas will generally have more independence on the job and be able to work on projects that they view as important.

Learning how to write strong grant proposals is an important skill for researchers and practitioners who are interested in advancing science. Writing grant proposals can be a daunting and scary task because it means expressing one's ideas for others to critique. Additionally, it requires time and energy. Writing grant proposals is a skill that can be learned and that improves with practice. Both the experienced and the first-time grant writer can learn how to enhance their grant-writing skills in order to make the process of writing proposals easier, more enjoyable, and more successful.

WHERE TO START

The successful grant proposal begins with a good idea that will be deemed worthy of funding. If you have determined a research idea, a few steps can help in turning it into a workable and fundable plan:

- **Clarify the plan.** Consider the idea and why it is important. Think about how you could go about implementing a test study for your idea. Think broadly about the contributions of your idea to science. But also think about the specifics, in order to ensure that your study will be feasible to implement and will truly address the research questions being explored. Thus, if you are interested in developing and evaluating a program to reduce risk of overweight in elementary school children, consider both how your approach is unique and will move the field of obesity prevention forward, and such specifics as the number of schools needed and how you will recruit participants. Come back to this step at several points in the grant-writing process in order to fully develop a clear research plan.

- **Review the literature.** Determine whether there is justification for the content area you wish to explore and for your proposed methods. See what work has been done in related areas and determine what the next step in the research chain of events needs to be. Ideally, some related studies have already demonstrated the importance of the topic, but weaknesses remain in the knowledge pool that can be filled by your study. With regard to the school-based obesity prevention idea, you would need to examine whether obesity is a topic worthy of being addressed and examine its prevalence, health implications, and amenability to change. You would also want to explore previous school-based obesity prevention interventions and their evaluations. You would further want to identify suitable target groups, novel intervention approaches, and appropriate evaluation strategies.
- **Talk with others.** Talk with people who have been successful in writing grant proposals. Listen to what they tell you. Experienced grant writers may tell you to refine your idea to increase its specificity and feasibility, and it is generally worthwhile to heed this advice. Also talk with people out in the field to get their insight. Thus, for the school-based obesity project, you might speak with other obesity prevention researchers (about the study design and the intervention), a statistician (about the number of participants that are needed for statistical purposes), school staff (about perceived needs and logistics within schools), and children (about their interests).
- **Explore funding possibilities.** Keep your eyes open for suitable funding agencies and grant opportunities related to your research plan. Read as much as you can about their guidelines and about previous projects they have funded. If you need more information, contact the funding agency. Prepare a clear, brief description of your plan, and call the contact person(s) at the funding agency to discuss your idea and assess its suitability for that funding agency. The

next section of this chapter addresses how to explore funding opportunities.
- **Go back and tweak your research ideas.** Incorporate what you have learned from reviewing the literature, talking with others, and gathering information from the funding agency into your plan.

LOOKING FOR FUNDS

Once you have a clear research idea, you will need to find a suitable funding agency. Online resources are listed at the end of this chapter. Although there are many useful resources, they can feel overwhelming. Try talking with others who have received funding in areas similar to the one you are interested in to learn about their experiences with different funding agencies. Consider the following possible sources of funding:

- **Institutional or in-house funds.** This is an excellent place to begin the grant-writing process, because institutes want to get their young investigators off to a good start. Often, these organizations make funds available to young investigators who are just getting started. Many times the aim of these funds is to help investigators with small, pilot studies that are likely to form the basis for larger grants down the road. Students are particularly encouraged to apply for in-house student awards for small research studies. Some graduate studies programs offer mechanisms for student research awards, and they are relatively easy to obtain.
- **Nonprofit and professional organizations.** The American Dietetic Association (ADA) or the American Heart Association often have grants for individuals at different levels of their careers, including students. Nonprofit and professional organizations offer funding opportunities to young investigators since they are interested in promoting research careers within their respective fields. For example, the National Eating Disorders Association has a small grant opportunity that is available only to investigators early in their careers who have not yet received a large research grant.
- **Foundations.** Foundations may provide funding to projects of local interest or within specific content areas. Foundations may address a particular topic area (eg, infant health) or may serve a local community. In contrast to other funding agencies, foundations

are often interested in funding projects that receive funds from multiple sources, thus demonstrating wider support for a project.

- **Industry.** Corporations often have foundations for research in areas that the company has identified as important. Usually, the funds are for a topic that will somehow be useful to the particular industry, although this is not always the case. Aside from their foundations, private sector businesses may have particular research interests of direct relevance to products they are developing. Food industry companies can be an excellent source for funding nutrition-related research, but it is important to clarify the conditions up front with regard to investigator independence in reporting study findings.

- **Government grants.** Federal, state, and other government agencies offer many grant opportunities. Grants may be available for all levels of researchers, and come in different amounts and from a wide variety sources. Topics of interest may be specified by the different funding agencies in the form of program announcements, priority areas, or specific requests for applications. Alternatively, researchers may submit their proposals for their own areas of interest. The largest funding agency for health-related research is the National Institutes of Health (NIH). Other significant federal agencies for nutrition-related research include the National Science Foundation, the US Department of Agriculture, and the Food and Drug Administration.

GRANT REVIEWS

Prior to writing the grant, consider who will review the proposal and how the review process works. The process will differ across funding agencies and particular grant mechanisms, but there are a number of similarities in the review process.

Review panels are often formed to review grant proposals. Reviewers on the panel read the proposals individually and then discuss them in a face-to-face meeting or via a telephone conference call. Review panels generally include researchers with some level of expertise in an area related to the content of each proposal. Grant proposals are distributed to reviewers, who prepare an evaluative summary of the proposal and give it a score. Sometimes all of the reviewers on a panel read the proposal and their scores get averaged to provide a summary score. More often, one or two primary reviewers will read the proposal and provide a description of the proposal and their evaluations to the larger panel of reviewers, the rest of whom have not read the proposal. The larger panel will contribute to the decision-making process regarding how the proposal should be scored based upon the primary reviewers' comments and the ensuing discussion.

Take the review process into account in writing a proposal. In particular, consider following points:

In general, individuals reviewing grant proposals do this work in addition to their regular work. Reviewers may read proposals in the evening after a full day of work, on a weekend, or even on an airplane. They appreciate encountering a clear, well-written research plan that addresses an important topic. Although it is the reviewers' job to do a thorough review of each proposal, it is your job to make the proposal leap out from the pile and to be as easy to read as possible. Thus, when writing a proposal, think about how best to get your ideas across to the reviewer. Tactics that can help a late-night reviewer include a clear, concise statement of the research questions and research plan at the beginning of the proposal; use of summaries and some repetition throughout the grant to emphasize major points; bolded subheadings to ease reading; effective diagrams to break up the text and clarify study designs and timelines; white space on the page between sections and at margins; short, clear sentences; and correct spelling and grammar. Good ideas may be lost in a poorly written proposal.

The expertise of the reviewers may be in a field related to the topic of the grant proposal, but not in the specific area being addressed. To increase your chance of getting a strong review, avoid assuming that the reviewer has a thorough understanding of the specific topic at hand, why it is important, and how it should be studied. Clearly lay out a justification for the topic being studied and the proposed research design. Building your proposal from basics will help the reviewer understand the importance of the research questions and the appropriateness of the research methods. It will also help the reviewer better explain the proposal to other members of the review panel if needed. Put yourself in the position of a reviewer in thinking about how your grant proposal will be read. The reviewer wants to come off in a positive light when presenting a review of your proposal to the other review panelists. The reviewer does not want to come across as not understanding the proposal or falsely judging its merit. Help your reviewer make an accurate presentation of what you are proposing and why it is important.

Give special attention to how the abstract and opening sections are framed. These first sections should clearly state what the study is about and why it is important. Make it easy for the primary reviewer to summarize the proposal in a succinct and convincing manner for other reviewers on the review panel and the funding agency. You should make it easy for the non-reader who sits on the review panel to take a quick look at the abstract and be enthused about the study.

GRANT PROPOSAL QUESTIONS

The format and length of grant proposals will differ by funding agency and grant mechanisms. Guidelines regarding the components to be included and their order of presentation will differ, and length limitations may range from 1 to 25 pages. But all proposals, regardless of format or length, need to address the following four questions (2):

- What is the proposed study about?
- Why is the study worth doing?
- Who is the research team and what makes them qualified to implement the study?
- How will the study be done and is the study plan the best one for addressing the research questions?

You are trying to sell both yourself and the research idea. You need to convince the reviewers and funding agency that the study needs to be done, that you are person to do the study, and that the proposed methods are the best way to get it done.

Grant applications for the NIH include four main sections that loosely correspond to the questions outlined earlier (2)

- Specific Aims—What?
- Background and Significance—Why?
- Preliminary Studies—Who?
- Research Design and Methods—How?

Each section's primary purpose is to address the question included in the parentheses following the section title, but there will still be overlap. For example, in the first section, the main purpose is to describe what the study is about, what the study's aims are, and why the study is important. Each of these four sections is described here.

Specific Aims—What?

The first section of an NIH grant application allows the applicant to immediately address the question "What?" "What is this study about?" It is helpful for the reviewer to learn what the proposed study aims to accomplish right at the beginning. In accordance with the type of study, the applicant may choose to utilize goals and specific aims, study objectives, research questions, and/or hypotheses. Reviewers generally like to see hypotheses; however, if the study is descriptive in nature, hypotheses may not be appropriate. Regardless of whether the research questions are framed as statements or questions, they need to be clear. A strong grant proposal will start with clear research questions and build upon them throughout the proposal (3).

Although the main point of the Specific Aims section is to describe what this study aims to achieve, it is also worthwhile to grab the reviewer's attention from the outset by stating why the proposed study is so important. Show how your specific research questions will help advance knowledge in the field by addressing a significant problem. Provide a succinct description of the study plan for addressing the research questions to give the reviewer a context for reading the proposal. Remember that this section may be the only section read by some review panelists, and it will be the first section read by all reviewers. Avoid too much detail; the details can come later, after you have convinced the reviewer of the importance of this study and helped the reviewer clearly understand what it is that the proposed study aims to achieve.

Background and Significance—Why?

The primary aim of this section is to address the question "Why?" Provide a clear justification for the proposed study, including both the topic being addressed and the proposed methodologies. Thus, for a nutrition intervention study, justify both the target of the intervention (eg, fruit and vegetable intake in children) and the methodologies being proposed to bring about increases in the targeted behavior (eg, increased availability in school cafeterias). A strong statement about how the proposed study will move the field forward and contribute to the advancement of science should be included at the end of this section.

This is your opportunity to demonstrate familiarity with the literature. The omission of a key study exploring a topic similar to that being addressed in this proposal will not be viewed favorably, particularly if the reviewer implemented the omitted study. You can show how your previous work has contributed to the topic being addressed in the proposal (and thus begin to address the question of "who?"). Remember that the purpose of this section is *not* to provide a thorough review of the literature, but rather to provide a justification for the proposed study. Common critiques from reviewers are that this section does not clearly justify a need for the proposed study and provides too much extraneous background information (4). A focus on justifying the proposed study rather than on reviewing the literature will make the applicant's work easier and lead to a more focused and successful proposal.

Preliminary Studies—Who?

The third section of an NIH application provides an opportunity for you to address the question "Who is the research team and why are they qualified to do the proposed study?" This section is often divided into two subsections. The first subsection describes the research team and their qualifications, whereas the second subsection describes relevant work by the research team that has led to the study being proposed. This section can be scary for young investigators with little writing experience. Young investigators should be encouraged to do the following:

- Begin with smaller grants to build up their record and demonstrate that they have the ability to successfully implement research studies.
- Apply for grants that are specifically intended for young investigators.
- Include more experienced investigators on their research team as either co-investigators or consultants.

Co-investigators are full-fledged team members who are involved in the study on an ongoing basis, whereas consultants are usually less involved but contribute their expertise in specific areas of need. If you experience difficulty in writing this section and cannot demonstrate adequate experience in areas related to the proposal's content, it may be worthwhile to consider adding additional investigators to the study or implementing a pilot study prior to embarking on the proposed study.

You need to convince the reviewer that the research team is highly qualified to implement the proposed study. This is not a time to be overly modest. It is best to use factual statements, rather than adjectives, to describe team members' expertise. For example, discuss each research team member's area of training, publication record, and previous research work. You should also discuss collaborative efforts by research team members to demonstrate that the team has worked successfully together in the past. Areas of complementary strengths should be emphasized. Finally, resources available to the research team that will help in the study's implementation should also be mentioned.

A description of relevant research and pilot work done by the research team should be described in this section of the proposal. Details of pilot studies, including what was done and what was learned should be included (4). A description of how the proposed study will build on previous work done by the research team can also be useful. The Preliminary Studies section provides a link to the following section of the proposal, in which the research design is laid out, by demonstrating the feasibility of the proposed study methodologies.

Research Design and Methods—How?

The longest and most detailed section of the grant proposal is the Research Design and Methods section. Here the details of how the study will be implemented are described. Study limitations and how they will be addressed should be discussed within the relevant subsections. Subsections of this portion of the application will differ with the specific study but will often include the following:

- **Overview.** A summarized introduction helps orient the reviewer to the detailed plan to follow. Often a diagram that presents the overall plan can be useful.
- **Research design.** Describe the research design and briefly justify its suitability for addressing the research questions (5).
- **Study population and recruitment.** Details on exclusion and inclusion criteria and how subjects will be recruited are absolutely essential (4). Concerns about problems such as bias or lack of ability to generalize from the study population should be addressed. A brief description of procedures for obtaining consent for study participation should be included, although there is a separate section of the application in which details on human subjects protections will be described.
- **Intervention.** If an intervention is part of the study, the theory underlying the intervention, components of the intervention, and differences between the intervention and control conditions should be described. A diagram of factors being addressed in the intervention and intervention components can be useful. Theoretical constructs being addressed in the intervention should be clear, and there should be consistency across the theoretical model, the intervention, and the evaluation plan.
- **Data collection procedures and tools.** Include details of how data will be collected and what the tools will look like. If a survey is being used, include a table

that describes the global constructs to be assessed, specific variables, questions for each variable, psychometrics of questions and scales, and sources of questions. A considerable amount of work goes into thinking about how best to design such a table, but given the need for detail, the limited time that a reviewer may spend on each proposal, and page limitations, tables can be a good way to provide information. Limitations of data collection tools (eg, collecting dietary data with one 24-hour recall or collecting self-reported data on height and weight) should be addressed in a manner that justifies the selection of these tools.

- **Timeline.** Provide a diagram that shows when different aspects of the study will be conducted. Adequate time should be allotted for recruitment of the sample, preparation of intervention materials and evaluation tools, data collection, data organization, data analysis, and manuscript preparation to disseminate the study's findings. See Figure 4.1 for an example of a timeline included in a grant proposal for a study on eating, activity, and weight in adolescents.
- **Statistical analyses.** Provide a clear plan for data analysis and justification for the sample size. Often

a statistician will assist in writing this section. It is crucial that the research questions be adequately addressed by the analysis plan.

- **Summary.** A brief summary can be provided to remind the reviewer about the strengths of the study and why it is worthwhile. Koren (6) indicates that it is important to remind the reviewers, who may have dozed off in the methods section, about the importance of the proposed study. A couple of sentences about the study's value allow the proposal to end on an upbeat tone.

You should provide a high level of detail in this section. It may seem logical to first see whether the proposal is going to get funded and work out the details later. Unfortunately, it does not work that way. Although the required level of detail may differ with the type of study, the length of the grant proposal, and the amount of funding being requested, the study plan always needs to be well-developed prior to learning whether the study will actually be funded. Even though this is a time-consuming project, it is far more efficient to invest the time in a strong grant proposal than to have to write numerous proposals because they do not get funded.

Study year / Calendar dates	Year 1 (9/07-8/08) Sep	Dec	Mar	Jun	Year 2 (9/08-8/09) Sep	Dec	Mar	Jun	Year 3 (9/09-8/10) Sep	Dec	Mar	Jun	Year 4 (9/10-8/11) Sep	Dec	Mar	Jun	Year 5 (9/11-8/12) Sep	Dec	Mar	Jun
Staff organization	▦																			
Literature review for surveys	▦																			
Revise data collection protocol	■				▨															
Annual mail contacts (tracking)	■										■				▦				▦	
School recruitment/approvals					▨	▨														
Survey revision/development		■				▨														
Focus groups and pilot testing			■					▨												
Survey prep for administration				■			▨													
Modify environ. tools/protocols		▦	▦	▦	▦	▦	▦													
Data collection						■	■	▨	▨											
Data organization									■	■	▨									
Scale construction/psychometrics										■	▨	▨								
Preparation of writing manual													▦	▦						
Nutrition/PA education													▦	▦						
Data analysis, writing papers													■	■		▨	▨			
Presentations at conferences															■	■	▨	▨		
Preparation of summary																				▦

Legend: General ▦ | Longitudinal ■ | Cross-sectional ▨

FIGURE 4.1   Example of a timeline included in a grant proposal.

Other Sections

The four sections just described are viewed as the main portion of the grant proposal, and page limitations are generally restricted to these four sections. However, there are a few other elements of a grant proposal that are worth mentioning.

The *title* of the grant is the first thing that reviewers will see. It can be challenging to find a title that is short, yet conveys the main message of the grant proposal and also generates some interest on the reviewer's part. The title may also guide the selection of an appropriate review panel for the proposal.

The *abstract* or summary page serves as a basis for assigning the proposal to a suitable review panel. It provides reviewers with their first look into what the proposal is about. It may be the only part read by some members of the review panel and often forms the basis for the review that the primary reviewer shares with the larger review panel. Although this section often gets written toward the end of the grant-writing process, be sure you have enough time to write a strong, convincing, and comprehensive abstract. *Appendixes* play an important role within grant proposals, but should be used judiciously. Material should be supplementary and not required reading, since not everyone on the review panel will receive them. Nevertheless, material such as scientific articles by research team members, copies of surveys, detailed information on survey questions, and letters of support should be included.

Other required sections include those dealing with issues of human subjects protection, the use of animals, the inclusion of women and minorities, and data safety monitoring. The guidelines for the completion of these sections will vary across funding agencies and should be followed closely.

BUDGET SECTION

The budget section includes a budget and budget justification. The budget usually includes three categories of costs:

- Personnel costs
- Other study-related costs
- Institutional overhead

Some of the costs typically included in a grant proposal for community-based nutrition intervention programs are outlined in Box 4.1. The actual items to be included in a budget vary from study to study. The presentation of the budget will also differ in accordance with the funding agency and the home institution from which the grant is being sent. Often a form will be provided to guide budget development and presentation. Carefully examine allowable expenses at both the institution and the funding agencies because there will be variations. For example, some funding agencies do not allow costs related to the principal investigator's time and others do not allow for institutional overhead charges.

BOX 4.1   Typical Budget Items for a Grant Proposal to Develop, Implement, and Evaluate a Community-Based Nutrition Intervention Program

Personnel Costs
- Principal investigator
- Co-investigators
- Statistician/programmer
- Study coordinator
- Interventionists
- Research assistants
- Secretary

Intervention Supplies
- Materials development and printing
- Supplies (eg, water bottles, pedometers)
- Food for meetings/tasting/distribution

Evaluation Costs
- Survey development and printing
- Purchase of computers/software (eg, 24-hour recall)
- Data entry/coding
- Participant incentives (recruitment, evaluation)

General Implementation Costs
- Mileage
- Office supplies, file cabinets, computers
- Rental of buses/vans
- Mailing costs
- Telephone
- Photocopying
- Translation of consent forms and other forms

Institutional Overhead
- Amount based on prior agreements between institution and funding agency
- May range from 0% to more than 50% of total study costs
- Covers costs such as building upkeep, rental space, heating, and administrative expenses related to grants and overall institution

Unless a study requires expensive equipment, the major costs of a study are usually personnel expenses. Personnel costs are typically presented as percentages of time (eg, 50% of time in year 1 and 100% of time in years 2 through 4). For personnel working on a part-time basis (eg, as interviewers) or as consultants on a grant, hourly rates may also be used. In developing a grant proposal, carefully consider all personnel you will need to work on the project, how much time they will realistically need, the types of background they should have, and how much they will cost. If you have specific people in mind, their names can be included in the budget justification.

The budget is generally followed by a budget justification that provides a more detailed explanation of how the funds will be used. For example, funds may be requested in the budget for a project director; an explanation of the roles of the project director will be explained in the budget justification.

A commonly asked question is "How much money should I ask for in my budget?" Ideally, the only question you will need to address in order to determine how much money to request is the following: "How much money is needed to implement the study as I would like?" In an ideal world, the project will determine the budget and you will find a funding agency (or a combination of funding agencies) willing to fund your study. In reality, however, your budget will also inform the study design. Prior to fully developing your study plan, explore potential funding agencies and examine how much money they typically award. If there is an upper limit, the study will need to be planned in accordance. The final budget should reflect the true costs. A budget that is padded with unnecessary costs will not be viewed favorably. A budget that is too low may be viewed as unrealistic and the author(s) may lose credibility. Reviewers and funding agencies generally have a good sense as to how much it costs to implement studies. That said, you might take on a study that is inadequately funded, either for ideological reasons or because you believe it is a necessary steppingstone to larger funding opportunities. In these cases, you will donate your own time and find interested students or young investigators who are willing to contribute their time in return for a valuable learning experience.

ADHERE TO THE PLAN

A grant proposal should be viewed as a contract between the principal investigator and the funding agency. The funding agency agrees to give the requested funds to the principal investigator, who agrees to do the research plan outlined in the grant proposal. However, things may change as the plan goes out into the field or to the lab. Usually, small changes in methodologies do not pose a problem and may be implemented at the discretion of the principal investigator and the research team. Small changes may include changes in proposed questions on a survey, staff reassignments, and minor modifications to the proposed intervention. However, large changes to proposed methodologies, and particularly changes that have implications for the key research questions, may not be permitted. If a need for modifying the original protocol arises, and it is not clear whether the proposed change constitutes a major change, it is a good idea to contact the project officer or liaison at the funding agency. Put major changes in writing to ensure mutual understanding, and document the agreement of the funding agency.

Sometimes a grant proposal will be approved for funding with a budget cut. In this case, determine if the study can be implemented as proposed at a lower cost or if protocol changes must be made to reduce study costs. If changes are required, these changes should be discussed with the contact person at the funding agency and put in writing. There may be a number of options for modifying the scope of work, and it is crucial to ensure that there is agreement on the best strategies.

IF THE GRANT DOES NOT GET FUNDED

An important component of being a successful grant writer is paying attention to the details discussed in this chapter; it is equally important to learn how to cope with rejection. If you write grant proposals, some will be rejected. Follow this advice for dealing with rejection:

- **Don't blame the reviewer.** Often the first reaction to a rejection is to blame the reviewer. You may think, "The reviewer didn't get it!" Or, "Didn't the reviewer see where I explained that part?" It may be more effective to think in terms of how to improve the proposal so the reviewer will understand the project's importance and the "missing" information will be more prominent in the proposal.
- **Don't take the rejection personally.** This can be tough after you've invested so much time and energy in a grant proposal. Try to avoid fatalistic thinking such as, "I don't have what it takes to be a good researcher." Or, "I'll never get funded." Instead, focus

on the limitations of the proposal and what needs to be done to turn it into a fundable project.

- **Develop a plan for resubmission.** Consider whether you should resubmit, what changes should be made, and where the revised proposal should go. Some funding agencies, such as the NIH, allow for resubmissions. In fact, at the NIH it is rare to be funded on a first submission, and resubmissions are encouraged. Before resubmitting your proposal, read the reviewers' comments carefully, convene your research group, and develop a plan for addressing the reviewers' concerns. Recognize that your natural tendency may be to defend your original position. Although you have the option of doing so, try to make the suggested modifications wherever possible. If you choose not to make a suggested change, justify your decision in a manner that demonstrates that you have carefully considered the reviewer's suggestion. In a resubmitted proposal, there may be pages allotted for a response to the reviewer. For NIH grants, three additional pages may be used to indicate how the grant was revised. You need to show how the grant was modified in response to each suggestion made by the reviewers. Take the time to carefully plan responses, and have others provide feedback on the content and the tone. In instances in which there is not an opportunity to resubmit to the same funding agency, look for other suitable funding agencies and tweak the proposal to ensure its suitability for its new audience. Although this can be a daunting task, particularly if you are feeling somewhat dejected, it is generally worth doing. It can be difficult to decide not to resubmit a proposal. If this is your decision, think about why your idea was not funded and what you need to do to get funded next time around. You might need to do some pilot studies to learn more about the field and prove the worthiness and feasibility of your research ideas. Think about the direction you want to go regarding content of research questions, research design issues, and writing styles. You may find that some of the text in the Background and Significance section can be used as a basis for a book chapter or a review article.

INCREASING THE LIKELIHOOD OF GETTING FUNDED

Because writing grant proposals is a time-consuming process, and no one likes to have their ideas rejected, it is crucial to consider ways to increase your chances for getting funded. The following suggestions are helpful when writing grant proposals. Try them out, find what works best for you, and then add your own ideas to the list.

- **Read and follow the directions carefully.** Grant proposals may be rejected because the font size was too small or the margins not wide enough. Read the directions carefully and know that there is no flexibility in abiding by them. Don't hesitate to contact the granting agency as you are developing your proposal if you have questions.

- **Give yourself a lot of time.** Developing a research idea, pulling together a team of investigators, writing a grant proposal, and editing and re-editing the proposal takes a lot of time and energy (6). Start the process early and allow yourself time to develop your thoughts. Leave time at the end for checking and rechecking. Try not to make any substantive changes immediately prior to submission; last-minute changes inevitably lead to careless mistakes and inconsistencies throughout the proposal. Write, get feedback, integrate feedback, rewrite, get more feedback, and rewrite. After you complete the grant proposal, take a little break to rejuvenate.

- **Work with a team.** Writing grant proposals can be a lonely experience. Your proposal will gain from the shared expertise of others. Add other investigators to your research team whose skills complement your own. Choose to work with individuals that are hardworking, will make valuable contributions to the study, and with whom you enjoy working. New investigators should consider adding more experienced investigators to their team to increase their likelihood of getting funded and to facilitate study implementation. Clarify roles and expectations with others on the team with open discussion; raising issues early in the process can decrease conflicts due to misunderstandings down the road.

- **Get feedback at different stages.** Have others review your proposal at different stages of its development for different types of feedback. At the beginning, have others review an outline or summary to get input on the big picture items such as the research questions and the proposed study plan. Have others review a near-final version at a stage when you still have enough time (and energy) to incorporate their suggestions. Keep in mind that the quality of the feedback that you get will be in line with the quality of the proposal that you are asking others to review. Thus, carefully check your proposal for sentence structure, grammar, spelling, and overall flow prior to asking others to take their time to review your proposal and provide meaningful feedback.

- **Start small and build on ideas.** Reviewers may be unlikely to grant a large sum of money to an inexperienced investigator or to an unexplored idea. Start small and build up (7). For example, a grant might be built on smaller projects implemented incrementally over a period of several years.
- **Make things easy for the reviewer.** Make it easy for the reviewers to understand why your study is worthwhile, to grasp your main ideas, and to read about the fine details. Although you want to include as much information as the funding agency's page limit allows, it may be counterproductive to submit a proposal with crowded pages. Put yourself in a reviewer's role and write accordingly.
- **Show that you have thought through the details.** Although it may be tempting to leave the details until after you have received the money, a lack of attention to detail will greatly decrease your chances of ever being funded.
- **Aim for study enthusiasm.** Remember that you are selling an idea. Although you don't want to come across as your own personal cheerleader, you need to convince the reviewer and the funding agency that the study being proposed is worth funding. You need to show that the idea is worth pursuing, that you are the best person to implement the study, and that your study design is the right way to go. Do this in a cautious and scientific manner, but don't get bogged down in the details and forget to convey enthusiasm for the topic.
- **Learn from the experience of others.** Talk with others who have written grant proposals to learn from their experiences. How do they come up with fundable research ideas? How do they budget their time? Read over other grant proposals. Participate in different grant-writing classes. There is no one correct way to go about writing grant proposals. By observing how different successful grant writers have gone about the process, you will begin to develop your own style.
- **Learn through first-hand experience.** Look for opportunities to get involved with grants that are being written. Help out by offering to conduct literature searches or read over different versions of the proposal. Request to be part of the meetings in which the grant proposal is being discussed in order to understand the big picture. Seek out opportunities to get involved in the grant review process. Although this can be time-consuming, serving as a reviewer

can help in understanding the review process and what constitutes a strong grant proposal.

ONLINE RESOURCES

The following Web sites can help you find funding:

- **Grants.gov** (http://www.grants.gov): The central site to find grants from government organizations. You may complete applications through this portal.
- **National Institutes of Health, Office of Extramural Research grants page** (http://grants1.nih.gov /grants/oer.htm): Includes links to funding opportunities (RFAs, PAs, and notices), research training, programs, forms, application materials, submission dates, resources, award data, and policies.
- **USDA National Agricultural Library Rural Information Center** (http://www.nal.usda.gov/ric): Provides information on different funding resources, links to funders and databases, and general guidelines.
- **Nonprofit Guides** (http://www.npguides.org/ links.htm): Grant-writing tools for nonprofit organizations, with general guidelines and links to funders and other grant-seeking resources.
- **US Department of Health and Human Services, Health Resources and Services Administration— Grants: Find, Apply, Review, Manage, Report** (http://www.hrsa.gov/grants/default.htm): Provides information on HRSA grant opportunities and information on getting funding.

CONCLUSION

Writing strong grant proposals is an important skill for RDs interested in contributing to the field of nutrition and in advancing their careers. A strong grant proposal begins with a good idea, which is transformed into a testable research question and a workable plan, and is pitched to a funding agency as a project worth investing in. A grant proposal should begin with clear research questions and build on them throughout the proposal. The aim is to get the reviewers and the funding agency excited about the project and to provide enough details to show that there is a well-developed and feasible implementation plan.

Writing grant proposals is both a daunting and rewarding task. Rejections are to be expected and can be difficult, but if the reviewers' comments are taken as good advice, and are not taken personally, they can help in improving future submissions. In order to be successful, it is usually best to start out with projects of a relatively small scope and gradually build upon them.

REFERENCES

1. Lusk SL. Developing an outstanding grant application. *West J Nurs Res.* 2004;26:367–373.
2. Eaves GN. Preparation of the research-grant application: opportunities and pitfalls. *Grants Mag.* 1984;7:151–157.
3. Bordage G, Dawson B. Experimental study design and grant writing in eight steps and 28 questions. *Med Educ.* 2003;37:376–385.
4. Inouye SK, Fiellin DA. An evidence-based guide to writing grant proposals for clinical research. *Ann Intern Med.* 2005;142:274–282.
5. Murray DM. *The Design and Analysis of Group-Randomized Trials.* New York, NY: Oxford University Press; 1998.
6. Koren G. How to increase your funding chances: common pitfalls in medical grant applications. *Can J Clin Pharmacol.* 2005;12:e182–185.
7. Penrod J. Getting funded: writing a successful qualitative small-project proposal. *Qual Health Res.* 2003;13:821–832.

5

Multidisciplinary Research

Madeleine Sigman-Grant, PhD, RD

Multidisciplinary research is best described by the old parable of the blind men and the elephant. Six blind men were led to different parts of an elephant. When asked "What sort of a thing is an elephant?" each provided a different answer. The one touching a leg said the elephant was a pillar; the one who touched the ear believed the elephant was a fan; the one who touched the tail was certain an elephant was a rope; no two of the men agreed. The men argued vehemently about what truly described an elephant. In reality, they were each right from their unique perspective, yet they were each wrong because they had only one perspective and none had explored the entire elephant. There are two morals to this tale: (a) it is only when all the pieces are put together that the complete picture is revealed, and (b) it is important to be tolerant and accepting of other viewpoints in order to see "the truth."

In a similar manner, one can ask, "What sort of thing is nutrition research?" Some might respond that it is the effect of nutrients on gene expression (biological and physiological research); others might say that it describes what people eat and why they make their choices (behavioral and psychological research); others might say that it is about communication (humanities and consumer research); another might say that it is about measuring the impact of supermarkets (environmental research); still others might describe the economic impact of food policy (economic research). Each response is correct, but is limited in perspective.

The complex interrelationship between the individual and the environment demands searching for answers in different ways and from different perspectives. However, as science becomes more specialized, it is easy to lose sight of the big picture. Multidisciplinary research expands knowledge, promotes innovation, provides a holistic view of "truth" and bridges the gap between research and practice. For example, if biological researchers determine that consumers should eat more of a particular nutrient, psychological researchers might track how consumers respond to this new information and agricultural economists could track economic effects. Having a multidisciplinary research team in place from the onset could ensure appropriate attention is paid to the varied, often unexpected and unintended social, moral, and ethical consequences of the initial research.

DESCRIPTION OF MULTIDISCIPLINARY RESEARCH

Multidisciplinary research can be defined as research that integrates theories, methods, and knowledge from multiple disciplines, while maintaining each discipline's distinctness (eg, a team composed of dietitians, sociologists, and economists) (1). Interdisciplinary research integrates the distinctly different disciplines (eg, nutrition, sociology, and economics) in such a way as to effectively form a new unified discipline (eg, women's health studies).

The Push behind Multidisciplinary Research

Multidisciplinary research has become more appealing as funding diminishes, the need for accountability rises, and knowledge expands. Probably the most pragmatic reason for establishing a multidisciplinary nutrition research team is the fiscal imperative, as more funding agencies are requiring a multidisciplinary approach (2). For example, the National Institutes of Health (NIH) has embraced the integration of basic social science scientific concepts and constructs with health research to define the etiology of disease and wellness in order to apply these concepts to treatment and prevention services (3–5).

Rewards of Multidisciplinary Research

Multidisciplinary research enhances understanding of complex issues, such as prevention of chronic disease, in ways that cannot be achieved by a single field of inquiry. Specialization leads to compartmentalization, which in turn limits knowledge of what is happening beyond the confines of one limited area. Hence, no longer can any one person or discipline be completely knowledgeable about a specific topic or method. Indeed, researchers can miss significant findings from other research fields that share common interests but are asking different questions or using different methods.

On the professional level, multidisciplinary teams can increase personal creativity and inspire complex thinking. They also strengthen collegiality, enhance flexibility, and stimulate intellectual exchange (2,6–9). Finally, multidisciplinary research can be the means to achieving one's goals that could not be achieved alone (6,7).

Challenges to Multidisciplinary Research

The task of changing from a single-discipline perspective to inclusion of multiple viewpoints does not come without inherent barriers (2,9–12). Some of these are personal, whereas others are fiscal (10). Perceived personal risks of entering into multidisciplinary research include concerns about promotion, tenure, publication records, and securing new positions (9). Multidisciplinary research can also be more expensive, requiring greater coordination and surveillance.

Nutrition researchers might need to collaborate with researchers from different departments within their institutions. Furthermore, nutrition researchers may need to work with others in different universities, in external organizations, and in public-private ventures. One way to mitigate differences would be to find colleagues who share a similar worldview and are familiar with the basic concepts of each other's discipline.

These interactions, in addition to the common frustrations that come from working with colleagues within one's own profession, create issues unique to cross-disciplinary collaboration. Often, working with those who are trained in a different lexicon, who follow a different set of values, or who respond to different incentives requires a period of adjustment before research can even begin. Conflict and loss of interest are two major barriers in creating and maintaining multidisciplinary research endeavors (2,8). Finally, scientists trained in quantitative methodologies may find it uncomfortable to accept qualitative methodologies when working with scientists trained in these approaches.

SUCCESSFUL MULTIDISCIPLINARY RESEARCH

Who Should Be Involved?

Frequently, nutrition researchers know which other disciplines to seek out for inclusion in a research project. In multidisciplinary research, nutrition researchers should include experts such as a biostatistician, an epidemiologist, or an economist at the proposal stage to design the study and data analysis. Psychologists may be included for research into eating disorders, whereas sociologists may be invited to join studies involving cultural differences in which understanding of the underlying relationships is needed.

For example, cancer studies have included diverse disciplines (4,13). Initial cancer research was restricted to biochemical and genetic research in animals and humans. Then epidemiologists and statisticians were required to further explain cancer incidence. Finally, cancer researchers acknowledged the need for understanding environmental and social factors (such as diet and lifestyle). The progressive inclusion of multiple disciplines has led to substantial advances in understanding the treatment and prevention of many types of cancer.

For those research questions for which the connections between disciplines are less obvious, Kostoff (12) suggests "text mining." This technique involves conducting a literature search in databases not normally used by the nutrition researcher, such as those in the social sciences, psychology, behavioral sciences, and humanities. The nutrition researcher interested in a particular issue (eg, obesity) enters keywords to identify papers and authors who are investigating the same issues in other disciplines. A librarian can be an excellent resource for help in text mining.

A similar technique was used to generate a list of disciplines needed to create a conceptual framework for understanding the complexity of unhealthful eating and physical inactivity (14). Initially, experts from the fields of nutrition and exercise physiology, the food industry and business conducted literature reviews. During brainstorming sessions, the final list of disciplines needed included sociology, anthropology, architecture and community building, economics, consumer research, food policy, transportation, geography, history, health care, and food and sensory sciences. The result produced an intricate schema depicting the relationships of various disciplines between individuals and the environment (15).

Decisions to Be Made

Once disciplines and specific people have been identified, a working relationship based on trust and mutual respect must develop over time. This is true for all collaborations. However, the time required for building multidisciplinary relationships may be substantially increased. For instance, when collaborators are from the same discipline, a common language allows them to immediately begin planning the project. With collaborators from distinctly different fields, even such a "simple" term as BMI (body mass index) may need to be defined. The necessary explanations can be achieved through informal conversations (8) and development of a glossary of terms.

For many research projects, proposals due dates often preclude lengthy preliminary interaction in which differences can be identified, discussed, and negotiated. When time for mutual exploration is not possible, exchange of basic readings will provide the perspective from each discipline to the problems at hand. From this exchange, researchers will be able to establish a common language, synergistic missions, and agreed-upon goals. It is essential to continue to refer to goals throughout the project; drifting away from these shared goals toward more familiar disciplinary work can occur, to the detriment of the collaboration.

Some decisions, such as who is responsible for daily management, who makes which decisions, who makes the final decision, and who communicates with the funding agency must be made initially and reviewed periodically as the research progresses. Continuity of leadership is essential. Investigators should exchange information about available resources and other time commitments, negotiate budgetary requirements, clarify contractual language, work out intellectual property rights, compare human subjects procedures, and coordinate statistical and other software packages. Attending to these issues is critical both at the proposal stage and throughout the research project. Although these matters arise for all collaborations, issues such as grant management, sharing of databases and analyses, and authorship may be drastically different between disciplines. Rather than assuming similarities, those involved with multidisciplinary research should query new colleagues to clarify how they handle each situation. This can be done as each portion of the grant application and study design is addressed.

Strategies for Working on a Multidisciplinary Team

Communication and mutual respect are the two main strategies consistently mentioned when describing multidisciplinary research (2,5,7–12). Face-to-face meetings are vital at all stages of the research (5). Budgets should include sufficient funds to support these meetings. Retreats provide a mechanism for providing an extended period of discussion and assimilation needed to create a common language, fuse methods, and nurture all members of the team (5).

Additional communication tools, which are especially useful when more than one site is involved, include the following: establishment and use of a central Web site, electronic chat rooms and bulletin boards, e-mail and Listservs, instant messaging, webcasting, newsletters, periodic updates, and conference calls. Other technological tools that might be helpful are those that manage and track task trajectories over time, tools that minimize information overload, software to schedule meetings and calls, similar referencing packages, and videoconferencing workshops (2). A single contact person should be appointed to coordinate these tools.

Personal Characteristics that Enhance Multidisciplinary Research

Persons who are successful working as part of a multidisciplinary research team are those who demonstrate strong, nonhierarchical mutual and personal respect for those with different opinions (8). Persons who approach conflict as a learning experience, who are self-confident within their own discipline, who value two-way communication as well as differences of opinions, and who can synthesize various perspectives including those of both senior and junior investigators make excellent partners. Trust, nurturance, understanding, tact, and thoughtfulness are characteristics that provide stability to the research team. Those persons who are less comfortable with compromise, role-blurring, and collective ownership of research may not be suited for multidisciplinary research.

CONCLUSION

Multidisciplinary nutrition research provides an opportunity to expand beyond the professional constraints of insufficient knowledge, tunnel vision, and limited perspective. Despite the challenges presented when working across distinctly different disciplines, the research results more closely approach the broader "truth." New, as well as established, researchers might consider incorporating at least one other discipline into their next project to determine the value of expertise beyond nutrition.

REFERENCES

1. Collins J. May you live in interesting times: using multidisciplinary and interdisciplinary programs to cope with change in the life sciences. *BioScience.* 2002;52:75–83.
2. Cummings J, Kiesler S. Collaborative research across disciplinary and organizational boundaries. *Soc Stud Sci.* 2005;35:703–722.
3. Bachrach C, Abeles R. Social science and health research: growth at the National Institutes of Health. *Am J Public Health.* 2004;94:22–28.
4. Forman M, Hursting S, Umar A. Nutrition and cancer prevention: a multidisciplinary perspective on human trials. *Annu Rev Nutr.* 2004;24:223–254.
5. Morgan G, Kobus K, Gerlach K, Neighbors C, Lerman C, Abrams D, Rimer B. Facilitating transdisciplinary research: the experiences of the Transdisciplinary Tobacco Use Research Centers. *Nicotine Tob Res.* 2003;5:S11–S19.
6. Bronstein L. Index of interdisciplinary collaboration. *Soc Work Res.* 2002;26:113–123.
7. Bronstein L. A model for interdisciplinary collaboration. *Soc Work.* 2003;48:297–306.
8. Creamer E. Collaborators' attitudes about differences of opinion. *J Higher Educ.* 2004;75:556–571.
9. Nissani M. Ten cheers for interdisciplinarity: the case for interdisciplinary knowledge and research. *Soc Sci J.* 1997;34:201–217.
10. Ellison P, Kopp C. A note on interdisciplinary research in developmental/behavioral pediatrics/psychology. *Pediatrics.* 1985;75:883–886.
11. Kezar A. Moving from I to we: reorganizing for collaboration in higher education. *Change.* 2005;37:50–57.
12. Kostoff R. Overcoming specialization. *BioScience.* 2002;52:937–941.
13. Jevning R, Biedebach M, Anand R. Cruciferous vegetables and human breast cancer: an important interdisciplinary hypothesis in the field of diet and cancer. *Fam Econ Nutr Rev.* 1999;12:26–30.
14. Hill J, Goldberg J, Pate R, Peters J. Introduction. *Nutr Rev.* 2001;59:S4–S9.
15. Booth SL, Sallis JF, Ritenbaugh C, Hill JO, Birch LL, Frank LD, Glanz K, Himmelgreen DA, Mudd M, Popkin BM, Rickard KA, St Jeor S, Hays NP. Environmental and societal factors affect food choice and physical activity: rationale, influences, and leverage points. *Nutr Rev.* 2001;59:S21–S39.

PART 3

—∿—

Descriptive Research

6

Descriptive Epidemiologic Research

Maureen Brady Moran, MPH, Sujata Archer, PhD, RD, and Linda Van Horn, PhD, RD

*E*pidemiology is defined as "the study of the distribution and determinants of disease frequency" (1). The epidemiologic methods for study design, data collection, and analysis provide the conceptual framework for describing the distribution of disease and for testing etiologic hypotheses for a disease or health consequence. This chapter focuses on descriptive epidemiologic research measurements and study designs applicable to nutrition and dietetics. The advantages and limitations of these measurements and designs are also presented.

TERMINOLOGY

Descriptive epidemiologic studies focus on the enumeration and description of subject characteristics of person, place, and time. These studies can be used to quantify the extent and location of nutrition problems within a population and suggest associations between diet and disease that can subsequently be evaluated in analytic research.

Personal characteristics can provide valuable insights into disease etiology. By examining who gets a disease, one can determine whether a particular age, gender, racial, or cultural group is more likely to be at risk. A wide variety of attributes that are associated with each individual person, such as socioeconomic status, family size, marital status, birth order, and personality traits, may be important to consider. For example, the personal attributes of family income and education both show a strong inverse association with the prevalence of iron-deficiency anemia in women of childbearing age (2).

Place-associated characteristics may also provide valuable insights about potential risk factors for nutrition-associated problems. Such data will lead researchers to investigate reasons for these differences to help identify possible risk factors. The importance of place can also be illustrated in that urban or rural living may affect the availability and price of food items. Even with today's food distribution system, the availability and price of highly nutritious, perishable foods such as fruits, vegetables, and fish vary dramatically by geographic region and based on whether a location is urban, suburban, or rural (3).

Time factors can also affect disease. Seasonal and interannual fluctuations in cumulative incidence, as well as secular trends, may indicate patterns that help elucidate causation. A cross-sectional observational study determined total vitamin D status in adolescent girls and elderly community-dwelling women in four northern European countries. The study reported that during winter the vitamin D status in the study participants was low (4). Timing and length of exposure to a risk factor, or the duration of the latency period, also may be important considerations. Multivitamin use may prevent colon cancer, but only after a long latency period. Recent use does not appear to be protective (5).

DISEASE FREQUENCY

Disease frequency measures the amount of disease or morbidity in a population and is expressed as incidence or prevalence. In practice, the amount of disease translates into risk of disease and becomes the foundation for all descriptive and comparative work. Knowledge of the frequency of a given disease in different populations can be used to compare the relative importance of this disease in these populations, or it may be used as a basis for comparing populations with different exposures to possible etiologic factors.

Measurement of Incidence

Cumulative incidence, or *incidence rate,* is the term used to describe disease frequency in a population. Cumulative incidence is the number of new cases of a disease that occur in a population at risk within a specified time interval. Frequently, the observed period is 1 year. It is defined as follows:

$$\text{Cumulative incidence} = \frac{\text{Number of new cases}}{\text{Population at risk}} \text{ In a time period}$$

Cumulative incidence is normally expressed as the number of cases per 100,000 population per year; it can also be expressed as the risk of disease (Box 6.1). The population at the midpoint in the study period is used as the population at risk.

BOX 6.1   Sample Calculation of Cumulative Incidence (CI): Colon Cancer CI Expressed as Risk of Disease

$$CI = \frac{\text{No. of persons in whom the disease develops}}{\text{Population at risk}} \times \text{Time period}$$

$$= \frac{\text{No. of new cases of colon cancer in county A}}{\text{Midyear population of county A}} \times 1 \text{ yr}$$

$$= \frac{20 \text{ new colon cancer cases in county A in 1991}}{995,000 \text{ population 7/1/91}} \times 1 \text{ yr}$$

$$= \frac{20}{995,000}$$

$$= \frac{2.01}{100,000}$$

or the risk of colon cancer in 1991 in county A is 0.002%.

When cumulative incidence is calculated, the denominator is based on population defined by geographic area. It can have an even more specific focus, such as a particular gender, age, or ethnic group, within the given area.

Cumulative incidence is useful for documenting the relative importance of a disease in a population and for tracking changes in the occurrence of a disease over time. Cumulative incidence can also provide etiologic clues. A comparison of the cumulative incidence for populations that have different age groupings, sex distributions, ethnicity, or geographic locations can identify population groups with low or high rates of disease. This identification of groups with a high incidence of disease can be used to target intervention programs where they are most needed.

A specific application of cumulative incidence for registered dietitians (RDs) is quantification of the attack rate of an outbreak of food poisoning. *Attack rate* is the term substituted for *cumulative incidence* when the period of observation is short. In this situation, the population would be at risk for a short time, and the study period would encompass the entire epidemic. Such a study reported a foodborne outbreak of *Shigella flexneri* serotype 2a infection associated with tomatoes. To determine restaurant-specific attack rates, the investigators divided the number of cases reported at each restaurant by an estimate of the number of meals served in the restaurant during the outbreak. In one of the restaurants 350 meals were served and 165 patrons became ill, for an attack rate of 47% (6).

Measurement of Prevalence

Prevalence is the *proportion* of the population that is affected by a certain disease or condition at a given time, and it includes both new and existing cases. Prevalence can be expressed either as point or period prevalence. *Point prevalence* depicts one point in time, as in a cross-sectional survey, and, unless otherwise specified, is how the term *prevalence* generally is defined. Point prevalence is calculated as follows:

$$\text{Point prevalence} = \frac{\text{Number of new, existing, and recurring cases}}{\text{Total population at risk}}$$

where the numerator and denominator are calculated at one point in time.

In contrast, *period prevalence* is calculated as follows:

$$\text{Period prevalence} = \frac{\text{Number of new, existing, and recurring cases during a given time period}}{\text{Total population at risk}}$$

Sometimes, incidence data are not available for a disease, so prevalence data are calculated. This alternative is acceptable as long as the person interpreting the numbers clearly understands that incidence is the number of new cases within a specified period and that prevalence is the number of both old and new cases within a period. A lack of understanding of the difference between incidence and prevalence is a common mistake in scientific writing (7).

Prevalence data are advantageous for assessing the frequency of diseases or conditions, such as obesity, that do not have an acute onset. A series of cross-sectional studies that document point prevalence can be used to track changes in the burden of a disease to a population. Prevalence is therefore useful for identifying people at greatest risk and for planning health services.

The difference between incidence and prevalence can introduce important sources of bias when evaluating the effect of a screening program in which both the identification of cases and the effectiveness of intervention need to be examined. By the nature of the definition of *prevalence*, it is obvious that chronic conditions such as hypertension would be more likely to be picked up in a survey than would short-term acute conditions such as influenza.

Reliability and Validity

Tests and tools used in descriptive epidemiologic research should be both reliable and valid. A reliable test gives the same results when the test is repeated on the same person several times. In other words, a reliable test gives reproducible results. A valid test measures what it is designed to measure.

Validity is used in epidemiologic studies to assess various methods of interest to RDs, such as dietary assessment and anthropometric measures. Epidemiologic studies using a quantitative food frequency questionnaire (FFQ) typically test the validity of the dietary instrument by comparing the resulting data with data obtained using other valid methods, such as multiple 24-hour dietary recalls. It is recommended that studies examine the validity and reliability of each dietary assessment method in choosing the best tool (8).

Increasingly, biochemical markers are being used as surrogates for dietary assessment measures because validation studies have shown that they provide an accurate assessment. One such study correlated biomarkers for glycemic control (HbA1c, plasma glucose, serum C-peptide, and serum insulin concentrations) with carbohydrate intake. Although carbohydrate intake was not associated with HbA1c, plasma glucose, or serum insulin, it was inversely associated with serum C-peptide concentrations (9).

Sensitivity and Specificity

Two parameters that are used to assess the validity of a test are sensitivity and specificity. Sensitivity is the proportion of persons who have the disease or condition who have positive test results. Specificity is the proportion of people who do not have the disease or condition who have negative test results. The higher the sensitivity, the more likely a person with disease will have a positive test result. These screening tests are schematically described in Figure 6.1.

Sensitivity and specificity are used to establish cutoffs or reference interval limits for a test. The goal is to maximize both sensitivity and specificity in order to minimize misclassification. Some people with positive test results do not truly have the disease. Conversely, some people with negative test results actually have the disease. Detsky and colleagues discuss how reference intervals are established to maximize sensitivity and specificity in their comparison of nutrition assessment techniques (10).

Predictive Value

The predictive value of a test is its ability to accurately distinguish people with or without the disease or condition. Thus, the positive predictive value is the probability of disease, given a positive test result. The negative predictive value is the probability of no disease, given a negative test result (Figure 6.2).

Predictive values are strongly affected by the prevalence of the condition or disease. Using a test with a given sensitivity and specificity, the differences in positive predictive values are notable as prevalence declines from 25% to 2.5% (Figure 6.3). If the condition of interest is rare, even a highly sensitive and specific test will produce results with a very low positive predictive value. In such a case, many of those who test positive do not truly have disease.

		Disease or Condition	
		Present	**Absent**
	Positive	a	b
Test			
	Negative	c	d

Sensitivity = Proportion of those with a disease who have a positive test

$$= \frac{a}{a + c}$$

Specificity = Proportion of those without a disease who have a negative test

$$= \frac{d}{b + d}$$

FIGURE 6.1   Schematic description of the screening test indexes sensitivity and specificity and their calculation.

Further testing (using a "gold standard") is necessary to distinguish true positives from false positives.

DESCRIPTIVE RESEARCH DESIGN

Descriptive studies are the simplest of all research designs. The most common types of descriptive studies include ecological studies, case reports or case series, cross-sectional designs, and surveillance systems. These types of studies simply report the characteristics of person, place, and time related to a disease or a condition of interest. They are used to identify patterns of a disease or condition. Such a study may report on countrywide populations, residents of small geographic areas, small groups of people, or individual subjects.

		Disease or Condition	
		Present	**Absent**
	Positive	a	b
Test			
	Negative	c	d

Positive predictive value = Proportion of those with a positive test who have a disease

$$= \frac{a}{a + b}$$

Negative predictive value = Proportion of those with a negative test who do not have a disease

$$= \frac{d}{c + d}$$

FIGURE 6.2   Schematic description of the predictive values of a screening test.

	Population = 4,000 Prevalence = 25%		Population = 4,000 Prevalence = 3.3%		Population = 4,000 Prevalence = 2.5%	
	Disease		**Disease**		**Disease**	
	+	−	+	−	+	−
Test Results +	980	150	392	180	98	195
−	20	2,850	8	3,420	2	3,705

Sensitivity $= \dfrac{980}{1,000} = 98\%$ $\dfrac{392}{400} = 98\%$ $\dfrac{98}{100} = 98\%$

Specificity $= \dfrac{150}{3,000} = 95\%$ $\dfrac{180}{3,600} = 95\%$ $\dfrac{195}{3,900} = 95\%$

Positive predictive value $= \dfrac{980}{1,130} = 86.7\%$ $\dfrac{392}{572} = 68.5\%$ $\dfrac{98}{293} = 33.4\%$

FIGURE 6.3   Comparison of positive predictive values in populations with differing prevalence of disease.

Descriptive studies are also valuable for identifying potential associations between risk factors and a disease. Frequently, descriptive studies are less expensive and take less time than analytic studies because they use precollected data, such as the National Food Consumption Survey; NHANES I, II, and III; vital statistics; or clinical records. Results from descriptive studies can form the basis of hypotheses for analytic research.

Ecological Studies

Ecological studies are beneficial for examining patterns relating a possible risk or causative factor to a disease. Often data from several countries are examined to identify these relationships. An ecological study examined the association between the magnitude of the income disparity between rich and poor in a country and diabetes mortality, obesity, and daily energy intake. Across 21 countries, greater income disparity was correlated with a higher prevalence of obesity, mortality from diabetes, and average energy intake (11).

It is important to note that ecological studies show only associations between a factor and a disease or condition. They do not show causation or the effect of potential confounding factors, and they certainly do not document the biological processes involved in a disease or condition.

Case Reports and Case Series

Unique experiences of one patient or a small group of patients with a similar diagnosis are reported as case reports or case series. These accounts can provide a basis for a more vigorous investigation using an analytic approach to examine the factors of interest. This brief documentation also alerts health care professionals to possible, but not proved, beneficial or life-threatening aspects of a disease or its treatment. To illustrate, pediatric neurologists identified a child who developed cardiomegaly and pulmonary edema while following a ketogenic diet for epilepsy. Cardiac status improved when the diet was discontinued. This led to an examination of 20 children at one medical center who were following a ketogenic diet; three were found to have similar cardiac abnormalities (12). Case reports or case series may also be used to document the beginning of an epidemic. Other uses for case reports include tracking toxicity reports of new foods.

A case series is of greater value than a single case report, because the former gives more documentation of evidence for the suggested hypothesis. Case reports or case series are never conclusive in establishing cause and effect, but they are useful for the initial descriptions of a new disease or for documenting the biological processes of a disease or condition.

Surveys

Surveys can provide a wide variety of descriptive information about a disease or condition, but their important contribution is in providing a view of the people studied at one point or period of time. Many national surveys have been done and are repeated periodically. Examples include the Continuing Survey of Food Intakes by Individuals and NHANES I, II, and III. Currently the Continuing Survey of Food Intakes by Individuals and the NHANES have been combined and are being conducted annually. These surveys have sophisticated sampling frames to provide representative information from all segments of the population or special high-risk population groups (13).

The Continuing Survey of Food Intake by Individuals conducted from 1994 to 1996 and the Supplemental Children's Survey conducted in 1998 have been used to examine the association between fast food consumption and dietary adequacy (14).

The primary advantage of surveys is that they can offer a representative overview of the health of the population (or cross-section). Their limitation is that the data cannot provide answers to questions about disease etiology. When a population is surveyed at one point in time, it may be difficult to determine whether exposure to a risk factor came before a disease unless questions about timing are included. For further discussion of surveys and using these large databases, see Chapter 13.

Surveillance

Surveillance is a systematic, *ongoing survey* designed to monitor specific health outcomes in a population over an extended period of time (15). Surveillance systems are used to identify and monitor public health problems.

Important components of a surveillance system include the cooperation and coordination of many individuals and groups, the collection of high-quality data, management of the data, and timely analysis and dissemination of the data for use.

Pertinent examples for RDs include the Pediatric Nutrition Surveillance System (PedNSS) and the Pregnancy Nutrition Surveillance System (PNSS), both of which are managed by the Centers for Disease Control and Prevention (16,17). The PedNSS monitors growth indicators, anemia status, and breastfeeding status of children and includes minimal demographic data. The PNSS monitors pre-pregnancy weight, pregnancy weight gain, anemia status, behavioral risk factors, birth outcome, and infant feeding status, and it includes demographic data. These systems include data on low-income women, infants, and children who participate in publicly funded health and nutrition programs in states that participate in these surveillance systems.

Measurement of Vital Statistics and Demographics

Vital statistics are based on data from records such as birth certificates, death certificates, and census data. Vital statistics are really a type of surveillance data, as they routinely monitor vital events. By law, birth and death certificates must be filed by the birth attendant or attending physician at the local town or city clerk's office; these data are also forwarded to county and state offices for compilation and reporting. At the beginning of each decade, the federal government collects population census data.

Birth and death certificate data are readily available from the vital records offices of counties or states. State vital statistics reports are published annually and can be obtained from the appropriate state records office. These reports are also available in the public documents area of public, college, or university libraries. National vital statistics reports are also available on the Internet from agencies such as the National Vital Statistics System (18). Examples of some data available are age-adjusted death rates for selected causes, such as diabetes mellitus or cardiovascular disease, by race and gender; data for births in the United States, according to maternal and demographic characteristics; and infant health status.

Vital statistics data are especially useful for documenting person, place, and time characteristics of a disease or condition, as well as for documenting the relative importance of a disease or health problem in a population. Cause-specific mortality rates can be used to identify the primary causes of deaths. This information can be used to target major problem areas, and in turn, as part of the follow-up, may lead to the development of intervention strategies to reduce the risk of death from a particular cause.

CONCLUSION

The two primary measures of disease frequency are incidence and prevalence. Cumulative incidence measures the rate of either the morbidity or mortality of a disease in a population over a specified period. Incidence density is similar to cumulative incidence, but it uses person-time as the denominator. In contrast, prevalence describes the burden of a disease to a population; it reflects the number of cases, both existing and new, at a specified point or period in time.

Screening tests are used to document the amount of disease that can be affected positively by early intervention. These tests must be reliable and valid. Specificity and sensitivity are used to evaluate validity. The predictive value of a test assesses its ability to accurately predict persons with and without a disease. Predictive values are strongly influenced by disease prevalence.

The major descriptive study designs include ecological studies, case reports and case series, surveys, and surveillance. The primary uses for descriptive studies are to provide information to develop priorities for health care planning and to generate hypotheses to be tested in analytic research.

REFERENCES

1. MacMahon B, Pugh TF. *Epidemiology: Principles and Methods.* Boston, Mass: Little, Brown; 1970.
2. Life Sciences Research Office, Federation of American Societies for Experimental Biology. *Third Report on Nutrition Monitoring in the United States: Volume 1.* Washington, DC: US Government Printing Office; 1995.
3. Pearson T, Russell J, Campbell MJ, Barker ME. Do "food desserts" influence fruit and vegetable consumption?—a cross-sectional study. *Appetite.* 2005:45:195–197.
4. Andersen R, Molgaard C, Skovgaard LT, Brot C, Cashman KD, Chabros E, Chazewska J, Flynn A, Jakobsen J, Karkkainen M, Kiely M, Lamberg-Allardt C, Moreiras O, Natri AM, O'Brien M, Rogalska-Niedzwiedz M, Ovesen L. Teenage girls and elderly women living in northern Europe have low winter vitamin D status. *Eur J Clin Nutr.* 2005;59:533–541.
5. Jacobs EJ, Connell CJ, Chao A, McCullough ML, Rodriguez C, Thun MJ, Calle EE. Multivitamin use and colorectal cancer incidence in a US cohort: does timing matter? *Am J Epidemiol.* 2003;158:621–628.
6. Reller ME, Nelson JM, Molbak K, Ackman DM, Schoonmaker-Bopp DJ, Root TP, Mintz ED. A large multiple-restaurant outbreak of infection with *Shigella flexneri* serotype 2a traced to tomatoes. *Clin Infect Dis.* 2006;42:163–169.
7. Flanders WD, O'Brien TR. Inappropriate comparisons of incidence and prevalence in epidemiologic research. *Am J Public Health.* 1989;79:1301–1303.
8. Kipnis V, Midthune D, Freedman L, Bingham S, Day NE, Riboli E, Ferrari P, Carroll RJ. Bias in dietary-reporting instruments and its implications for nutritional epidemiology. *Public Health Nutr.* 2002; 5(6A):915–923.
9. Yang EJ, Kerver JM, Park YK, Kayitsinga J, Allison DB, Song WO. Carbohydrate intake and biomarkers of glycemic control among US adults: the Third National Health and Nutrition Examination Survey (NHANES III). *Am J Clin Nutr.* 2003;77:1426–1433.
10. Detsky AS, Baker JP, Mendelson RA, Wolman SL, Wesson DE, Jeejeebhoy KN. Evaluating the accuracy of nutritional assessment techniques applied to hospitalized patients: methodology and comparisons. *JPEN J Parenter Enteral Nutr.* 1984;8: 153–159.
11. Pickett KE, Kelly S, Bruner E, Lobstein T, Wilkinson RG. Wider income gaps, wider waistbands? An ecological study of obesity and income inequality. *J Epidemiol Comm Health.* 2005;59:670–674.
12. Best TH, Franz DN, Gilbert DL, Nelson DP, Epstein MR. Cardiac complications in pediatric patients on the ketogenic diet. *Neurology.* 2000;54:2328–2330.
13. Centers for Disease Control and Prevention, National Center for Health Statistics. National Health and Nutrition Examination Survey Web site. Available at: http://www.cdc.gov/nchs/nhanes.htm. Accessed February 28, 2007.
14. Bowman SA, Gortmaker SL, Ebbeling CB, Pereira MA, Ludwig DS. Effects of fast-food consumption

on energy intake and dietary quality among children in a national household survey. *Pediatrics.* 2004;113:112–118.

15. Teutsch SM, Churchill RE. *Principles and Practice of Public Health Surveillance.* New York, NY: Oxford University Press; 1994.

16. Centers for Disease Control and Prevention. *Pediatric Nutrition Surveillance: 1997 Full Report.* Atlanta, Ga: US Department of Health and Human Services, Centers for Disease Control and Prevention; 1998.

17. Centers for Disease Control and Prevention. *Pregnancy Nutrition Surveillance: 1996 Full Report.* Atlanta, Ga: US Department of Health and Human Services, Centers for Disease Control and Prevention; 1998.

18. Centers for Disease Control and Prevention, National Center for Health Statistics. National Vital Statistics Systems Web site. Available at: http://www.cdc.gov/nchs/nvss.htm. Accessed February 28, 2007.

FURTHER READING

Abramson JH. *Making Sense of Data.* 3rd ed. New York, NY: Oxford University Press; 2001.

Weiss NS. *Clinical Epidemiology: The Study of the Outcome of Illness.* New York, NY: Oxford University Press; 2006.

The Philosophy, Role, and Methods of Qualitative Inquiry in Research

Cheryl L. Achterberg, PhD, and Susan W. Arendt, PhD, RD

Qualitative research has always been an integral part of cross-cultural comparisons and descriptions of food habits in the nutrition and anthropology literature (1–3). It also offers a great deal of insight into nutrition and dietetics. Registered dietitians (RDs) in both research and practice can use various qualitative approaches, and can benefit from the types of information that are produced from qualitative works. The purpose of this chapter is to define qualitative research, to describe when and why it should be conducted, to review its methods, and to address its limitations. Examples of qualitative research in a broad range of nutrition topics are examined, including clinical nutrition, community nutrition, and foodservice management. Different approaches to data collection and data analysis are included, along with a discussion of computer-assisted data analysis programs.

QUALITATIVE RESEARCH

Qualitative research may be defined as any data-gathering technique that generates open-ended, narrative data or words rather than numerical data or numbers (4,5). For example, a qualitative approach to research on individuals' definition of the words *healthy eating* generated a large number of definitions in the individuals' own words (6). This might vary greatly from a quantitative approach that used a small set of closed-ended definitions generated by RDs in a multiple-choice survey questionnaire. The primary

caveat in qualitative research is that the words must reflect the point of view of the study participant, not the researcher (7,8). Qualitative research is based on the assumption that findings about human interaction, thinking, and behavior are better understood and more scientifically valid when seen from the inside out than when seen from the outside in (9–14).

COMPARING AND CONTRASTING QUALITATIVE AND QUANTITATIVE APPROACHES

Qualitative and quantitative research approaches have a shared view that the world can be known through systematic, empirical observation. However, the appropriateness, fit, and scope of the data produced by qualitative or quantitative studies vary according to the particular issue of interest. For example, qualitative approaches are seldom appropriate in evaluating blood lipids, but they are often appropriate in the study of social behavior (eg, food choices made alone or in groups of peers) (15).

Both qualitative and quantitative approaches may be descriptive, evaluative, theory building, and context-sensitive. The qualities of the two approaches can be viewed along a continuum; at the extreme ends are the major differences between the research approaches, but in between are the numerous similarities. Although qualitative researchers start out with words, they may end up using numbers to describe their results in a quantifiable way.

Likewise, quantitative researchers may start out with numbers, but often they use words to describe their results. Thus, researchers from both traditions use both words and numbers, and both use interpretive analyses in one form or another. One of the advantages of qualitative research is that qualitative data can be analyzed as such. These data (words) can also be converted subsequently to quantitative data for future analysis—for example, by simply ranking or counting the number of statements within each of a set of categories. Quantitative data rarely, if ever, exhibit the converse versatility. Box 7.1 illustrates the similarities and differences between qualitative and quantitative research.

BOX 7.1　General Similarities and Differences between Qualitative and Quantitative Research

> **Similarities**
>   Descriptive
>   Evaluative
>   Context-sensitive
>   Viewed on continuum
> **Differences**
>   Data
>   Sample size
>   Data collection techniques
>   Terminology

Additional differences are noted in sample size, terminologies, and data collection techniques. Sample size in quantitative research is predetermined and important to establish statistical significance of data. The focus shifts in qualitative research to the depth of participant information. For example, in a study by Sleigh (16), 10 primary caregivers for children with cerebral palsy were interviewed, and in another study, two anorexic participants were studied (17).

In qualitative research, terminologies including participants/informants, meaningfulness, and inductive approach are used rather than subjects, validity, and deductive approach respectively. Data differences include methods of collection and analysis as noted later in this chapter. Use of field notes, observations, and artifacts are common in qualitative research.

According to the traditional or purist perspective, an investigator can use only one approach or the other because the fundamental differences between qualitative and quantitative philosophies make it impossible to combine methods from the two traditions without violating the principles unique to each one (9). This chapter broadens the purists'

view, because nutrition and dietetics are applied sciences, and therefore are more interested in identifying what works than in defending a particular methodology on philosophical grounds alone. Mixed methodologies that incorporate both quantitative and qualitative approaches are not only permissible, but are to be encouraged, in our view. Of course, the final methodology also must be sufficiently rigorous to earn credibility for the results it produces.

REASONS TO DO QUALITATIVE RESEARCH

The American Dietetic Association's (ADA) research philosophy states, "Dietetics professionals are responsible to incorporate research into all areas of practice" (18).

Answering New, Different, or Old Questions

The most common reason investigators do qualitative research is that it "enables researchers to ask new questions, answer different kinds of questions and readdress old questions" (19). The aim is to yield data that are richer in description and presumably, deeper in insight and understanding than closed-ended quantitative measures. Tukey is quoted by Lincoln and Guba (9) as saying that it is better to have "an appropriate answer to the *right* question, which is often vague, than an *exact* answer to the wrong question, which can always be made more precise." In these situations, qualitative methods can be used to discover pertinent questions, variables, concepts, and problems, as well as to generate hypotheses or even theories that are more pertinent to the practitioner-researcher (20,21).

The most common situations in which investigators choose a qualitative research approach follow:

- Traditional quantitative approaches are inadequate to improve practice or understanding of a problem issue.
- The researchers are as interested in process variables as they are in outcome variables. Examples of each type of variable will help to clarify this. When studying obesity in children, a researcher may decide to look at certain outcome variables such as a child's weight, stature, and energy expenditure. However, process variables that lead to the outcome variables can also be important. These process variables may include a child's perceptions of weight and exercise, parents' perceptions of weight and exercise, and how parents convey these perceptions to their children.

- Evaluators wish to know both how and why a given outcome happens. For example, RDs may want to know why some clients adhere to a recommended diet plan and others do not.
- The evaluation needs to be extremely audience-specific or very detailed in nature. An example might be a needs assessment for a group of women with both diabetes mellitus and bulimia.
- The researcher needs data on social context, structure, and interactions within which a particular behavior pattern can be understood. These data may be particularly important in understanding aberrant dietary behavior expressed by either individuals or groups, such as anorexia, nonorganic failure to thrive, over-consumption in elementary school-aged children, or binge drinking.

Difficulty Collecting Quantitative Data

In some cases, quantitative survey data may be difficult to collect from certain groups of people, such as young children (22), people who speak English as a second language (23), or those who are unfamiliar with the testing procedures (24). Other people may refuse to answer survey questionnaires because they distrust questionnaires, the source of the questionnaire (eg, private industry or government), or researchers in general. Yet all of these groups may readily participate in the more intimate and interactive data collection procedures offered by qualitative methodologies.

A small, in-depth qualitative study may also provide more useful information than a large-scale quantitative study during formative evaluations (ie, during the design and development testing of new products or programs), when the details provide insight as to how a future intervention program or product might be developed or improved before further investments of time, personnel, and money are made. This kind of study can result in an economy of effort in the long run, whether the product is a new gastric tube, hospital menu, pamphlet, or weight-loss program.

One of the main reasons the interest in qualitative research has grown in community settings is that the more traditional, quantitative methods are often impractical; hospitals and clinics have neither the staff, resources, nor expertise to mount a study with a sample size of thousands or with controls sufficient to detect statistical significance. Even with sufficient resources, problems in practice may arise. For example, people cannot be randomly assigned to different clinics in different communities to assess the impact of a new educational or counseling intervention.

Qualitative methods often present a more pragmatic approach to conducting research in a natural setting.

THE RANGE OF QUALITATIVE RESEARCH IN NUTRITION AND DIETETICS

Qualitative research has become routine in food product development and sensory evaluation (25,26), food and nutrition marketing (27), materials development (28,29), program evaluation (30,31), dietary intake assessment (32), nutrition education (33–35), and dietetics education (36,37). Additional qualitative research has emerged in the areas of food insecurity (38–41), food choice (42), and feeding routes (43,44).

Theory and Designs

No qualitative researcher is able to observe from a blank slate, and no quantitative researcher should be blind to unanticipated data produced by a given experiment or study. The theory-generation value of both qualitative and quantitative studies depends on the questions posed, particular data in hand, previous work done in the field, and the researcher's insight and creativity.

Theory Differences

Theoretical research relies on theory to guide study design, interpretation of results, or both. The theory provides a conceptual framework for approaching the research problem, choosing the hypotheses, understanding the results, and relating them to the real world. Research can be performed atheoretically in both qualitative and quantitative inquiries. In the atheoretical approach, the underlying theory is not made explicit before or after the study, and thus is not open to verification, analysis, discussion, or development (45). Each study is designed and interpreted independently, with no common ground on which to base generalization. For example, when no comprehensive theory exists as to why diet, smoking, stress, gender, age, and even beard growth are related to serum cholesterol levels and heart disease, it is not surprising that the results vary from study to study (46).

Design Differences

Qualitative and quantitative research designs also have an important major difference. In qualitative research, the investigator retains the right to modify or alter the study design in the field according to the need to reassess issues that become apparent only in the field (12). The quantitative research design, in contrast, is seldom if ever altered, regardless of circumstances.

DATA COLLECTION

Participant Selection (Sampling)

In qualitative research, sampling may relate to people, settings, times, events, and processes (47). According to Morse and Field (48), two principles guide qualitative sampling to increase the trustworthiness of data. The first is appropriateness, or the extent to which the sample includes all relevant perspectives (eg, people, settings, times) that can inform the study or question in hand. The second is adequacy, or the extent to which enough data are available to provide a rich description of the phenomenon and the context in which it occurs from each relevant perspective. Adequacy is achieved when results get repetitive or redundant (49) and additional interviews fail to provide fresh insights.

Decisions regarding sample size in qualitative research often rest on a compromise that balances the scope of topics and perspectives explored against the depth to which each topic or perspective is studied. Studies that encompass a broad number of topics and perspectives are not likely to afford researchers the opportunity to explore each topic or perspective in depth with each participant or group. In contrast, studies that address issues in depth with each participant or group may need to be limited in the number of topics or perspectives covered and the number of subjects involved because of the usual constraints of time and money.

Three types of qualitative sampling have been described by Coyne (50): selective, purposeful, and theoretical. Selective sampling occurs when the researcher identifies the people, times, and places to be sampled in advance of study commencement. Selection is based on preconceived notions of when, where, and from whom the most fruitful data might come.

Purposeful sampling is similar, but it occurs after data collection and analysis have begun (51). Purposeful sampling is an ongoing process based on analysis of data gathered to date. Results from one round of data gathering and analysis are used to determine when, where, and from whom to collect the next round of data based on the needs of the study.

Theoretical sampling is purposeful in the sense that it occurs after data collection and analysis have commenced. It differs from purposeful sampling, however, in that theoretical sampling focuses on filling information gaps that hinder theory development. Subjects are selected solely on the basis of their ability to provide information needed to develop, expand, and refine nascent theory emerging from data already collected and analyzed. Theoretical saturation occurs when the addition of subjects, times, or places fails to offer new insights on the theory undergoing construction (52).

In sampling for group interviews, additional considerations related to group dynamics may apply. It is often advisable to assemble relatively homogeneous (eg, homogeneous with respect to age, educational background, ethnic group, status, or income) groups so that participants are comfortable expressing their views in front of other members of the group (53). For example, if studying breastfeeding perceptions, the researcher may separate men from women to alleviate discomfort and encourage participants to freely discuss the topics in their respective groups. If a variety of perspectives is required, additional groups may be formed, each representing a different perspective. By the same token, it may be best for group members to be strangers to one another so that the social liability of candid discussion is minimized (54).

Approaches and Collection Techniques

Individual interviews, group interviews, and analysis of material culture (newspaper stories, reports, diaries, photographs, films, transcripts of speeches, stories, and other narratives) are basic qualitative research methods available to RDs. An exhaustive list of methods and all their variations would fill this chapter and many more. It would also be dated, because new methods are always being developed. Therefore, this section is intended only to introduce you to fundamental methods in the hopes of encouraging further exploration of qualitative strategies that can be used to inform the practice of dietetics.

Two primary methods of qualitative data collection are *observations* and *interviews* (55). In their classic form, these methods are applied in naturalistic settings, where study participants live, work, and play in everyday life. Naturalistic settings are important because qualitative research hinges on the fundamental notion that events and observations can be understood only within the context in which they occur (56). Examples of naturalistic settings relevant in dietetics include hospitals, skilled care and assisted living facilities, outpatient nutrition clinics, soup kitchens, supermarkets, restaurants and fast-food outlets, school cafeterias, home kitchens, and family dinner tables.

Observation

Observation can help researchers explore and understand the apparent gap between what people know or say and what they actually do (57). For example, Weber and Dalton (58) used participant observation to study the food habits of terminally ill men, and Matheson and Achterberg (59) collected observational data to explore children's use of a computer nutrition education program. Tools used by the researcher may include observational forms to record what is being seen, videotapes for review after observation is completed, and field notes to record observations and researcher's thoughts.

Ethnography

The terms *participant observation, field research,* and *field studies* have been used synonymously with ethnography (60). Ethnographic studies allow the researcher to understand social behavior and gain insights into people's lives. The researcher becomes part of the study and is able to learn more through firsthand experiences by participating themselves. Ethnography occurs over an extended period of time, during which the researcher becomes immersed in the culture of a family, ethnic group, or other community.

In one such study (61), researchers spent 22 months in an aboriginal community in an effort to develop prevention strategies for type 2 diabetes in an urban aboriginal population. The study used a mixed methodology (combining both qualitative and quantitative methods). Ethnography was the more qualitative portion of the study. A risk factor survey was used for the more quantitative portion of the study.

Case Studies

Qualitative case studies involve a detailed description of a particular circumstance, event, activity, or program. Case studies are addressed in detail in Chapter 2.

Interviews

Interviews are planned interactions in which one person systematically obtains information from one or more other people via questioning and discussion (62). Studies may vary widely with respect to the amount of time spent per interview and the number of interviews conducted with each individual or group (63).

Individual interviews.   The most common individual interviews are one-to-one verbal exchanges guided by open-ended questions from the interviewer (64). Individual interviews have been used in dietetics to uncover perceptions of foodservice personnel in relation to school lunch programs (65); understand satisfactions and challenges of dietetics and nutrition professionals living in New York state (66); explore self-image among overweight adolescent girls (67); develop insights about food- and nutrition-related issues specific to Hispanic audiences (68); and describe beliefs about diet and health, weight perceptions, and weight-loss practices among Lakota Indians (69). In-depth interviews usually require multiple, extended sessions to explore issues in detail. For example, in one study, researchers interviewed 23 women three times each to evaluate continuity and change in dietary behavior (70).

Most individual interviews consist of guided conversations, but they may also involve specially designed activities such as cognitive response tasks. Cognitive response tasks use stimulus cues, often in the form of persuasive messages or illustrations, to elicit thoughts. These thoughts are labeled *cognitive responses* and are presumed to mediate the persuasive impact of the message via the content and structure of memory (71). Shepherd and Sims (72) used the cognitive response task to explore women's mental reactions to a brochure encouraging the moderation of dietary fat and cholesterol. Rayner and coworkers (73) used a similar approach to investigate subjects' thoughts as they shopped "normally" and as they shopped "healthily" for foods on a predetermined list.

Group interviews.   Group interviews include the focus group interview, nominal group process, and Delphi process. Focus group interviews are designed to stimulate and facilitate topic- or product-relevant discussion among small groups of representatives of the target audience (53). Group dynamism is used to help draw out information about behaviors, attitudes, and opinions that may not be divulged as readily in one-to-one interviews (54). A number of "how to" guides exist that readers can refer to for more detailed guidance (53).

The focus group interview is probably qualitative research technique the most widely used in dietetics. Typically, focus groups are used as a part of audience assessment in planning nutrition education materials and programs. For example, Conners et al (74) conducted focus group interviews with elementary schoolchildren to explore cafeteria factors that influence their milk-drinking behavior. Other investigators have used focus group techniques to explore the views of adolescents in relation to the family meal (75), to explore barriers to healthy eating at school (76), to conduct needs assessment and establish instructional goals for a multimedia nutrition education program for adults (77), and to elicit perspectives related to support of breast-feeding by low-income fathers (78). Focus group research may be conducted with one interview per group or repeated interviews with groups that serve as panels (79). For an especially creative application of focus groups in nutrition education, see Balch et al (80).

Researchers may also use projective techniques in an attempt to reveal deep seated emotions by introducing "highly ambiguous, novel tasks" and severely limiting the response time so participants have little chance to formulate rational responses or censor their thoughts (81–82). For example, A projective technique was used by McCashion (83) to explore emotions underlying meal planning and preparation. Women in focus groups were asked to draw spontaneous pictures depicting what dinnertime meant to them. The resulting artwork reflected intense frustration, feelings of helplessness, and emotional exhaustion in relation to the chore of coming up with ideas for dinner, shopping for dinner, and preparing it. These insights were used to drive the development of Ready, Set, Dinner computer software.

The nominal group process is a group method of soliciting and consolidating opinions using a highly structured consensus-generating technique where each participant expresses opinions in writing, shares opinions with the facilitator one by one, reacts individually to all suggestions grouped by the facilitator according to some common characteristic, privately reevaluates personal opinions in light of what others have said, discusses differences within the group, and repeats the cycle until agreement is reached (84).

The Delphi process, a similar technique, is conducted by mail rather than in a group meeting. For examples of the Delphi process in action, see Gregoire and Sneed (85,86).

Figure 7.1 depicts the continuum of qualitative research; approaches are presented from "pure" in the traditional, unstructured, open-ended sense to "less pure" approaches associated with a relatively more structured or semi-quantitative approach. The left side of the continuum, starting with ethnography, represents a more purist approach. Data sources for ethnographic study include researchers' diaries, artifacts, and photos as is illustrated in work by Thompson, Gifford, and Thorpe (61). On the right side of the continuum are qualitative research approaches considered less pure but still valuable. Formal content analysis work by Byrd-Bredbenner, Finckenor, and Grasso (87) would be an example of this type of research.

They identified health-related content in television shows targeting 2- to 11-year-olds.

Data Analysis

Despite the growing number of texts on qualitative research methods, advice on how to analyze data produced by these methods remains relatively scarce (88). Qualitative data analysis begins with the research question (89). It can proceed both inductively (moving from particular cases to generalizations) and deductively (moving from general cases to the particular). In addition, (a) qualitative data analysis may be theory driven, theory generating, or both, and (b) analysis lies on a continuum that ranges from purely qualitative to more quantitative (refer to Figure 7.1).

Content Analysis

Content analysis is a method in which the researcher systematically identifies and examines characteristics of written documents, audiotapes, or videotapes with the goal of making inferences (54). Examples include works identifying factors influencing fruit and vegetable intake among low-income black youth (90), analyzing television advertising nutrition claims during African-American programs (91), and assessing breastfeeding beliefs and attitudes among Turkish women (92).

Historical research employs content analysis to interpret past events, drawing data from documents such as diaries, letters, poetry, music, and prose created at the time of the event (48). For example, Liquori (93) examined administrative reports, faculty writings, and dissertations from a large academic nutrition department to explore the changing dimensions of science and practice in the nutrition profession over a 55-year period. Individual interviews with subjects who taught or studied in the graduate program from 1937 to 1992 were used to complement the document analysis.

In most cases where researcher-subject encounters are electronically recorded, a written transcript is subsequently produced. Transcripts are usually verbatim accounts designed to preserve, as much as possible, everything that was said during the encounter. Transcripts, however, do not preserve nonlinguistic data such as emphasis, mood, tone of voice, and other descriptive information that can be so crucial in elaborating meaning (94,95). Because of this problem, Jones (95) warns against the temptation to let reading transcripts become a substitute for listening to tapes. It is also critical that the original interviewer edit each typed transcript carefully to check

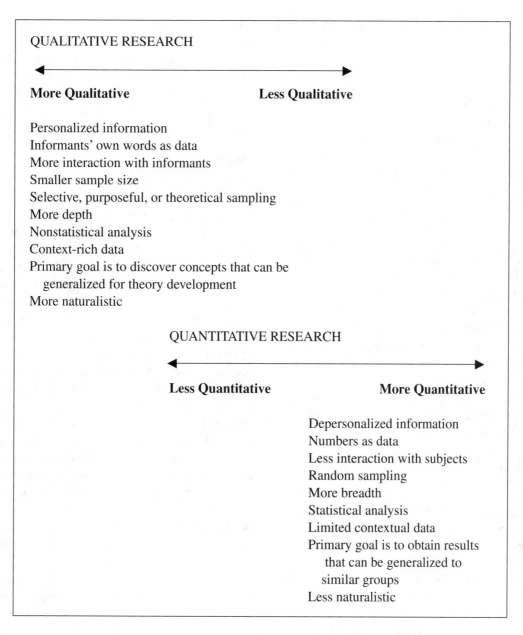

FIGURE 7.1   The continuum of qualitative research approaches and related data sources, ranging from more open-ended (less structured) to less open-ended (more structured).

for accuracy, to fill in the gaps using notes taken during and after the interview, and to annotate the transcript appropriately. Annotations may be needed to clarify ambiguous situations (eg, "the numerous, intermittent comments regarding this issue were provided by a single respondent who kept repeating her position, rather than several different respondents in consensus"). MacLean, Meyer, and Estable (96) offer additional suggestions for improving accuracy of transcripts.

Transcribing tapes is very time-consuming and there-fore costly. Miles (97) estimates that a 60- to 90-minute tape

takes approximately 6 to 8 hours to transcribe. Morton-Williams (94) offers a rule of thumb of 4 to 6 hours per transcript for individual in-depth interviews or group inter-views. One single interview can result in 20 to 40 pages of single-spaced text (98).

Voice recognition software, an automated form of dictation and transcription, is a relatively new technologi-cal tool that qualitative researchers might consider using in their work. It converts verbalizations into text via auto-mated dictation. The advantages and disadvantages of voice recognition software have been noted (99). Two current competing products are Naturally Speaking by Dragon Dictate and ViaVoice by IBM.

Unitizing

Unitizing is a step in the coding process whereby a recorded stream of verbalization (in the form of a transcript or document) is segmented into units of analysis that can be categorized (55,100). It is employed primarily in cases where qualitative data are destined for quantitative analysis (100). Units may be defined in terms of time (eg, 20-second units for the analysis of television commercials), speaker (eg, all statements made by one speaker while holding the floor), or content (eg, each word, phrase, statement, or group of statements that express a single, coherent thought). Pilot testing should help determine which type of unit is the most appropriate for a given project and how the units will be recorded. Recording of units should always include cross-references that trace each unit back to its original location in the transcript so that the surrounding context may be revisited as the need arises. Context is often needed to clarify the intent of ambiguous comments. Moreover, preserving and emphasizing context is a fundamental principle of qualitative research that makes it unique in its contribution to the body of knowledge.

Coding

Coding facilitates the organization, management, and retrieval of qualitative data and helps the investigator extract meaning from the data in a systematic way, uncovering patterns or themes that might otherwise be obscured by the sheer mass of information.

Coding schemes may be developed inductively from the data themselves or be driven by existing theory in a deductive manner.

The mechanical aspects of organizing or coding data involve a creative process that varies from researcher to researcher and from project to project. There is no particular formula; however, pilot work is needed to refine the system and make sure that it works. An investigator may start with an elaborate coding scheme, only to find it too cumbersome to be practical. In contrast, an investigator may begin with a very simple scheme but find that it fails to cover or describe certain types of data adequately (101). In either case, adjustment or refinement of the coding system is necessary.

One way to maximize objectivity in qualitative data analysis is to use two or more independent analysts who can serve as cross-checks for one another (54). A subset of the data might be subjected to analysis by multiple, independent coders when researchers need some indication of interrater agreement but cannot afford to use multiple coders for the entire data set. The important point is that researchers must have a firm rationale for coding or organizing data, foster consistency in the coding process (100) and expose the process to personal and peer scrutiny, increasing the confirmability of the work.

Once a coding system has been established, it may be judged according to two criteria outlined by Guba (102): internal homogeneity and external heterogeneity. The former refers to the extent to which all data within a category reflect the concept represented by that category. That is, do the data within each category follow the rules of inclusion for that category (55)? The latter refers to the extent to which the categories are mutually exclusive. In other words, are the differences between categories consistent?

Other researchers, such as Berg (54) state that when a passage mentions or relates to more than one theme, it should be shown under both themes. Codes or categories can be nested or may be overlapped (51). For example, in coding a transcript for misconceptions about the Food Guide Pyramid, the following comment was categorized as a misconception about the grain group and a misconception about the vegetable group: "Shouldn't potatoes be here with the other fatty starches in the bread group?" To classify the quotation as one or the other (a misconception about the grain group or a misconception about the vegetable group) would have resulted in a considerable loss of information. However, a redefinition of categories would have been unwarranted, especially given that each category had already been used extensively, and this verbalization was the only one that satisfied both. As always, the important point is that the researcher be explicit about the criteria for multiple coding and be consistent in applying that criteria.

Intercoder Reliability

Extensive pilot testing of the coding process is recommended to generate a well-defined set of instructions that can increase the reliability of the processes. When the units of analysis are to be counted, ranked, or subjected to statistical analyses, or all three, reliability of the coding process should be firmly established. Several methods for assessing intercoder agreement are available (103–105). When the units of analysis are not counted, ranked, or subjected to statistical analysis, consensus strategies are often used to code data. Members of the research team work together to assign codes to observations or verbalizations. In this case, intercoder reliability is not an issue.

Computer Analysis of Qualitative Data

The use of computers to manage qualitative data has become commonplace (106). Commercial software is available; however, advantages and cautions should be considered when using software for qualitative data analysis (98,107,108). Examples of dedicated software include ATLAS/ti, NVivo, HyperRESEARCH, and The Ethnograph. Researchers share dedicated software, along with support and information on the use of commercial software, through a networking project commonly referred to as Computer Assisted Qualitative Data Analysis Software (CAQDAS) (109).

Displaying Data

Data display is a way to summarize data in a visual fashion to facilitate analysis and reporting (110). Some examples of data displays are matrices, diagrams, flowcharts, and concept maps. Data displays can help researchers spot connections and relationships that might otherwise be obscured (89). They can also help researchers report data in ways that enhance understanding (51).

Data displays may be an important strategy for improving qualitative data analysis and reporting, but they are subject to drawbacks. For example, it is tempting to select quotations that are particularly colorful, but selection on this basis alone can be misleading if the quotations reflect the views of only one participant. As with coding, investigators working on data displays are advised to record and report decision rules used to selectively display data so that the process remains open to review.

Interpreting Data and Verifying Interpretation

This chapter separated data analysis from interpretation for the sake of discussion. In reality, however, the two often proceed simultaneously to some extent. Indeed, preliminary interpretation may provide direction for further data collection and analysis. It is important, however, to remember that the final interpretation must rest on a comprehensive evaluation of all the data.

Interpretation of results is valid to the extent that it accurately reflects the reality represented by data (111). Interpretations are verified by actively scrutinizing the data for evidence of disconfirmation (rather than confirmation). Miles (97) and Miles and Huberman (110) provide some tactics for applying this scrutiny that remain useful today:

- **Look for concomitant variation, and assess conditions that create greater or lesser concomitant variation.** Does the pattern of variation observed in one part of the data hold true across all the data and/or across data reported by other researchers? If not, what are the circumstances (for example, settings, sources, or occasions) under which the pattern of variation seems to hold most consistently? What are the circumstances under which the pattern of variation is weaker or not observed?
- **Look for negative cases.** Are there data that seem to contradict a conclusion? If so, what is the extent and relative trustworthiness of these data?
- **Rule out spurious or confounding factors.** What are possible alternative explanations for the data? Are the alternative explanations supported by the data in part or in whole?
- **Look for intervening variables.** Are there potential intervening variables without which patterns of concomitant variation would evaporate?
- **Make predictions and search for violations.** What else would be true if this prediction were correct? Is the prediction true according to the data? What would not be true if this prediction were correct?
- **Get feedback from informants.** Does the interpretation ring true to the people who provided the data? According to Maykut and Morehouse (55, p 176), "The validity of findings ultimately rests on whether the participants or people who know them will see a recognizable reality" in the results. The key question as posed by Greenhalgh and Taylor (112, p 742) is, "How comprehensible would this explanation be to a thoughtful participant in the setting?"

Interpretation is considerably easier if a variety of data collection strategies and analytic techniques have been used and yield similar conclusions. This concept, obtaining data from a variety of sources and using various techniques of analysis, is known as *triangulation* (assuming the use of at least three different techniques), and it is probably the best defense against criticism of investigator bias or subjectivity in qualitative research (113).

EVALUATING QUALITATIVE RESEARCH

The merit of qualitative research depends on the trustworthiness of its results and conclusions. Four distinct aspects of trustworthiness defined in the literature are dependability, credibility, confirmability, and transferability (114,115).

Dependability is the extent to which participant's meanings are accurately understood by the researchers. It can be strengthened by the judicious use of follow-up questions and probes to clarify and confirm the meaning of what an interviewee says. Dependability can also be strengthened by member checks, in which participants are asked to review data summaries to see if they ring true from the insider perspective.

Credibility is the extent to which the phenomenon of interest has been adequately described. Data are credible when they provide a rich description of the phenomenon from a variety of perspectives rather than merely describing its surface features from a limited number of critical vantage points.

Confirmability is the extent to which findings and conclusions are supported by evidence from the data. Confirmability can be enhanced by documenting the emergence and evolution of concepts and linking them with the data from which they are derived at each stage of the evolution. This process may be facilitated by the use of study diaries.

Transferability is the extent to which findings from a qualitative study are useful in understanding how people experience the target phenomenon in other settings or under other conditions. Transferability of findings is determined after the fact by subsequent research with different audiences in different circumstances.

In quantitative research, the confidence placed in results and conclusions rests largely on the validity and reliability of measurement instruments used to collect data. In qualitative research, confidence rests on trustworthiness (116). Further information on evaluation along with a list of relevant questions to ask when assessing a qualitative piece can be found in Mays and Pope (117).

LIMITATIONS AND CONCERNS WITH QUALITATIVE RESEARCH

Qualitative research has its own limitations. Perhaps the most obvious is that generalizations cannot be made from any one data set to larger populations. Also, it is often difficult to compare qualitative studies because they are context bound. In addition, qualitative data do not at present lend themselves to meta-analysis, although researchers are pursuing ways to solve this problem. Data collection is very dependent on personnel (as opposed to equipment and statistical software), and data quality subsequently depends entirely on the quality and training of personnel. Data analysis tends to be time-consuming and

tedious. In fact, when qualitative and quantitative methods are used together, it is sometimes difficult to complete the qualitative analysis in time to be useful to the quantitative process.

CONCLUSION

Human events are far too complex to be viewed or analyzed from any single perspective (118–120). RDs, therefore, should explore the variety of methodologies offered by the qualitative approach to research, especially to develop and evaluate interventions or programs in clinical or community environments. Qualitative studies are becoming increasingly important, particularly in nutrition education and intervention. The National Institutes of Health now encourages grant application for qualitative research projects (121).

Qualitative research includes ethnographic studies, case studies, individual interviewing, focus groups, and other approaches. The benefits in using qualitative research include a deeper understanding to improve dietetics practice while yielding significant findings. In sum, qualitative research is a viable means of problem-solving in our field.

REFERENCES

1. Pelto PJ, Pelto GH. *Anthropological Research: The Structure of Inquiry.* 2nd ed. Cambridge, UK: Cambridge University Press; 1999.
2. Wilson CS. Food custom and nurture. *J Nutr Educ.* 1979;11(suppl):211.
3. Lefèvre P, Suremain CÉ, Celis ER, Sejas E. Combining causal model and focus group discussions experiences lcarned from a socio-anthropological research on the differing perceptions of caretakers and health professionals on children's health (Bolivia/Peru). *Qual Rep.* 2004;9:1–17.
4. Knafl KA, Howard MJ. Interpreting and reporting qualitative research. *Res Nurs.* 1984;7:17.
5. Miles MB, Huberman AM. Drawing valid meaning from qualitative data: toward a shared craft. In: Fetterman DM, ed. *Qualitative Approaches to Evaluation Education: The Silent Scientific Revolution.* New York, NY: Praeger; 1988:222.
6. Falk LW, Sobal J, Biscogni CA, Connors M, Devine CM. Managing healthy eating: definitions, classifications, and strategies. *Health Educ Behav.* 2001;28:425–439.

7. Rose K, Webb C. Analyzing data: maintaining rigor in a qualitative study. *Qual Health Rep.* 1998;8: 556–562.

8. Kirk J, Miller ML. *Reliability and Validity in Qualitative Research.* Beverly Hills, Calif: Sage Publications; 1986:1.

9. Lincoln YS, Guba EG. *Naturalistic Inquiry.* Beverly Hills, Calif: Sage Publications; 1985:338.

10. Jacob E. Qualitative research traditions: a review. *Rev Educ Res.* 1987;57:1.

11. Taylor SJ, Bogdan R. *Introduction to Qualitative Research Methods: A Guidebook and Resource.* 3rd ed. New York, NY: John Wiley and Sons; 1998.

12. Bulmer M. Concepts in the analysis of qualitative data. *Soc Rev.* 1979;27:65.

13. Sandelowski M. The problem of rigor in qualitative research. *ANS Adv Nurs Sci.* 1986;27–37.

14. Denzin NK, Lincoln YS. *The SAGE Handbook of Qualitative Research.* 3rd ed. Thousand Oaks, Calif: Sage Publications; 2005.

15. Bisogni CA, Connors M, Devine CM, Sobal J. Who we are and how we eat: a qualitative study of identities in food choice. *J Nutr Educ Behav.* 2002;34:128–139.

16. Sleigh G. Mothers' voice: a qualitative study on feeding children with cerebral palsy. *Child Care Health Dev.* 2005;31:373–383.

17. Chan ZCY, Ma JLC. Anorexic eating: two case studies in Hong Kong. *Qual Rep.* 2002;7(4). Available at: http://www.nova.edu/ssss/QR/QR7-4/chan.html. Accessed April 9, 2006.

18. American Dietetic Association. ADA's research philosophy. Available at: http://www.eatright.org/cps/rde/xchg/ada/hs.xsl/career_916_ENU_HTML.htm. Accessed February 28, 2007.

19. Fetterman DM. Qualitative approaches to evaluating education. *Educ Res.* 1988;17–23.

20. Strauss A, Corbin J. *Basics of Qualitative Research.* Newbury Park, Calif: Sage Publications; 1998.

21. Reeder LG. Social epidemiology: an appraisal. In: Jaco EG, ed. *Patients, Physicians, and Illness.* 3rd ed. New York, NY: Free Press; 1979:97–101.

22. Goodwin RA, Brulé D, Junkins EA, Dubois S, Beer-Borst S. Development of a food and activity record and a portion-size model booklet for use by 6- to 17-year-olds: a review of focus group testing. *J Am Diet Assoc.* 2001;101:926–928.

23. Achterberg CL, Van Horn B, Maretzki A. Evaluation of dietary guideline bulletins revised for a low literature audience. *J Ext.* 1994;32(4). Available at:

http://www.joe.org/joe/1994december/rb2.html. Accessed June 20, 2006.

24. Shatenstein B, Claveau D, Ferland G. Visual observation is a valued means of assessing dietary consumption among older adults with cognitive deficits in long-term care settings. *J Am Diet Assoc.* 2002;102:250–252.

25. Marlow P. Qualitative research as a tool for product development. *Food Technol.* 1987;74,76.

26. Kennedy OB, Stewart-Know BJ, Mitchell PC, Thurnham DI. Consumer perceptions of poultry meat: a qualitative analysis. *Nutr Food Sci.* 2004;34:122–129.

27. Kraak V, Pelletier D. How marketers reach young consumers: implications for nutrition education and health promotion campaigns. *Fam Econ Nutr Rev.* 1999;11(4):31–41.

28. Borra A, Kelly L, Tuttle M, Nevelle K. Developing actionable dietary guidance messages: dietary fat as a case study. *J Am Diet Assoc.* 2001;101:678–684.

29. Crockett S, Lytle L, Elmer P, Finnegan J, Luepker R, Laing B. Formative evaluation for planning a nutrition intervention: results from focus groups. *J Nutr Educ.* 1995;27:127–132.

30. Marino D, White C. Interviewing participants key to dietetic students' understanding of emergency food needs. *J Nutr Educ.* 1999;31:119A.

31. Cargo M, Salsberg J, Delormier T, Desrosiers S, Macaulay AC. Understanding the social context of school health promotion program implementation. *Health Educ.* 2006;106:85–97.

32. Shankar AV, Gittelsohn J, Stallings R, West KP, Gnywali T, Dhungel C, Dahal B. Comparison of visual estimates of children's portion sizes under shared-plate and individual plate conditions. *J Am Diet Assoc.* 2001;101:47–52.

33. Matheson D, Achterberg C. Description of a process evaluation model for nutrition education computer-assisted instruction programs. *J Nutr Educ.* 1999; 31:105–113.

34. Mitchell K, Branigan P. Using focus groups to evaluate health promotion interventions. *Health Educ.* 2000;100:261–268.

35. Chambers DH, Higgins MM, Roeger C, Allison AA. Nutrition education displays for young adults and older adults. *Health Educ.* 2004;104:45–54.

36. Kruzich LA, Anderson J, Litchfield RE, Wohlsdorf-Arendt S, Oakland MJ. A preceptor focus group approach to evaluation of a dietetic internship. *J Am Diet Assoc.* 2003;103:884–886.

37. Arendt SA, Gregoire MB. Barriers when teaching leadership through group work: hospitality management and dietetics students' perspectives. *J Fam Consum Sci Educ.* 2006;98:32–43.

38. Connell CL, Lofton KL, Yadrick K, Rehner TA. Children's experiences of food insecurity can assist in understanding its effect on their well-being. *J Nutr.* 2005;135:1683–1690.

39. Kempson KM, Keenan DP, Sadani PS, Ridlen S, Rosato NC. Food management practices used by people with limited resources to maintain food sufficiency as reported by nutrition educators. *J Am Diet Assoc.* 2002;102:1795–1799.

40. Tarasuk V, Eakin JM. Charitable food assistance as symbolic gesture: an ethnographic study of food banks in Ontario. *Soc Sci Med.* 2003;56:1505–1515.

41. Tarasuk V, Eakin JM. Food assistance through "surplus" food: insights from an ethnographic study of food bank work. *Agric Human Values.* 2005;22:177–186.

42. Devine CM, Connors MM, Sobal J, Bisogni CA. Sandwiching it in: spillover of work onto food choices and family roles in low-and moderate-income urban households. *Soc Sci Med.* 2003;56:617–630.

43. Orrevall Y, Tishelman C, Herrington MK, Permert J. The path from oral nutrition to home parenteral nutrition: a qualitative interview study of the experiences of advanced cancer patients and their families. *Clin Nutr.* 2004;23:1280–1287.

44. Pasman HRW, The BAM, Onwuteaka-Philipsen BD, Ribbe MW, van der Wal G. Participants in the decision making on artificial nutrition and hydration to demented nursing home patients: a qualitative study. *J Aging Stud.* 2004;18:321–335.

45. Achterberg CL, Novak JD, Gillespie AH. Theory-driven research as a means to improve nutrition education. *J Nutr Educ.* 1985;17:179.

46. Dean K. Nutrition education research in health promotion. *J Can Diet Assoc.* 1990;51:481–484.

47. Johnson JC. Research design and research strategies. In: Bernard HR, ed. *Handbook of Methods in Cultural Anthropology.* Walnut Creek, Calif: Altamira Press; 1998:131–153.

48. Morse JM, Field PA. *Qualitative Research Methods for Health Professionals.* 2nd ed. Thousand Oaks, Calif: Sage Publications; 1995.

49. Lincoln YS, Guba EG. *Naturalistic Inquiry.* Beverly Hills, Calif: Sage Publications; 1985.

50. Coyne IT. Sampling in qualitative research. Purposeful and theoretical sampling: merging or clear boundaries? *J Adv Nurs.* 1997;26:623–630.

51. Coffey A, Atkinson P. *Making Sense of Qualitative Data: Complementary Research Strategies.* Thousand Oaks, Calif: Sage Publications; 1996.

52. Glaser BG, Strauss AL. *The Discovery of Grounded Theory: Strategies for Qualitative Research.* New York, NY: Aldine de Gruyter; 1967.

53. Krueger RA, Casey M. *Focus Groups: A Practical Guide for Applied Research.* 3rd ed. Thousand Oaks, Calif: Sage Publications; 2000.

54. Berg BL. *Qualitative Research Methods for the Social Sciences.* 3rd ed. Boston, Mass: Allyn and Bacon; 1998.

55. Maykut P, Morehouse R. *Beginning Qualitative Research: A Philosophic and Practical Guide.* Washington, DC: Falmer Press; 1994.

56. Evans JF. Changing the lens: a position paper on the value of qualitative research methodology as a mode of inquiry in the education of the deaf. *Am Ann Deaf.* 1998;143:246–254.

57. Marshall C, Rossman GB. *Designing Qualitative Research.* Newbury Park, Calif: Sage Publications; 1989.

58. Weber CD, Dalton A. A case study: the food habits of three terminally ill men. *Top Clin Nutr.* 1992;7:30–36.

59. Matheson D, Achterberg C. Ecologic study of children's use of a computer nutrition education program. *J Nutr Educ.* 2001;33:2–9.

60. Esterberg KG. *Qualitative Methods in Social Research.* Boston, Mass: McGraw-Hill; 2002.

61. Thompson SJ, Gifford SM, Thorpe L. The social and cultural context of risk and prevention: food and physical activity in an urban Aboriginal community. *Health Educ Behav.* 2000;27:727–743.

62. Lipchik E. *Interviewing.* Rockville, Md: Aspen; 1988.

63. Sobal J. Sample extensiveness in qualitative nutrition education research. *J Nutr Educ.* 2001;33:184–192.

64. Fontana A, Frey JH. The interview: from structured questions to negotiated text. In: Denzin NK, Lincoln YS, eds. *Handbook of Qualitative Research.* 2nd ed. Thousand Oaks, Calif: Sage Publications; 2000:645–672.

65. Gittelsohn J, Toporoff EG, Story M, Evans M, Anliker J, Davis S, Sharma A, White J. Food perceptions and dietary behavior of American-Indian children, their caregivers, and educators: formative assessment findings from Pathways. *J Nutr Educ.* 2000;32:2–13.

66. Devine CM, Jastran M, Bisogni CA. On the front line: practice satisfactions and challenges experienced by dietetics and nutrition professionals working in community setting in New York State. *J Am Diet Assoc.* 2004;104: 787–792.

67. Neumark-Sztainer D, Story M, Faibisch L, Ohlson J, Adamiak M. Issues of self-image among over-weight African-American and Caucasian adolescent girls: a qualitative study. *J Nutr Educ.* 1999;31:311–320.

68. Gans KM, Lovell HJ, Fortunet R, McMahon C, Carton-Lopez S, Lasater TM. Implications of qualitative research for nutrition education geared to selected Hispanic audiences. *J Nutr Educ.* 1999;31:331–338.

69. Harnack L, Story M, Rock BH, Neumark-Sztainer D, Jerrery R, French S. Nutrition beliefs and weight loss practices of Lakota Indian adults. *J Nutr Educ.* 1999;31:10–15.

70. Paquette M, Devine CM. Dietary trajectories in the menopause transition among Quebec women. *J Nutr Educ.* 2000;32:320–328.

71. Wright P. Message-evoked thoughts: persuasion research using thought verbalizations. *J Consum Res.* 1980;7:151.

72. Shepherd SK, Sims LS. Employing cognitive response analysis to examine message acceptance in nutrition education. *J Nutr Educ.* 1990;22:215–228.

73. Rayner M, Boaz A, Higginson C. Consumer use of health-related endorsements on food labels in the United Kingdom and Australia. *J Nutr Educ.* 2001;33:24–30.

74. Conners P, Bednar C, Klammer S. Cafeteria factors that influence milk-drinking behaviors of elementary school children: grounded theory approach. *J Nutr Educ.* 2001;33:31–36.

75. Neumark-Sztainer D, Story M, Ackard D, Moe J, Perry C. The family meal: views of adolescents. *J Nutr Educ.* 2000;32:329–334.

76. Meyer MK, Conklin MT, Lewis JR, Marshak J, Cousin S, Turnage C, Wood D. Barriers to healthy nutrition environments in public school middle grades. *J Child Nutr Manag.* 2001;25(2):66–71.

77. Carlton DJ, Kicklighter JR, Jonnalagadda SS, Shoffner MB. Design, development, and formative evaluation of "Put Nutrition Into Practice," a multi-media nutrition education program for adults. *J Am Diet Assoc.* 2000;100:555–563.

78. Schmidt MM, Sigman-Grant M. Perspectives of low-income fathers' support of breastfeeding: an exploratory study. *J Nutr Educ.* 1999;31:31–37.

79. Shepherd SK, Sims LS, Davis CA, Shaw A, Cronin FJ. Panel versus novice focus groups: reactions to content and design features of print materials. *J Nutr Educ.* 1994;26:10–14.

80. Balch GI, Loughrey K, Weinberg L, Lurie D, Eisner E. Probing consumer benefits and barriers for the national 5-A-Day campaign: focus group findings. *J Nutr Educ.* 1997;29:178–183.

81. Walker R. *Applied Qualitative Research.* London, UK: Gower Publishing; 1985.

82. Braithwaite A, Lunn T. Projective techniques in social and market research. In: Walker R, ed. *Applied Qualitative Research.* London, UK: Gower Publishing; 1985.

83. McCashion L. Ready, set, dinner: how the National Potato Promotion Board leveraged its nutrition education program for maximum results. *J Nutr Educ.* 1996;28:47D.

84. Jones J, Hunter D. Consensus methods for medical and health services research. In: Mays N, Pope C, eds. *Qualitative Research in Health Care.* London, UK: BMJ Publishing Group; 1996:46–58.

85. Gregoire MB, Sneed J. Barriers and needs related to procurement and implementation of dietary guidelines. *School Food Service Res Rev.* 1993;17:46–49.

86. Gregoire MB, Sneed J. Standards for nutrition integrity. *School Food Service Res Rev.* 1994;18:106–111.

87. Byrd-Bredbenner C, Finckenor M, Grasso D. Health related content in prime-time television pro-gramming. *J Health Commun.* 2003;8:329–341.

88. Morse JM. Validity by committee. *Qual Health Res.* 1998;8:443–445.

89. Mason J. *Qualitative Researching.* Thousand Oaks, Calif: Sage Publications; 1996.

90. Molaison EF, Connell CL, Stuff JE, Yardrick KM, Bogle M. Influences on fruit and vegetable consumption by low-income black American adolescents. *J Nutr Educ Behav.* 2005;37:246–251.

91. Henderson VR, Kelly B. Food advertising in the age of obesity: content analysis of food advertising on general market and African American television. *J Nutr Educ Behav.* 2005;37:191–196.

92. Bramhagen AC, Axelsson I, Hallström I. Mother's experiences of feeding situation-an interview study. *J Clin Nurs.* 2006;15:29–34.

93. Liquori T. Food matters: changing dimensions of science and practice in the nutrition profession. *J Nutr Educ.* 2001;33:234–246.

94. Morton-Williams J. Making qualitative research work: aspects of administration. In: Walker R, ed. *Applied Qualitative Research.* Brookfield, Vt: Gower Publishing; 1985.

95. Jones S. The analysis of depth interviews. In: Walker R, ed. *Applied Qualitative Research.* Brookfield, Vt: Gower Publishing; 1985:56.

96. MacLean LM, Meyer M, Estable A. Improving accuracy of transcripts in qualitative research. *Qual Health Res.* 2004;14:113–123.

97. Miles MB. Qualitative data as an attractive nuisance: the problem of analysis. *Adm Sci Q.* 1979;4:590.

98. Pope C, Ziebland S, Mays N. Qualitative research in health care: analysing qualitative data. *BMJ.* 2000;320:114–116.

99. Park J, Zeanah AE. An evaluation of voice recognition software for use in interview-based research: a research note. *Qual Res.* 2005;5:245–251.

100. Ericsson KA, Simon HA. *Protocol Analysis: Verbal Reports as Data.* Cambridge, Mass: MIT Press; 1984.

101. Atkinson P, Coffey A. Analyzing documentary realities. In: Silverman D, ed. *Qualitative Research: Theory, Method, and Practice.* Thousand Oaks, Calif: Sage Publications; 1997:45–62.

102. Guba EG. *Toward a Methodology of Naturalistic Inquiry in Educational Evaluation.* Los Angeles, Calif: UCLA Center for the Study of Evaluation; 1978.

103. Geutzkow H. Unitizing and categorizing problems in coding qualitative data. *J Clin Psychol.* 1950;6:47–51.

104. Folger JP, Hewes DE, Poole MS. Coding social interaction. In: Dervin B, Voight M, eds. *Progress in Communication Sciences.* Norwood, NJ: Ablex Publishers; 1984:4.

105. Tinsley HEA, Weiss DJ. Interrater reliability and agreement of subjective judgments. *J Couns Psychol.* 1975;22:358.

106. Miles MB, Huberman AM. *Qualitative Data Analysis: An Expanded Sourcebook.* Thousand Oaks, Calif: Sage Publications; 1994.

107. Miles MB, Weitzman EA. 1996 . . . the state of qualitative data analysis software: what do we need? *Curr Sociol.* 1996;44:207–224.

108. Conrad P, Reinharz S. Computers and qualitative data: editors' introductory essay. *Qual Sociol.* 1984;7:3.

109. CAQDAS Networking Project Web site. Available at: http://caqdas.soc.surrey.ac.uk. Accessed February 28, 2007.

110. Miles MB, Huberman AM. Drawing valid meaning from qualitative data: toward a shared craft. In: Fetterman DM, ed. *Qualitative Approaches to Evaluation in Education: The Silent Scientific Revolution.* New York, NY: Praeger; 1988:222.

111. Hirschman EC. Humanistic inquiry in marketing research: philosophy, method, and criteria. *J Mark Res.* 1986;23:237.

112. Greenhalgh T, Taylor R. Papers that go beyond numbers (qualitative research). *BMJ.* 1997;315:740–743.

113. Achterberg CL. Qualitative methods in nutrition education evaluation research. *J Nutr Educ.* 1988;20:244.

114. DePoy E, Gitlin LN. *Introduction to Research.* London, UK: Mosby; 1994.

115. Leininger M. Evaluation criteria and critique of qualitative research studies. In: Morse JM. *Critical Issues in Qualitative Research Methods.* Thousand Oaks, Calif: Sage Publications; 1994;95–115.

116. Ambert A, Adler PA, Adler P, Detzner DF. Understanding and evaluating qualitative research. *J Marriage Fam.* 1995;57:879–893.

117. Mays N, Pope C. Assessing quality in quantitative research. *BMJ.* 2000;320:50–52.

118. Bronfenbrenner U. *The Ecology of Human Development.* Cambridge, Mass: Harvard University Press; 1979.

119. Hamilton JA. Epistemology and meaning: a case for multimethodologies for social research in home economics. *Home Econ Forum.* 1989;4:12.

120. Morgan DL. Practical strategies for combining qualitative and quantitative methods: applications to health research. *Qual Health Res.* 1998;8:362–376.

121. National Institutes of Health, Office of Behavioral and Social Sciences Research. Qualitative Methods in Health Research: Opportunities and Considerations in Application and Review. Available at: http://obssr.od.nih.gov/Publications/Qualitative.PDF. Accessed April 9, 2006.

PART 4

—◊◊◊—

The Conduct of Observational and Experimental Research Studies

8

Analytic Nutrition Epidemiology

Monica E. Yamamoto, DrPH, RD, FADA

Nutrition epidemiology, a subdiscipline of epidemiology, addresses the fundamental question, does diet or nutrition make a difference to health and disease? The term *diet* refers to items ingested, and *nutrition* refers to the nutrient results of those ingested items. *Epidemiology,* the investigative basic science for health, studies "the distribution and determinants of health-related states or events and applies these to control health problems" (1). Operationally, epidemiologic studies can be categorized as either descriptive or analytic. Descriptive epidemiology studies the frequency, distribution, and pattern of health-related states or events (2). Analytic epidemiology examines whether a factor is a source of risk or directly causes a health or disease effect. Descriptive epidemiology findings, while not definitive for disease associations or causal relationships, are key sources for causal (etiologic) hypotheses that are the focus of analytic epidemiologic work. Analytic nutrition epidemiology investigates whether diet exposures are significantly associated with, or have a causal linkage with, health or the risk, progression, or prognosis of disease.

This chapter provides an introduction to analytic nutrition epidemiology. First, an overview of analytic epidemiology discusses analytic goals and measures. Next, key issues in designing and implementing analytic nutrition epidemiologic studies are discussed. Finally, analytic epidemiology study designs are examined, including their uses, advantages, limitations, implementation

issues, analytic considerations, findings, and diet and nutrition examples.

WHAT IS ANALYTIC NUTRITION EPIDEMIOLOGY?

Analytic nutrition epidemiology seeks to explain the described occurrence of disease or disease-related phenomena (3,4) in relation to diet and nutrition. It investigates diet and nutrition as potential determinants of population disease patterns (3,5,6). Researchers use analytic nutrition epidemiology to ask, If and/or what diet and nutrition factors independently contribute to, or are likely to cause, the pattern of health or disease identified in the population?

Analytic epidemiologic observational designs study potential health-related relationships as they occur in nature (4) and examine evidence to explain why diseases are distributed the way they are (4). Types of designs include cross-sectional studies, surveillance studies, cohort studies, and case-control studies. Descriptive epidemiology also uses cross-sectional and surveillance designs but use these to report characteristics of occurrences (eg, time, place, and individual traits). Additionally, analytic epidemiology employs experimental (etiologic) studies where the investigator intervenes and then examines the effect of the intervention on one or more specific health or disease outcomes. Experimental analytic epidemiology designs include

BOX 8.1   Measures of Association

$$\text{Relative Risk (RR)} = \frac{\text{Cumulative Incidence in the Exposed}}{\text{Cumulative Incidence in the Nonexposed}}$$

$$\text{Attributable Risk (AR)} = \left[\begin{array}{c}\text{Cumulative Incidence}\\ \text{in the Exposed}\end{array}\right] - \left[\begin{array}{c}\text{Cumulative Incidence}\\ \text{in the Nonexposed}\end{array}\right]$$

$$\text{Population Attributable Risk (PAR)} = \left[\begin{array}{c}\text{Cumulative Incidence}\\ \text{in the Population}\end{array}\right] - \left[\begin{array}{c}\text{Cumulative Incidence}\\ \text{in the Nonexposed}\end{array}\right]$$

$$\text{Odds Ratio (OR)} = \frac{\text{Exposed Cases} \times \text{Nonexposed Controls}}{\text{Unexposed Cases} \times \text{Exposed Controls}}$$

randomized controlled trials (RCTs), group-randomized trials, and multicentered RCTs.

Analytic nutrition epidemiology observational investigations examine whether health risks are significantly associated with diet and nutrition exposures (3,5). Analytic nutrition experimental investigations test whether diet or nutrition exposures are causally linked with health or disease outcomes. Finally, all analytic epidemiology studies include four groups: subjects who have the disease (or high risk of disease), subjects who do not have the disease (or are not at high risk), subjects with a particular exposure, and subjects without a particular exposure (5).

GOALS OF ANALYTIC EPIDEMIOLOGY

Analytic epidemiology has two specific goals:

- Establish whether a significant association exists between a specific factor and a disease outcome
- Examine or test evidence for a causal effect of a specific factor on a disease outcome

Establishing Association

What Is an Association?

The first step in identifying a factor's importance to health or disease is to examine whether an association exists between this specific factor and the disease in question (1). The analysis tests whether the risk associated with a particular disease is significantly different based on the presence or level of the factor. In other

words, it studies whether the specific risk factor is associated with a higher-than-normal or lower-than-normal risk of having a particular disease, disease prognosis, or disease progression.

What Are Measures of Association?

Epidemiology expresses disease association as risk of disease (see Box 8.1). This risk can be an overall risk or a risk specific to a particular exposure. Terms that express overall risk include *risk difference, relative risk,* and *odds ratio* (or *relative odds*). *Risk difference* is the proportion in the unexposed group with the disease as compared to the proportion in the exposed group (7). *Relative risk* is the proportion of subjects with the disease who have been exposed compared to the proportion not exposed. The *odds ratio,* or *relative odds,* is an estimate of relative risk that is calculated when the disease is rare. For example, the risk of heart disease, a common disease, is expressed as a relative risk, whereas the risk of esophageal cancer, a relatively rare disease, is represented as an odds ratio. *Odds ratio* is also used to express risk estimates generated from case-control studies because these estimates derive from "constructed" populations rather than natural ones. Terms that focus on the impact (7) of specific risk exposures (factors) include *etiologic fraction, attributable risk,* and *population attributable risk*. The *etiologic fraction* is the proportion of subjects exposed (exposed-unexposed/exposed) to a particular factor who have the disease. *Attributable risk* is the amount of risk that can be assigned to a particular factor. *Population attributable risk* is the proportion of the disease incidence in a population (both exposed and nonexposed) that can be associated with a specific exposure (1).

What Study Designs Are Used to Study Associations?

Observational study designs, used to study associations, collect observations of subjects and do not include interventions. Epidemiologic observational designs include cross-sectional studies, surveillance studies, cohort studies, and case-control studies. Cross-sectional studies are those completed at one point in time (eg, the National Health and Nutrition Examination Surveys (NHANES); those completed at designated intervals typically for monitoring purposes (eg, surveillance studies such as the Pediatric Nutrition Surveillance System [PedNSS] and the Pregnancy Nutrition Surveillance System [PNSS]); those that examine the same group of individuals repeatedly over time (eg, cohort studies such as the Prostate, Lung, Colorectal, and Ovarian Cancer Screening Trial [PLCO]); and case-control studies. Observational studies compare exposed and nonexposed groups for case status (cohort studies), compare cases and noncases (case-control studies) for potential risk factors, or study populations for both case status and potential risk factors (cross-sectional studies and surveillance studies) (1). Measures of association are derived from these analyses. For example, the 1999–2002 NHANES, a cross-sectional study, was examined for associations between chronic disease status and nutrient levels (8). The PedNSS was examined for an association between breastfeeding and reduced risk of being an overweight child (9).

Establishing Causation

What Is Causation?

Etiologic epidemiologic studies (ie, studies of disease causation) build on evidence for a significant association between a specific factor and a disease outcome where a possible causal relationship has been suggested. An experimental study tests whether a causal relationship actually exists between the factor and the disease.

Criteria for Causation

For ethical as well as logistic reasons, epidemiologic studies are not "pure experimental studies." Specific causal criteria have been suggested for epidemiologic studies. The eight classical criteria, commonly called Hill's criteria, are frequently cited for this purpose (Box 8.2) (5). Hill's first criterion is consistency of the association. Similar associations are found in a variety of studies (with different populations, study designs, and statistical methods). His second criterion is strength of the association. The magnitude of the association between the factor and the

disease is significant. As illustrated in Figure 8.1, a relative risk of 1 indicates that the risk of a disease outcome is the same as expected. A relative risk with factor exposure substantially greater or less than 1 indicates that the disease outcome is likely to be associated with the factor. Hill's third criterion is specificity of association. A single cause results in a single outcome. With the fourth criterion, the temporal relationship, the exposure or factor precedes the disease outcome. The fifth criterion is evidence for a biological gradient. A dose relationship is seen with a specific threshold, or an increased effect is seen with an increased dose. The sixth criterion is biological plausibility. There is biological evidence from relevant experiments (eg, in vitro cell systems, animal models, or human metabolic and clinical studies). Hill's seventh criterion is coherence. The causal relationship is congruent with existing knowledge about the disease or condition (5). The final criterion is evidence from experimentation where specific evidence is provided through controlled experiments, including laboratory studies, animal models, and randomized clinical trials (5).

BOX 8.2   Hill's Criteria for Causation

---

1. Association's consistency*
2. Association's strength*
3. Association's specificity*
4. Association's temporality
5. Biological gradient (dose/response)*
6. Biological plausibility*
7. Coherence*
8. Experimental evidence

*Reduced criteria for diet and nutrition studies agreed upon by both Potischman and Weed (10) and the Committee on Diet and Health, Food and Nutrition Board, National Research Council (11).

Source: Data are from reference 4.

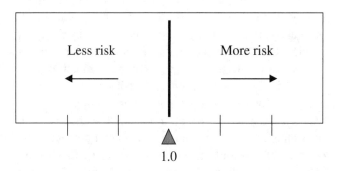

FIGURE 8.1   Relative risk.

EXAMPLE.   A highly significant relationship between salt intake and rise in blood pressure has been widely reported (strength of association). This is found regardless of the population studied (consistency of association). This association has been found regardless of other potential confounding influences, such as obesity or hypertensive vs normal blood pressure (specificity of association). Higher salt intakes at an earlier point have been shown to lead to later higher blood pressures, and reduced salt intakes have been shown to lead to subsequent lower blood pressures (temporal relationship). A dose-response relationship has been shown with salt intakes, with higher intakes resulting in higher blood pressures and lower intakes resulting in lower blood pressures (biological gradient). Several well-known mechanisms for this relationship have been documented (biological plausibility). This association and its underlying mechanisms fit well with existing knowledge about blood pressure response (coherence). Finally, there is a large body of experimental evidence from animal studies and human clinical trials that has documented this relationship (evidence from experimentation). An important caveat to this summary is that several key questions remain unresolved regarding the relationship between salt intake and blood pressure (12). For example, the precise mechanism underlying the salt and blood pressure relationship has not been definitively established (13). Also, susceptible subgroups who elicit an even larger blood pressure response with salt need to be identified (14).

Diet and nutrition studies pose unique challenges in applying causal criteria (10,11). Evaluation of associations for causal effects in diet and nutrition studies (3) is complex because frequent exceptions to the Hill criteria are encountered. Diet and nutrition factors have built-in measurement difficulties (eg, measurement error, possible lack of intake variation in population, and intake distributions unrelated to disease processes). Measurement problems can lead to serious underestimates of causal effects or produce "evidence" for causal effects that do not exist. Because everyone eats (ie, dietary exposures are common), somewhat small relative risks of 0.7 to 1.5 could be important (3). In contrast, exposures from environmental contaminants or occupation would be "uncommon" because they would involve only a subset of the population. It should be noted that there is considerable debate regarding the size of relative risk that should be considered important. Some

epidemiologists argue that risks less than 3.0 (ie, three times expected levels) are likely to be spurious. Others argue that relative risks as low as 0.2 (ie, 20% greater than expected levels) may be important if the factor has widespread exposure and is likely to have significant measurement error. Diet exposures would fit that description.

Absolute consistency of findings is not a realistic expectation (3), and perfect specificity of associations is rare (11). This imperfect consistency and specificity could be due to the complexity of the disease process, the imprecision of diet measures, or the specific effects of diet components on organ systems or the disease processes (11). Dose-response relationships are likely to be "nonlinear or almost any shape depending on the starting point on a hypothetical spectrum of exposure" (3). Thus, typical analytic approaches may not detect underlying relationships. Also, a clear dose-response relationship might easily be the result of bias or confounding (3).

Arguments supporting biological plausibility that are developed "post hoc, should be viewed cautiously because they can usually be developed for most observations, including those that are later refuted" (3). There is a lack of well-defined mechanisms for most cancers and many other chronic diseases (3). This fact hampers the ability of chronic disease researchers to meet criteria for biological plausibility and coherence. Finally, experimental studies, particularly in humans, might provide key evidence for causal relationships. However, practical considerations (eg, time and money constraints) and ethical considerations limit such investigations.

In light of these many concerns, it has been strongly suggested (10,11) that the Hill criteria are too stringent to apply to diet and nutrition studies. Instead, a minimum set of causal criteria has been recommended. This minimum set would include consistency of findings, strength of association, dose response, biological plausibility, and temporality. This reduced set of criteria was used by the Committee on Diet and Health (Food and Nutrition Board of the National Academy of Sciences) for its landmark publication *Diet and Health: Implications for Reducing Chronic Disease Risk* (refer to Box 8.2) (11).

EXAMPLE.   The Food and Drug Administration reviewed evidence for the relationship between periconceptional folic acid intake and neural tube defects (NTDs) in the early 1990s and subsequently implemented a policy for folic acid fortification of flours and cereals in the United States. Evidence from case-control studies and a prospective cohort study supported a consistent and strong association between occurrence of NTD and lower folic acid intakes, status, or both. A dose-response relationship was supported for prevention of NTD in both women who have never had a child with NTD and women who previously delivered a child with NTD. The temporality criterion was met because folic acid supplementation appeared effective only when given during the specific critical neural tube fetal developmental period. Some experimental data were available from two human studies (one British, one Chinese). Both provided credible evidence that folic acid supplementation in the periconceptional period significantly reduced the occurrence of NTD in women with previous NTD deliveries (the British study) and those without such a history (the Chinese study). Although a 1996 (15) critique pointed to shortcomings in these experiments, newer, randomized double-blind supplement studies of folic acid alone are unlikely to be done because of ethical considerations (13). Nonetheless, evidence supporting biological plausibility for folate and NTDs (15) has continued to mount (16). Also, positive outcomes in the wake of folate fortification have been substantial. These include evidence for a reduction in the US prevalence of folate deficiencies (17,18) and a substantial reduction in NTDs (19).

Study Designs to Study Causation

Like other scientific disciplines, epidemiology uses experimental designs to study causation. Here, the investigator randomly assigns individuals to treatment or no treatment (control group). General study designs (and relevant issues) for examining causation are discussed in detail in Chapters 2 and 9. Epidemiologic investigations also include designs with multiple study centers and extended follow-up, and designs that randomly assign groups rather than individuals to treatment or control status. In the case of multicentered studies with long-term follow-up, disease outcomes are compared for each randomization group controlled for center-specific effects. In the case of studies that randomly assign groups, disease outcomes are compared for each group rather than for each individual.

ISSUES IN ANALYTIC NUTRITION EPIDEMIOLOGIC STUDIES

Issues relevant to any analytic nutrition epidemiology study design include the analytic question, the choice of diet and/or nutrient exposures, problems resulting from poor exposure measurements, potential for other biases, and potential for confounding and multivariate relationships between diet and disease.

The Analytic Nutrition Epidemiology Question

From an epidemiologic perspective, diet and nutrition can be viewed as key factors potentially influencing health and disease or as a specific health/disease outcome. Nutrition studies often examine diet/nutrition as an outcome and analyze data for determinants of those outcomes. In epidemiologic studies, diet and nutrition are commonly studied as independent contributing factors (association) or independent etiologic factors (causation) of health/disease outcomes.

Diet and/or Nutrient Exposure

The term *exposure* refers to a factor's dose (ie, amount and concentration along with duration of that exposure). To determine exposure, a method of measurement is needed that will sufficiently capture differences that truly exist (1). The method needs to capture measurements of potential active agents and their doses. Dietary exposure measurements are challenging and have been an active area of research for more than four decades. Investigations of food safety problems can use food information from one point in time. Investigations of chronic diseases, which are major causes of debilitation and death, require diet and/or nutrient exposures that capture an extended period of intake behavior. The term *usual intake* is often used to connote this type of diet exposure. "Usual" intake is difficult to capture in the heterogeneous US population, given its rapidly changing food marketplace and Americans' enthusiasm for food choice change. Given existing measurement problems, investigators are encouraged to include more than one dietary assessment method and/or use other related measures of exposure, such as biological (eg, blood or urine) or molecular (eg, genetic) markers (20). Newer approaches are being developed and studied. Various aspects of measurement methods for diet and/or nutrient exposures are discussed in Chapter 6.

The exposure measurement is meant to provide a reliable, accurate, and valid measurement of diet and/or nutrient exposure. Reliability is the characteristic in which repeated measurements done in a steady-state period yield similar results. Accuracy indicates that systematic error is minimized in the measurement (21). Validity is the degree to which a test is capable of measuring what it is intended to measure (21). None of these qualities can be corrected by increased sample size. To increase confidence in the reliability of the test, each subject can be tested at least twice (5). Random error may be mitigated through careful measurement and large sample size. However, even then, random error cannot be completely eliminated and may be due to individual biological variation, residual sampling or measurement error (21).

Other diet and/or nutrient exposure considerations are important to the study design. Evidence for sufficient variation in the diet or nutrient intake is needed. If everyone ate the same way, no outcome differences with diet would be detected (1). The latency period between diet exposure and disease is important. A negative result from a 5-year cohort study might be due to a latency period of 10 years or longer between diet exposure and disease outcome. Also, there may be a critical exposure period for a particular diet-disease relationship. For example, the critical period may be in childhood, with the disease manifesting itself in adulthood (3). Finally, the effects of diet and/or nutrient exposure may be acute and transient rather than long-term. For example, a double-blind placebo-controlled study found a significant lowering of blood pressure in the group supplemented with potassium compared with the placebo group after 6 weeks, but no blood pressure differences were found at 12 weeks (22).

Choice of Nutrition Exposure Variable(s)

Nutrition can be represented as a single food or nutrient, components of these (eg, bioactive food element or active nutrient metabolite), groups of foods or nutrient classes, combinations of these groupings (either investigator determined or derived with statistical grouping methods), a score or scores based on specific criteria, or a marker that indicates that a particular critical diet/nutrient threshold has been met (ie, a biomarker). The decision of which exposure variable to investigate is pivotal because this choice can largely determine whether any true effect can be detected (23).

Diet assessments are important but problematic because they can be complex, difficult, and imperfect. However, standardized collection methodology, research quality food-nutrient databases, standardized coding and data processing mitigate some of these problems. Additionally, ongoing biometric advances have generated methods for performing adjustments to facilitate estimation of diet influences (24–28).

Brief diet assessment methods, such as the food frequency questionnaire (FFQ), enjoy wide usage in epidemiologic studies because they minimize collection expense and participant burden and many are formatted for automated scanners. However, FFQs have intrinsic challenges (29,30). Several FFQs have been constructed and are in use (30). The FFQ's fit to the population to be studied is essential. For example, if that population includes an important subgroup that has unique food choice behaviors, the question of whether and how much to tailor the FFQ is important. Also important is whether the tailored FFQ should be validated. Pilot data are important to answer these questions. Companion calibration studies are recommended for studies using FFQs (29). The calibration studies collect detailed dietary intake information from a subgroup to adjust FFQ intake estimates. Alternatively or in addition, blood markers of nutrient intakes and biomarkers related to nutrient intakes are recommended (6,31). Finally, improvements in collected dietary data have been achieved through training and cognitive insights developed from research in these areas (32).

Regardless of the method used to generate diet/nutrition data, the underlying problem is that the role of diet/nutrition in particular disease outcomes is still under study as are mechanisms for disease outcomes themselves. Illustrative of this are supplement studies of single nutrients with strong evidence from observational studies and with well-defined mechanisms. Surprisingly, the supplemented nutrients have not consistently shown predicted protective action with their associated disease processes. For example, in a large beta carotene supplement study of smokers, the supplemented group had a greater risk of developing lung cancer than the control group (33). In another large study, increased dietary fiber intakes did not reduce the risk of recurring adenomatous colon polyps, a precursor lesion to colon cancer (34). Some researchers have suggested that the nutrients or food components investigated in these studies were not the active players or had minor roles compared to others that were not studied. For example, recent analyses suggest that risk of colon cancer may be more strongly associated with folate intake than with fiber intake (35). Alternatively, the nutrient or food component that was analyzed could be part of a group that in concert represents the "active" unit. In the case of the dietary fiber study, recent analyses from the aforementioned study have identified dried beans as the potential "active" unit (36). Another possibility is that the tested nutrient or food component is effective only in a subgroup. For example, in one report, the protective effect of dietary fiber on colon cancer risk was seen only in men (37).

Interest in the technique of diet patterning has reemerged (38) with positive findings from diet pattern trials such as those testing the Mediterranean Diet and the Dietary Approaches to Stop Hypertension (DASH) pattern.

The patterns approach, therefore, may have an increased likelihood of capturing "active" diet/nutrition elements. The concept behind diet patterning is that empirically derived, objective, distinct food choices can be discerned with statistical techniques (39). The method attempts to examine the effect of the diet as a whole rather than to examine the effect of a particular food/nutrient or food/nutrient component. Techniques such as factor analysis, principal components, and cluster analyses have been used for this purpose. The approach is appealing given the background of failed trials of single nutrients and diet components; the multiplicity of foods and/or nutrients associated with a single disease entity; and the variety of foods consumed by subjects with low or high disease risk. Finally, proponents of these patterning methods suggest a future where healthful eating patterns may be derived through use of these techniques (40). Patterns reports to date, however, have received mixed reviews. Some critics argue that these studies have not generated any new hypotheses (41) but rather identify patterns very similar to ones that might be constructed from general healthful eating advice. Other researchers suggest that the approach may be more productive than more traditional methods (40). Because renewed diet patterning efforts are relatively recent, future advances in application of these techniques may provide additional insights.

Problems Resulting from Poor Exposure Measurements

In analytic epidemiology studies, poor measures in both comparison groups make it impossible to detect existing associations. Poor measures in one of the groups can lead to findings of an association where none exists or association in the opposite direction (20). Diet and disease studies have inherent problems. Because of the limited range of variation in the diet within most populations, in combination with the inevitable error in measuring intake, very modest relative risks (0.5 to 2.0) are usually found for diet effects. Because dietary intakes are an obligatory human behavior (ie, everyone eats), even small risks associated with diet should be important (3). If risks were large, less precise exposure measures would capture those differences. However, smaller risks would require more refined exposure measures. Willett (3) notes that typical dietary intake differences between cases and controls is only about 5%, and even a systematic error of 3% to 4% would seriously distort such a relationship. Furthermore, measurement errors would dilute or conceal any

effect of diet on health/disease outcomes in experimental studies.

Potential for Other Biases

Systematic errors are also possible in epidemiologic studies through selection bias, other measurement bias, and analytic bias. Systematic errors are errors that occur regularly, are in the same direction, and are reproducible. Methodological sources of bias can obscure an existing relationship (3). Selection bias occurs when there is a systematic difference between the characteristics of people chosen for the study and people who are not chosen. For example, having some diseases may reduce a person's chance of being selected for a study (15). Several other subject selection biases are possible. The healthy-workers bias can be encountered in occupational epidemiology studies, where workers are likely to be healthier than people not working. There may be an increased likelihood of healthier and/or health-conscious and motivated individuals agreeing to participate in studies (volunteers' bias). An incidence-prevalence bias (Neyman's bias [3]) can also occur. This bias occurs where there is a loss of cases (by death or recovery) due to significant periods of time between exposure and development of the disorder. Finally, spurious differences between exposure and the disease can be due to differential hospitalization of cases and those without the disease with the exposure (Berkson's bias [3]).

Measurement bias occurs when individual measurements or classifications of disease or exposure are inaccurate. Measurement bias that occurs equally in the groups being compared (nondifferential bias) almost always results in an underestimate of the true strength of the relationship (15). Recall bias can occur when the subject is aware of the study hypothesis. An information bias can occur where different quality and/or extent of information is obtained from exposed versus nonexposed subjects (1). A related problem is the Hawthorne effect (5), where the subject's performance changes because he or she is being studied. Measurement implementation problems can also occur (eg, quality control bias and nonstandardized measurement bias) (5). Blinding (where subjects and research staff are unaware of whether subjects are assigned to the treatment or the control group) is used in experimental studies to obviate subject measurement bias. Because knowledge about exposure status may bias assessment, outcome assessors may also be blinded to subject assignments or exposure status (1).

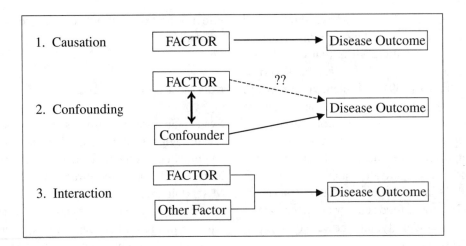

FIGURE 8.2   Comparison of predictive values.

Bias may also be encountered in the analysis phase. Unintentional bias may occur in the data analyses and in interpretations of study findings if the investigators have strong study preconceptions (1).

Potential for Confounding

As illustrated in Figure 8.2, confounding relationships are relationships where the factor of interest is related to another factor that is also influencing the outcome of interest. With confounding, the association can be explained by another factor associated with both the exposure and the disease (20). Confounding is not strictly a type of bias because it does not result from systematic error in research design (21). Confounding occurs when a nonrandom distribution of risk factors in the source population also occurs in the study population. For example, smoking can confound a relationship between coffee drinking and a disease outcome because people who drink coffee are also more likely to smoke (1). Confounders can obscure or exaggerate existing associations (5). Another possibility is that an unmeasured third variable was related to the exposure and disease in an opposite direction, resulting in negative confounding (3).

The inability to control for confounding is a major limitation of descriptive epidemiologic studies. Analytic studies can be designed to consider potential confounding factors when testing associations or causal relationships between key factors and disease outcomes. Analytic studies accomplish this goal through design features (eg, randomization, restriction, and matching) and analysis strategies (eg, stratification and statistical modeling). In experimental studies, randomization can be used to randomly distribute confounders to treatment and control groups. Restriction limits the study to people who have particular characteristics. Matching used in case-control studies selects controls to match cases by potential confounding factors to ensure that confounders are evenly distributed in the two groups being compared (21).

Potential for an Effect Modifier

An effect modifier (ie, an interaction) is a third variable that alters the association between an exposure and a disease outcome (refer to Figure 8.2) (42). With effect modification, the exposure may not have the same effect in all settings or subgroups of the population (20). For example, diet studies often separate gender and age groups because diet may have a different effect on a particular outcome for these subgroups. Gender and age, in these cases, are considered effect modifiers. Another effect modifier may be genetic factors. A design strategy would be to randomly assign subjects to ensure that groups are balanced or to match controls on effect modifier variables (5). In large studies control for confounding is usually done in the analytic phase. Stratified analyses are performed where relationships of interest are examined in well-defined and homogeneous categories (strata) of the confounding variable (21). Diet and/or nutrition variables can also be effect modifiers. For example, drug treatment of a disease might be enhanced or diminished as the result of diet or nutrition. A study discussing folate, alcohol, and breast cancer presented later in this chapter shows diet as an effect modifier.

EXAMPLE. The following study examines a potential interaction between smoking and serum carotenoids in relation to diabetes. A subset (4,493) of subjects from the Coronary Artery Risk Development in Young Adults (CARDIA) study (43) was examined. CARDIA was a large (*n* = 5,115), 15-year, multicenter, prospective, epidemiologic study of black and white young adults that examined the development of cardiovascular disease risk. The analysis subset had baseline data on smoking status, serum carotenoids, plasma glucose, and known confounding factors; had completed follow-up surveys; and did not have diabetes at baseline. During the 15 years of follow-up, 8 were diagnosed with diabetes. After adjusting for race, sex, study center, age, education, systolic blood pressure, ethanol intake, energy intake, energy expenditure, vitamin supplement use, and serum lipid levels, researchers found that serum carotenoid levels were significantly inversely related to diabetes incidence, but only in nonsmokers.

Multivariate Relationship of Diet and Disease

Willett (3) cautions that diet and disease relationships are likely to be "extremely complex for both biologic and behavioral reasons." Food and nutrients are biologically complex. Nutrients are largely provided by foods, and foods typically contain a variety of nutrients. Not surprisingly, specific nutrients tend to be intercorrelated. There are nutrient-to-nutrient interactions where the effect of one nutrient depends on the level of another. What we eat and the quantity eaten are also related to other health-related, nondiet factors such as age, gender, occupation, and behaviors (eg, smoking and exercise). All these can distort, modify, or confound relationships of diet and disease.

Multivariate methods are needed to tease out and clarify the effect of diet and nutrition on outcomes. Nonetheless, these effects can be complicated. Willett (3) points to the example of the effect of obesity on cardiovascular disease. When obesity is examined in a multivariate model that includes serum lipids, blood pressure, glucose tolerance, and body fat, the effect of obesity on cardiovascular disease is diminished because obesity is likely to be also acting through the other factors. In other words, because of inherent data problems, multivariate methods are not foolproof in discerning diet/nutrient effects. Rather, new study designs and future developments are needed.

ANALYTIC EPIDEMIOLOGIC STUDY DESIGNS

Observational Study Designs for Examining Associations: Cross-Sectional Studies

Cross-sectional epidemiologic studies, also called *prevalence studies* or *surveys* (44), are those where subjects are measured at approximately the same point in time. Both the exposure to a particular risk factor and disease outcome (case status) are determined at the same time (1,5). Although generally used for descriptive studies, they can also provide suggestive analytic information. Cross-sectional study data are commonly used to provide evidence for possible risk factors for disease outcomes (1).

Advantages and Disadvantages of Cross-Sectional Studies

The key advantage of cross-sectional studies is that they are relatively simple and inexpensive because neither follow-up measures nor treatment are required (5).

However, because of several inherent problems, cross-sectional studies are of limited utility in studying causal inference (44). Because measurements are made only at one point, the temporal relationship between exposure and disease outcomes cannot be tested (1). The problem of reverse causality bias can occur (44) where the disease outcome appears to precede the exposure in time (44). Furthermore, cross-sectional studies are likely to include survivors and new cases (1), with early disease-related deaths missed.

Cross-Sectional Study Implementation Issues

Key challenges in implementing cross-sectional studies include the ability to ensure and verify reasonable sample representativeness (3), the ability to capture "cases" (those with the disease outcome of interest) (1), and the ability to capture adequate variation in key exposure variables (4). Several analytic cautions are needed in examining cross-sectional data. Associations found may be related to survival rather than to disease development (1). Furthermore, because early disease-related deaths would result in lost "cases," there would be a reduced ability to find significant relationships between exposure and disease outcome.

Types of Findings in Cross-Sectional Studies

Associations between exposures or risk factors and disease outcomes can be suggested. In such studies, individuals with and without the disease can be examined in relation to exposures, other potential risk factors, or both. Cross-sectional studies identify factors that may affect the level of a risk factor (6). The NHANES series are examples of cross-sectional studies.

EXAMPLE.   Cross-sectional studies can also be multi-centered. The International Study of Salt and Blood Pressure (INTERSALT), conducted in 52 population samples worldwide, tested whether salt intake (as assessed by urinary sodium levels) was associated with higher blood pressure (45). INTERSALT found a linear positive relationship between sodium and blood pressure regardless of whether the individual was normotensive or hypertensive. Also, it found that blood pressure increased with age in only those with higher salt intakes.

Suggestive evidence for the influence of other nutrients (eg, protein) on blood pressure led to the subsequent International Population Study on Macronutrients and Blood Pressure (INTERMAP). INTERMAP (46) was a population-based epidemiologic investigation in 20 diverse samples from four countries (Japan, China, the United Kingdom, and the United States) from men and women aged 40 to 59 years. Two sets of consecutive 2-day 24-hour recalls were collected for each participant and dietary supplement intake was recorded in detail from patient interviews and supplement labels. Also collected were 24-hour urine samples coinciding with day 2 of each recall pair. INTERMAP found that vegetable protein intakes were associated with lower blood pressures and animal protein intakes with higher blood pressures (47). Further, analyses have shown that lower education, which has frequently been associated with higher blood pressure, was also associated in INTERMAP with dietary intakes that typically lead to higher blood pressures (48).

Observational Study Designs for Examining Associations: Cohort Studies

Cohort studies track health information of individuals over a period of time (49). They focus on disease development (21) and allow the study of the natural history of disease (44). An important feature of the cohort design is its time perspective on exposures. Concurrent cohort designs assess exposures as they occur during the study, but this kind of study is the most expensive (1). Retrospective studies examine exposures backward in time, and prospective studies look forward in time for exposures. A combined approach determines past exposure and provides follow-up of future exposures (1). Cohort studies are feasible for the study of common diseases where the exposure to risk factor(s) results in a measurable disease outcome within a reasonable time following the exposure. For practical reasons, cohort studies are not suitable for diseases with long latency periods (eg, 20 years) or for rare diseases requiring extraordinarily large sample sizes (49).

Advantages and Disadvantages of Cohort Studies

Cohort studies offer several advantages. They can examine whether there is a temporal relationship between exposure and the disease. They can provide direct information on the temporal sequence of events (20) and can establish timing and directionality of events (5). Prospective cohort studies enable the measurement of diet before disease onset (3). Cohort studies are easier and may be less costly to conduct than experimental studies (5). Finally, cohort studies can evaluate many diseases and exposures simultaneously (49). Cohort study designs have several disadvantages. Although they are less complex and costly than experimental studies, cohort studies are nonetheless expensive, resource intensive, and difficult because they require the monitoring of large numbers of subjects over an extended period (49). Additionally, they are ill suited for studies with of disease conditions with long latency periods (41).

Cohort selection and recruitment is challenging, with the selection of a random sample for the cohort being particularly tricky (5). People who refuse to volunteer may have particular characteristics, and their nonparticipation may bias the results (6). It may be difficult to find "nonexposed" individuals if exposure is widespread. (5). Groups may differ at the beginning of the study (the problem of confounding) (44). Over the course of the study, subjects may change their behavior because they are being studied, or their exposure to the factor of interest may change (49). With long studies, subject nonresponse and loss to follow-up are likely problems (1). If the loss to follow-up is correlated with disease, risks associated with exposure will be diminished. If this loss is correlated with exposure, risk estimates will be biased (6).

Cohort Study Implementation Issues

Cohort studies are warranted when there is sufficient evidence that exposure leads to disease (clinical observations, case-control studies, and so on) and a relatively short interval between exposure and development of disease (1).

However, there may be disagreement regarding what constitutes strong evidence, and diseases of interest may have low rates of occurrence (1). To obviate problems with participant recall of exposures (49,50), retrospective studies are possible if there are appropriate and adequate past records (1). There are practical limits, however, because even common diseases such as heart disease require a cohort size in the thousands (3).

It is becoming increasingly common for large intervention studies to mount postintervention follow-up studies of participants after the main studies have been completed. Examples of these types of cohort studies include the Multiple Risk Factor Intervention trial, the Modification of Diet in Renal Disease study, and the Trials of Hypertension Prevention study. For example, 7 years after the completion of the Trials of Hypertension Prevention phase 1 study, Baltimore investigators (51) recontacted Baltimore participants and ascertained their hypertension status; measured their blood pressure, heights, and weights; and collected 24-hour urine samples for sodium and creatinine measurement. About 40% had developed hypertension. However, the investigators found that previous weight-loss and sodium-reduction participants had lower odds of developing hypertension compared with controls (odds ratio = 0.23 and 0.65). Approximately 19% of weight-loss participants and 22.4% of sodium-reduction participants had developed hypertension (51).

Among the analytic considerations in cohort studies, assessment of the disease outcome and the selection of the nonexposed comparison group are key. Because there may be changes over time in relevant criteria and methods of assessment, ensuring comparability of repeated measures is crucial (1). Key information on subjects lost to follow-up (eg, disease occurrence or death) is important to capture. Specific analyses are required to account for such losses.

Types of Findings in Cohort Studies

In cohort studies, exposed and nonexposed groups measured at baseline and followed over time are compared for disease incidence or deaths. Data are collected at two or more distinct time points (at baseline and in follow-up) (52). Subjects presumably are comparable from one period to the next (52). Data are compared between and among these periods (52), specifically for the incidence of disease (or new occurrence of the disease outcome) in those individuals exposed and not exposed to the risk factors of interest. Measurements generated express the proportion of the exposed who get the disease (or die) compared with those not exposed (1). These measurements can be in terms of relative risks, odds ratios, and attributable risk ratios (1). Cohort studies are usually prospective (ie, follow-up is forward in time) but can also be retrospective (ie, prior history is examined). The following example describes a prospective nutrition epidemiology study (53); (for an example of a retrospective nutrition epidemiology cohort study refer to the Vitamin and Lifestyle [VITAL] study [54]).

EXAMPLE. An example of a prospective cohort study is the Prostate, Lung, Colorectal, and Ovarian Cancer Screening trial (PLCO) (53). This cohort, recruited from 1993 to 2001 from 10 centers, was formed to study whether screening for those cancers would reduce their incidence and mortality. Enrollees were 55 to 74 years of age, had never had any of the four cancers, had no recent screenings, and were not undergoing treatment for other cancers except nonmelanoma skin cancer. They were randomly assigned to screening or usual medical care. Because only intervention subjects completed dietary assessments, this report examined whether dietary folate intakes and alcohol use had an association with incident breast cancers in women participants assigned to screening. Excluded from the analyses were subjects with incomplete or implausible dietary data. Analyses were done for 25,400 women, of whom 691 were subsequently diagnosed with breast cancer. Median follow-up time was 4.9 years.

In the PLCO cohort study, food folate intakes were not related to incident breast cancers. However, folate supplement use seemed to increase the risk of this cancer in these postmenopausal women. Similar to the findings from other studies, an increased risk with higher alcohol consumption was found in women with low food folate intakes. Investigators discussed biological plausibility of their folate supplement finding as well as possible study limitations that would require further studies to elucidate whether this finding holds up over time.

Observational Study Designs for Examining Associations: Case-Control Studies

Popular among epidemiologists examining diet and nutrition questions, the case-control design examines cases (individuals with disease) and controls (those without disease) for risk factor or prior exposure differences (1,5,49). Controls are matched with cases on characteristics correlated with possible disease causes. These characteristics are not independent causes but are involved in the pathway through which the possible causes of interest lead to disease. As compared with the cohort study, which starts with exposure, the case-control study starts with identification of diseased individuals. Case-control studies compare diseased and nondiseased individuals, whereas cohort studies examine exposed and nonexposed individuals. Case-control studies are well suited for studies of rare disorders and studies where the lag time between exposure and outcome is long (44).

Advantages and Disadvantages of Case-Control Studies

Case-control studies offer several advantages. They are relatively quick and inexpensive, and they require smaller sample sizes than cross-sectional or cohort studies. Because investigators can set the criteria for selecting controls, they can untangle potential confounding factors and interactions more precisely (1,49,50). Matching increases reliability and decreases the costs of study (50).

Case-control studies have a number of disadvantages. By design, case-control studies can investigate only one disease outcome (49). Information about relevant exposures may be problematic. There may be significant differences in quality of information with cases researched more thoroughly (49). Cases and controls are likely to have different recall of specific exposures and events relevant to the studied disease outcome (18). For example, illness can affect recall of diet (3). Reliance on records to determine exposure may be equally inadequate for exposure determination (49). Furthermore, because case-control studies do not involve a time sequence, it would not be possible to demonstrate temporal causality between specific exposures and disease outcomes (49).

Other disadvantages of case-control studies arise from their intrinsic complexity. The selection of cases and controls, although seemingly straightforward, is challenging. Case-control studies can suffer from bias error, given the problem of sampling of controls (49). The selection of controls is an ongoing area of methodological concern (44). Finding suitable control matches is especially difficult where multiple matching factors are required. Here the matching variable is related to the risk factor or disease under study but is not a true confounder or is so highly correlated with other matching variables as to be superfluous. Overmatching results in loss of efficiency and may also result in bias (49).

Another disadvantage is that specific complex analyses are required for case-control data. Data analysis for matched analyses is more complex to compute and understand. Furthermore, any variable used as a matching variable cannot be estimated (1,49). For example, if controls were matched on age and race, it would not be possible to examine the effect of age or race on the disease studied.

Case-Control Study Implementation Issues

The selection of cases and controls for case-control studies is a critical but complex issue. Given the problem of case misclassification, investigators need to specify how cases are identified or ascertained (1,50). Case selection should be based on a formulated, precise disease definition (49) with inclusion and exclusion criteria specified to increase the likelihood of exposure to the risk factor of interest (1,49). New (incident) cases are preferred because the risk factor being studied may be avoided by individuals who already have the condition (ie, existing cases). For example, diet changes may occur following diagnosis. Additionally, cases may be lost before or soon after being diagnosed, and cases found may reflect survival rather than sickness (1,49).

A reliable source for cases must be identified (49). Potential sources include hospitals, primary care practices, clinics, and health maintenance organizations. Disease-specific patient registries are an additional case source. However, case selection from a single source can be problematic. The patient population is likely to reflect referral patterns or other local factors and limit the ability to generalize study findings to other individuals with that disease. For example, cases from a hospital that is a tertiary care facility may be severely ill (1), whereas other individuals may be less ill or have less complicated illnesses.

Controls are defined as individuals who had an equal chance of exposure to a risk factor and had some potential for getting the disease but do not have the disease (49). Ideally, controls are similar to cases in all respects other than having the disease in question. Conceptually, controls are representative of people without the disease from the same population as the cases. Controls are selected to "match" specific characteristics of cases, such as age, race, gender, or socioeconomic status (1). The purpose of matching is to adjust for potential confounding. There may be many differences between cases and controls besides exposure. Matched characteristics are those that potentially influence the disease outcome and are also related to the exposure being studied. For example, age and gender are commonly used matching factors because they often influence disease status. Controls are selected to match case characteristics that are of concern. Matching, by direct control of confounders, may reduce the required sample size or would support the use of a shorter exposure period for a risk factor.

Ideally, the selection of controls would be a probability sample (ie, a random sample representative of the population). Recruitment can be resource intensive because only 60% to 70% of control eligibles are likely to complete study interviews (3). In practice, controls are recruited from various sources. Hospital controls and controls drawn from patient care lists are convenient, inexpensive, and presumably can provide comparable medical data. However, this source is not foolproof, given the likelihood of differential rates of hospitalization (Berkson's bias [3]) and potentially similar exposure to risk factors with different diseases (49)—for example, the use of antioxidant supplements for cardiovascular disease and cancer.

Community controls are recruited from the same population as cases. Sources include school rosters, selective service lists, and insurance company lists. Random-digit dialing is frequently used because the first three digits of telephone numbers generally match neighborhood boundaries. However, the random-sampling frame is difficult to obtain, and it is expensive and time-consuming (49). Whatever recruitment frame is used, volunteers tend to be health-conscious (3) and therefore are not actually representative of the population. A "best friend" control is usually similar in age and other demographic and social characteristics. Alternatively, spouses or siblings (genetic controls) are sometimes used.

Some studies use multiple controls per case. These controls can be all of the same type or different types (1). In general, the greater number of controls per case, the greater precision in estimates and tests (1). Power (one measure of precision) increases as the number of controls increases for a fixed number of cases (20). Nonetheless, precision improvements are small beyond a case-to-control ratio greater than 1:4. Controls of a different type may be used for specific analyses (1). For example, the investigator may use hospital controls to control for the effect of hospitalization while using neighborhood controls to control for social and/or environmental influences.

Alternate Case-Control Study Designs

Other approaches to the case-control design have been used, including the nested case-control study and the frequency matching approach. In the nested case-control study design, cases are identified from an ongoing cohort study, with controls drawn from that same study. Cases and controls, therefore, are identified from the same cohort (49). Baseline and follow-up data on exposures, risk factors, and disease status are collected from the cohort study. Cases are identified during the course of follow-up, and controls are selected from the cohort (1). This design combines the efficiencies and strengths of both the cohort and case-control designs. The Harvard studies (the Physicians' Health study, the Nurses' Health study, and the Health Professionals' Health study) and other cohort studies (eg, the Western Electric study and the Cardiovascular Health study) have used the nested case-control design with their cohorts.

Technically, frequency matching is not a case-control design. As such, it does not require the stringent analytic procedures of that type of design. This approach ensures that the control sample and the case sample have a similar makeup (49). Control matching is done so that the proportion with a certain characteristic is similar among cases and controls (group or frequency matching)—for example, women comprise 50% of both cases and controls (1). With this type of matching, controls are selected after all of the cases are identified (1).

Analytic Considerations in Case-Control Studies

The drawback to matching is that the matching factor's effect on the outcome cannot be estimated. For example, if marital status is a matching factor, distribution of marital status between cases and controls would be the same. Specific techniques for the analysis of case-control data are detailed in several texts on epidemiology methods. Schlesselman's text, listed in Further Reading at the end of this chapter, is the standard reference for case-control studies. The reader is referred to these for in-depth instructions in performing more advanced analyses beyond general odds ratios.

Types of Findings in Case-Control Studies

The case-control analysis generates an estimate of the odds ratio for having the disease with a specific exposure level or risk factor. Additionally, this type of analysis can provide an estimate of the attributable risk associated with the specific exposure level or risk factor (44).

An example of a case-control study with hospital cases and population-based controls (55) is presented next. Refer to Kelemen et al (56) for an example of a case-control study where both cases and controls are drawn from the population. Refer to Chasan-Taber et al for an example of a nested case-control study (57).

EXAMPLE. In a case-control study, investigators used an FFQ to examine a series of hospital cases with age-matched (within 5 years) and sex-matched controls randomly selected from residence rolls from the patients' town (population-based controls) (55). The cases were 239 patients with myocardial infarctions (MIs) who were admitted to six local hospitals. Controls were 282 individuals without a history of MI or angina. After controlling for age and energy intake, the highest quintile (compared with the lowest quintile) of *trans* fatty acid intakes was associated with a significantly higher risk of coronary heart disease (CHD) (odds ratio = 2.4; confidence interval = 1.4 to 4.2). This relationship was still significant after controlling for other CHD risk factors and other dietary variables, including other fats, dietary cholesterol, vitamins C and E, carotene, and fiber. Because the intakes of cases were assessed after the patients had been hospitalized, the authors assessed the possibility that the hospitalization and MI diagnosis influenced recall of the "usual" diet. The investigators excluded cases who reported that they had "high cholesterol" before their MI, those who had changed their intake of butter to margarine in the previous 10 years, and those who were on a "special diet."

Etiologic Study Designs for Examining Causation: Randomized Controlled Trials

The RCT is the most efficient design for investigating a causal relationship between a treatment and its effect and is considered the gold standard for testing the effectiveness of clinical and public health therapeutic and preventive measures (1). Its essential features are the planned allocation of subjects to treatment (ie, randomization) (49) and the experimenter-controlled level of exposure (5). Randomization is used to overcome selection bias and to ensure that confounders are equally distributed among groups. In other words, randomization's goal is to ensure that the observed difference at the study's end can be directly attributable to the study factor (44), that is, the experimental treatment. Other specific features of the

RCT are discussed in Chapter 9 and elsewhere in this monograph.

Etiologic Study Designs for Examining Causation: Group-Randomized Trials

Group-randomized trials are clinical trials that allocate identifiable groups, rather than individuals, to treatment or control conditions (49,50,58). More trials of this type are likely to be fielded as effective prevention strategies are identified through usual RCT methodology. In the 1980s, three well-designed community trials for heart disease prevention were conducted in the United States: the Minnesota Heart Health Trial, the Stanford Five-City Project, and the Pawtucket Heart Health Program. Each of these trials included a comprehensive intervention focusing on established risk factors and using state-of-the-art behavioral strategies (59). The risk factors included cigarette smoking, hypertension, and elevated serum cholesterol levels. In the early 1990s, physician practice–based RCTs for heart disease prevention were conducted (60,61). Neither the community trials (62) nor the physician practice–based trials (60,61) showed significant treatment effects. Building on that experience, substantial methodological research on group-randomized trials has accelerated (58) and continues to be pursued. Issues needing more study include special sampling, outcome measures, and statistical techniques that may be required for this type of study.

Advantages and Disadvantages of the Group-Randomized Trial

The group-randomized trial design allows the investigator to examine the effects of interventions that operate at the group level, where the physical or social environment is manipulated or cannot be delivered to individuals (58). For example, the physician practice–based trials previously mentioned tested the efficacy of heart disease prevention interventions delivered by randomly selected physician practice groups as compared with control practice groups. The group-randomized trial provides the opportunity to directly test the experimental treatment in its "natural" environment. Thus, group-randomized trials are more likely to provide key information on the generalizability of the intervention (ie, its external validity). External validity refers to the ability of the study's conclusions to be applicable to other people at other locations and at other times. They offer an experimental framework to test public health strategies.

Although group-randomized trials seem simple and straightforward, recent methodological work has uncovered serious pitfalls in carrying them out. Important among these pitfalls are design and analysis issues. Given its inherent statistical properties, the group-randomized trial requires a larger sample size, careful attention to potential subgroups and outcomes, and a sophisticated analysis plan. Because of these previously underappreciated complexities, studies with null findings are common. Additionally, there is a need for stronger interventions that can produce detectable significant effects. Pooled analysis of the three community-based trials previously mentioned found that results were still below expectations even when adequate power was available (62). Results below expectations were also found in subsequent group-randomized studies with strong design and analytic plans (eg, the Child and Adolescent Trial for Cardiovascular Health) (58,63).

Statistical Issues in Group-Randomized Trials

The specific statistical considerations for group-randomized trials are crucial. However, they are beyond the scope of this chapter. Instead, the reader is referred to Murray's seminal textbook (58) and the current literature in this area. Finally, although most research design and implementation would benefit from statistical advice, this type of input is a requirement for group-randomized trials because of the complexity and evolving nature of this method.

More research is needed to understand the best approaches to collecting outcome data that are likely to capture significant differences. Some investigators have suggested the use of end point data at the community level (indicators) rather than measurements at the expensive individual level. Another approach is the use of more frequent, small surveys of randomly selected samples of the population or subgroups rather than infrequent, large surveys to capture end point trends (58).

Rooney and Murray (64) found that stronger intervention effects were detectable in studies with greater methodological rigor. These studies were characterized by the use of appropriate group-randomized trial methods—that is, they were planned from the start to use the assignment unit for the analysis unit, they used a sufficient number of randomized assignment units for each condition, they adjusted for baseline differences in important confounding variables, they had extended follow-up, and

they limited drop out levels and loss to follow-up. Also, smaller identifiable groups for assignment units (eg, work sites, physician practices, schools, and churches) may be better for detecting intervention effects. This makes sense because it is likely to be more difficult to change the "health behavior and risk profile of an entire heterogeneous community rather than in smaller identifiable groups" (58).

EXAMPLE. The Child and Adolescent Trial for Cardiovascular Health (CATCH) was a multicentered group-randomized trial (63) conducted in four field sites (San Diego, Houston, New Orleans, and Minneapolis) over a 3-year period. Each site recruited 24 eligible schools with 56 of the 96 schools randomized to intervention. Half of these received school-based intervention alone and the other half received both a school-based intervention and a family intervention. The study's primary end points were individual serum cholesterol levels and, at the school level, amounts of fat and sodium in school lunches and time spent by students in vigorous physical activity. A baseline survey was completed of 60.4% of eligible third graders ($n \approx 5,000$ students) in the CATCH schools. Follow-up individual measures were done when these children completed the third, fourth, and fifth grades, with about 80% completing final measurements. School measurements for school lunches and physical activity were completed at the same intervals. CATCH found a significant improvement in school measurements and a nonsignificant improvement in individual serum cholesterol measurements. The intervention group with additional family intervention showed greater dietary knowledge but were otherwise similar to the other intervention group. The investigators suggested that the limited time and resources for the intervention resulted in a weaker-than-desirable effect (58,63).

Etiologic Study Designs for Examining Causation: Multicentered Randomized Controlled Trials

The essential and obvious difference between the standard single-center RCT and the multicentered RCT is the number of involved centers. The multicentered RCT offers the ability to study questions that would be impractical for a single-center RCT due to sample size or resource limitations and for which there is an adequate pool of interested and qualified investigators (65). The questions addressed by multicentered RCTs arise from observational, basic science and evidence from small clinical trials, especially if these data are inconclusive or conflicting and indicate the need for a larger and/or more diverse subject pool (65).

Advantages and Disadvantages of the Multicentered Randomized Controlled Trial

Multicentered RCTs have several advantages. They can efficiently examine questions that require a larger number of subjects and/or study groups or subgroups (eg, they can allow for minority inclusions, geographic spread, and rural/urban residence). They offer greater possibility for a more heterogeneous study population, thereby providing a broader basis for generalization of findings. Multiple centers are able to expedite the recruitment and follow-up of eligible subjects to meet trial requirements. Also, economies of scale are offered. Multicentered RCTs can afford central laboratory and reading centers, as well as dedicated resource centers for quality control, performance monitoring, and data analysis (eg, a data-coordinating center). Overall, these RCTs result in less cost per patient.

The multicentered RCT has several disadvantages. Multicentered RCTs require larger sample sizes than single-center RCTs, and the more heterogeneous sample that characterizes the multicentered RCT makes it is more difficult to detect treatment differences. Multicentered RCTs are administratively complex involving multiple principal investigators, a steering committee, a data-coordinating center, an external safety-monitoring board, and specific central laboratory and other measurement reading and coding centers. A complex organizational and communication structure is needed to link these components. (Web-based communications are now widely used to facilitate linkages.) These administrative complexities are cumbersome but essential.

Although less costly per subject, the overall cost of these studies is large, particularly for participant recruitment. Data publication may be slowed or facilitated depending on the particular study teams and oversight committees.

Other Multicentered Randomized Controlled Trial Implementation Issues

The RCT is collaborative and requires cooperative work, which is not easily accomplished when study personnel are located at various centers. It is necessary to maintain communications and decision-making structures because the study requires uniformity in study procedures. Performance of study methods and procedures requires supervision and documentation. Quality control requires standard application of measurements and intervention in multiple sites with many staff over several years.

Multicentered Randomized Controlled Trial Findings and Analyses Issues

In multicentered RCTs, issues of findings and analyses are similar to those of the single-centered RCT. The one exception is the likely need to adjust for center-specific effects in the analyses.

EXAMPLE.   The Trials of Hypertension Prevention (TOHP), a multicentered RCT, was comprised of ten geographically dispersed centers. It recruited 2,182 participants aged 35 years to 54 years with high-normal blood pressures (diastolic blood pressure of 80 mm Hg to 89 mm Hg). In TOHP phase 1, control subjects were compared with those on interventions. Interventions were 18 months of weight loss, sodium reduction, or stress reduction) or 6 months of nutrient supplements (potassium, calcium, magnesium, and fish oil). In the intervention groups, mean weight loss of 3.2 kg was associated with a significant decrease in blood pressure of 2.9 mm Hg diastolic and 2.4 mm Hg systolic, and a sodium reduction of 44 mmol was associated with a significant decrease of 2.1 mm Hg diastolic and 1.2 mm Hg systolic. Neither stress reduction nor supplement use was associated with significant short-term decreases in blood pressure reduction. TOHP Phase 2 tested sodium reduction and weight loss alone and in combination against a control group for their long-term effects on blood pressure (22,66).

CONCLUSION

Analytic nutrition epidemiology provides a framework and tools to test whether diet and/or nutrition make a statistically significant difference to health or disease outcomes. The tools provide tests for risk (association) and etiology (causation). Diet and/or nutrient exposure is a critical element in nutrition epidemiology studies, and considerable care is needed when choosing exposures for these studies. Analytic nutrition epidemiology studies consider health and disease outcomes from a multivariate perspective and examine potential risk factors such as diet and nutrition, taking into account potential confounding and effect modifiers.

Analytic nutrition epidemiology uses two general types of study design: observational and experimental. Observational studies include cross-sectional studies, cohort studies, and case-control studies. In experimental studies RCTs are considered the gold standard for etiologic investigations. Observational studies attempt to develop evidence for risk (association) of diet and nutrition on health or disease outcomes. Each type of design has its advantages and disadvantages. The choice of design should be based on the study question, the existing body of evidence relevant to the study question, and the available study resources.

REFERENCES

1. Gordis L. *Epidemiology*. Philadelphia, Pa: WB Saunders; 2004.

2. Merrill RM, Timmreck TC. *Introduction to Epidemiology*. 4th ed. Boston, Mass: Jones and Bartlett Publishers; 2006.

3. Willett W. Overview of nutritional epidemiology. In: *Nutritional Epidemiology*. 2nd ed. New York, NY: Oxford University Press; 1998:3–17.

4. Kelsey JL, Petitti DB, King AC. Key methodologic concepts and issues. In: Brownson RC, Petitti DB, eds. *Applied Epidemiology*. New York, NY: Oxford University Press; 1998:35–70.

5. Streiner DL, Norman GR. *PDQ Epidemiology*. 2nd ed. St. Louis, Mo: Mosby; 1996.

6. Freudenheim JL. A review of study designs and methods of dietary assessment in nutritional epidemiology of chronic disease. *J Nutr.* 1993;123:401–405.

7. Gerstman BB. Measures of association and potential impact. In: *Epidemiology Kept Simple: An Introduction to Traditional and Modern Epidemiology*. 2nd ed. Hoboken, NJ: Wiley-Liss; 2003:164–166.

8. Guallar E, Silbergeld EK, Navas-Acien A, Malhotra S, Astor BC, Sharrett AR, Schwartz BS. Confounding of the relation between homocysteine and peripheral arterial disease by lead, cadmium and renal function. *Am J Epidemiol.* 2006;163:700–708.

9. Grummer-Strawn LM, Mei Z. Centers for Disease Control and Prevention Pediatric Nutrition Surveillance System. Does breastfeeding protect against pediatric overweight? Analysis of longitudinal data from the Centers for Disease Control and Prevention Pediatric Nutrition Surveillance System. *Pediatrics.* 2004;113:81–86.

10. Potischman N, Weed DL. Causal criteria in nutritional epidemiology. *Am J Clin Nutr.* 1999;69 (suppl):S1309–S1314.

11. Committee on Diet and Health. Methodologic considerations in evaluating the evidence. In: Food and Nutrition Board, Commission on Life Sciences, National Research Council, eds. *Diet and Health: Implications for Reducing Chronic Disease Risk.* Washington, DC: National Academy Press; 1989:23–40.

12. Chobanian AV, Hill M. *Summary Report: The NHLBI Workshop on Sodium and Blood Pressure: A Critical Review of Current Scientific Evidence.* Bethesda, Md: National Institutes of Health, NHLBI; 1999.

13. Blaustein MP, Zhang J, Chen L, Hamilton BP. How does salt retention raise blood pressure? *Am J Physiol.* 2006;290:R514–R523.

14. Swift PA, Markandu ND, Sagnella GA, He FJ, MacGregor GA. Modest salt reduction reduces blood pressure and urine protein excretion in black hypertensives: a randomized control trial. *Hypertension.* 2005;46:308–312.

15. Rayburn WF, Stanley JR, Garrett E. Periconceptional folate intake and neural tube defects. *J Am Coll Nutr.* 1996;15:121–125.

16. Tamura T, Picciano MF. Folate and human reproduction. *Am J Clin Nutr.* 2006;83:993–1016.

17. Dietrich M, Brown CJ, Block G. The effect of folate fortification of cereal-grain products on blood folate status, dietary folate intake and dietary folate sources among adult non-supplement users in the United States. *J Am Coll Nutr.* 2005;24:266–274.

18. Pfeiffer CM, Caudill SP, Gunter EW, Osterloh J, Sampson EJ. Biochemical indicators of B vitamin status in the US population after folic acid fortification: results from the National Health and Nutrition Examination Survey 1999–2000. *Am J Clin Nutr.* 2005;82:442–450.

19. Honein MA, Paulozzi LJ, Mathews TJ, Erickson JD, Wong LY. Impact of folic acid fortification of the US food supply on the occurrence of neural tube defects. *JAMA.* 2001;285:2981–2986.

20. Brownson RC. Epidemiology: the foundation of public health. In: Brownson RC, Petitti DB, eds. *Applied Epidemiology*. New York, NY: Oxford University Press; 1998:3–34.

21. Beaglehole R, Bonita R, Kjellstrom T. *Basic Epidemiology*. Geneva, Switzerland: World Health Organization; 1993.

22. Whelton PK, Kumanyika SK, Cook NR, Cutler JA, Borhani NO, Hennekens CH, Kuller LH, Langford H, Jones DW, Satterfield S, Lasser NL, Cohen JD. Efficacy of nonpharmacologic interventions in adults with high-normal blood pressure: results from phase 1 of the Trials of Hypertension Prevention. The Trials of Hypertension Prevention Collaborative Research Group. *Am J Clin Nutr.* 1997;65(suppl): S652–S660.

23. Fraser GE. A search for truth in dietary epidemiology. *Am J Clin Nutr.* 2003;78(3 suppl):521S–525S.

24. Kaaks R, Ferrari P, Ciampi A, Pummer M, Riboli E. Uses and limitation of statistical accounting for random error correlations, in the validation of dietary questionnaire assessments. *Public Health Nutr.* 2002;5:969–976.

25. Freedman LS, Midthune D, Carroll RJ, Krebs-Smith S, Subar AF, Troiano RP, Dodd K, Schatzkin A, Bingham SA, Ferrari P, Kipnis V. Adjustments to improve the estimation of usual dietary intake distribution in the population. *J Nutr.* 2004;134: 1836–1843.

26. Subar AF, Dodd KW, Guenther PM, Kipnis V, Midthune D, McDowell M, Tooze JA, Freedman LS, Krebs-Smith SM. The food propensity questionnaire: concept, development and validation for use as a covariate in a model to estimate usual food intake. *J Am Diet Assoc.* 2006;106:1556–1563.

27. Tooze JA, Midthune D, Dodd KW, Freedman LS, Krebs-Smith SM, Subar AF, Guenther PM, Carroll RJ, Kipnis V. A new statistical method for estimating the usual intake of episodically consumed foods with application to their distribution. *J Am Diet Assoc.* 2006;106:1575–1587.

28. Kevin W, Dodd KW, Guenther PM, Freedman LS, Subar AF, Kipnis V, Midthune D, Tooze JA, Krebs-Smith SM. Statistical methods for estimating usual intake of nutrients and foods: a review of the theory. *J Am Diet Assoc.* 2006;106:1640–1650.

29. Kushi LH. Gaps in epidemiologic research methods: design considerations for studies that use food frequency questionnaire. *Am J Clin Nutr.* 1994;59 (1 suppl):180S–184S.

30. Subar AF, Thompson FE, Kipnis V, Midthune D, Nurwitz P, McNutt S, McIntosh A, Rosenfeld S. Comparative validation of the Block, Willett and National Cancer Institute food frequency questionnaires: the Eating at America's Table Study. *Am J Epidemiol.* 2001;154:1089–1099.

31. Bingham SA. Biomarkers in nutritional epidemiology. *Public Health Nutr.* 2002;5:821–827.

32. Thompson FE, Subar AF, Brown CC, Smith AF, Sharbaugh CO, Jobe JB, Mitti B, Gibson JT, Ziegler RG. Cognitive research enhances accuracy of food frequency questionnaire reports: results of an experimental validation study. *J Am Diet Assoc.* 2002;102: 212–225.

33. Omenn GS. Chemoprevention of lung cancer: the rise and demise of beta-carotene. *Ann Rev Public Health.* 1998;19:73–99.

34. Schatzkin A, Lanza E, Corle D, Lance P, Iber F, Caan B, Shike MK, Weissfeld J, Burt R, Cooper MR, Kikendall JW, Cahill J. Lack of effect of a low-fat, high-fiber diet on the recurrence of colorectal adenomas. Polyp Prevention Trial Study Group. *N Engl J Med.* 2000;342:1149–1150.

35. Bingham S. The fibre-folate debate in colo-rectal cancer. *Proc Nutr Soc.* 2006;65:19–23.

36. Lanza E, Hartman TJ, Albert PS, Shields R, Slattery M, Caan B, Iber F, Kikendal JW, Lance P, Daston C, Schatzkin A. High dry bean intake and reduced risk of advanced colorectal adenoma recurrence among participants in the poly prevention trial. *J Nutr.* 2006;136:1896–1903.

37. Jacobs ET, Lanza E, Alberts DS, Hsu CH, Jiang R, Schatzkin A, Thompson PA, Martinez ME. Fiber, sex, and colorectal adenoma: results of a pooled analysis. *Am J Clin Nutr.* 2006;83:343–349.

38. Hu F. Dietary pattern analysis: a new direction in nutritional epidemiology. *Curr Opin Lipidol.* 2002;13:3–9.

39. Newby PK, Tucker KL. Empirically derived eating patterns using factor or cluster analysis: a review. *Nutr Rev.* 2004;62:177–203.

40. Jacques PF, Tucker KL. Are dietary patterns useful for understanding the role of diet in chronic disease? *Am J Clin Nutr.* 2001;73:1–2.

41. Kant AK. Dietary patterns and health outcomes. *J Am Diet Assoc.* 2004;104:615–635.

42. Freudenheim JL. Study design and hypothesis testing: issues in the evaluation of evidence from research in nutritional epidemiology. *Am J Clin Nutr.* 1999;69(suppl):S1315–S1321.

43. Hozawa A, Jacobs DR Jr, Steffes MW, Gross MD, Steffen LM, Lee DH. Associations of serum carotenoid concentrations with the development of diabetes and insulin concentration: interaction with smoking. The Coronary Artery Risk Development in Young Adults (CARDIA) Study. *Am J Epidemiol.* 2006;163:929–937.

44. Gerstman BB. Types of epidemiologic studies In: *Epidemiology Kept Simple: An Introduction to Classic and Modern Epidemiology.* New York, NY: Wiley-Liss; 2003:173–178.

45. Stamler J. The INTERSALT Study: background, methods, findings, and implications. *Am J Clin Nutr.* 1997;65(suppl):S526–S642.

46. Stamler J, Elliott P, Dennis B, Dyer AR, Kesteloot H, Liu K, Ueshima H, Zhou BF, INTERMAP Research Group. INTERMAP: background, aims, design, methods, and descriptive statistics (non-dietary). *J Hum Hypertens.* 2003;17:591–608.

47. Elliott P, Stamler J, Dyer AR, Appel L, Dennis B, Kesteloot H, Ueshima H, Okayama A, Chan Q, Garside DB, Zhou B. Association between protein intake and blood pressure: the INTERMAP Study. *Arch Intern Med.* 2006;166:79–87.

48. Stamler J, Elliott P, Appel L, Chan Q, Buzzard M, Dennis B, Dyer AR, Elmer P, Greenland P, Jones D, Kesteloot H, Kuller L, Labarthe D, Liu K, Moag-Stahlberg A, Nichaman M, Okayama A, Okuda N, Robertson C, Rodriguez B, Stevens M, Ueshima H, Horn L Van, Zhou B. Higher blood pressure in middle-aged American adults with less education—role of multiple dietary factors: the INTERMAP study. *J Hum Hypertens.* 2003;17:655–775.

49. Woodward M. Fundamental issues. In: *Epidemiology: Study Design and Data Analysis.* Boca Raton, Fla: Chapman & Hall/CRC; 1999:1–30.

50. Friedman GD. *Primer of Epidemiology.* 4th ed. New York, NY: McGraw-Hill; 1994.

51. He J, Whelton PK, Appel LJ, Charleston J, Klag MJ. Long-term effects of weight loss and dietary sodium reduction on incidence of hypertension. *Hypertension.* 2000;35:544–549.

52. Sempos CT, Liu K, Ernst ND. Food and nutrient exposures: what to consider when evaluating epidemiologic evidence. *Am J Clin Nutr.* 1999;69 (suppl):S1330–S1339.

53. Stolzenberg-Solomon RZ, Chang S-C, Litzmann MF, Johnson KA, Johnson C, Buys SS, Hoover RN, Ziegler RG. Folate intake, alcohol use, and post-menopausal breast cancer risk in the Prostate, Lung, Colorectal, and Ovarian Cancer Screening Trial (PLCO). *Am J Clin Nutr.* 2006;83:895–904.

54. Gonzalez AJ, White E, Kristal A, Littman AJ. Calcium intake and 10-year weight change in middle-aged adults. *J Am Diet Assoc.* 2006;106: 1066–1073.

55. Ascherio A, Hennekens CH, Buring JE, Master C, Stampfer MJ, Willett WC. Trans fatty acids intake and risk of myocardial infarction. *Circulation.* 1994;89:94–101.

56. Kelemen LE, Cerhan JR, Lim U, Davis S, Cozen W, Schenk M, Colt J, Hartge P, Ward MH. Vegetables, fruit and antioxidant-related nutrients and risk of non-Hodgkin's lymphoma: a National Cancer Institute-Surveillance, Epidemiology, and End Results population-based case-control study. *Am J Clin Nutr.* 2006;83:1401–1410.

57. Chasan-Taber L, Selhub J, Rosenberg IH, Malinow MR, Terry P, Tishler PV, Willett W, Hennekens CH, Stampfer MJ. A prospective study of folate and vitamin B6 and risk of myocardial infarction in US physicians. *J Am Coll Nutr.* 1996;15:136–143.

58. Murray DM. *Design and Analysis of Group-Randomized Trials.* New York, NY: Oxford University Press; 1998.

59. Shea S, Basch CE. A review of five major community-based cardiovascular disease prevention programs. Part I. Rationale, design, and theoretical framework. *Am J Health Promot.* 1990;4:203–213.

60. Caggiula AW, Watson JE, Kuller LH, Olson MB, Milas NC, Berry M, Germanowski J. Cholesterol-lowering intervention program. Effect of the step I diet in community office practices. *Arch Intern Med.* 1996;156:1205–1213.

61. Keyserling TC, Ammerman AS, Davis CE, Mok MC, Garrett J, Simpson R Jr. A randomized controlled trial of a physician-directed treatment program for low-income patients with high blood cholesterol: the Southeast Cholesterol Project. *Arch Fam Med.* 1997;6:135–145.

62. Winkleby MA, Feldman HA, Murray DM. Joint analysis of three US community intervention trials for reduction of cardiovascular disease risk. *J Clin Epidemiol.* 1997;50:645–658.

63. Luepker RV, Perry CL, McKinlay SM, Nader PR, Parcel GS, Stone EJ, Webber LS, Elder JP, Feldman HA, Johnson CC. Outcomes of a field trial to improve children's dietary patterns and physical activity: The Child and Adolescent Trial for Cardiovascular Health (CATCH). *JAMA.* 1996;275:768–776.

64. Rooney BL, Murray DM. A meta-analysis of smoking prevention programs after adjustment for errors in the unit of analysis. *Health Educ Q.* 1996;23:48–64.

65. Meinert CL, Tonascia S. *Clinical Trials: Design, Conduct, and Analysis.* New York, NY: Oxford University Press; 1986.

66. The Trials of Hypertension Prevention Collaborative Research Group. Effects of weight loss and sodium reduction intervention on blood pressure and hypertension incidence in overweight people with high-normal blood pressure. The Trials of Hypertension Prevention, phase II. *Arch Intern Med.* 1997;157: 657–667.

FURTHER READING

Heber D, ed. *Nutritional Oncology.* Boston, Mass: Elsevier-Academic Press; 2006.

Kelemen LE. Nutrition epidemiology. In: Talley NJ, Locke GR III, Saito YA, eds. *GI Epidemiology.* London, England: Blackwell Publishing; 2007.

Schlesselman JJ. *Case-Control Studies: Design, Conduct, Analysis.* New York, NY: Oxford University Press; 1982.

Weaver CM, Heaney RP, eds. *Calcium in Human Health.* Totowa, NJ: Humana Press; 2006.

9

Designing, Managing, and Conducting a Clinical Nutrition Study

Amy E. Griel, PhD, Tricia L. Psota, BS, and Penny M. Kris-Etherton, PhD, RD

Clinical nutrition research is an overarching term that encompasses research conducted with human participants using many different experimental designs, participant populations, and methods, including the delivery of the treatment diet(s). The central focus of controlled clinical nutrition studies is to evaluate the effects of a dietary modification on one or more end point(s).

Clinical nutrition studies have provided crucial evidence that serves as the basis for dietary guidance issued for health promotion and disease prevention, as well as the treatment and management of a wide variety of clinical conditions. In addition, findings from clinical nutrition studies have been central to defining nutrient requirements that are the basis for Dietary Reference Intakes (DRIs) issued by the National Academy of Science. Thus, the ongoing process of revising dietary recommendations depends on high-quality clinical nutrition research studies. An exciting new frontier in clinical nutrition research is the elucidation of the effects of bioactive compounds and foods on a multitude of established and emerging biomarkers of health and disease. The underlying impetus is to develop dietary guidance that advances our ability to promote health and well-being and to build upon current medical nutrition therapy guidelines for the treatment and prevention of disease.

The study design, subject population, and methods to employ in clinical nutrition research are determined by the research question(s) to be addressed. Studies can vary from small (small-scale clinical studies with just a few participants) to large clinical trials involving thousands of participants and multiple research sites. Clinical nutrition studies also vary by length of study time, and they range from acute (hours to days) to longer term (weeks to months) to studies that span years. The participant population may target specific population groups, such as children or the elderly; focus on specific disease states, such as hypertension or inflammatory bowel disease; or be representative of the population at large. The diet(s) used in clinical nutrition research studies are inherently variable because of the vast array of dietary factors that can be evaluated, including single nutrients/bioactive components, multiple nutrients/ bioactive components, single and multiple foods/food groups/beverages, and dietary patterns.

This chapter presents a basic overview and guidelines for the conduct of clinical nutrition research and describes the important factors that must be considered and implemented to appropriately answer the experimental question(s). For more comprehensive information about the design and conduct of clinical nutrition research, refer to the resources listed in Box 9.1. See Box 9.2 for a summary of a study protocol for a controlled clinical nutrition study.

IDENTIFYING IMPORTANT CLINICAL RESEARCH NEEDS

Many resources provide information about important and timely clinical nutrition research needs. Some provide information about research topics of interest, and others are

BOX 9.1   Resources for Conducting Clinical Nutrition Research Studies

- Dennis BH EA, Obarzanek E, Clevidence BA, eds. *Well-Controlled Diet Studies in Humans: A Practical Guide to Design and Management.* Chicago, Ill: American Dietetic Association; 1999.
- Kay CD, Kris-Etherton PM, Psota TL, Bagshaw DM, West SG. Clinical nutrition studies: maximizing opportunities and managing the challenges. In: *Berdanier's Handbook of Nutrition and Food Science.* Boca Raton, Fla: CRC Press (in review).
- Carey VJ, Bishop L, Charleston J, Conlin P, Erlinger T, Laranjo N, McCarron P, Miller E, Rosner B, Swain J, Sacks FM, Appel LJ. Rationale and design of the Optimal Macro-Nutrient Intake Heart Trial to Prevent Heart Disease (OMNI-Heart). *Clin Trials.* 2005;2:529–537.
- Allison DB, Gadde K, Ryan D, Pi-Sunyer FX. *Design, Analysis, and Interpretation of Randomized Clinical Trials in Obesity* (video proceedings of a National Institutes of Health–funded conference held in Newark, NJ, December 2006). Available at: http://main.uab.edu/shrp/default.aspx?pid=97738.

BOX 9.2   Protocol for a Controlled Clinical Nutrition Study

Study Preparation
- Justification of the study
- Defined protocol
- Hypotheses/Objectives
- Resources

Subjects
- Inclusion and exclusion criteria
- Recruitment
- Screening procedures

Diet
- Precisely defined diet, menu(s), and feeding protocol

Methods
- Study design
- Randomization
- Monitoring, compliance, retention, termination
- Measurements, methods

Statistics/Data
- Sample size calculations
- Data variables
- Data collection
- Error and bias
- Analyses

agencies that fund clinical nutrition research. Examples of resources that identify research needs include workshop proceedings and task force reports, such as the *Third Report on Nutrition Monitoring in the United States* (1), publications from the National Academies (2–5), and *Healthy People 2010* (6); position papers from the American Dietetic Association (ADA); science advisories/statements from the American Heart Association and the American Diabetes Association; and publications from the Centers for Disease Control. In addition, the ADA Evidence Analysis Library provides summaries (for ADA members) of the best available research on many dietetics and nutrition topics. Clinical nutrition research questions also can be identified via the Food and Drug Administration (FDA) Web site. Specifically, petitions for health claims that have been filed can help identify timely issues.

The Agency for Healthcare Research and Quality is another valuable resource to use for identifying clinical nutrition research needs on timely topics. The National

Institutes of Health *Guide for Grants and Contracts,* published weekly and available on-line, identifies research topics of interest and funding opportunities. Similar information is available from the US Department of Agriculture. The Community of Science is a comprehensive funding resource, which sends weekly e-mails to registered researchers regarding funding opportunities in their field.

In an effort to reduce the selective reporting of results from clinical research trials, the International Committee of Medical Journal Editors has created a policy that any study submitted for publication must be registered as a clinical trial in the public registry (7). This registry informs researchers about clinical nutrition studies that are being conducted or those that have been completed and may not be published. Because it is sometimes difficult to publish papers that show no effect, this registry will be a useful resource to researchers in identifying research questions that merit studying. See Chapter 31 for more details on this registry.

STUDY HYPOTHESES AND OBJECTIVES

Hypothesis-driven research is a foundation of clinical nutrition research. It is always linked to specific objectives that robustly test the study hypothesis (or hypotheses). The objectives of a clinical nutrition trial generally are presented quantitatively so specific end points can be measured precisely. Hypotheses are designed to evaluate the effect of the test diet intervention(s) on some number of end points. This can be done in one or more population groups. Thus, the hypotheses determine the experimental design, methods to be implemented, and subsequent statistical analyses. Statistical tests are performed on the null hypothesis (that no association or difference exists). Examples of hypotheses and null statements are shown in Table 9.1.

Many clinical nutrition studies test primary and secondary hypotheses. The primary hypotheses are the most important to the researchers and involve the outcome variables for which the study has been powered. Secondary hypotheses can answer questions related to the primary hypotheses. These additional questions may provide information about mechanisms of action, as well as information about the effects of the diet intervention(s) on any number of other end points, all of which could generate valuable scientific information and possibly a novel discovery.

When defining the hypotheses and objectives of a clinical nutrition study, it is important to determine whether the expected response to the test diet will be evaluated in a very controlled setting or a free-living setting. The distinction will shape the study design. Using a controlled study design, the *efficacy* of the treatment can be evaluated (ie, the maximum response achievable for the treatment given under tightly controlled conditions). The *effectiveness* can be evaluated using a free-living study design (ie, the response observed to an experimental design that mimics what can be implemented in a real-world setting).

If there is little evidence in the literature about the expected response to a specific level (dose) of nutrient/dietary constituent, dose-response studies are a prerequisite to the implementation of a larger clinical nutrition study. Not only is dose important, but the timeline of end point collection has to be established. For example, it is conceivable that the response could be missed because samples were not collected on an appropriate timeline.

STUDY DESIGN

When designing a clinical nutrition study, researchers must consider the scope of the study, the time needed to detect a meaningful result, the level of intensity or dietary control required, and the demands that are placed on the participants enrolled in the study. The randomized controlled trial (RCT) study design is considered the "gold standard" for clinical nutrition research. RCTs employ a comparative design that involves an intervention with one or more treatments; each participant is assigned to a group based on a formal randomization procedure (8).

Within any RCT, the length of the treatment period must be sufficient to adequately test the treatment effects.

TABLE 9.1   Examples of Hypotheses and Null Statements

	Hypothesis	**Null Statement**
Single nutrient example	*Trans* fatty acids increase the TC:HDL-C ratio vs saturated fatty acids.	*Trans* fatty acids do not increase the TC:HDL-C ratio more than saturated fatty acids.
Bioactive compound example	Plant stanol/sterol esters decrease absorption of fat-soluble vitamins.	Plant stanol/sterol esters do not decrease absorption of fat-soluble vitamins.
Specific food and nutrient profile example	A diet high in α-linolenic acid from walnuts decreases inflammatory status as measured by CRP level.	A diet high in α-linolenic acid from walnuts does not decrease inflammatory status as measured by CRP level.
Multiple nutrient manipulation example	Replacing dietary carbohydrate with dietary protein decreases plasma triglycerides.	Replacing dietary carbohydrate with dietary protein does not decrease plasma triglycerides.
Dietary pattern example	A diet that meets the food-based recommendations of the US Dietary Guidelines, 2005, significantly decreases blood pressure and LDL-C in individuals with stage 1 hypertension and hypercholesterolemia.	A diet that meets the food-based recommendations of the US Dietary Guidelines, 2005, does not decrease blood pressure and LDL-C in individuals with stage 1 hypertension and hypercholesterolemia.

Abbreviations: CRP, C-reactive protein; HDL-C, high-density lipoprotein cholesterol; LDL-C, low-density lipoprotein cholesterol; TC, total cholesterol.

For example, it is well established that serum lipids stabilize following 3 weeks of a particular dietary intervention. Consequently, in this situation, each diet period should be at least 3 weeks, and preferably 4 or more to ensure that the end point measurements are accurate. It may be necessary to conduct a pilot study to determine the length of the treatment period needed to ensure that the response has stabilized. Another determinant of the duration of the clinical study is the number of diets studied. Thus, the time required to see a treatment effect, the number of diets studied, and the length of the washout periods or breaks between treatments are factors that affect the duration of the study.

In a parallel design RCT, participants are randomly assigned to a particular treatment group and remain on this treatment throughout the study. In a crossover design study, each participant serves as his or her own control. In the simplest example, a two-period crossover design, each participant would receive either intervention or control (A or B) in the first period and the alternative treatment (A or B) in the second period. One of the major advantages of the crossover design is that "variability is reduced because the measured effect of the intervention is the difference in an individual participant's response to intervention and control" (8). The decrease in variance allows researchers to use a smaller sample size than that used in a parallel design RCT. Although a crossover design study is generally longer than a parallel design study, there is an advantage in that each participant is "exposed" to all treatments tested in the study. This design is particularly powerful in controlling for variation associated with hyper- and hypo-responders because they participate in each type of intervention, which reduces interparticipant variation.

When using the crossover design, researchers presume that there are no carryover effects from the first to subsequent periods. However, the validity of this assumption must be evaluated in each study. The need to avoid carryover effects rules out the use of a crossover design in many different circumstances. For example, if the intervention during the first period cures the disease, the participant would obviously receive no benefit from the treatment or control in the second period. Frequently, a crossover design has a washout period or compliance break that separates the different periods within the study design. After the completion of a crossover design study, statistical analyses can be completed to test for any possible carryover effects (9).

The use of a factorial study design allows the researcher to address multiple objectives within one study. In factorial designs, the factor is the major independent variable, with two or more levels as a subdivision of each factor. For example, in a study designed to test whether increased carbohydrate intake increases triglyceride levels, researchers could also test whether the quality of the carbohydrate (ie, the amount of fiber) has an effect on triglyceride levels. Using a factorial design, researchers would use the following groups to test the aforementioned objectives: (a) high carbohydrate/low fiber, (b) high carbohydrate/high fiber, (c) low carbohydrate/low fiber, and (d) low carbohydrate/high fiber. In this example, carbohydrate amount has two levels and fiber content has two levels; thus, it is a 2×2 factorial design. This is the simplest form of the factorial design. In this notation, the number of numbers indicates how many factors there are and the number values denote how many levels there are. In a 3×4 factorial design, there are two factors, one factor with three levels and the other with four levels. The number of different treatment groups in any factorial design can easily be determined by multiplying through the number notation (eg, a 3×4 factorial study has 12 treatment groups).

A free-living clinical nutrition study in which participants self-select their diet based on advice from the study personnel involves less control than an RCT. This type of free-living, self-selected diet study design often is used for weight-loss trials (10). The general population frequently considers the results of free-living clinical nutrition studies more achievable than the results of studies that employ a greater level of dietary control. This is because the free-living interventions have already been tested in a real-world setting. Free-living, self-selected clinical nutrition studies can be especially successful with close participant monitoring. However, such monitoring is not always possible when free-living individuals go about their daily routines.

Postprandial studies enable researchers to evaluate the acute effects of a specific nutrient, food, or mixed meal on an end point(s) of interest. Although many biomarkers typically are studied in the fasting state, there is growing interest in identifying what occurs during the postprandial period. This is because many individuals are in the postprandial period for as long as 12 to 14 hours each day. Researchers have used postprandial studies to evaluate the acute effects of specific nutrients, foods, or nutrient profiles that have been tested chronically. For example, researchers have studied the postprandial effects of components of the Mediterranean diet on endothelial function (11).

Postprandial studies can build on the results of in vitro studies as well as in vivo studies of longer durations. For example, based on the results of a chronic feeding study, a recent study evaluated the effects of consuming particular tomato components and quantified in vitro antiplatelet activity and ex vivo platelet function (12). These studies can provide valuable information about the mechanisms associated with the diet-related pathophysiology of disease processes.

Dose-response studies provide information about the range of biological effects in response to different doses of nutrients/dietary constituents evaluated. Implicit to this type of study is the assumption that the maximally effective dose can be established. Consequently, all of this information is used to make dietary recommendations for prevention and treatment of diseases. For example, evidence from dose-response studies was used to support the recommendation that specific dietary intake levels of stanol and sterol esters can lower low-density lipoprotein cholesterol (13).

Before issuing a health claim for a food or nutrient, the FDA and other government agencies require that dose-response studies establish the appropriate nutrient levels or amounts of food for those claims. You may refer to numerous resources for guidelines for conducting clinical nutrition research aimed at qualifying a food or nutrient for a health claim (14–17).

RESOURCES

Sufficient resources are essential for the conduct of a clinical nutrition study. Self-selected diet studies require facilities for instruction, cooking demonstrations, and diet assessment; office space; and computer support. At the other end of the spectrum, well-controlled feeding studies need facilities for food storage, preparation, serving, and cleanup. Studies that do not involve feeding participants on-site must have a facility for the storage of meals, foods, or supplements that are picked up by, or delivered to, the participants. Location, accessibility, and ambience of the feeding site or the facility where participants pick up meals, foods, or supplements are important factors in the recruitment and retention of study participants. Interventions employing supplements must have facilities for preparation and packaging, either in-house or through contractual arrangement with the manufacturer.

Most clinical nutrition studies collect clinical and/or biochemical end point measurements. These can range from simple measurements, such as body weight and skin fold thickness, to more complex procedures involving biochemical analyses of body fluids, tissue samples, whole-body procedures such as DEXA, and even nutrigenomics. Investigators must have resources for carrying out these measurements or make contractual arrangements with other reputable laboratories.

All studies need personnel, funding, and an adequate population from which to recruit. Nonessential resources, such as participant incentives and exploratory end point measurements, can enhance the overall implementation of a study. If the budget allows for them, additional study end points should be included. For example, researchers may wish to collect additional biological samples that can be assayed at a later time; add a questionnaire that could be administered easily and inexpensively; collect information about physical activity level (eg, using a step counter); or gather additional anthropometric data (eg, waist circumference in the supine position).

BUDGET

A budget that will sufficiently cover all study costs is essential. Although the actual cost depends on the design, scope, and duration of the study, there are some general budgeting guidelines. The major budget categories are personnel, supplies (including food costs), laboratory assays and procedures (which may be contracted out), equipment, and, sometimes, participant stipends. In most cases, budgets must include an institution-specified percentage of the direct cost of the project to cover overhead. The research and grants office of the sponsoring institution provides this information.

Senior professional personnel are responsible for scientific decisions and control of the budget. They also have an important role in compliance and building and sustaining staff and participant morale over the course of the study. Consistent day-to-day management by a study coordinator is necessary to supervise kitchen operations (where applicable), laboratory procedures, and data collection. Studies involving diet instruction need registered dietitians (RDs) to provide the intervention. Feeding studies need personnel to prepare food and food aliquots for assay. During the course of the study, work assignments may change; therefore, some staff members should be prepared to assume various job responsibilities.

Well-controlled feeding studies require additional expenses, especially if food is prepared and served on-site. These may include the costs of leasing kitchen and dining facilities and renting food storage and freezer space. A study may need to budget for high-precision scales for weighing food, high-powered blenders for preparing food aliquots for chemical analysis, and other specialized equipment. In general, food is the most expensive item in controlled feeding studies. See Dennis et al (18) for more on resources required to conduct-controlled feeding studies.

Most studies also will require equipment and supplies for clinical, anthropometric, and laboratory measurements and may need to budget for shipping costs for laboratory samples. The budget should cover the cost of statistical and computer capabilities, including specialized software, to manage and analyze data. Clerical activities to cover in the budget include preparation of recruitment materials, completing forms, handling communication, scheduling potential recruits, and preparation of reports. Miscellaneous expenses include forms, duplicating costs, monetary incentives for the participants, transportation, parking for participants, social activities, and closeout costs.

STUDY PARTICIPANTS

Selection of the Participant Population

Investigators should define the study population in advance to include specific inclusion and exclusion criteria. These criteria set parameters that more clearly define the study population. The hypotheses to be tested should guide the selection of the participant population. In some cases, if a diet treatment is being tested to evaluate changes in a biological end point, the participants must be outside the range of normal if investigators are to identify a diet response. When a value measured is normal at the beginning of the study this may indicate that these participants will not be responsive to the dietary intervention. For example, in a study of blood pressure responses to a diet intervention, the test diet may have little or no effect in normotensive participants but elicit a significant blood pressure–lowering effect in participants with hypertension. Likewise, a high-fiber diet may have no effect on C-reactive protein (CRP), a marker of inflammation, in participants who have low (ie, normal) values, whereas in participants with elevated CRP levels, a high-fiber diet would be expected to decrease CRP.

On the other hand, if the abnormal end point value is due to participants having various comorbidities, it is essential to know this and exclude these participants from the study because they could have a different diet response than would be expected. Thus, it is best to test the study hypothesis without the interference of underlying physiological conditions that may overpower the effects of the diet intervention. For example, in a study of the effects of dietary interventions on elevated blood cholesterol levels, a potential participant who has hypercholesterolemia due to hypothyroidism should not be included with other participants whose hypercholesterolemia is caused by habitual consumption of an atherogenic diet. The excluded participant's comorbid condition would potentially prevent a response to the experimental diet. This participant's response (or lack of one) would increase the variability in the study results beyond what was originally estimated and create possible problems with the analyses of the data.

Researchers must also decide whether more than one group of participants should be studied. Based on the results of previous studies, it may be known that certain groups of individuals have a distinctive response to an intervention diet. For example, individuals with elevated baseline triglyceride levels have decreased clearance of postprandial triglyceride-rich lipoproteins following a high-fat meal, compared with individuals with normal baseline levels. Thus, a study that includes both groups of individuals may evaluate different population group responses to the diet intervention. The inclusion of multiple groups of individuals (eg, from different ages, genders, races, classes, or geographic locations) may also allow for the generalization of study results to a greater proportion of the general population.

Sample Size

Researchers must take appropriate precautions to ensure that a study sample is large enough to detect differences between groups or treatments. Thus, study design must include calculations of sample sizes that offer adequate levels of significance and power. When choosing the data to perform sample size calculations, researchers must be precise and choose not only a design but also outcome data that closely resemble the study in question. Although calculating sample size is an integral component of any study design, researchers must understand that these calculations provide only an estimate of the needed size of a study sample. Once an estimate is obtained, it is necessary to account for other factors, such as dropout rates in clinical trials. A review of prior studies that are similar in design and length will provide information about the potential for dropouts or withdrawals from a study. In determining the final sample size for the study, investigators should err on the side of being conservative, within the monetary bounds of the design.

Participant Recruitment

Once the study population is defined, successful recruitment relies on a careful plan with multiple strategies (8). Early in the planning stages of a study, the investigators must evaluate the likelihood that a sufficient number of study participants can be obtained within an appropriate time frame and geographical area. If an important aspect of the study design and/or hypothesis is differential effects on diverse population groups, multiple sites may be required for the study to meet the recruitment goals. For example, in designing a study to evaluate the effects of a dietary intervention on high blood pressure, it may be desirable to recruit a population of African Americans because this population is at higher risk for developing hypertension. If a study such as this were based in a community with a small African-American population, investigators might need to include a second site, from which more African Americans could be recruited.

The recruitment process often begins with an advertisement placed in a local newspaper or alternative media source (eg, Listserv or Web site posting). The recruitment advertisement should include pertinent inclusion/exclusion criteria and a method for interested individuals to contact the study personnel (eg, a toll-free telephone number).

Participant Screening

Screening ensures that participants meet eligibility criteria and understand what participation in the study entails. Participants can either be randomly allocated to treatment and control groups or be assigned to different groups based on predetermined characteristics to create balanced or similar groups at the beginning of the study. In general, a rigorous screening process is critical to the success of the study. In addition to ensuring that potential participants meet eligibility criteria, screening provides an opportunity to evaluate subjective data, such as attitude, behavior, interest, commitment, and maturity, which are important attributes to understand when seeking to retain participants and maintain compliance.

The complexity of the screening process depends on the specificity of participants' exclusion criteria. Some studies require only a simple questionnaire, whereas others may require anthropometric, dietary, and laboratory data, as well as information on lifestyle practices, such as smoking and physical activity behavior, and a medical examination to rule out underlying disease. It is particularly important that the screening process not prompt participants to make any behavior changes before the study begins. If possible, the interval between screening and the commencement of the study should be brief. Baseline assessments at the beginning of the study may determine whether individuals have changed behavior between the screening

and the start of the study. In addition, baseline measurements assess all participants at a similar time point, whereas the screening process could take months to complete.

When the screening phase is a multiple-step process that eliminates ineligible individuals in the early steps, it is more efficient and less costly. The first stage in the screening process often includes questionnaires, which may be completed during telephone interviews, during personal interviews, or on the participants' own time. During this initial step, researchers should explain to participants what will be expected of them if they decide to participate. At this step investigators should also ask questions to determine whether the individuals' medical histories meet the study's inclusion criteria. After the initial phase, if individuals meet the eligibility requirements, they proceed to a more in-depth screening appointment, which may include a clinic visit and the collection of relevant anthropometric and laboratory measurements. For example, investigators for a blood pressure–lowering study must establish that interested individuals are hypertensive.

Participant Randomization

Participant randomization is used to remove systematic error and selection bias in clinical trials. In the most prevalent form of randomization, simple randomization, each participant is assigned to a treatment without regard for assignments made to other participants. The main disadvantage of simple randomization is that it may lead to an imbalance in terms of participant characteristics that are known to be related to the variables under study (eg, more males in one group; lower or higher mean values for a key baseline variable in one group) and thereby affect study results.

In stratified randomization, investigators construct strata based on variables of interest and perform a randomization scheme separately within each stratum. For example, for a study designed to evaluate the effects of a treatment in older vs younger individuals, participants would be assigned to either a "younger" group or an "older" group, then members of each group would be randomly assigned for treatment. In this way, stratified randomization ensures balance between the treatment groups with respect to various combinations of specific end point measures.

Constrained, or blocked, randomization is used to avoid imbalance in the number of participants assigned to each group (19). Within this randomization scheme, a sequence of blocks contains a prespecified number of treatments in a random order. This balances the randomization scheme at the completion of each block. For example, if groups of 10 participants are enrolled in a study every 3 weeks, a constrained randomization would evenly distribute the treatment allocations across each enrollment group.

In a nonrandomized concurrent control study, the control group and the treatment group are not necessarily "treated" at the sample time. For example, a study may compare survival results of patients treated at two different institutions, with one institution using a new experimental procedure and the other practicing traditional medical care. The major weakness of the nonrandomized design is that the intervention and control groups may not be strictly comparable, making it difficult to elucidate effects of the treatment(s) in question.

Incentives

Incentives are important for participation in a clinical nutrition study. Although monetary incentives can be effective, other types of tangible incentives also encourage participation in the research process and may provide benefits to participants. When designing a study that provides the participants with nutrition information/education, investigators should present this as an incentive and convey the lasting influences that participation in the study could provide. Low-cost nutrition-related incentives include dietary assessment analysis, nutrition counseling sessions, chronic disease risk profiles, pedometers, and recipes.

Incentives facilitate participant recruitment and retention. Thus, investigators should choose incentives that will appeal to the population from which participants will be drawn. For example, in some studies, incentives should be age- and gender-specific.

Incentives should be appropriate for the time and effort required to participate in the screening process and research study. Incentives should not be so grandiose that they encourage people with no intention of being study participants to participate in the screening process, and they should not imply or be perceived as coercion. However, incentives that are perceived as "worthless" by the participants could have unintended consequences. Undesirable incentives could contribute to selection bias and a lack of participant commitment to the study.

Researchers should recognize a distinction between incentives for recruitment and incentives for retention. Incentives that are given throughout the study, such as recipes or laboratory results, can have a big impact because they demonstrate the effectiveness of the nutrition

intervention to the participants. Although incentives may be given periodically throughout the study, the bulk should be reserved for participants who successfully complete the study. If monetary incentives are provided, rates may be prorated depending on the level of completion achieved by each individual, with the bulk of the payment received upon completion of the entire study. Many Institutional Review Boards mandate that participants are compensated for the time they spend in the study.

Participant Monitoring

Investigators must adequately monitor participants enrolled in a study. The level of monitoring is often a function of the overall intensity of the study design. For example, in an RCT feeding study, participants may be required to fill out daily and weekly monitoring forms in which they would have the opportunity to report any lack of compliance with the study protocol. These monitoring forms can prompt participants to report any study food they did not eat or any food not included in their experimental diet plan that they consumed. The forms can also ask participants to report changes in activity levels, medication usage, or alcohol intake if such changes may interfere with study outcomes.

Although monitoring forms are a tool to monitor compliance, the study staff also should take time to interact with participants and make note of any inconsistencies that are reported in conversations. In a free-living study where study personnel may not interact with participants for a period of weeks or months, a more formal monitoring system may need to be implemented, such as weekly phone calls or e-mails. Participants who are actively involved in the research process are more likely to be committed to the project and comply with the study protocol.

Informed Consent

Researchers must obtain informed consent from human participants, giving them all the information they need to make an informed decision about whether they want to participate in the study. Informed consent implicitly requires that researchers clearly and accurately describe what the clinical trial entails. In addition, all information must be provided in writing. Informed consent documents must be written at a level that can be understood by all potential participants (approximately fifth-grade reading level) and contain information in lay, rather than scientific, terms. For example, the amount of blood taken should be stated in household measures, such as tablespoons, instead of milliliters. Participants are then given the opportunity to review the information and ask as many questions as needed. Once all questions have been answered, participants acknowledge their willingness to participate in the study by signing the informed consent document. Investigators must give individuals a copy of the signed informed consent document to refer to throughout the study should they have questions (see Box 9.3).

BOX 9.3   Important Components of an Informed Consent Form*

- Title of the project (including recognition of institutional review board [IRB] approval)
- Contact information for the principal investigator and pertinent study personnel
- Instructions to participant
- Purpose of the study
- Procedures involved in the study
  - Screening procedure
  - Active study period (ie, diet periods/weight-loss periods)
  - Follow-up measurements
- Research testing
  - Blood sampling
  - Additional physical measurements (eg, exercise testing, DEXA scans, anthropometric measurements, blood pressure measurements)
  - Dietary assessment
  - Questionnaires (if applicable)
- Compliance with study protocol (list any conditions for dismissal from the study)
- Discomforts and risks (to the subject)
  - Include for each measure outlined in "research testing" section
- Benefits (to the subject)
- Potential benefits to society
- Statement of confidentiality
- Right to ask questions
- Compensation
- Injury statement
- Voluntary participation
- Signature and date of participant signature
- Signature of witness (study personnel)

*The contents of an informed consent may vary by institution.

The inherent rights of all human participants who participate in a clinical nutrition study include the right to join or leave a research study whenever they wish to do so. Individuals should never be pressured or coerced to join or leave a study. Individuals cannot lose access to their regular medical care, and they have the right to know about alternative care options. The increasing complexity of the health care system has led to more rigorous regulations from institutional review boards and more detailed informed consent documents. For example, genetic testing is included in many clinical nutrition studies, and this has drawn more attention to the disclosure of research findings and the linking of biological outcomes to personal identifiers of human participants. Individuals must therefore understand that they will likely not receive genetic testing information at the conclusion of the study. When informed consent procedures are implemented appropriately, participants' confidence in the study is bolstered.

Participant Retention and Compliance

Adequate resources are needed to retain participants and ensure excellent compliance over the course of the study. Investigators must develop protocols defining retention policies and activities. Likewise, studies need protocols for dealing with compliance issues, policies for acceptable deviations from study protocols, and criteria for participant dismissal. The policy for participant dismissal must be shared with participants. Meticulous screening of potential participants will help identify those who will be cooperative and committed to all aspects of the study. The level of staff support provided to participants will vary depending on the design of the study. For example, controlled feeding studies tend to involve more personal interactions between staff and participants than free-living studies have.

To meaningfully interpret treatment effects, investigators must assess compliance with the experimental protocol (20). In some studies, the treatment effect may be biased by noncompliance. All studies must evaluate compliance in the final data analysis. For example, if a clinical study is designed to evaluate the effects of iron supplementation on measures of iron status and half of the treatment group takes 50% of their prescribed supplement, this must be quantified and considered in interpretation of the data analyses. A common approach to analysis of clinical trials is called *intent to treat*. In this analysis, all data that are available for an individual are evaluated, even if the individual drops out early or is noncompliant. This analysis tests the effect of the mode of intervention but not the factors that could explain the effect.

To assess compliance, researchers must consider several variables that vary as a function of the type and design of the investigation. In some studies, measurement of compliance may entail a simple, straightforward approach, whereas other studies may depend on measuring a biological variable that requires a complex assay. For example, platelet phospholipid fatty acids are required to assess adherence to test diets high in certain fatty acids. Likewise, the methods selected for assessing compliance may range from very sensitive (measuring a urinary metabolite) to relatively insensitive (participants' self-assessment of compliance). Another consideration is whether compliance is assessed objectively or subjectively. Subjective assessment can be as simple as asking participants if they are adhering to the protocol. This approach is successful when the investigator and participants have established a trusting relationship. Often, investigators can effectively ascertain compliance from participants' attitudes and behavior (eg, level of participation, punctuality). If investigators suspect that participants are not complying with the experimental protocol, they need to address this concern promptly and in a nonconfrontational manner. If noncompliance is an issue that may affect the study outcome, the participant must be dismissed from the study.

Perfect compliance (ie, no deviation from the experimental protocol) is the goal of all clinical nutrition studies, but it is essential in metabolic studies. Not only must the participants consume all the allotted food (and not lose any through emesis), they also must refrain from consuming any other food or substances that might bias the results of the study. However, it is seldom feasible to maintain study participants in an enclosed, supervised environment 24 hours a day for an extended period. Therefore, proxy measures often are employed with varying degrees of sensitivity.

Once energy equilibrium has been established, body weight changes may signal compliance problems. These changes, however, are a gross indicator of noncompliance. This method would not differentiate between noncompliant food intake and changes in energy expenditure, nor would it detect small deviations in food intake that could have a large effect if certain foods were systematically omitted or consumed outside the protocol.

When a complete collection of excreta are obtained, metabolites and other substances may be assayed. For example, a constant sodium intake should be reflected in a constant sodium excretion (21). The validity of using urine and fecal biomarkers as an index of intake depends, of course, on the completeness of the collections. Complete 24-hour collections with a diet of constant composition are useful in determining urinary creatinine excretion (22); *p*-aminobenzoic acid administered in tablet form has been used to assess the completeness of urine collections (23) and, added to food, to monitor dietary compliance (24).

A detailed description of various methods for assessing compliance is beyond the scope of this chapter. For more information, the reader is referred to Bingham (25). Finally, it is important to note that given human frailties and social needs, compliance is most likely not going to be perfect. It can be enhanced if overall morale is high and the protocol allows some free choices (eg, diet beverages may be consumed at social gatherings).

DIETARY INTERVENTION

The Experimental Diet

Clinical nutrition studies can be designed to evaluate the effects of a single nutrient, individual foods, or dietary patterns on end points of interest. Studies may provide single nutrients by supplements (eg, eicosapentaenoic acid and docosahexaenoic acid) (26) or individual foods (eg, fatty fish) (27). Some studies have provided bioactive components via foods such as dark chocolate (flavan-3-ols, procyanidins) (28) and processed tomato products (lycopene) (29). In some instances, investigators have used individual foods, such as peanuts and peanut products or walnuts, to manipulate the nutrient profile of the diet (30–32).

In some cases, multiple nutrient manipulations are studied. For example, the OmniHeart study evaluated diets with different macronutrient profiles on cardiovascular end points (33). In other instances, investigators focus on the effects of dietary patterns on end points of interest. Examples of this type of study include the Dietary Approaches to Stop Hypertension study (34) and the Portfolio Diet study (35).

Thus, there are many different options to consider when planning clinical nutrition studies and the choice of the experimental diet to be tested will depend on the hypothesis being evaluated. Figure 9.1 shows how dietary control varies across a spectrum and provides examples of studies of varying dietary control.

To achieve optimum adherence by study participants, the menus for delivering the test diets should include popular, well-liked foods. A variety of foods on the menus helps researchers to avoid situations where specific food dislikes deter potential participation in the study. Depending on the

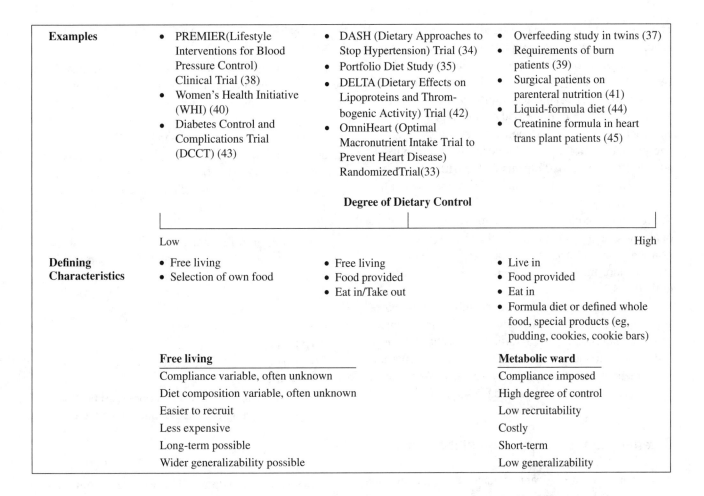

FIGURE 9.1   Studies of varying dietary control.

study purpose, single foods on the menu can sometimes be substituted for others with similar nutrient content.

Researchers must select the number of days in a menu rotation. A shorter menu cycle (eg, 3 days) may have less nutrient variability than a longer menu rotation. However, if the cycle length is too short, participants may experience food "fatigue," especially in studies of longer duration, and this can compromise adherence to the study protocol. To avoid serving the same meal on the same day each week, do not use a 7-day menu cycle. A 6-day menu cycle offers sufficient variety and can elicit good participant adherence over several months of a controlled feeding study (32).

Test Diet Implementation Strategies

When designing the intervention, the researcher must consider a number of trade-offs. The greater the dietary control, the more costly the study and the less attractive it is to potential participants. Formula diets or synthetic

mixtures provide the greatest degree of consistency, because each mouthful swallowed has the same composition. However, the results may be of limited relevance to investigators seeking to understand the effects of natural foods. At the other end of the scale, studies that are more feasible, in terms of cost and recruitment, are more difficult to interpret because the results are confounded by issues of compliance and the variability in dietary composition. As noted previously, the objectives of the study must be clearly formulated and, if necessary, revised to meet the limitations imposed by feasibility and reality. Once this is done, the investigator can decide whether the attainable objectives justify doing the study.

Estimating Energy Requirements

In controlled feeding studies, investigators must assess the energy requirements of the participants to ensure weight maintenance or promote a defined rate of weight change.

This assessment will affect the quantity of food needed and, hence, the budget. Energy requirements can be estimated using various methods (36). Many studies use the Harris-Benedict formula to calculate an individual's basal energy expenditure (BEE), and then multiply the result by an activity factor to determine total energy expenditure. This approach may provide a good estimate of participants' energy needs; however, the energy estimate must be adjusted for some participants (37). Mifflin et al have reported an equation that predicts energy needs better than the Harris Benedict formula (38). In fact, the Mifflin–St Jeor equation has provided the most accurate estimate of actual resting metabolic rate in the largest percentage of nonobese and obese individuals (39). However, this method, too, may not provide reliable estimates for all individuals.

Because equations can produce only "best estimates" of participants' energy needs, participants should be weighed daily and staff should monitor participants' feelings of hunger and fullness. In studies where weight maintenance is the goal, these feelings are better short-term indicators of whether energy needs are being met with the test diet.

Determining the Composition of the Diet

Many commercial software packages are available that can estimate the nutrient composition of foods. Nutrient databases, however, are derived from mean composition values, which may not reflect what actually is being consumed. For some nutrients, the content of these nutrients in foods can vary greatly, which reinforces the need to chemically analyze the test diets, especially for the nutrients being studied. For studies in which free-living participants choose from food selection groups, approximate nutrient values may be sufficient. However, as the study design moves toward greater control of the diet, the need for analytic values increases. A good plan is to analyze aliquots of the calculated diets and to make adjustments, if necessary, before the study starts. If differences are identified between calculated and assayed values, the food sources that account for the error must be identified and modified. If possible, aliquots should be collected and analyzed periodically throughout the study. Refer to Phillips and Stewart (40) for additional details on sampling and preparation of composites. Valuable resources for selection of a food analysis laboratory are the Association of Official Analytical Chemists and the American Oil Chemists' Society (AOCS) (41). The AOCS examination board provides a list of AOCS-certified laboratories.

POTENTIAL PROBLEMS: RANDOM ERROR AND BIAS

Although careful attention to detail helps eliminate the systematic error present in a clinical trial, random error (also known as *random fluctuations* or *random variability*) cannot be controlled in the same manner. The heterogeneity of the human population generally leads to substantial random variation in clinical trials; however, the impact of random error can often be minimized by increasing the sample size. Other examples of random error in clinical trials are changes associated with seasonality or circadian rhythms.

In addition to random error, clinical bias can yield point estimates that differ significantly from the true values. Sources of bias in clinical trials include the following:

- Selection bias
- Procedure selection bias
- Postentry exclusion bias
- Bias due to selective loss of data
- Assessment bias
- Bias due to retroactive definitions (post hoc analysis wherein subgroups are defined after the data are analyzed)
- Statistical bias

Such biases can diminish the external validity of the study and render the data and outcomes invalid.

QUALITY ASSURANCE

No study is better than the quality of its data (8). Quality assurance is an ongoing process of assessment and evaluation according to predetermined criteria, feedback, and correction. A well-designed quality assurance system incorporates quality control procedures at every point in the study where information is transferred. Quality control is part of an overall management strategy that includes written and oral progress reports, budget monitoring, and morale building of staff and participants.

Quality assurance begins with the selection of the most accurate and precise methods attainable. Whenever possible, studies should set methodological standards and routinely monitor them for accuracy. (An internal quality control system allows for reanalysis of samples at different times.)

Quality assurance includes training of personnel, regular maintenance and calibration of equipment, monitoring of the performance of personnel and equipment,

TABLE 9.2   Quality Assurance Considerations in a Clinical Study

Aspects of the Study	Recommended Quality Control Procedures
Methods	• Validate for accuracy • Establish performance standards
Training staff and monitoring	• Establish protocols
Performance	• Establish written procedures • Determine performance standards • Provide staff feedback
Forms	• Design forms • Pilot test forms for validity and reliability
Subjects	• Complete daily and/or weekly monitoring forms • Receive feedback from staff who reviewed monitoring forms
Data	• Verify accuracy of data and data entry • Adjudicate questionable data

application of data editing criteria, and documentation of the quality of corrective feedback throughout the collection and processing of data. A well-trained staff can help ensure that data are collected and managed without bias and minimal variability.

Training, however, is only the first step; regular monitoring is also necessary. Subtle changes in procedures over time can cause considerable drift, which could bias the results. Similarly, equipment must also be regularly monitored.

Investigators develop the tools for quality assurance, such as the protocol, procedure manuals, forms for data collection, and data management, in the planning phase. Data management incorporates documentation of data quality, including protocol violations and missing and spurious values. As the data are collected, the research team must visually inspect completed forms, follow the ranges for acceptable values, use logic, and perform consistency checks so problems can be detected and corrected early (see Table 9.2). Ideally, the quality assurance program prevents problems before they occur.

DATA MANAGEMENT

Without quality data, meaningful conclusions cannot be made. Three main problems associated with data collection are missing data, incorrect data, and excess variability (8). Investigators can prevent such problems with proper organization and training of study personnel. Quality control measures should be in place to avoid data management errors. For example, when performing anthropometric measurements on study participants, the most robust data are generated from multiple measurements performed by at least two different members of the research team. Implicit to this is that the measurements obtained by different staff members have minimal variance.

DATA ANALYSIS: PRIMARY AND SECONDARY

Accurate data analysis is required for the appropriate interpretation of the outcome variables of clinical trials. Treatment comparisons can be between-participant factors or within-participant factors. Between-participant factors test the effect on different groups, with each participant providing one response associated with a single level of the treatment factor. In contrast, within-participant factors test the effect of two or more treatments on each individual participant. Each participant provides multiple responses, with one response associated with each level of the treatment factor. Thus, a parallel design study tests between-participant factors, whereas a crossover design can test within-participant factors. As discussed previously, other factors within the model (eg, order and period/treatment interactions) can be used to test for carryover effects in a crossover design study.

Investigators must pay close attention when analyzing data that includes repeated measures because correlation of the data may occur over time or under different conditions. The simplest form of repeated measures data is paired data (eg, pre- and posttreatment measures). A more complicated method of handling repeated measures uses the repeated measures analysis of variance (ANOVA). ANOVA includes a "time" factor in the model, accounting for the fact that measurements taken on the same participant are not independent.

TRANSLATION

Researchers are obliged to communicate their study findings to the scientific community and the general public. Peer-reviewed papers published in the scientific literature are usually the best way to communicate study results to the scientific community. Other communications include abstracts, articles in the non-peer-reviewed professional literature and the popular press, and the final report. In addition, presentations at scientific meetings and conferences can rapidly communicate study findings. A body of scientific evidence, not one study, is usually the basis for setting or modifying nutrition policy. Whereas one study may produce a novel discovery that greatly influences subsequent research efforts, these new efforts, in turn, add to the evidence base for making dietary recommendations to promote health and treat diseases and conditions. See Chapter 30 for more details.

CONCLUSION

The number and sophistication of clinical nutrition studies have increased rapidly in recent years. However, key fundamental concepts remain the core for designing and conducting all clinical nutrition studies. The guidance presented herein, and elsewhere in the literature, provides a road map for all the necessary steps that have to be taken to carry out high-quality clinical nutrition research. Justified hypotheses guide the key aspects of studies. Critical considerations are the study and diet designs, strategy for delivering the experimental diet(s), statistical power, evaluation of the appropriate study population, appropriate statistical analyses, and all logistics that pertain to carrying out all aspects of the study in a high-quality manner, and, importantly, communicating the study results. The success of a clinical nutrition study depends on a skilled and well-trained clinical staff, all of whom are adaptive and effective in interacting with study participants. All study staff and participants must be deeply committed to carrying out the study.

RDs have many opportunities to be involved in all aspects of clinical nutrition research. Given their knowledge and expertise, RDs understand the nutrition research needs that will advance clinical practice and health promotion efforts. We encourage RDs to be more proactive in seeking out leadership roles in clinical nutrition research and, thereby, contribute substantively to the ongoing evolution of nutrition recommendations for health and treatment of disease.

REFERENCES

1. Federation of American Societies for Experimental Biology. Third Report on Nutrition Monitoring in the United States: executive summary. In: Office LSR, ed. *Prepared for the Interagency Board for Nutrition Monitoring and Related Research.* Washington, DC: US Government Printing Office; 1995.

2. Rouse T, Davis DP. *Exploring a Vision: Integrating Knowledge for Food and Health.* Washington, DC: National Academies Press; 2004.

3. Otten J, Hellwig JP, Meyer LD. *Dietary Reference Intakes: The Essential Guide to Nutrient Requirements.* Washington, DC: National Academies Press; 2006.

4. Institute of Medicine. *Informing the Future: Critical Issues in Health.* 2nd ed. Washington, DC: National Academies Press; 2003.

5. Institute of Medicine. *Informing the Future: Critical Issues in Health.* 3rd ed. Washington, DC: National Academies Press; 2005.

6. US Department of Health and Human Services and National Heart, Lung, and Blood Institute. *Healthy People 2010: Understanding and Improving Health.* 2nd ed. Washington, DC: US Government Printing Office; 2000.

7. DeAngelis CD, Drazen JM, Frizelle FA, Haug C, Hoey J, Horton R, Kotzin S, Laine C, Marusic A, Overbeke AJ, Schroeder TV, Sox HC, Van Der Weyden MB; International Committee of Medical Journal Editors. Clinical trial registration: a statement from the International Committee of Medical Journal Editors. *JAMA.* 2004;292: 1363–1364.

8. Friedman LM, DeMets DL. *Fundamentals of Clinical Trials.* 3rd ed. Ann Arbor, Mich: Springer-Verlag; 1998.

9. Grizzle JE. The two-period change-over design and its use in clinical trials. *Biometrics.* 1965;21:467–480.

10. McManus K, Antinoro L, Sacks F. A randomized controlled trial of a moderate-fat, low-energy diet compared with a low fat, low-energy diet for weight loss in overweight adults. *Int J Obes Relat Metab Disord.* 2001;25:1503–1511.

11. Vogel RA, Corretti MC, Plotnick GD. The postprandial effect of components of the Mediterranean diet on endothelial function. *J Am Coll Cardiol.* 2000;36:1455–1460.

12. O'Kennedy N, Crosbie L, van Lieshout M, Broom JI, Webb DJ, Duttaroy AK. Effects of antiplatelet components of tomato extract on platelet function in vitro and ex vivo: a time-course cannulation study in healthy humans. *Am J Clin Nutr.* 2006;84: 570–579.

13. National Cholesterol and Education Program. Executive summary of the Third Report of the National Cholesterol Education Program (NCEP) Expert Panel on Detection, Evaluation, and Treatment of High Blood Cholesterol in Adults (Adult Treatment Panel III). *JAMA.* 2001;285: 2486–2497.

14. Arvanitoyannis IS, Van Houwelingen-Koukaliaroglou M. Functional foods: a survey of health claims, pros and cons, and current legislation. *Crit Rev Food Sci Nutr.* 2005;45:385–404.

15. Ferrari CK. Functional foods, herbs and nutraceuticals: towards biochemical mechanisms of healthy aging. *Biogerontology.* 2004;5:275–289.

16. Halsted CH. Dietary supplements and functional foods: 2 sides of a coin? *Am J Clin Nutr.* 2003;77 (suppl):1001S–1007S.

17. Hasler CM. Functional foods: benefits, concerns and challenges—a position paper from the American Council on Science and Health. *J Nutr.* 2002;132: 3772–3781.

18. Dennis B, Ershow AG, Obarzanek E, Clevidence BA. *Well-Controlled Diet Studies in Humans: A Practical Guide to Design and Management.* Chicago, Ill: American Dietetic Association; 1999.

19. Hill AB. The clinical trial. *Br Med Bull.* 1951;7: 278–282.

20. Windhauser MM, Evans MA, McCullough ML. Dietary adherence in the Dietary Approaches to Stop Hypertension trial. DASH Collaborative Research Group. *J Am Diet Assoc.* 1999;99(suppl):S76–S83.

21. Schachter J, Harper PH, Radin ME, Caggiula AW, McDonald RH, Diven WF. Comparison of sodium and potassium intake with excretion. *Hypertension.* 1980;2:695–699.

22. Jackson S. Creatinine in urine as an index of urinary excretion rate. *Health Phys.* 1966;12:843–850.

23. Bingham S, Cummings JH. The use of 4-aminobenzoic acid as a marker to validate the completeness of 24 h urine collections in man. *Clin Sci* (Lond). 1983;64:629–635.

24. Roberts SB, Morrow FD, Evans WJ. Use of p-aminobenzoic acid to monitor compliance with prescribed dietary regimens during metabolic balance studies in man. *Am J Clin Nutr.* 1990;51:485–488.

25. Bingham S. The dietary assessment of individuals; methods, accuracy, new techniques and recommendations. *CAB Int.* 1987;57:705–774.

26. Dietary supplementation with n-3 polyunsaturated fatty acids and vitamin E after myocardial infarction: results of the GISSI-Prevenzione trial. Gruppo Italiano per lo Studio della Sopravvivenza nell'Infarto miocardico. *Lancet.* 1999;354:447–455.

27. Burr ML, Fehily AM, Gilbert JF. Effects of changes in fat, fish, and fibre intakes on death and myocardial reinfarction: diet and reinfarction trial (DART). *Lancet.* 1989;2:757–761.

28. Keen CL, Holt RR, Oteiza PI, Fraga CG, Schmitz HH. Cocoa antioxidants and cardiovascular health. *Am J Clin Nutr.* 2005;81(suppl):298S–303S.

29. Dutta-Roy AK, Crosbie L, Gordon MJ. Effects of tomato extract on human platelet aggregation in vitro. *Platelets.* 2001;12:218–227.

30. Griel AE, Eissenstat B, Juturu V, Hsieh G, Kris-Etherton PM. Improved diet quality with peanut consumption. *J Am Coll Nutr.* 2004;23: 660–668.

31. Kris-Etherton PM, Pearson TA, Wan Y. High-monounsaturated fatty acid diets lower both plasma cholesterol and triacylglycerol concentrations. *Am J Clin Nutr.* 1999;70:1009–1015.

32. Zhao G, Etherton TD, Martin KR, West SG, Gillies PJ, Kris-Etherton PM. Dietary alpha-linolenic acid reduces inflammatory and lipid cardiovascular risk factors in hypercholesterolemic men and women. *J Nutr.* 2004;134:2991–2997.

33. Appel LJ, Sacks FM, Carey VJ. Effects of protein, monounsaturated fat, and carbohydrate intake on blood pressure and serum lipids: results of the OmniHeart randomized trial. *JAMA.* 2005;294: 2455–2464.

34. Appel LJ, Moore TJ, Obarzanek E. A clinical trial of the effects of dietary patterns on blood pressure. DASH Collaborative Research Group. *N Engl J Med.* 1997;336:1117–1124.

35. Jenkins DJ, Kendall CW, Faulkner D. A dietary portfolio approach to cholesterol reduction: combined effects of plant sterols, vegetable proteins, and viscous fibers in hypercholesterolemia. *Metabolism.* 2002;51:1596–1604.

36. St Jeor S, Stumbo PJ. Energy needs and weight maintenance in controlled feeding studies. In: Dennis B, Ershow AG, Obarzanek E, Clevidence BA, eds. *Well-Controlled Diet Studies in Humans: A Practical Guide to Design and Management.* Chicago, Ill: American Dietetic Association; 1999.

37. Lin PH, Proschan MA, Bray GA. Estimation of energy requirements in a controlled feeding trial. *Am J Clin Nutr.* 2003;77:639–645.

38. Mifflin MD, St Jeor ST, Hill LA, Scott BJ, Daugherty SA, Koh YO. A new predictive equation for resting energy expenditure in healthy individuals. *Am J Clin Nutr.* 1990;51: 241–247.

39. Frankenfield DC, Rowe WA, Smith JS, Cooney RN. Validation of several established equations for resting metabolic rate in obese and nonobese people. *J Am Diet Assoc.* 2003;103: 1152–1159.

40. Phillips K, Stewart, KK. Validating diet composition by chemical analysis. In: Dennis B, Ershow AG, Obarzanek E, Clevidence BA, eds. *Well-Controlled Diet Studies in Humans: A Practical Guide to Design and Management.* Chicago, Ill: American Dietetic Association; 1999.

41. American Oil Chemists' Society. *Official Methods and Recommended Practices of the American Oil Chemists; Society.* Champaign, Ill: American Oil Chemists' Society; 1987–1988.

10

Interpretation and Use of Data from the National Nutrition Monitoring and Related Research Program

Ronette R. Briefel, DrPH, RD, and Karil Bialostosky, MS

The National Nutrition Monitoring and Related Research Program (NNMRRP), previously referred to as the National Nutrition Monitoring System, is composed of interconnected federal and state activities that provide information about the dietary and nutritional status of the US population, conditions that affect the dietary and nutritional status of individuals, and relationships between diet and health (1–4). *Nutrition monitoring* has been defined as "an ongoing description of nutrition conditions in the population, with particular attention to subgroups defined in socioeconomic terms, for purposes of planning, analyzing the effects of policies and programs on nutrition problems, and predicting future trends" (5). This chapter provides an overview of the uses of nutrition-monitoring data, the program's surveys and surveillance systems, research activities, and the resources available to registered dietitians (RDs) and other nutrition professionals. These resources include published reports, data sets for secondary data analysis, and applied research methodologies. This chapter also provides information on uses and limitations of nutrition-monitoring data, tips for the proper interpretation of the data, and sources of further information.

The NNMRRP is considered one of the best nutrition-monitoring systems in the world. A complete history of the program has been described elsewhere (1–4,6,7). The National Nutrition Monitoring and Related Research Act of 1990 (3) called for the development of a Ten-Year Comprehensive Plan, which was published for public comment in 1991 (6). The plan was finalized in 1993 (7) and included three primary goals:

- Provide for a comprehensive NNMRRP through continuous and coordinated data collection
- Improve the comparability and quality of data across the NNMRRP
- Improve the research base for nutrition monitoring

These national goals are complemented by state and local objectives to strengthen data collection capacity; to improve the quality of state and local data; and to improve methodologies to enhance the comparability of NNMRRP data across national, state, and local levels. Despite numerous efforts to gain support for reauthorization, the nutrition monitoring legislation was not renewed in 2002 (1,2). Monitoring activities are continuing, as described here, but without the support and guidance of a federal coordinating group or legislative mandate.

The program aims to study the relationship between food and health through data collection in five measurement component areas:

- Nutrition and related health measurements
- Food and nutrient consumption
- Knowledge, attitudes, and behavior assessments
- Food composition and nutrient databases
- Food supply determinations

Nutrition-monitoring data collected at the national, state, and local levels are used directly and indirectly to assess the contributions that diet and nutritional status make to the health of the American people, and to learn about the factors affecting dietary and nutritional status.

PURPOSES AND RESEARCH USES OF NUTRITION MONITORING DATA

Nutrition monitoring is vital to policy making and research (1,2,4,6–9). The nutrition-monitoring measurement components also provide information to help establish research priorities (1,2,9). Nutrition research provides data for policy making and for identifying nutrition-monitoring needs (7–10). For example, nutrition-monitoring data have been used to evaluate progress toward achievement of the *Healthy People 2010 Objectives for Improving Health* (11); to develop guidelines for prevention, detection, and management of nutrition conditions (12–14); and to evaluate the impact of food assistance programs (15,16) and nutrition initiatives for military feeding systems (17).

National data are used to develop reference standards for nutritional status. For example, the Centers for Disease and Control and Prevention (CDC) Growth Charts (18) now include charts for infants through adolescents 19 years of age, as well as new charts for body mass index by age and gender. The charts are included in NutStat, a nutrition anthropometry program in the computer software package Epi Info, which calculates both z scores and percentiles (19). Monitoring also provides information for public policy decisions related to nutrition education programs, such as the US Dietary Guidelines for Americans (20); public health programs, such as the National Cholesterol Education Program (12); and federally supported food assistance programs, such as the Special Supplemental Nutrition Program for Women, Infants, and Children (WIC) and school meals (9,15,16,21,22) and the Thrifty Food Plan (23).

Nutrition-monitoring data are also used to make public policy decisions related to the regulation of fortification, safety, and labeling of the food supply (24–26); food production and premarketing approvals; and food safety programs (10,26,27). Regulatory agencies have used data to provide dietary exposure estimates for nutrient and nonnutrient food components (10,26–28). In the early 1990s, the US president's science adviser identified the need for human nutrition research "that is ultimately aimed at promoting health, preventing disease, and reduc-

ing health care costs" (29). The NNMRRP supports research on the nutrient requirements throughout the life cycle and the development of the Dietary Reference Intakes (DRIs) and their applications (30), research on food composition and nutrient content and bioavailability (31–34), nutrition education research (8,11,14,35), research on the relationship of knowledge and attitudes to dietary and health behavior (36,37), and research on the economic aspects of food consumption (38,39). Data have also provided information about the role of nutrition in the etiology, prevention, and treatment of chronic diseases and conditions (11,14,15,30) and have been used to identify food and nutrition research priorities of significance to public health (11,30).

Applied nutrition research is conducted to improve survey methods (1,7,8,10,34), to interpret dietary intake and nutritional status (40,41), to measure food security (42–44), and to increase the capability to capture state and local nutrition information (7,45–47). For example, a Federal Working Group developed an 18-item household food security measure for national monitoring and a comparable six-item scale for use in state and local monitoring (42,43). An expert panel of the Institute of Medicine reviewed the 18-item measure and made specific recommendations on the concepts, definitions, and labeling of food security and hunger outcomes, and research needed to improve the measurement of the frequency and duration of food insecurity (44).

COMPONENTS OF NUTRITION-MONITORING MEASUREMENT

The first national dietary surveys were carried out in the 1930s. Since then, more than 40 surveys and surveillance systems have evolved in response to the information needs of federal agencies and other nutrition-monitoring data users. Chronological listings of past nutrition-monitoring surveys and activities have been published (1,2,6,7). The major data collection activities are briefly summarized in Table 10.1 and this chapter. More detailed descriptions can be found in *Nutrition Monitoring in the United States: The Directory of Federal and State Nutrition Monitoring and Related Research Activities* (47), as well as previous publications (1,7,48). The directory includes a section on nutrition-monitoring research activities, but it has not been updated since 2000. Therefore, federal agencies' Web sites are the best source of current nutrition-monitoring surveys and surveillance and research activities.

TABLE 10.1 Major Federal Nutrition Monitoring Surveys and Surveillance Activities in 2007 [a, b]

Date Initiated	Department	Agency	Survey	Target US Population	Sample Size and Type	Response Rate[c]	Comments
Nutrition and related health measurements							
Continuous (1915)	HHS	CDC/NCHS	National Vital Registration System	Total US population	All births and deaths in the US	—	Complete coverage
Annual (1957)	HHS	CDC/NCHS	National Health Interview Survey (NHIS)	Civilian, noninstitutionalized household population	98,649 individuals, 39,509 households	87% household; 69% adult; 78% children	2005 survey
1999- (1971)	HHS, USDA	CDC/NCHS, ARS for dietary component (beginning in 2002)	National Health and Nutrition Examination Survey	Civilian, noninstitutionalized individuals. Oversampling of African Americans, Mexican Americans, persons ages 12-19 y and ≥ 60 y (and in 1999-2003, pregnant women).	~5,000/y examined; 21,004 interviewed and 19,759 examined in 1999-2002; 10,122 interviewed and 9,643 examined in 2003-2004	Interview response rate: 80% in 2001-2002 and 79% in 2003-2004; examination response rate: 76% in 2003-2004	Data are released in 2-year cycles (1999-2000; 2001-2002; 2003-2004, etc)
Continuous (1973)	HHS	CDC/NCCDPHP	Pregnancy Nutrition Surveillance System (PNSS)	Low-income, high-risk pregnant women	856,123 records (women)	—	2004; coverage reflects no. of women participating in programs in a given year in 25 states and 6 tribal governments
Continuous (1973; continuous since 1978)	HHS	CDC/NCCDPHP	Pediatric Nutrition Surveillance System (PedNSS)	Low-income, high-risk children, birth–age 20 y	10,630,483 records and 6,822,769 children ages < 5 y (most children are < 5 y)	—	2004; coverage reflects the no. of clinic visits in participating programs in 40 states and DC, Puerto Rico, and 6 tribal governments
Food and nutrient consumption							
Continuous (1917)	DOD	USARIEM	Nutritional Evaluation of Military Feeding Systems and Military Populations	Enlisted personnel of the Army, Navy, Marine Corps, and Air Force; limited cadet population	20-240 individuals, depending on study focus	90%-99%	
Continuous (1980)	DOL	BLS	Consumer Expenditure Survey (expenditures on food purchases)	Civilian, noninstitutionalized population and a portion of the institutionalized population	7,500 households per/quarter; 6,000 individuals per y	85% for households; 87% for individuals	Quarterly interview survey of consumer units; Diary survey of consumer units kept for 2 consecutive 1-week periods

(Continued)

TABLE 10.1   (Continued)

Date Initiated	Department	Agency	Survey	Target US Population	Sample Size and Type	Response Rate[c]	Comments
Biennial 2004 (1992)	USDA	FNS	Study of WIC Participants and Program Characteristics	WIC participants identified using mail surveys of state and local WIC agencies, record abstractions at local WIC service sites	8,016,918 records in 2002	—	Near census of WIC participants
2005 (1992)	USDA	FNS	School Nutrition Dietary Assessment Study III	School-age children in grades 1-12 in 48 conterminous states and DC	Approx 300 schools and 2,300 students in 2005; 1,576 schools in 2002	80% for schools and 88% for menu survey in 2002	2002 survey focused on meals offered and interviews of 1,075 cafeteria managers for the menu survey; 2005 survey also included students' 24-hour dietary intakes, heights, and weights
Annual supplement (Annually since 1995)	BLS, CB, USDA	FNS, ERS	Current Population Survey (CPS), Supplement on Food Security	Civilian, noninstitutionalized US population age ≥16 y	~55,500 for CPS	85% for 2003 supplement	
Knowledge, attitudes, and behavior assessments							
Periodic 2004 (1982)	HHS	FDA; NIH/NHLBI	Health and Diet Survey	Civilian, noninstitutionalized individuals in households with telephones, age ≥18 y, living in 50 states and DC	2,000 planned for 2004; 2,743 in 2002	41% in 2002	
Continuous (1984)	HHS	CDC/NCCDPHP	Behavioral Risk Factor Surveillance System (BRFSS)	Individuals age ≥18 y residing in households with telephones in participating states, DC, Puerto Rico, US Virgin Islands, and Guam	2,000-4,000 per state	80% in 1995	
Food composition and nutrient data bases							
Continuous (1892)	USDA	ARS	National Nutrient Data Bank Food Composition Laboratory	—	1,000 key foods; 3,000 foods in the Primary Nutrient Data Set; 80 nutritional components; 65	—	

					nutrients in Standard Reference File	
Annual (1961)	HHS	FDA	Total Diet Study	Representative diets of specific age-sex groups	280 foods	2003 market basket survey
Continuous (1977)	USDA	ARS	Food and Nutrient Database for Dietary Studies and Survey Nutrient Database for Trends Analysis; Pyramid Servings and Servings Database	Used for CSFII and NHANES and other dietary studies	—	—
Continuous (1999)	HHS, USDA	NIH, ARS	Dietary Supplement Ingredient and Labeling Database	Dietary supplements	—	—
Food supply determinations						
Annual (1909)	USDA	ERS, ARS, CNPP	US Food and Nutrition Supply Series: Estimates of Food Available and Estimates of Nutrients	—	400 commodity foods	100 key foods, energy and 60 nutrients/components
Annual (1909)	DOC	NOAA/NMFS	Fisheries of the United States	Civilian residents, US population	—	—
Continuous (1985)	USDA	ERS, CNPP	AC Nielsen SCANTRACK (scanned data in supermarkets) and Homescan Consumer Panel	Supermarkets in 52 major markets for SCANTRACK; households in 23 major markets for the consumer panel	4,800 supermarkets; 61,500 households (15,000 for fresh foods)	85% for households in Homescan

[a]Note that listings are in chronologic order based on date of inception (in parentheses).

[b]ARS, Agricultural Research Service; BLS, Bureau of Labor Statistics; CB, Census Bureau; CDC, Centers for Disease Control and Prevention; CNPP, Center for Nutrition Policy and Promotion; DOC, Department of Commerce; DOD, Department of Defense; DOL, Department of Labor; ERS, Economic Research Service; FDA, Food and Drug Administration; FNS, Food and Nutrition Service; HHS, Department of Health and Human Services; HRSA, Health Resources Services Administration; NA, not available; NCCDPHP, National Center for Chronic Disease Prevention and Health Promotion; NCHS, National Center for Health Statistics; NHLBI, National Heart, Lung, and Blood Institute; NIH, National Institutes of Health; NMFS, National Marine Fisheries Service; NOAA, National Oceanic and Atmospheric Administration; USARIEM, US Army Research Institute of Environmental Medicine; USDA, US Department of Agriculture; WIC, Special Supplemental Nutrition Program for Women, Infants, and Children.

— = Not applicable.

[c]Percentage of sample population that responded.

Nutrition and Related Health Measurements

Nutrition and related health data have a wide variety of applications to policy making, research, health and nutrition education, medical care practices, and reference standards. The cornerstone of this NNMRRP measurement component, the NHANES, provides national data on the nutritional status, dietary intake, and numerous health indexes of the US population (1–3,7,8,48–51). It also provides national population reference distributions, national prevalences of diseases and risk factors, and trends in nutrition and health status over time. The design for the third NHANES (1988 to 1994) emphasized producing reliable national estimates for the total US noninstitutionalized population, as well as Mexican Americans, African Americans, older persons, and children younger than 6 years (52). Physical measurements, such as body measurements, blood pressure, findings of dental examinations, and results of biochemical and hematologic tests, allow for studying the relationships among diet, nutrition, and health. Beginning in 1999, the NHANES had a continuous, annual design and oversampled Mexican Americans, African Americans, older persons, adolescents, and pregnant females (in 2000, it also began oversampling low-income persons) (49–51). (*Oversampling* occurs when certain groups are sampled with higher probabilities than others to provide adequate sample sizes for reliable estimates for these groups.) NHANES follow-up studies allow epidemiologic investigations of the relationships of nutrition and health to risk of death and disability.

The National Health Interview Survey (NHIS) annually provides information about self-reported health conditions. It periodically provides information about special nutrition and health topics, such as vitamin/mineral supplement use, youth risk behavior, aging, food program participation, diet and nutrition knowledge, cancer, disabilities, and food preparation. Other special supplements relate to the tracking of US health and nutrition objectives (53). Large sample sizes enable data to be reported for the major racial/ethnic subgroups in the US population in addition to age group, gender, and income level.

A number of other surveys and surveillance systems, primarily conducted by the CDC, also contribute nutrition-related health information, particularly for low-income pregnant women, infants, and children who participate in publicly funded health, nutrition, and food assistance programs (45,47,54). These surveillance systems provide data representative of the participating populations in participating states and include physical measurements such as height, weight, hemoglobin levels, and hematocrit levels but

also information such as breastfeeding status and TV and video watching habits of children who participate in WIC.

For example, the Pediatric Nutrition Surveillance System (PedNSS), which has been sponsored since 1973, is used to monitor indicators of nutritional status (eg, anemia, birth weight, weight) among low-income, high-risk infants and children who participate in publicly funded health, nutrition, and food assistance programs (47,54,55). The Pregnancy Nutrition Surveillance System (PNSS), sponsored since 1973 and in continuous operation since 1978, tracks nutrition-related problems and behavioral risk factors associated with low birth weight among high-risk prenatal populations (47,54,55).

Food and Nutrient Consumption

Food and nutrient consumption measurements include estimates of individuals' intakes of foods and beverages (nonalcoholic and alcoholic) and nutritional supplements, as well as levels of nonessential nutrients, such as dietary fiber. The Continuing Survey of Food Intakes by Individuals (CSFII) of the USDA and the NHANES of the US Department of Health and Human Services (HHS), the two cornerstone NNMRRP surveys, were established to provide national estimates of food and nutrient intakes in the general US population and subgroups. The CSFII (which was integrated within the NHANES in 2002) emphasized the food and nutrient intake of the general population and the low-income population (1,10,34,56,57). It collected data on dietary intake on two independent days and captured information on economic variables, such as where food was purchased and where food was eaten. The NHANES III collected information on one day of intake and on a second day on a subsample. Prior to their integration, both surveys covered intake for all days of the week and all the seasons. In the NHANES, dietary intake is related to health status in the same individuals; in addition, racial-ethnic determinants of health are emphasized. These surveys also can be used to compare intake with Food Guide Pyramid food groups; to assess adherence to the Dietary Guidelines using the Healthy Eating Index; and to assess nutrient adequacy and excess using the DRIs (30). In addition to, and together with, the FDA's Total Diet Study (58), these studies provide the potential to assess levels of additives and pesticides in diets consumed. NHANES III data were used to prepare methylmercury intake estimates for the 1997 US Environmental Protection Agency *Mercury Study Report to Congress*, which looked at human exposure to mercury from fish and shellfish intake (28).

As noted, the NHANES and CSFII were integrated within the continuous NHANES framework as *What We Eat in America,* and the CSFII is no longer conducted (10,50,51,57). Prior to the integration, the HHS and the USDA jointly implemented improvements in sample design, dietary methodologies, and related survey questionnaires. The survey now includes a nationally representative annual sample of African-American, white, and Mexican-American persons for all-income and low-income households, as well as a common dietary data collection and processing system, the Automated Multiple Pass Method (AMPM) (34,51). Beginning in 2002, the NHANES included two days of intake per examined person (one day in person and a second on the telephone) for the estimation of usual nutrient intake and a food propensity questionnaire for the estimation of usual food intake (10,49–51). The National Cancer Institute (NCI) developed the food propensity questionnaire to assess infrequently consumed foods to augment the two dietary recalls (59).

Periodic assessments of food and nutrient consumption have been conducted for specific subgroups of the population that were not adequately covered in national surveys—military populations, American Indians, children, and low-income populations (17,47). A Supplemental Children's Survey was conduced by the USDA from 1997 to 1998 specifically to assess pesticide exposure in the diets of infants and young children (56). Since 1995, a special yearly supplement to the US Census Bureau's Current Population Survey (CPS) has been devoted to measuring the extent of food insecurity and hunger among people living in US households (42,44). In addition, the NHANES (beginning in 1999), the Survey of Program Dynamics, and the US Department of Education's Early Childhood Longitudinal Study (kindergarten cohort in 1998 and birth cohort in 2000) have incorporated the measure.

Evaluations of the USDA nutrition and food assistance programs are routinely conducted. For example, the Adult Day Care Program Study and the Early Childhood and Child Care Study each determined the characteristics and dietary intakes of their participants and of the day-care centers participating in the Child and Adult Care Food Program. A number of studies have been conducted to evaluate the nutrition and health effects of participating in WIC; to provide current participant and program characteristics; and to describe the infant feeding practices of WIC participants, including breast-feeding initiation and duration, formula feeding, and the introduction of supplementary foods (21,46,47). The first School Nutrition Dietary Assessment Study assessed the diets of American schoolchildren and the contribution of the National School Lunch Program to overall nutrient intake in 1992 (60). A second study was conducted to compare changes in the food and nutrient content of USDA school meals and food service operations (22). A third study in 2005 (not yet published) collected measures of students' heights and weights and diets and information on the school food environment, including the availability of foods and beverages in vending machines and school stores (61).

Knowledge, Attitude, and Behavior Assessments

National surveys that measure knowledge, attitudes, and behavior about diet and nutrition and how they relate to health were added to the nutrition-monitoring program in the mid-1980s. In general, the Health and Diet Survey, sponsored by numerous agencies, focuses on people's awareness of relationships between diet and risk for chronic disease, on health-related knowledge and attitudes, and on weight-loss practices (62,63). The Diet and Health Knowledge Survey (initiated by the USDA in 1989 and last conducted in 1994–1996) focused on the relationship of individuals' knowledge and attitudes about dietary guidance and food safety to their food choices and nutrient intakes (56). There are plans to collect similar information in a future NHANES module.

Surveys addressing specific topics have been periodically conducted to meet specific data needs, such as NCI's 5-A-Day for Better Health Baseline Survey in collaboration with the food industry to assess knowledge, behavior, and attitudes about fruits and vegetables; the FDA's study of consumer food-handling practices and awareness of microbiological hazards; and FDA studies to evaluate the features and usability by consumers of the Nutrition Facts label (50).

The Behavioral Risk Factor Surveillance System (BRFSS), initiated in 1984, focuses on personal behavior (such as diet, physical activity, and weight-loss practices) and nutritional and health status. It has been used by state health departments to plan, initiate, and guide health promotion and disease prevention programs, as well as to monitor their progress over time (37,45,64,65). In 2002, BRFSS data became available for prevalence estimates of metropolitan and micropolitan statistical areas, allowing the CDC to make county estimates to assist local public health planners and program evaluators (37,64). The Youth Risk Behavior Survey monitors priority health risk behaviors such as smoking, diet, physical activity, and weight-loss practices among adolescents through national, state, and local surveys (66,67).

Food Composition and Nutrient Databases

Since 1892, the USDA has operated the National Nutrient Data Bank to derive representative nutrient values for more than 6,000 foods and as many as 80 components consumed in the United States. Data are obtained from the food industry, USDA-initiated analytic contracts, and the scientific literature. Values from the data bank are released as part of the USDA Nutrient Data Base for Standard Reference, which is updated annually to reflect changes in the food supply and in analytic methodology. These values are used as the core of most nutrient databases developed in the United States for special purposes, such as databases used in the commercially available dietary analysis programs (31,33,34,68).

The FDA's Total Diet Study (58) provides annual food composition analysis based on the foods consumed most frequently in the CSFII and the NHANES. Representative foods are collected from retail markets, prepared for consumption, and analyzed individually for nutrients and other food components at the Total Diet Laboratory to estimate consumption of selected nutrients, minerals, and organic and elemental contaminants.

Food Supply Determinations

Since 1909, US food supply estimates have indicated levels of foods and nutrients available for consumption. These data, updated and published annually by the USDA as the US Food and Nutrient Supply Series, are used to assess the potential of the US food supply to meet the nutrition needs of the population and changes in the food supply over time. The data are also used to evaluate the effects of technological alterations and marketing changes on the food supply over time; to study the relationships between food and nutrient availability and nutrient-disease associations; and to facilitate the management of federal marketing, food assistance, nutrition education, food enrichment, and fortification policy. Conducted annually by the National Marine Fisheries Service, the Fisheries of the United States survey provides annual estimates of fish and shellfish disappearance in the distribution system (47).

Since 1985, monthly and annual proprietary sales data purchased from AC Nielsen Company have been used to measure grocery store sales of all scannable packaged food products (47,69), as well as fruits and vegetables and many prepared foods from the supermarket. Supermarket scanner data (SCANTRACK) do not reflect some prepared foods from the supermarket, or foods from restaurants or other food outlets. Households participating in the Homescan

Consumer Panel transmit data on scanned purchases, including fresh foods, weekly through a telephone line.

NUTRITION-MONITORING RESOURCES AVAILABLE TO RESEARCHERS

Published Scientific and Technical Reports

A number of scientific and technical reports have been periodically produced under the guidance of the Interagency Board for Nutrition Monitoring and Related Research (1,47,48,70–72). Scientific reports provide summary statistics on the dietary and nutritional status of the American population, as well as recommendations to improve the program. Research summaries and full reference citations can be found in the *Third Report on Nutrition Monitoring in the United States* (48). *Nutrition Monitoring in the United States: The Directory of Federal and State Nutrition Monitoring and Related Research Activities* (47) provides information on the multitude of surveys, surveillance systems, and selected research activities completed or under way in 2000 at the federal level, as well as some state-level surveys. The online publication provides hypertext links to Web sites that describe each activity in more detail (47).

Technical reports on applied research methods have been published to standardize the data collection and reporting of data from the program. Examples include reports on sociodemographic indicators (71) and dietary assessment methods (41,72,73). These reports have improved the coordination of nutrition-monitoring and research activities across the program and have documented national survey methods so that state and local researchers can use common data collection methods to compare state and local data with national data.

Progress has been made in using electronic bulletin boards to announce or distribute survey data, survey reports, and nutrition-monitoring publications and to distribute data in various electronic forms. In addition, increased efforts are being directed toward instructing users on how to access, process, and interpret data appropriately via the provision of training manuals, survey documentation on methods and quality control procedures, data user conferences at national and regional levels, and the use of Listservs.

One widely used training tool is the interactive CDC Growth Chart Training for health care professionals (74). The training modules include background information on the 2000 CDC Growth Charts, guidance on how to use and interpret the growth charts, and clinical applications of the charts (74). The *NHANES III Anthropometric Procedures Video* enables RDs and other nutrition professionals to collect data comparable to national data (75). It demonstrates the standardized anthropometric procedures that were used to collect body measurements. This allows others to follow the NHANES anthropometric methodology and enable researchers to compare data collected in local clinics and other population-based studies with national reference data.

Other Sources of Information on Nutrition Research

The Internet has greatly facilitated access to information (see Box 10.1). Research abstracts and, in many cases, the actual reports of findings can be found on-line. For example, the federal Human Nutrition Research and Information Management system database maintained by the National Institutes of

Health (NIH) is a searchable database that includes national nutrition-monitoring research and applied methodologies supported in whole or in part by the federal government.

A useful guide on NIH research activities is found in a periodic report entitled *National Institutes of Health Program in Biomedical and Behavioral Nutrition Research and Training*. Other health resources at the NIH include consumer health publications, information on clinical trials, health hotlines, Grateful Med, and the NIH Health Information Index (refer to Box 10.1). The NIH Health Information Index is a subject-word guide to diseases and conditions under investigation at NIH and helps users find the NIH institute that supports research related to a given health concern.

At the CDC, NCHS data systems include data on vital statistics, as well as information on health status, lifestyle, exposure to unhealthy influences, the onset and diagnosis of illness and disability, and the use of health care. The

BOX 10.1   Sources of Federal Information on Nutrition Research, Surveys, and Data Sets

---

Centers for Disease Control and Prevention: http://www.cdc.gov
- National Center for Chronic Disease Prevention & Health Promotion: http://www.cdc.gov/nccdphp
- National Center for Environmental Health: http://www.cdc.gov/nceh
- National Center for Health Statistics: http://www.cdc.gov/nchs
- National Health and Nutrition Examination Survey: http://www.cdc.gov/nchs/nhanes.htm
- Nutrition Monitoring Directory: http://www.cdc.gov/nchs/data/misc/direc-99.pdf
- Prevention Research Centers: http://www.cdc.gov/prc
- Publications and Products: http://www.cdc.gov/doc.do/id/0900f3ec8021ee7a

Federal Electronic Research and Review Extraction Tool (FERRET): http://www.cdc.gov/nchs/datawh/ferret/ferret.htm

Food and Drug Administration Center for Food Safety and Applied Nutrition: http://vm.cfsan.fda.gov

National Institutes of Health: http://www.nih.gov
- Dietary and nutrition measurements: http://dietary-supplements.info.nih.gov
- Health Information Index, Health Hotlines, clinical trials: http://www.nih.gov/health
- Human Nutrition Research and Information Management: http://hnrim.nih.gov
- Internet Grateful Med: http://www.nlm.nih.gov/services/igm.html
- MEDLARS: http://www.nlm.nih.gov/bsd/mmshome.html
- MEDLINE, PubMed: http://www.pubmed.gov

National Marine Fisheries Service surveys: http://www.nmfs.noaa.gov

US Department of Agriculture: http://www.usda.gov
- AGRICOLA: http://www.nal.usda.gov
- Agricultural Research Service (ARS): http://www.ars.usda.gov/main/site_main.htm?modecode=12-35-50-00
- Center for Nutrition Policy and Promotion: http://www.cnpp.usda.gov
- Economic Research Service: http://www.ers.usda.gov/briefing
- Food and Nutrition Service: http://www.fns.usda.gov/oane
- Food Surveys Group (ARS): http://www.ars.usda.gov/Services/docs.htm?docid=7787

National Center for Chronic Disease Prevention and Health Promotion carries out surveillance and behavioral research and demonstration projects on maternal and child health, as well as chronic disease prevention, and the National Center for Environmental Health covers public health surveillance and applied research (eg, epidemiologic studies, laboratory analyses, statistical analyses, and behavioral interventions). CDC's Network of Prevention Research Centers includes academic researchers, public health agencies, and community members that conduct applied research in disease prevention and control.

The FDA's Center for Food Safety and Applied Nutrition Web site includes publications pertaining to scientific research and regulatory programs. Many of the published studies have had a direct impact on consumer protection, such as the development of methods for monitoring contaminants in foods.

The USDA Food and Nutrition Service Web site provides information on published reports and ongoing research in the areas of child nutrition programs, the Food Stamp Program, food security, and WIC. The Center for Nutrition Policy and Promotion links policy with research. As a result, the center publishes information on the Dietary Guidelines for Americans and USDA's MyPyramid. The Economic Research Service (ERS) publishes food and nutrition assistance programs reports and information on research-funding opportunities, and these can be downloaded at the ERS Web site. (Refer to Box 10.1.)

Thousands of scientific journals contain information about federal and nonfederal nutrition research. To find the most current listing of journals, researchers are encouraged to use the Internet to search MEDLINE/PubMed and AGRICOLA (AGRICultural OnLine Access) (refer to Box 10.1). AGRICOLA gives citations for journal articles, monographs, theses, audiovisual materials, and technical reports relating to all aspects of agriculture, whereas MEDLINE is a biomedical database with citations from journal articles only. Both databases can be used to retrieve journal abstracts. The use of a database requires the development of a search strategy. A search strategy contains the key words, phrases, or terms of interest; synonyms for these terms; and how they should be combined.

Data Sets for Secondary Data Analysis

The surveys of the National Nutrition Monitoring Program generate a large amount of data. For selected surveys, agencies produce data sets for public use and publish survey findings in government and peer-reviewed reports. Many agencies offer information on CD-ROMs or on-line along with documentation on sampling methods, survey design, sample sizes, and survey instruments and questionnaires. Consult the survey Web sites for agency-specific information on ways to obtain data sets.

On-line data tables can also be found at many Web sites. NCHS releases short reports and Health-E Stats and the CDC publishes the Morbidity and Mortality Weekly Report (MMWR) online. ARS posts numerous dietary intake data tables on its survey Web site. The Web sites for the major surveys and surveillance systems have been included as references in this publication. In other cases, agencies provide data for a cost. Some agencies make data sets available through the National Technical Information Service. Other reports and documents are available from the US Government Printing Office.

The Federal Electronic Research and Review Extraction Tool (FERRET), a government-developed computer search tool, enables users to access and manipulate large demographic and economic data sets over the Internet. FERRET provides one-stop access to statistics from the CPS, the Survey of Income and Program Participation, and NCHS data systems. FERRET allows users to quickly locate current and historical information from these sources, get tabulations for specific information they need, make comparisons between different data sets, create simple tables, and download large amounts of data from the Internet to computers for custom reports.

For agency-specific information on ways to obtain data sets, see agency Web sites. Many agencies that conduct national nutrition surveys maintain lists of peer-reviewed research articles or bibliographies of survey findings. These references can be found by visiting the surveys' home pages.

Limitations and Other Factors in Survey and Surveillance Data Analysis

When analyzing survey and surveillance data, one must consider whether the data are suitable for the questions being asked. The design of the survey, the strengths and weaknesses of the methods used, and the introduction of bias must all be considered. Bias in survey or surveillance data can arise from errors in the sampling process and coverage of the target population, from the lack of response to the survey by respondents and/or particular groups of respondents, and from measurement error. Chapter 3 describes four types of research errors that can lead to biased results: sampling, noncoverage, nonresponse, and measurement errors. For purposes of this chapter and the consideration of whether survey and surveillance data may be biased, errors are described for two areas: (a) *sampling bias,* which includes sampling and noncoverage errors, and (b) *nonsampling bias,* which includes nonresponse and measurement errors as well as data processing errors. Researchers must learn to evaluate surveys and surveillance data to assess whether bias has been introduced, and if so, what can be done to minimize its effects on the analysis and interpretation of the data.

Sampling Bias

Examples of sampling bias include frame bias and consistent sampling bias. A *frame* is the sampling list used when the listing of the sampling units in the population is too difficult or tedious. Frame bias can be caused by the use of an incomplete list. For example, a sample based on a listing of telephone numbers for a particular city or geographic area would include only those households that have telephones or telephone numbers in a directory. The sample would therefore be biased in two directions: neither households without telephones nor households with unlisted numbers would be represented. The sample would likely underrepresent low-income households and people who prefer unlisted numbers.

Consistent sampling bias can be introduced by the mechanical procedures used to select units from the frame into the sample. In the telephone survey example, a consistent sampling bias could arise if the sample of telephone numbers were contacted from 9 AM to 5 PM on weekdays. Employed persons and students would be unlikely to be at home during those hours.

Decisions are sometimes made to narrow the areas covered in area probability samples to reduce the costs associated with collecting the data. These decisions can lead to noncoverage bias (ie, the failure to include elements in the sample that would properly belong in the sample). For example, the exclusion of areas with a low Hispanic population from the Hispanic Health and Nutrition Examination Survey resulted in a slight underrepresentation of more affluent Hispanics in the sample (76).

Nonsampling Bias

Nonsampling bias arises from systematic errors related to nonresponse, measurement, or data processing. Nonresponse bias results from the failure to obtain observations on some elements selected and designated for the sample. This bias occurs because people are not at home despite repeated attempts to contact them, they refuse to participate, or they are incapacitated and unable to participate. This bias

also occurs because of lost data, such as lost interviews and laboratory accidents. Incomplete reporting is a potential for bias in survey and surveillance data. Missing data elements should be excluded from analyses.

Statisticians frequently use the survey response rate as an overall indicator of the quality of a survey. When a substantial proportion of the sample selected for a survey does not participate, a potential for bias exists if the nonrespondents differ from the respondents in some systematic way. The greater the nonresponse, the greater the potential for bias.

Even when a substantial proportion of the original sample does not participate in the survey, the sample may not be biased, and studies of nonresponse bias can be performed. These types of studies have been performed for some of the national surveys (48). Nonresponse bias analyses to examine whether there were systematic differences between samples interviewed but not examined and the examined samples were performed for the NHANES I, II, and III and found no evidence of bias (77–79).

Measurement bias or *measurement error* refers to consistent errors arising in the interview or laboratory method used to obtain the data. In 24-hour dietary recalls, measurement bias can be introduced through the interview methods (eg, when probing for amounts of fat or alcoholic beverage consumption), coding assumptions (eg, rules for assigning default codes), errors in the food composition database used to estimate nutrient levels, or selection of days of the week to conduct the interviews. Systematic bias with respect to underreporting energy intake with the 24-hour recall method is well-established (30,80,81), and its impact on the interpretation of national dietary intakes has been studied (41,57,69,81).

Sample Weights and Design Effects

The statistical technique used to identify survey samples introduces complexities into the analysis of the data. In area probability sampling, some trade-offs are made in the randomness of the sample to minimize the costs of the survey. The technique is multistage, and at each stage, sample elements with a known probability are selected. In the NHANES, the stages of selection are defined as counties, areas within counties (called *segments*), households, and household members. To produce the estimates for the nation based on observations from individuals, the data for individuals must be inflated by their probability of selection, adjusted for nonresponse, and then poststratified to bring the population estimate into close agreement with the US Census Bureau estimates. To make these procedures easier for the users of the survey data, sample weights incorporating the three levels of adjustments appear on the public-use data files. For weighted analyses, analysts can work with special computer software packages that use an appropriate method for estimating variances for complex samples, such as SUDAAN (82), WesVarPC (83), and STATA (84).

Area probability samples are not simple random samples, and the assumptions of simple random sampling do not apply when hypothesis testing is performed with survey data. Data sets distributed by the NCHS and other sources describe special computer programs that take into account the complex nature of the sample and the design effect in the calculation of test statistics (49,85). Many national surveys, such as the NHANES, have a complex survey design and use clustered sampling rather than simple random sampling. The design effect is the ratio of the true variance of a statistic (taking the complex sample design into account) to the variance of the statistic for a simple random sample with the same number of cases. Design effects differ for different subgroups and different statistics; no single design effect is universally applicable to any given survey or analysis. The design effect can be used to adjust estimates and statistics computed by using assumptions of simple random sampling for the complexities in the sample design (86).

Determining whether a subsample is free of bias involves comparing the subsample with the overall sample for characteristics related to the subject of inquiry. Whenever analyses of this type are performed, it is essential that the analytic subsample be examined for bias and that the sample weights and design effects be used in the analysis.

Program Participation Data

Surveillance data collected on women and children participating in publicly funded food assistance, nutrition, or health programs involve a self-selected population and thus are not representative of the community at large. Factors that differentiate members of this group from the general population include their meeting the income eligibility level, having a nutritional or health risk, and having the personal initiative or knowledge to participate in available programs. The PedNSS and PNSS involve primarily low-income populations and have overrepresentation by racial and ethnic minority populations in comparison with the general population (55). Although the surveillance population does not represent all women and children in the state, the data can be representative of program participants and thus be useful for planning public health and nutrition programs and evaluating the impact of these programs on the nutrition and health status of the target populations (54,55). Eligibility criteria can vary from state to state and

over time, making comparisons across states and time difficult. Knowledge of program enrollment criteria and changes in criteria over time is important for appropriately interpreting nutrition surveillance data.

Quality of Data

Nutrition surveillance data are collected in more than 4,000 public health clinics across the country, and each data set has its own quality issues. Clinic staff members have a wide range of expertise in nutrition assessment and data collection. Calibrated equipment, periodic training of staff, and quality control and assurance programs are important aspects of maintaining high-quality surveillance data. Consultation, training, and written protocols are available from the CDC (45,55). In recent years, emphasis has been placed on improving the quality control of data collected in the surveillance systems.

National surveys that collect physical measurements, such as the NHANES, have extensive quality control and assurance programs, as well as well-documented data collection and laboratory protocols (47,49). However, data quality may be a concern with national survey methods. Researchers should review the survey methods and quality control procedures and data prior to their analysis and interpretation of the data.

Survey and surveillance data collected through personal or proxy interviews are self-reported data and thus subject to error. Inaccuracy may be related to poor recall; sensitivity to, or lack of understanding of, the question; or lack of knowledge to answer the question. For example, it has been shown that self-reported heights and weights are biased; men report being taller than they are, and women report weighing less than they actually do (87). Parents' reporting of their children's heights and weights has also been shown to be inaccurate (88); however, maternal recall of infant birth weight has been validated and shown to be accurate (89). Interviewer training on how to ask sensitive questions and elicit responses can improve the quality of self-reported data.

GETTING STARTED ON YOUR OWN RESEARCH

What Is Your Area of Interest, and How Will Your Research Be Put to Use?

Before you begin your research, it is important to ask yourself certain questions: What is my outcome of interest? Is it, for example, nutrition and food security of people who participate in one of the food assistance programs? Is it how effectively knowledge and attitudes about nutrition translate into action? Is the purpose of the study to determine whether an intervention has had an impact on health status (eg, whether it has lowered blood cholesterol levels or blood pressure)? The purpose could also be to determine whether participation in a given program has saved health care dollars or lives. Perhaps you are interested in the general population, children, older Americans, a particular racial or ethnic group, people with low incomes, or pregnant women.

Nutrition-monitoring information may be used in several ways: for analysis of raw survey data to answer your research questions about trends in diet and nutritional status or about national incidences or estimates, to study relationships of diet and health, to investigate the contribution of diet and supplements to total nutrient intake, to cite published findings or reference data, or to use national methods in your own research study. If you are designing your own study, you may want to use national data collection and survey tools to allow data comparisons.

Before starting your research, it is important to decide what practical applications it will have. In other words, will you be enhancing the pool of knowledge, and will the findings be useful to you and others? Perhaps the research will be used to develop educational programs. Alternatively, it might be used to develop a tool to evaluate a program or to evaluate an intervention. Research you conduct might be used to develop new food products or test their attributes. It might be used to set reference standards or to promulgate policy.

What Resources and Data Sets Are Available and Relevant?

Once you decide in what nutrition-monitoring measurement area your interests lie, it is useful to go to key sources, such as survey Web sites, journals, and reference reports, and determine whether a certain survey or surveillance system includes variables of interest. Journal articles and federal agency Web sites provide information on recent studies that may be pertinent to your area of research (49–55,85). Reference materials provide information on normal values or targets to which your findings can be compared.

Remember, too, that there are benefits and trade-offs when using a public-access data set, as opposed to collecting your own data. For example, surveys such as the NHANES provide a nationally representative sample, do not require that you spend time and money collecting data, and are recognized as credible sources of data. However, in using these survey results, you might be limited to the use of variables that did not exactly meet your needs, and you might not get information about your particular population of interest.

Who Is Your Audience?

Before beginning your research, you will need to decide whether it can be translated for use by its intended audience. Therefore, knowledge of your beneficiaries is important. Perhaps your research will benefit consumers who are looking for information to make decisions about their nutrition and health. Public and private policy makers might use research findings as a basis for creating dietary guidance materials and programs to enhance the nutritional quality of food supplies, provide food assistance, and evaluate policies. Health educators might make use of your findings to develop a framework for population subgroups and disease prevention guidelines. Physicians and other health professionals might use your research to keep abreast of current knowledge or to provide dietary recommendations to patients. Food, nutrition, and health associations may use knowledge gleaned from your study to set policy or to educate their constituencies. The media might use your research as an educational tool or for background information. Finally, trade associations and people in industry might use it to develop guidelines for product improvement.

What Are Your Resources and Level of Expertise?

Before embarking on your research project, you should know your financial and staffing resources and constraints. Do not underestimate the financial, human, and labor resources that are required to conduct research. You will need to determine whether your staff has the expertise and ability to analyze survey data that use a complex design. Depending on resources and appropriateness, you may decide to conduct one of the different types of studies described in Chapters 2, 6, and 8, or you may decide to analyze data from one of the surveys or surveillance activities described in this chapter. Another consideration is the sample size required to obtain estimates of interest (see Chapter 27). The length of time you have to conduct your research might also influence your study design and other options. If you are collecting dietary intake data, NCI provides a review of dietary methods and research studies and considerations for selecting a dietary method to meet your data needs (90). Other publications can help you apply the DRIs to group dietary data (30).

CONCLUSION

The national nutrition surveys and state surveillance systems offer a broad array of information for policy making and research opportunities for RDs and other nutrition professionals. For example, survey data can be used to study the relationship between dietary intake and nutritional status and obesity among high-risk groups, or the effect of changes in food fortification on the nutrient status of target groups. Surveillance data can be used to track dietary behaviors among population subgroups over time in relation to assessing or planning health promotion activities. Nutrition monitoring data sets may not include adequate sample sizes for some population groups of interest or local areas, but they do provide a reference population for comparison to other research studies.

Surveys and surveillance systems are also a source of well-tested survey instruments, methods, and data collection protocols that can be used or adapted for data collection in research studies. Care must be taken when analyzing the data, from both a statistical and an interpretive standpoint (76). Careful interpretation of trends in diet, nutritional status, or health in the population involves consideration of changes and improvements in data collection and laboratory methods (91). A number of resources are available on federal agency Web sites to assist with locating this information.

REFERENCES

1. Briefel RR. Nutrition monitoring in the United States. In: Bowman B, Russell R, eds. *Present Knowledge in Nutrition.* 9th ed. Washington, DC: ILSI Press; 2006.

2. Woteki CE, Klein RR, Klein CJ, Jacques PF, Kris-Etherton PM, Mares-Perlman JA, Meyers LD. Nutrition monitoring: summary of a statement from an American Society for Nutritional Sciences Working Group. *J Nutr.* 2002;132:3782–3783. (Data supplement available at: http://www.nutrition.org/cgi/data/132/12/3782/DC1/1.)

3. US Congress. *National Nutrition Monitoring and Related Research Act of 1990.* Washington, DC: 101st Congress; 1990. Pub L 101–445.

4. Ostenso GL. National Nutrition Monitoring System: a historical perspective. *J Am Diet Assoc.* 1984;84:1181–1185.

5. Mason JB, Habicht J-P, Tabatabai H, Valverde V. *Nutritional Surveillance.* Geneva, Switzerland: World Health Organization; 1984.

6. US Department of Health and Human Services and Department of Agriculture. *Proposed Ten-Year Comprehensive Plan for the National Nutrition Monitoring and Related Research Program.* Washington, DC: US Government Printing Office; 1991. Publication 91-25967:SS 716-55767.

7. US Department of Health and Human Services and US Department of Agriculture. *Ten-year Comprehensive Plan for the National Nutrition Monitoring and Related Research Program.* Washington, DC: US Government Printing Office; 1993. Publication 58:32752–32806.

8. Woteki CE. Integrated NHANES: Uses in national policy. *J Nutr.* 2003;133(suppl):582S–584S.

9. Sims LS. Research aspects of public policy in nutrition generating research questions to determine the impact of nutritional, agricultural, and health care policy and regulations on the health and nutritional status of the public. The Research Agenda for Dietetics Conference Proceedings. *J Am Diet Assoc.* 1992;92:25–38.

10. Murphy SP. Collection and analysis of intake data from the integrated survey. *J Nutr.* 2003;133(suppl):585S–589S.

11. US Department of Health and Human Services. *Healthy People 2010: Understanding and Improving Health.* 2nd ed. Washington, DC: US Government Printing Office; 2000. Available at: http://www.healthypeople.gov. Accessed February 13, 2007.

12. National Cholesterol Education Program. *Third Report of the National Cholesterol Education Program (NCEP) Expert Panel on Detection, Evaluation, and Treatment of High Blood Cholesterol in Adults (Adult Treatment Panel III).* Bethesda, Md: National Heart, Lung, and Blood Institute; 2002. NIH publication 02-5215.

13. Centers for Disease Control and Prevention. Recommendations to prevent and control iron deficiency in the United States. *MMWR Morb Mortal Wkly Rep.* 1998;47(RR-3):1–29.

14. National Heart, Lung, and Blood Institute. *Seventh Report of the Joint National Committee on Prevention, Detection, Evaluation, and Treatment of High Blood Pressure (JNC 7).* Washington, DC: US Department

of Health and Human Services; 2004. DHHS publication 04-5230.

15. Fox MK, Hamilton W, Biing-Hwan L. *Effects of Food Assistance and Nutrition Programs on Nutrition and Health.* Vol 4: Executive Summary of the Literature Review. Washington, DC: Economic Research Service, USDA; 2004. Food Assistance and Nutrition Research Report No. 19-4.

16. Committee on National Statistics. National Research Council. Institute of Medicine. *Evaluating Food Assistance in an Era of Welfare Reform. Summary of a Workshop.* Washington, DC: National Academies Press; 1999.

17. Poos M, Costello R, Carlson-Newberry SJ. Institute of Medicine, Food and Nutrition Board. *Committee on Military Nutrition Research Activity Report 1994–1999.* Washington, DC: National Academies Press; 1999.

18. Kuczmarksi RJ, Ogden CL, Grummer-Strawn LM, et al. *CDC Growth Charts: United States.* Washington, DC: National Center for Health Statistics; 2000.

19. Centers for Disease Control and Prevention. What Is Epi Info? Available at: http://www.cdc.gov/epiinfo. Accessed February 13, 2007.

20. US Department of Health and Human Services and Department of Agriculture. *Dietary Guidelines for Americans, 2005.* 5th ed. Washington, DC: US Government Printing Office; 2005. HHS publication HHS-ODPHP-2005-01-DGA-A. USDA Home and Garden Bulletin No. 232.

21. Bartlett S, Bobronnikov E, Pacheco N, et al. WIC Participant and Program Characteristics 2004. Summary. Alexandria, Va: Food and Nutrition Service; 2006. Available at: http://www.fns.usda. gov/NU/Published/WIC/FILES/pc2004.pdf. Accessed February 13, 2007.

22. Fox MK, Crepinsek MK, Connor P, Battaglia M. *School Nutrition Dietary Assessment Study-II. Final Report.* Alexandria, Va: Food and Nutrition Service; 2001.

23. Carlson A, Kinsey J, Nadav C. Revision of USDA's low-cost, moderate-cost, and liberal food plans—Center Reports—United States Department of Agriculture. *Fam Econ Nutr Rev.* Spring 2003.

24. Lewis CJ, Crane NT, Wilson DB, Yetley EA. Estimated folate intakes: data updated to reflect food fortification, increased bioavailability, and dietary supplement use. *Am J Clin Nutr.* 1999;70:198–207.

25. US Department of Health and Human Services, Food and Drug Administration. Notice of final rule:

food labeling: health claims and label statements; dietary fiber and cardiovascular disease; dietary fiber and cancer. *Federal Register.* January 5, 1993; 2552–2605.

26. Anderson SA, ed. *Estimation of Exposure to Substances in the Food Supply.* Bethesda, Md: Life Sciences Research Office; 1988.

27. Institute of Medicine. *Estimating Consumer Exposure to Food Additives and Monitoring Trends in Use.* Washington, DC: National Academy Press; 1992.

28. US Environmental Protection Agency, Office of Air Quality Planning & Standards and Office of Research and Development. *Mercury Study Report to Congress.* Washington, DC: Environmental Protection Agency; 1997. EPA-452/R-97-003.

29. Office of Science and Technology Policy, Executive Office of the President. *Meeting the Challenge. A Research Agenda for America's Health, Safety, and Food.* Washington, DC: US Government Printing Office; 1996.

30. Institute of Medicine, Food and Nutrition Board. *Dietary Reference Intakes: Applications in Dietary Assessment.* Washington, DC: National Academies Press; 2001.

31. Haytowitz DB, Pehrsson PR, Smith J, Gebhardt SE, Matthews RH, Anderson BA. Key foods: setting priorities for nutrient analyses. *J Food Comp Analysis.* 1996;9:331–364.

32. Schakel SF, Buzzard IM, Gebhardt SE. Procedures for estimating nutrient values for food composition databases. *J Food Comp Analysis.* 1997;10:102–114.

33. Anderson E, Perloff B, Ahuja JKC, Raper N. Tracking nutrient changes for trends analysis in the United States. *J Food Comp Analysis.* 2001;13:287–294.

34. Raper N, Perloff B, Ingwersen L, Steinfeldt L, Anand J. An overview of USDA's dietary intake data system. *J Food Comp Analysis.* 2004;17: 545–555.

35. Randall B, Sprague K, Connell DB, Golay J. WIC Nutrition Education Demonstration Study: Prenatal Intervention. Alexandria, Va: Food and Nutrition Service, US Department of Agriculture; 2001. Available at: http://www.fns.usda.gov/oane/MENU/ Published/WIC/FILES/WICNutEdPrenatal.pdf. Accessed February 13, 2007.

36. Wooden J, Oakland MJ, Jensen HH, Kissack P. Food label use by older Americans: data from the Continuing Survey of Food Intakes by Individuals 1994–96. *J Nutr Elderly.* 2004;24:35–52.

37. Centers for Disease Control and Prevention. Health Risks in the United States: Behavioral Risk Factor Surveillance System. At a Glance 2006. Available at: http://www.cdc.gov/nccdphp/publications/aag/brfss.htm. Accessed February 13, 2007.

38. Lu N, Samuels ME, Huang KC. Dietary behavior in relation to socioeconomic characteristics and self-perceived health status. *J Health Care Poor Underserved.* 2002;13:241–257.

39. Putnam JJ, Allshouse JE. *Food Consumption, Prices, and Expenditures, 1970–97.* Washington, DC: US Department of Agriculture; 1999. Statistical Bulletin No. 965. Available at: http://www. ers.usda.gov/publications/sb965/sb965a.pdf. Accessed February 13, 2007.

40. Briefel RR. Assessment of the US diet in national nutrition surveys: national collaborative efforts and NHANES. *Am J Clin Nutr.* 1994;59(suppl): S164–S167.

41. Briefel RR, Sempos CT, McDowell MA, Chien S, Alaimo K. Dietary methods research in the third National Health and Nutrition Examination Survey: underreporting of energy intake. *Am J Clin Nutr.* 1997;65(suppl):S1203–S1209.

42. Economic Research Service. Food Security in the United States. Available at: http://www.ers.usda.gov/briefing/foodsecurity. Accessed February, 13 2007.

43. Blumberg SJ, Bialostosky K, Hamilton WL, Briefel RR. The effectiveness of a short form of the Household Food Security Scale. *Am J Public Health.* 1999;89:1231–1234.

44. National Research Council. Panel to Review the US Department of Agriculture's Measurement of Food Insecurity and Hunger. *Food Insecurity and Hunger in the United States. An Assessment of the Measure.* Washington, DC: National Academies Press; 2006.

45. Centers for Disease Control and Prevention. Behavioral Risk Factor Surveillance System. State Information. State-by-State Listing of How Data Are Used. Available at: http://www.cdc.gov/ brfss/dataused.htm. Accessed February 13, 2007.

46. National Research Council. Committee on National Statistics. *Summary of Workshop on Food and Nutrition Data Needs.* Washington, DC: National Academies Press; 2004.

47. Bialostosky K, ed. *Nutrition Monitoring in the United States: The Directory of Federal and State Nutrition Monitoring and Related Research Activities.* Hyattsville, Md: National Center for Health Statistics; 2000. DHHS publication 00-1255. Available at: http:// www.cdc.gov/nchs/data/misc/direc-99.pdf. Accessed July 16, 2006.

48. Life Sciences Research Office, Federation of American Societies for Experimental Biology. *Third Report on Nutrition Monitoring in the United States: Volumes 1 and 2. Prepared for the Interagency Board for Nutrition Monitoring and Related Research.* Washington, DC: US Government Printing Office; 1995.

49. National Center for Health Statistics. National Health and Nutrition Examination Survey. Available at: http://www.cdc.gov/ nchs/nhanes.htm. Accessed February 13, 2007.

50. National Center for Health Statistics. DHHS-USDA Survey Integration—What We Eat in America. Available at: http://www. cdc.gov/nchs/about/major/nhanes/faqs.htm. Accessed February 13, 2007.

51. Agricultural Research Service, Food Surveys Research Group. What We Eat in America. Available at: http://www.barc.usda.gov/bhnrc/foodsurvey/home.htm. Accessed February 13, 2007.

52. US Department of Health and Human Services, National Center for Health Statistics. *Third National Health and Nutrition Examination Survey, 1988–94, Reference Manuals and Reports* [survey on CD-ROM]. Hyattsville, Md: Centers for Disease Control and Prevention; 1996.

53. National Center for Health Statistics. National Health Interview Survey. Available at: http://www.cdc.gov/nchs/nhis.htm. Accessed February 13, 2007.

54. Polhamus B, Thompson D, Dalenius K, Borlande E, Smith B, Grumer-Strawn L. Pediatric Nutrition Surveillance. 2004 Report. Centers for Disease Control and Prevention; 2006. Available at: http://www.cdc.gov/pednss/pdfs/PedNSS_2004_Summary.pdf. Accessed February 13, 2007.

55. Centers for Disease Control and Prevention. *Pediatric and Pregnancy Nutrition Surveillance System.* Available at: http:// www.cdc.gov/pednss. Accessed February 13, 2007.

56. Tippett KS, Enns CW, Moshfegh AM. Food consumption surveys in the US Department of Agriculture. *Nutr Today.* 1999;34: 33–46.

57. Dwyer J, Picciano MF, Raiten DJ, Members of the Steering Committee. Estimation of usual intakes: What We Eat in America–] NHANES. *J Nutr.* 2003;133(suppl):609S–623S.

58. Pennington JAT, Capar SC, Parfitt CH, Edwards CW. History of the Total Diet Study (Part II). *J AOAC Int.* 1996;79:163–170.

59. National Cancer Institute. Risk Factor Monitoring and Methods. How Is NCI Supporting the NHANES? Available at: http://www. riskfactor.cancer.gov/ studies/nhanes. Accessed February 13, 2007.

60. Burghardt JA, Devaney BL, Gordon AR. The School Nutrition Dietary Assessment Study: summary and discussion. *Am J Clin Nutr.* 1995;61(suppl): S252–S257.

61. Food and Nutrition Service. The School Nutrition Dietary Assessment Study III Overview. http://www.fns.usda.gov/oane/menu/SNDAIII/ SNDAIIIOverview.pdf. Accessed April 25, 2007.

62. Heaton AW, Levy AS. Information sources of US adults trying to lose weight. *J Nutr Educ.* 1995;27:182–190.

63. Lin C-TJ, Choiniere C. FDA Health and Diet Survey—2004 Supplement. Fats and Carbs: A Snapshot of Consumer Knowledge from a Recent FDA Survey. Available at: http://www. cfsan.fda.gov/~comm/crnutri2.html. Accessed February 13, 2007.

64. Centers for Disease Control and Prevention. Behavioral Risk Factor Surveillance System. Available at: http://www.cdc.gov/brfss. Accessed February 13, 2007.

65. Figgs LW, Bloom Y, Dugbatey K, Stanwyck CA, Nelson DE, Brownson RC. Uses of Behavioral Risk Factor Surveillance System data, 1993–1997. *Am J Public Health.* 2000;90:774–776.

66. Kann L, Kinchen SA, Williams BI, et al. Youth Risk Behavior Surveillance—United States, 1997. State and local YRBS coordinators. *J Sch Health.* 1998;68:355–369.

67. Centers for Disease Control and Prevention. Assessing Health Risk Behaviors among Young People: Youth Risk Behavior Surveillance System. At a Glance 2004. Available at: http://www.cdc.gov/ nccdphp/publications/aag/yrbss.htm. Accessed February 13, 2007.

68. Agricultural Research Service. Welcome to the Nutrient Data Laboratory Home Page. Available at: http://www.ars.usda.gov/main/ site_main.htm?modecode=12354500. Accessed February 13, 2007.

69. National Research Council. Panel on Enhancing the Data Infrastructure in Support of Food and Nutrition Programs, Research, and Decision Making. *Improving Data to Analyze Food and Nutrition Policies.* Washington, DC: National Academies Press; 2005.

70. Ervin B, Reed D, eds. *Nutrition Monitoring in the United States. Chartbook I: Selected Findings from the National Nutrition Monitoring and Related Research Program.* Hyattsville, Md: Public Health Service; 1993. DHHS publication (PHS) 93-1255-2.

71. Survey Comparability Working Group. *Improving Comparability in the National Nutrition Monitoring and Related Research Program: Population Descriptors.* Hyattsville, Md: National Center for Health Statistics; 1992.

72. National Center for Health Statistics. Wright J, Ervin B, Briefel R, eds. *Nutrition Monitoring and Tracking the Year 2000 Objectives.* Hyattsville, Md: National Center for Health Statistics; 1994.

73. Briefel RR. Assessment of the US diet in national nutrition surveys: national collaborative efforts and NHANES. *Am J Clin Nutr.* 1994;59(suppl): S164–S167.

74. Centers for Disease Control and Prevention. CDC Growth Chart Training. Available at: http://www.cdc.gov/nccdphp/dnpa/ growthcharts/ index.htm. Accessed February 13, 2007.

75. National Center for Health Statistics. *NHANES III Anthropometric Procedures* [videotape]. Washington, DC: US Government Printing Office; 1996. Stock Number 017-022-01335-5.

76. Woteki CE, Wong FL. Interpretation and utilization of data from the National Nutrition Monitoring System. In: Monsen ER, ed. *Research: Successful Approaches.* Chicago, Ill: American Dietetic Association; 1992:204–219.

77. Landis JR, Lepkowski JM, Eklund SA, Stehouwer SA. *A Statistical Methodology for Analyzing Data from a Complex Survey: The First National Health and Nutrition Examination Survey.* Washington, DC: US Government Printing Office; 1992. DHHS publication 82-1366. Vital and Health Statistics, Series 2, No. 92.

78. Forthover RN. Investigation of nonresponse bias in NHANES II. *Am J Epidemiol.* 1983;117: 507–515.

79. Khare M, Mohadjer LK, Ezzati-Rice TM, Waksberg J. An evaluation of nonresponse bias in NHANES III (1988–91). *1994 Proc Section Survey Research Methods, Am Stat Assoc.* 1995;2: 949–954.

80. Bingham SA. The dietary assessment of individuals: methods, accuracy, new techniques, and recommendations. *Nutr Abst Rev.* 1987;57:705–742.

81. Institute of Medicine. Food and Nutrition Board. *Dietary Reference Intakes: Energy, Carbohydrate, Fiber, Fat, Fatty Acids, Cholesterol, Protein, and Amino Acids.* Washington, DC: National Academies Press; 2004.

82. Shah BV, Barnwell BG, Bieler GS. *SUDAAN User's Manual: Software for Analysis of Correlated Data. Release 6.04.* Research Triangle Park, NC: Research Triangle Institute; 1995.

83. Westat Inc. *A User's Guide to WesVarPC.* Rockville, Md: Westat; 1996.

84. Stata Corporation. *STATA Statistical Software for Professionals. Release 9.* Available at: http://www.stata.com. Accessed February 13, 2007.

85. National Center for Health Statistics. Current NHANES Web Tutorial. Available at: http://www.cdc.gov/nchs/tutorials/currentnhanes/index.htm Accessed April 25, 2007.

86. Rust KF, Rao JN. Variance estimation for complex surveys using replication techniques. *Stat Methods Med Res.* 1996;5:283–310.

87. Rowland ML. Self-reported weight and height. *Am J Clin Nutr.* 1990;52:1125–1133.

88. Davis H, Gergen PJ. Mexican-American mothers' reports of the weights and heights of children 6 months through 11 years old. *J Am Diet Assoc.* 1994;94:512–516.

89. Gayle HD, Yip R, Frank MJ, Nieburg P, Binkin NJ. Validation of maternally reported birthweights among 46,637 Tennessee WIC program participants. *Public Health Rep.* 1988;103:143–147.

90. National Cancer Institute. Risk Factor Monitoring and Methods. Dietary Intakes: What We've Learned: Measuring Intakes. Available at: http://riskfactor.cancer.gov/diet/learned/measure.html. Accessed February 13, 2007.

91. Briefel R, Johnson C. Secular trends in dietary intake in the United States. *Annu Rev Nutr.* 2004;24:401–431.

PART 5

Integrative and Translational Research

11

—ᴍ—

Meta-analysis in Nutrition Research

Judith Beto, PhD, RD

This chapter introduces the concept of meta-analysis, with a focus on the practical application both as a research technique and as a clinical practice component. The strengths and limitations of meta-analysis are presented. Comparisons are made with traditional narrative and newer systemic review formats found in the scientific literature.

TERMINOLOGY

Meta-analysis is a formal, defined data system to combine results of numerous small independent studies. By using the statistical power of a larger merged sample size, the combined results mathematically and theoretically represent the estimated outcome as if the merged data set originally existed as a single larger study. Meta-analysis seeks to merge the reported results of similar research studies to mathematically answer specific, quantitative questions.

Glass originally used the term *meta-analysis* in 1976, to describe the technique used to systematically examine the relationship between class size and student achievement (1). Chalmers brought the term into the field of medical science and health care evaluation (2). Others followed with statistical methods to address the challenges of more heterogeneous data sets (3–5). The methods continue to evolve as researchers strive to create mathematical models to address variations in study design, quality of study data reported, and/or baseline population differences. For

example, the effect of initial body weight needs to be considered when combining trials on weight reduction. The effect of a 25-pound weight loss on cardiovascular risk would be dramatically different if a patient's baseline study weight was 125 pounds compared with 325 pounds.

The validity of a meta-analysis should be judged based on identical standards used to ensure quality and rigor in traditional research evaluation. Researchers should clearly state their hypothesis to define the research question. They should clearly outline specific inclusion-exclusion criteria before searching for studies and provide a stepwise methods section to help the reader understand the process used to pool and analyze the final set of studies. Without these steps, readers will be unable to understand whether the reported results apply to their own practice situations.

Nutrition is a relatively recent topic for meta-analysis. This is primarily because randomized interventions with placebo controls are not common in nutrition studies. (Many nutrition studies examine long-term intake patterns within uncontrolled lifestyle settings.) Table 11.1 lists selected meta-analyses of nutrition-related studies (6–18).

Several of the meta-analyses listed in Table 11.1 also include a systematic review of the literature within the same publication (12,18). A systematic review provides an organized, narrative evaluation of a cohort of studies without a mathematical evaluation. Authors may include the "leftover" studies in this manner. This is most commonly done when insufficient data are available to perform a meta-analysis (eg, when only three studies in a subgroup

TABLE 11.1 Examples of Nutrition Research Meta-analyses Using Both Traditional Methodology of Randomized Clinical Trials and Less Traditional Use of Observational Epidemological Databases

Year Published	Authors	Meta-analysis Research Topic
2003	Huncharek M et al (6)	Dietary cured meat and risk of adult glioma
2003	Rand WM et al (7)	Nitrogen balance studies for estimating protein requirements in healthy adults
2004	Opperman AM et al (8)	Health effects of using the glycemic index in meal planning
2004	He K et al (9)	Fish consumption and incidence of stroke
2004	Etminan T et al (10)	Role of tomato products and lycopene in the prevention of prostate cancer
2005	Cohen JT et al (11)	Prenatal intake of n-3 polyunsaturated fatty acids and cognitive development
2005	Martin RM et al (12)	Breastfeeding and childhood cancer
2005	Harder T et al (13)	Duration of breastfeeding and risk of overweight
2005	Stratton RJ et al (14)	Enteral nutritional support in prevention and treatment of pressure ulcers
2005	Peter JV et al (15)	Treatment outcomes of early enteral vs early parenteral nutrition in hospitalized patients
2006	Pavia M et al (16)	Association between fruit and vegetable consumption and oral cancer
2006	He FJ et al (17)	Fruit and vegetable consumption and incidence of stroke
2006	Akobeng AK et al (18)	Effect of breastfeeding on risk of celiac disease

meet similar criteria). The terms *systematic review* and *meta-analysis* are not interchangeable (see Table 11.2). Although systematic reviews are an organized and methodical way to write a narrative review, they do not require the rigor and objective mathematical testing required in a meta-analysis (19).

The Cochrane Collaboration is a not-for-profit international organization that provides up-to-date information on a variety of health care topics. More than 13,000 people from over 100 countries have created more than 2,500 current reviews, and more than 1,000 planned reviews are in progress. Recently, the concept of "cumulative" meta-analysis has

TABLE 11.2 Comparison of Meta-analysis and Systematic Review Methodology

Initial Research Question	Meta-analysis Required	Systematic Review Required
Detailed research protocol	Required; needs narrow research question scope	May be less stringent or wider in research question scope
Inclusion/exclusion criteria	Required; tight definition limits inclusion to studies that theoretically could have been one original single multicenter trial	Less stringent; can combine a greater diversity of study designs, participants, research questions, and outcome variables
Exhaustive literature search	Required; usually limited to peer-reviewed published data	Required; may include wider variety of study designs
Data extraction	Studies must share common design and outcome measure	Studies may have variable design and outcome measures
Design of studies	Must use similar design; randomized studies cannot be combined with observational cohort	Study design can be used as a grouping variable for result summary
Mathematical or other quantitative comparison measure	Required; size of study is reflected in weighted variance giving larger effect to larger studies	Not required; percentages and defined outcomes by study groupings replace simple "vote counting"
Evaluating statistical validity for comparison (heterogeneity of data)	Requires use of meta-analysis software or standardized estimate of effect models programmed into spreadsheets; funnel plots or Q statistics used to illustrate symmetry of data	No standardized mathematical formulas are used; no accepted visual or graphic representation of study homogeneity
Insufficient studies for comparison	Cannot be done unless sufficient data to analyze; only studies meeting strict criteria can be combined	Can be done with any amount of data; all studies can be grouped and treated in narrative nonmathematical summary
Scientific rigor	High rigor	Less rigor
Results presentation	Graphic presentation of odds ratios, effect sizes	Tabular form of studies with data

been introduced. Author groups are expected to continually survey clinical studies as they are published and recalculate effect sizes. The goal of this cumulative procedure is to theoretically accumulate evidence until the benefit (or lack of benefit) is objectively known and no further clinical trials are required to establish the research conclusions. Free access is provided to all peer-reviewed summaries. The Cochrane Collaboration also provides downloadable software (RevMan/Review Manager, Version 4.2.8, Cochrane Collaboration, 2006) to promote research interest in combining data (20).

META-ANALYSIS TECHNIQUE

A carefully executed meta-analysis follows a predefined rigorous protocol similar to traditional research. The key features are as follows (21,22):

- Following a defined stepwise procedure to search for, limit, and evaluate all data available
- Providing an objective and quantitative measure of evidence extracted from each study using a standardized data format
- Merging data of common outcome measures using established mathematical formulas to create a stronger statistical estimate through larger sample size
- Examining heterogeneity or differences among individual studies through use of statistical and graphic method
- Presenting results as measurable outcomes that can be translated into clinical practice through performance indicators such as number to treat or absolute risk differences

Meta-analysis research is conducted in the same manner as an original clinical trial. Investigators begin by writing a detailed research protocol, which is used as a template to search, collect, and analyze data. The components of the protocol are identical to those of traditional research (23). (See Chapter 9 for more information about specific components of research design, protocol writing, and implementation.)

Formulating the Research Question

Questions that lend themselves to meta-analysis usually involve comparison of two or more treatments or theories within a common disease or condition or within areas of practice where controversy exists. However, meta-analysis cannot answer all research questions. For example, it would be difficult to perform a successful meta-analysis of self-prescribed herbal therapies for fatigue. The outcome, fatigue, lacks a commonly accepted, clinically measurable definition (unlike blood pressure or body weight). Also, the dose and timing of various herbal treatments are not standardized.

A meta-analysis should begin with a clear, focused research question that seeks to resolve an issue or identify an area of unknown cause and probable effect. Strictly defined inclusion and exclusion criteria are essential to promote the combining of studies that are as similar in design and content as possible.

Completing an Exhaustive Literature Search

Initially, analysts should perform an exhaustive literature search. Chapter 12 covers this topic in detail. Meta-analyses traditionally include only published peer-reviewed studies, although initial identification of non-peer-reviewed literature and unpublished data can provide larger pools of potential publications.

Study Limitations and Data Extraction

All studies retrieved are evaluated against the strict inclusion and exclusion criteria. Studies that do not meet the criteria are documented for exclusion cause and removed from the analysis process. Studies that meet the criteria continue through the meta-analysis, moving to the step of data extraction using a standardized form. Most investigators create their own forms using a simple computer spreadsheet or checklist format tailored to the research question and outcome measures. Basic demographic data and other background information should be collected to describe the study population as part of the results. Reliability and validity of data should also be evaluated. For example, is the food frequency questionnaire (FFQ) used in one study comparable in content to the FFQ used in another study? Were the FFQs administered in a similar manner (eg, self-administered or interview-assisted, in person or by mail)? Were any validation studies done, such as comparing a 3-day food diary during the study to an earlier FFQ?

Meta-analyses usually include an additional step to assess study quality. A wide array of checklists, scales, and methods are used, and opinions about this process vary (24,25). Typically, more than one investigator completes both the data extraction and quality assessment procedures.

The investigators' data are compared, and discrepancies are resolved between them or by a third observer.

Computation of Study Effects

Next, the investigators transfer extracted data to a spreadsheet format. Examples of data are milligrams of vitamin C consumed per kilogram of body weight, presence or absence of a disease state such as diabetes, or a fasting serum glucose level. The researchers use appropriate meta-analysis techniques to combine the data by weighting each study outcome by the size of the study (number of participants) and the variability in the data reported within each study (standard deviation of mean). Because of the sample size, smaller studies will typically show more variability within a sample than larger studies (26,27). To help readers assess where true effects lie, the meta-analysis must give statistics for individual studies, grouped studies, and overall effects. Several computer programs can help generate the meta-analysis statistics, but the statistics also can be created with basic spreadsheets. In either case, the investigator must have a thorough understanding of the theory behind the meta-analysis models to make appropriate data decisions and use the correct statistical tests to test relationships. For example, a meta-analysis may show a 2% risk reduction in colon cancer incidence with a daily multivitamin supplement compared with no supplement. The 2% absolute risk difference is significant, but it may not be large enough to warrant a change in current practice.

Whenever possible, investigators are encouraged to translate the effect sizes found into implications for clinical practice. Absolute risk differences that compare two or more treatments with percentage changes may not be meaningful. In meta-analyses such as the example of colon cancer and multivitamins described earlier, it may be helpful to include the number needed to treat (NNT). In the colon cancer example, the NNT represents the number of patients who would need to receive the multivitamin supplement for the specified period of time to prevent one incidence of colon cancer (22).

Evaluation of Study Bias

Even when an exhaustive literature search is conducted, researchers must consider the possibility of study bias. Studies with positive results tend to be published far more frequently than studies showing negative or neutral results. Smaller studies may tend to report biased effects because of more diverse participants (28,29). Mathematical computations can be used to generate a heterogeneity index to rate the probability that the data could have existed as a single clinical trial and infer how reliably the data can be viewed when combined. Newer visual methods of funnel plots can show effect sizes of individual studies and look for symmetry patterns to estimate potential bias (30,31).

Presentation and Discussion of Results

As with any research study, the results should be presented in comprehensive tables and figures. The meta-analysis should provide tables summarizing the demographics and characteristics of the studies included in the analysis. The discussion should describe both the strengths and the limitations of the analysis.

CONCLUSION

Meta-analysis is an objective quantitative method to combine a body of similar clinical studies to increase the strength of the belief in the observed effect. It is comparable to a clinical trial in traditional research methodology and rigor. A randomized clinical trial with a comparison placebo-control group is the gold standard for inclusion in meta-analysis. Meta-analyses can provide evidence upon which to base practice patterns. Meta-analyses can help identify what new clinical studies need to be conducted to provide the missing evidence and then updated to incorporate new data.

More recent meta-analyses in nutrition have included cohort and observational studies to examine the effect of long-term intake of foods over time while correlating their effect to disease incidence. The use of these less controlled populations may result in observed trends rather than clear cause-effect relationships. Meta-analyses should be evaluated with the same concerns of general research for reliability, validity, and appropriate statistical techniques used in the execution of the research question.

REFERENCES

1. Glass GV. Primary, secondary and meta-analysis of research. *Educ Res.* 1976;5:3–8.
2. Maclure M. Dr. Tom Chalmers, 1917–1995: the tribulations of a trialist. *Can Med Assoc.* 1996;155:986–988.

3. Hedges LV, Olkin I. *Statistical Methods for Meta-analysis.* San Diego, Calif: Academic Press; 1985.

4. D'Agostino RB, Weintraub M. Meta-analysis: a method for synthesizing research. *Clin Pharmacol Ther.* 1995;58:605–616.

5. Egger M, Smith GD, Phillips AN. Meta-analysis: principles and procedures. *BMJ.* 1997;315:1533–1537.

6. Huncharek M, Kupelnick B, Wheeler L. Dietary cured meat and the risk of adult glioma: a meta-analysis of nine observational studies. *J Environ Pathol Toxicol Oncol.* 2003;22:129–137.

7. Rand WM, Pellett PL, Young VR. Meta-analysis of nitrogen balance studies for estimating protein requirements in healthy adults. *Am J Clin Nutr.* 2003;77:109–127.

8. Opperman AM, Venter CD, Oosthuizen W, Thompson RL, Vorster HH. Meta-analysis of the health effects of using the glycaemic index in meal-planning. *Brit J Nutr.* 2004;92:367–381.

9. He K, Song Y, Daviglus ML, Liu K, Van Horn L, Dyer AR, Goldbourt U, Greenland P. Fish consumption and incidence of stroke: a meta-analysis of cohort studies. *Stroke.* 2004;35:1538–1542.

10. Etminan T, Takkouche B, Caamano-Isorna F. The role of tomato products and lycopene in the prevention of prostate cancer: a meta-analysis of observational studies. *Cancer Epidemiol Biomarkers Prev.* 2004;13:340–345.

11. Cohen JT, Bellinger DC, Connor WE, Shaywitz BA. A quantitative analysis of prenatal intake of n-3 polyunsaturated fatty acids and cognitive development. *Am J Prev Med.* 2005;29:366–374.

12. Martin RM, Middleton N, Gunnell D, Owen CG, Smith GD. Breast-feeding and cancer: the Boyd Orr cohort and a systematic review with meta-analysis. *J Natl Cancer Inst.* 2005;97:1446–1457.

13. Harder T, Bergmann R, Kallischnigg G, Plagemann A. Duration of breastfeeding and risk of overweight: a meta-analysis. *Am J Epidemiol.* 2005;162:397–403.

14. Stratton RJ, Ek AC, Moore Z, Rigby P, Wolfe R, Elia M. Enteral nutritional support in prevention and treatment of pressure ulcers: a systematic review and meta-analysis. *Ageing Res Rev.* 2005;4:422–430.

15. Peter JV, Moran JL, Phillips-Hughes J. A meta-analysis of treatment outcomes of early enteral versus early parenteral nutrition in hospitalized patients. *Crit Care Med.* 2005;33:213–220.

16. Pavia M, Pileggi C, Nobile CG, Angelillo IF. Association between fruit and vegetable consumption and oral cancer: a meta-analysis of observational studies. *Am J Clin Nutr.* 2006;83:1126–1134.

17. He FJ, Nowson CA, MacGregor GA. Fruit and vegetable consumption and stroke: meta-analysis of cohort studies. *Lancet.* 2006;367:320–326.

18. Akobeng AK, Ramanan AV, Buchan I, Heller RF. Effect of breastfeeding on risk of coeliac disease: a systemic review and meta-analysis of observational studies. *Arch Dis Child.* 2006;91:39–43.

19. Mullen PD, Ramierz G. The promise and pitfalls of systematic reviews. *Annu Rev Public Health.* 2006;27:81–102.

20. The Cochrane Collaboration. Available at: http://www.cochrane.org. Accessed June 10, 2006.

21. Schultze R. *Meta-analysis: A Comparison of Approaches.* Toronto, Canada: Hogrefe and Huber; 2004.

22. Riegelman RK. *Studying a Study and Testing a Test: How to Read the Medical Evidence.* 5th ed. Philadelphia, Pa: Lippincott Williams and Wilkins; 2005.

23. Leedy PD, Ormrod JE. *Practical Research: Planning and Design.* 8th ed. New York, NY: Prentice-Hall; 2004.

24. Chalmers TC, Smith H Jr, Blackburn B, Silverman B, Schroeder B, Reitman D, Ambroz A. A method for assessing the quality of a randomized control trial. *Control Clin Trials.* 1981;2:31–49.

25. Moher D, Jadad AR, Nichol G, Penman M, Tugwell P, Walsh S. Assessing the quality of randomized controlled trials: an annotated bibliography of scales and checklists. *Control Clin Trials.* 1995;16:62–73.

26. Ades AE, Lu G, Higgins JP. The interpretation of random-effects meta-analysis in decision models. *Med Decision Making.* 2005;25:646–654.

27. Laird NM, Mosteller F. Some statistical methods for combining experimental results. *Int J Technol Assess Health Care.* 1990;6:5–30.

28. Dickersin K, Chan S, Chalmers TC, Sacks HS, Smith H Jr. Publication bias and clinical trials. *Control Clin Trials.* 1987;8:343–353.

29. Dickersin K. The existence of publication bias and risk factors for its occurrence. *JAMA.* 1990;263:1385–1389.

30. Hayashino Y, Noguchi Y, Fukui T. Systematic evaluation and comparison of statistical tests for publication bias. *J Epidemiol.* 2005;15:235–243.

31. Terrin N, Schmid CH, Lau J. In an empirical evaluation of the funnel plot, researchers could not visually identify publication bias. *J Clin Epidemiol.* 2005;58:894–901.

12

—ᴍ—

Systematic Reviews to Support Evidence-Based Practice

Esther F. Myers, PhD, RD, FADA, Patricia L. Splett, PhD, RD, FADA,
and Suzanne Brodney Folse, PhD, RD

The relationship between research and practice in dietetics is a two-way interaction. Research findings are translated into dietetics practice, and dietetics practice identifies questions that need to be researched. This dynamic relationship has become even more evident with the widespread adoption of evidence-based medicine (EBM), also called evidence-based practice (EBP). Evidence relative to a specific practice question is brought together through the process of a systematic review that includes searching for, selecting, critically evaluating, synthesizing and grading the reports, and disseminating the systematic review results. The resulting document represents a summary and synthesis of the best available data, which is then used to develop evidence-based recommendations and to aid practice decisions. Documents summarizing systematic reviews are intended to inform and guide choices made by health care practitioners and policy makers. The procedures used in the evidence analysis process must be explicit, transparent, and rigorous in terms of scientific methodology.

The American Dietetic Association (ADA) has embraced the concept of EBP and defined and identified key considerations of evidence-based dietetics practice (EBDP) (1,2): "Evidence-Based Dietetics Practice is the use of systematically reviewed scientific evidence in making food and nutrition practice decisions by integrating best available evidence with professional expertise and client values to improve health outcomes."

To fulfill this commitment, the ADA supports a specific system for evaluating and grading the evidence, and provides recommendations for medical nutrition therapy (MNT) protocols, practice guidelines, and other guides for dietetics practice. The ADA now uses a specific process to prepare the guides for clinical practice, known as *Evidence-Based Nutrition Practice Guidelines,* and has created reference manuals to support the development of evidence-based practice guidelines (1,3,4). Both practitioners and researchers make critical contributions to EBDP by identifying what questions are faced in clinical practice, by having knowledge of and ability to access a relevant body of research, by developing the ability to critically evaluate published research and other data sources, and by synthesizing best available evidence into summary documents.

This chapter provides an overview of EBDP and the systematic review process used to evaluate and present evidence. It includes examples or describes worksheets and the resulting summary documents from the EAL. The final section describes how various associations of health professionals and institutions use systematic reviews to support EBP.

EVIDENCE-BASED PRACTICE: AN OVERVIEW

In the 1980s, EBP began appearing in the medical literature; it became common terminology in the 1990s, and is an expectation of practice today (5). Two major applications of EBP are especially relevant to dietetics practice: (a) the review and synthesis of the best available evidence to create recommendations for a defined area of practice (guidelines development and health policy making), and (b) the search for scientific evidence to answer a specific question related to care for a specific patient or subgroup of patients (clinical decision making).

Evidence-based practice is guided by two fundamental principles. First, there is a hierarchy of strength of evidence behind recommendations. Second, the clinician uses judgment when weighing the trade-offs associated with alternative management strategies, including consideration of patient values and preferences as well as societal values (6,7).

The methodology for accessing, reviewing, and summarizing research has evolved, and several distinct methods are now acknowledged in the medical literature and widely used (6–14). The Agency for Healthcare Research and Quality (AHRQ; formerly called the Agency for Health Care Policy and Research) funded an evidence report/technology assessment to evaluate the systems used to rate the strength of scientific evidence (15). The report identified three important domains that should be addressed by systems to grade the strength of the evidence:

- **Quality**—how the system aggregated the quality ratings for individual studies and determined the extent to which bias was minimized in the body of research.
- **Quantity**—how the systems evaluated the magnitude of the effect, the number of research studies available, and the sample size/power of the research studies.
- **Consistency**—how the system ensured consistency in reporting similar findings from various research study designs.

Thirty-four evidence grading systems, in addition to systems being used by the six evidence practice centers of AHRQ, were evaluated in 2002. Seven systems were identified that fully addressed these three domains (7,12,14,16–19).

Many associations of health professionals, expert panels, and institutions have established mechanisms for conducting evidence reviews and producing clinical practice guidelines based on those reviews (8,9,20,21). The terminology and concepts of EBP are widely accepted and integrated into health care policy and academic curriculums despite the limitations of the current practice of grading the evidence used to develop recommendations for practice, and of inadequate documentation of the impact of the resulting clinical practice guidelines (20,22–24). Through

AHRQ Center for Practice and Technology Assessment, 12 evidence-based practice centers (EPCs) are funded to conduct evidence-based reviews on selected topics (25). The World Health Organization recently committed to a systematic evidence-based approach as the way to determine the upper intake levels for nutrients (26). The US Dietary Guidelines published in 2005 also noted the need to have a truly evidence-based approach to reviewing the research as the basis for establishing the US Dietary Guidelines and the Food Guidance system (27). Currently, evidence-based reviews are being conducted by clinicians in response to specific questions they face in practice. Groups of practitioners and researchers also conduct systematic reviews in important areas of practice and make the summary documents available. Practitioners and policymakers can then turn to these preprocessed reviews for information to guide decisions. Conducting systematic reviews has become an area of research in its own right, with research being conducted on the various methods involved in conducting systematic reviews (28).

Some critics of EBP consider it impossible to fully implement because of time demands and the lack of strong research in many areas of practice. Other critics contend that EBP is a dangerous innovation perpetrated to serve those desiring to cut costs and suppress freedom in clinical decision-making (29–33). Proponents have addressed these concerns and have clarified that evidence used in EBP is not limited to randomized trials and meta-analyses (7).

SYSTEMATIC REVIEWS USED IN EVIDENCE-BASED DIETETICS PRACTICE

EBDP relies on systematic reviews of the best available evidence. A systematic review is a form of research that provides a summary of medical reports on a specific clinical question, using explicitly defined methods to search, critically evaluate, and synthesize the world literature systematically (28). The key to this process is critical evaluation of available published research studies and other sources of data. Following are the essential steps of the process of systematically reviewing the evidence:

1. Identifying a specific problem or area of uncertainty
2. Formulating the problem as a question
3. Finding and selecting relevant evidence
4. Evaluating the research reports
5. Synthesizing the evidence and grading the evidence

6. Forming recommendations or making decisions using the best available evidence
7. Disseminating the findings

The difference between a traditional narrative review or review of literature and a systematic review is that the publication of a systematic review requires that the formal search strategy, formal method of evaluating the research reports, and formal methods of grading the research and making recommendations are clearly described. A traditional narrative review is usually based on a question, uses some method of searching and evaluating relevant evidence, and includes synthesis and potentially recommendations. A systematic review with data pooling and new statistical analysis is called a meta-analysis (see Chapter 11).

Various groups have organized the process of systematic review of evidence into four to eight steps or components (8,34–36). However, all descriptions incorporate the items in the seven listed steps, which will be discussed in this chapter. A basic requirement of the systematic review process used in EBDP is that a protocol—the methodology—must be articulated before the evidence search, review, and synthesis begins. In establishing the protocol, the reviewers must balance several objectives, some of which may conflict.

Identifying a Specific Problem or Area of Uncertainty

The process begins with identifying an area to be explored. This step is commonly driven by questions and uncertainties identified by practitioners or raised by other parties, such as payers. Following are types of general questions about nutrition services:

- Does MNT given by a registered dietitian (RD) result in changes in patients' levels of dietary fat, saturated fat, serum cholesterol, and cardiac risk factors?
- What is the optimal duration and frequency of follow-up visits for hypercholesterolemia by an RD using MNT?
- Do additional MNT visits with an RD result in further reductions in total and low-density lipoprotein cholesterol (LDL-C)?

Formulating the Question

EBDP focuses on the art of asking specific questions that can be answered using existing data, and that are relevant to clinical decision making. Questions about basic biological processes or background questions are not appropriate for EBDP; such questions would be better answered by appropriate texts on the topics (37). Craig et al provide a method for framing questions dealing with diagnosis, harm/etiology, prognosis, and intervention, all of which have a slightly different format for design of the question (37). The key components identified by Craig et al are:

- Patient population of concern
- Intervention
- Outcome
- Comparator
- Best feasible primary research study design
- Best MEDLINE search term for study type

Most questions in dietetics deal with treatment or prevention interventions, and these questions should include the following four components: (a) a population with the specific clinical problem; (b) an intervention, procedure, or approach (eg, the type, amount, or timing of MNT); (c) the comparator intervention (other approaches to care for the same clinical problem); and (d) the outcome of interest.

For example, a question using this format could be written as follows: "For adult patients with disorders of lipid metabolism, is including sterols and stanols in a cardioprotective diet more effective than a cardioprotective diet without sterols and stanols for reducing LDL-C and mortality?" The four components are addressed:

- **Patient population of concern:** Adult patients with disorders of lipid metabolism
- **Intervention:** Including sterols and stanols in a cardioprotective diet
- **Comparator:** A cardioprotective diet without sterols and stanols
- **Outcome:** Reducing LDL-C and mortality

In many instances, the systematic research protocol may start with a broad overarching question, such as the one above about stanols and sterols, which is then answered by several more specific subquestions that address various aspects of the overall question (3,36). Analytic frameworks may also be constructed to visually show how the subquestions relate to the overarching question (3). Following are examples of some of the pertinent subquestions that answer the broad question about whether to include stanols and sterols in a cardioprotective diet. In these cases, the "for adult patients with disorders of lipid metabolism" is presumed because the questions are located in the disorders of metabolism for adults topic area.

- What effect does the intake of plant sterols and stanols have on total cholesterol and LDL-C?
- How do sterols and stanols compare in terms of their efficacy in lowering LDL-C?
- How do esterified and non-esterified forms of stanols and sterols compare in terms of their cholesterol-lowering ability?
- How are the effects of stanols and sterols on cholesterol levels altered when eaten as part of a cholesterol-lowering (cardioprotective) diet?
- Can plant stanols further reduce LDL-C and total cholesterol in people receiving statin therapy?
- Can statin dose be reduced through the use of stanols and sterols?
- Are there any unintended adverse effects of consuming stanols and sterols?

Finding and Selecting the Relevant Evidence

After formulating the question that is the basis for the review, a search plan or protocol must be developed to identify all evidence in relevant research studies and other reports to ensure an unbiased review. The search plan should identify the databases to be searched and initial key search terms as well as the criteria a research report must meet to be included in the systematic review.

Searching for Evidence

The search plan usually starts with electronic databases. Some search strategies may also include hand searching of relevant resources (38). For example, the search protocol reported by the Cochrane Collaboration for nutrition supplementation after hip fracture included studies found using specified electronic databases (BIOSYS, CABNAR, CINAHL, EMBASE, HEALTHSTAR, and MEDLINE), reference lists in clinical trial reports and other relevant articles, investigators and experts, and a hand search of four nutrition journals.

Other search strategies may include other common databases such as CENTRAL database, LILAC, or CRISP database (3,36). The search plan should also specify whether the keyword must be in the title, abstract, or the text when using electronic databases, as well as the hand search methodology. Avenell et al concluded that if a researcher relied on just one of the most popular electronic databases, such as MEDLINE, only approximately half the studies would have been identified (39). Another source for identifying research reports is conference abstracts.

In 2003, Scherer et al reviewed more than 29,000 abstracts and estimated that 52.6% were published within 9 years of presentation as abstracts published in conference proceedings (40). Publication was linked to positive results (eg, defined as a result favoring the experimental treatment). The Cochrane Library also includes the CENTRAL database, which includes a comprehensive listing of randomized controlled trials (RCTs) and controlled clinical trials (41). In addition to the databases to be searched, the key search terms are identified in the search plan. Search terms need to be specific to the databases being searched (3).

Selecting the Evidence

In addition to identifying how to find the literature, the search plan includes explicit a priori criteria, called *inclusion and exclusion criteria*, that guide the filtering process to select the research reports to be included in the systematic review. Criteria should include the definition of the levels of evidence and preferred types of studies accepted for purposes of the review. Box 12.1 (6) shows the types of

BOX 12.1   Hierarchy of Strength of Evidence for Treatment Decisions

N of 1 randomized clinical controlled trial (RCT)*
Systematic review of randomized trials
Single randomized trial
Systematic review of observational studies addressing patient-important outcomes
Single observational study addressing patient-important outcomes
Physiologic studies
Unsystematic clinical observations

*The N of 1 RCT refers to a study design where patients undertake pairs of treatment periods in which they receive a target treatment in 1 period of each pair and a placebo or alternative in the other. Both patients and clients are blinded and the order of target and control treatment are randomized and study is continued until both patient and clinician conclude the benefit or lack of benefit of the target intervention. There are limited circumstances when this study design is feasible.

Source: Guyatt GH, Haynes RB, Jaeschke RZ, Cood DJ, Green L, Naylor CD, Wilson MC, Richardson WS. Users' Guides to the Medical Literature: XXV. Evidence-based medicine: principles for applying the Users' Guides to patient care. Evidence-Based Medicine Working Group. *JAMA.* 2000;284:1290–1296. Used with permission from American Medical Association. Copyright 2000 American Medical Association. All rights reserved.

studies used to make treatment decisions, arranged in a hierarchy according to strength of evidence. Although most search strategies limit eligible evidence to published peer-reviewed research, and favor evidence toward the top of the hierarchy, some institutions take a more liberal approach. For example, Goode reported that the University of Colorado model includes nine nonresearch sources of evidence in the multidisciplinary practice model: benchmarking data; clinical expertise; cost-effective analysis; pathophysiology; retrospective or concurrent chart review; quality improvement and risk data; international, national, and local standards; infection control data; and patient preferences (42).

In some cases, a protocol may indicate that the review will include only a specific number (eg, six) of the most important studies relevant to the question rather than listing all available studies (14). Limitation to a set number of research reports early in the process has a great potential for introducing bias. The careful implementation of a sound search plan is critical to a high-quality systematic review. Introducing bias in the selection of the research to be reviewed will seriously flaw the final systematic review. Cooper and Zlotkin described the importance of the filtering process used to apply the criteria in the selection of the research articles to be reviewed (43). Processes usually include at least two independent reviews of the article to determine whether it should be included in the review. The Cochrane Collaboration recommends using one expert and one non-expert in this process. Decisions about the types of research reports allowed and the search plan must be explicitly defined in the protocol, implemented as defined, documented, and described in the final summary document (3).

After articles and reports that contain potential evidence are located, each one must be carefully read to determine whether it meets the established criteria for inclusion (as defined in the protocol) and provides relevant evidence to answer the research question. The following are examples of the search plans for nutrition-related studies defined by the Cochrane Collaboration and by the ADA EAL.

Selection Criteria for Study of Hyperlipidemia by the Cochrane Collaboration

Randomized trials (44) of dietary advice given by an RD were compared with advice given by another health professional or self-help resources. The main outcome was differences in serum cholesterol levels between groups receiving RD advice and each of the other intervention groups. The following selection criteria were used:

- **Age**—Studies of individuals at least 18 years old.
- **Gender**—Both males and females.

- **Health**—Studies of patients with or without existing heart disease or previous myocardial infarction.
- **Setting**—Free-living subjects recruited from primary care settings, workplaces, outpatient clinics, and other community settings. Studies of patients who are hospitalized or living in institutions will be excluded.
- **Follow-up**—At least 6 weeks from the baseline visit.
- **Types of interventions**—Dietary advice primarily related to food intake rather than dietary supplements will be included. Advice may be about food preparation, shopping, and what foods to eat or avoid. Interventions are provided by health professionals. Self-help forms of dietary education will be included. Studies that include provision of meals and trials of lipid-lowering drugs where drugs are given to the intervention group only will not be included.
- **Primary outcomes**—Will be net change in serum cholesterol level. Secondary outcomes will be change in LDL-C, HDL-C, body mass index, and blood pressure. Data on patient satisfaction will also be examined.

The ADA's Search Plan for Stanols and Sterols on Adults with Disorders of Lipid Metabolism

The ADA Evidence Analysis Library includes the search plan that identified the research report inclusion and exclusion criteria, databases searched, and search terms used (45). (Refer to Box 12.2.)

Evaluating the Research Reports

The evaluation of each research report involves two processes: data abstraction and quality evaluation. Data from each of the eligible research reports are extracted according to the protocol. Some methodologies suggest that the abstraction process should vary depending on whether the question to be answered falls into the category of prognosis, diagnosis, treatment, or economic issues (8,18). The following types of data are usually extracted for each research report evaluated: author and date, methodology/type of study, number and characteristics of study participants, intervention, outcome measures, findings, and author's conclusions.

In addition to extracting information, various methods are used to evaluate the quality of each individual research report. The quality of each research report is evaluated using criteria relevant to the particular study design. The two instruments used to evaluate research by the ADA are included in Figures 12.1 and 12.2 (3).

The instruments used by the ADA include 10 validity questions based on the AHRQ domains for research studies. Subquestions are listed under each validity question that identify important aspects of sound study design and execution relevant to each domain (15). Some subquestions also identify how the domain applies to specific research designs. The quality criteria are applied based on the study design type.

QUOROM (Quality of Reports of Meta-analyses of Randomized Controlled Trials) has proposed a standard for the review and monitoring of systematic reviews and meta-analysis of randomized trials (46). In addition there are companion standards that suggest common evaluation criteria for clinical trials (CONSORT), for observational studies (STROBE), for meta-analysis of observational studies (MOOSE), and for studies of diagnostic accuracy (STARD) (47–50). Each of these documents consists of a checklist and flow diagram outlining the process. Although the QUORUM checklist is targeted for meta-analysis, many of the suggested criteria apply to systematic reviews that do not include meta-analysis. The criteria are similar to those included in the quality checklist for review articles used by the ADA (refer to Figure 12.2). The process of evaluating the quality of the evidence should have all the rigor of other scientific methods to ensure solid recommendations for clinical practice (35).

Synthesizing and Grading the Body of Evidence

Two related processes form the next step in the systematic review: the process of synthesizing the body of evidence and the process of grading the strength of the evidence.

Synthesizing the Body of Evidence

After the research reports have been evaluated individually, the body of research must be synthesized. Various methods are used. In the ADA's system, an Evidence Analysis Summary Table, Evidence Summary, and Conclusion Statement are prepared. Up until the synthesis of the body of evidence, the evidence-analysis process for EBDP is similar to meta-analysis. In a meta-analysis following a systematic review, data from individual studies may be pooled quantitatively and reanalyzed using established statistical methods. However, instead of combining the results data statistically, as is done in meta-analysis (refer to Chapter 11), the EBDP process synthesizes the body of evidence into supporting materials and a conclusion statement with a grade that is used to reflect the strength of the body of evidence that supports the conclusion statement.

The ADA uses several documents to show this synthesis. The first is an Evidence Summary Table, which extracts the key data from each study that relates to the question being answered (see Table 12.1). At the same

---

BOX 12.2   Example of Search Inclusion and Exclusion Criteria

Date Searched: March 2004
Inclusion Criteria
- English only
- Published after 2001
- Human subjects
- Sample > 10 in each treatment group
- Drop-out < 20%
- Must report lipids
- Must report dietary composition
- Must report plasma carotenoids measured

Exclusion Criteria
- Not in English
- Any study that does not have humans as subjects (eg, genetic, cellular, animal)
- Published before 2001 (for update); published before 1991 (for original guide)
- Sample size fewer than 10 in each treatment group
- Drop-out rate was > 20%

Search Terms
 sterol AND hyperlipidemia, sterol AND cholesterol, stanol AND hyperlipidemia, stanol AND cholesterol, phytosterol AND hyperlipidemia, phytosterol AND cholesterol, phytostanol AND hyperlipidemia, phytostanol AND cholesterol

Electronic Databases
 PUBMED MEDLINE database, the Database of Abstracts of Reviews of Effects (DARE), and the Agency for Healthcare Research and Quality (AHRQ) database.

Source: Reprinted with permission from American Dietetic Association Evidence Analysis Library. Disorders of Lipid Metabolism, Stanols and Sterols. Available at http://www.adaevidencelibrary.com/topic.cfm?cat=1059. Accessed February 10, 2007.

VALIDITY QUESTIONS				
1. Was the *research question* clearly stated?	Yes	No	Unclear	N/A
2. Was the *selection* of study subjects/patients free from bias?	Yes	No	Unclear	N/A
3. Were *study groups comparable*?	Yes	No	Unclear	N/A
4. Was method of handling *withdrawals* described?	Yes	No	Unclear	N/A
5. Was *blinding* used to prevent introduction of bias?	Yes	No	Unclear	N/A
6. Were *intervention*/therapeutic regimens/exposure factor or procedure and any comparison(s) described in detail? Were *intervening factors* described?	Yes	No	Unclear	N/A
7. Were *outcomes* clearly defined and the *measurements valid and reliable*?	Yes	No	Unclear	N/A
8. Was the *statistical analysis* appropriate for the study design and type of outcome indicators?	Yes	No	Unclear	N/A
9. Are *conclusions supported by results* with biases and limitations taken into consideration?	Yes	No	Unclear	N/A
10. Is bias due to study's *funding or sponsorship* unlikely?	Yes	No	Unclear	N/A

MINUS/NEGATIVE (−)
If most (six or more) of the answers to the above validity questions are "No," the report should be designated with a minus (−) quality rating symbol on the Evidence Quality Worksheet.

NEUTRAL (∅)
If the answers to validity criteria questions 2, 3, 6, and 7 do not indicate that the study is exceptionally strong, the report should be designated with a neutral (∅) quality rating symbol on the Evidence Quality Worksheet.

PLUS/POSITIVE (+)
If most of the answers to the above validity questions are "Yes" (including criteria 2, 3, 6, 7 and at least one additional "Yes"), the report should be designated with a plus quality rating symbol (+) on the Evidence Quality Worksheet.

FIGURE 12.1   Quality criteria checklist: primary (original) research—validity questions. Reprinted with permission from ADA Evidence Analysis Manual. Available at: http://www.adaevidencelibrary.com. Accessed February 10, 2007.

time, a narrative Evidence Summary (Box 12.3) is created to summarize the trends and data. The last step of the synthesis is to answer the question in the Conclusion Statement (Box 12.4).

Grading the Conclusion Statement

The Conclusion Statement is graded to indicate the strength of the evidence that supports the statement. Table 12.2 shows the process that the ADA uses for determining the grades assigned to conclusion statements (3). The conclusion grade reflects the types of research in the hierarchy of evidence, the quality of the studies, and consistency and magnitude of effect.

Other systems are used by other organizations to determine levels of evidence that represent the same concept as the grade assigned to a conclusion statement used in the ADA system. The most widely used alternative system was one that evolved from the Canadian Task Force on the Periodic Health Examination, which proposed one of

the first hierarchies for rating or grading levels of evidence (Table 12.3) (8).

Formulating Recommendations

Over the past 20 years, information on the science of synthesizing research results has expanded. However, methods for linking evidence to recommendations for practice are less well developed than methods for synthesizing evidence. When formulating recommendations based on the evidence, it is helpful to have a logical approach to identifying and mapping out a chain of hypothesized causal relationships among the determinants, interventions, and intermediate and ultimate health outcomes (3,12,51). The ADA differentiates recommendations for practice from evidence analysis conclusion statements. Evidence-based guides for dietetics practice result from an explicit translation process, and focus on clinical application and consideration of other patient and dietary factors.

VALIDITY QUESTIONS				
1. Was the question for the review clearly focused and appropriate?	Yes	No	Unclear	N/A
2. Was the search strategy used to locate relevant studies comprehensive? Were the databases searched and the search terms used described?	Yes	No	Unclear	N/A
3. Were explicit methods used to select studies to include in the review? Were inclusion/ exclusion criteria specified and appropriate? Were selection methods unbiased?	Yes	No	Unclear	N/A
4. Was there an appraisal of the quality and validity of studies included in the review? Were appraisal methods specified, appropriate, and reproducible?	Yes	No	Unclear	N/A
5. Were specific treatments/interventions/exposures described? Were treatments similar enough to be combined?	Yes	No	Unclear	N/A
6. Was the outcome of interest clearly indicated? Were other potential harms and benefits considered?	Yes	No	Unclear	N/A
7. Were processes for data abstraction, synthesis, and analysis described? Were they applied consistently across studies and groups? Was there appropriate use of qualitative and/or quantitative synthesis? Was variation in findings among studies analyzed? Were heterogeneity issues considered? If data from studies were aggregated for meta-analysis, was the procedure described?	Yes	No	Unclear	N/A
8. Are the results clearly presented in narrative and/or quantitative terms? If summary statistics are used, are levels of significance and/or confidence intervals included?	Yes	No	Unclear	N/A
9. Are conclusions supported by results with biases and limitations taken into consideration? Are limitations of the review identified and discussed?	Yes	No	Unclear	N/A
10. Was bias due to the review's funding or sponsorship unlikely?	Yes	No	Unclear	N/A
MINUS/NEGATIVE (−) *If most (six or more) of the answers to the above validity questions are "No," the review should be designated with a minus (−) quality rating symbol on the Evidence Quality Worksheet.*				
NEUTRAL (∅) *If the answer to any of the first four validity questions (1–4) is "No," but other criteria indicate strengths, the review should be designated with a neutral (∅) quality rating symbol on the Evidence Quality Worksheet.*				
PLUS/POSITIVE (+) *If most of the answers to the above validity questions are "Yes" (must include criteria 1, 2, 3, and 4), the report should be designated with a plus quality rating symbol (+) on the Evidence Quality Worksheet.*				

FIGURE 12.2   Quality criteria checklist: review articles—validity questions. Reprinted with permission from ADA Evidence Analysis Manual. Available at: http://www.adaevidencelibrary.com. Accessed February 10, 2007.

Official recommendation statements usually are accompanied by a rating that indicates the strength of the recommendation. Table 12.4 shows various popular methods of characterizing the strength of the recommendations that can be made from a body of evidence (3,52). Box 12.5 is an example of a recommendation from the ADA EAL. Table 12.5 defines the terms and ratings assigned to recommendations that reflect the graded evidence in the ADA EAL that support the recommendation. This table also summarizes the implications for practitioners as they apply the recommendation (4).

Disseminating Findings

The process and findings of a systematic review are reported in a variety of formats, including peer-reviewed publications, technical reports, professional presentations, continuing education opportunities, and online reference sites. If the review is submitted for publication in a peer-reviewed journal, this may result in a long time delay and reach a limited audience. There are two different points at which the findings from the ADA evidence analysis process can be disseminated: after the

TABLE 12.1 Sample Evidence Summary Overview: Stanols and Sterols and Hyperlipidemia Overview Table

Author	Design (All Randomized Controlled Trials)	Dietary Comp. of Groups Reported	What Food Was Provided?	Sterol Dose	Stanol Dose	Change Lipids	Change Carotenoids	Corrected for LDL	Other
Examined Lipids and Carotenoids Non Carotenoid-fortified Foods									
Davidson 2001	Parallel	Yes	Low-fat salad dressing + margarine	0,3,6,9 g	0	5%–9% LDL	Yes, but in normal ref range	Yes	4 levels sterols, 8 wk
Hendriks 2003	Parallel	Yes	Low-fat spread given	1.6 g	0	4% TC, 6% LDL	Decrease but not after adj for LDL	Yes	1 year
Ntanios 2002	Crossover	Yes	Spread	1.8 g	0	6% TC, 10% LDL	Decrease, even after adj	Yes	Examined high versus low baseline TC
Mensink 2001	Parallel	Yes; FFQ	3 c yogurt w/stanols, margarine and shortening		2.98 g	7% TC, 8% LDL	Yogurt: decreases carotenoids; Margarine/shortening: increase tocopherols	Yes	
Maki 2001	Parallel	Yes, diet record	Reduced fat spread	1.1 or 2.2		4% TC, 5% LDL	Decreased; For atherosclerosis: most still within reference range	Yes	Asked to follow low-fat
Nestel 2001	Crossover	3 day food, some data: SF, chol, fib.	Cereal, bread, margarine w/compounds	2.4 g	2.4 g nonesterified		Sterols: no dec. in carotenoids	No?	
Homma 2003	Parallel	Yes	Spread	0	2 g or 3 g	2:6% TC 10% LDL Nutrition: 3.6% C 7% LDL	Dec alpha-toco, other no	No?	Japanese people—low-fat diet
Volpe 2001	Crossover	Yes, 3-d food records	Drink-yogurt based	1g; 2g (phase2)		Lowered	Not lowered	No	Vit A/E/D only assessed in 11 patients in an open-label phase 2
Christiansen 2001	Parallel	Yes, 7 day food diaries	Spread	1.5 or 3.0	Lowered		Not lowered	No	
Carotenoid Fortified or Asked to Consume Foods Rich in Carotenoids									
Quilez 2003	Parallel	Yes	muffins, croissant	3.2 g	0	Decrease	Carotenoids unfortified, decreased	Yes	Not mar garine
Noakes 2002	Crossover	Yes	Spread, suggested increased PO carotenoids	2.3 g	2.5 g	8%–9% LDL	Carotenoids, fortified, increased dec vs control but not compared to baseline	Yes	Examined high vs low baseline TC 3 w, low-fat spread and a high-fat spread

Source: Reprinted with permission from American Dietetic Association Evidence Analysis Library. Specific Foods and Disorders of Lipid Metabolism: Plant Sterols/Stanols. Available at: http://www.adaevidencelibrary.com/topic.cfm?cat=1059. Accessed August 25, 2006.

BOX 12.3   Sample Evidence Summary

The evidence summary for the topic of stanols and sterols in Disorders of Lipid Metabolism includes the following sections:

- **Background:** description of chemical compounds, normal intake, mechanisms of action and level of intake necessary to produce reductions in total and LDL cholesterol
- **Effectiveness in normocholesterol subjects:** Narrative brief summary of key aspects of the four Western and two Japanese studies
- **Effectiveness in hypercholesterol subjects:** Narrative brief summary of key aspects of the eight studies (organized by type of study)

The full evidence summary can be viewed at: http://www.adaevidencelibrary.com/topic.cfm?/cat=1059.

Source: Adapted with permission from American Dietetic Association Evidence Analysis Library. Specific Foods and Disorders of Lipid Metabolism: Plant Sterols/Stanols. Available at: http://www.adaevidencelibrary.com/topic.cfm?cat=1059. Accessed August 25, 2006.

BOX 12.4   Sample Conclusion Statement

What effect does the intake of plant sterols and stanols have on total cholesterol and LDL cholesterol?

Plant sterols and stanols are potent hypocholesterolemic agents and a daily consumption of 2–3 g (through margarine, lowfat yogurt, orange juice, breads, and cereals) lowers TC concentrations in a dose dependent manner by 4%–11% and LDL cholesterol concentrations by 7%–15% without changing HDL cholesterol or triacylglycerol concentrations.

Grade I

Grade Levels: I—good/strong; II—fair; III—limited/weak; IV—expert opinion only; and V—grade not assignable.

Source: Reprinted with permission from American Dietetic Association Evidence Analysis Library. Specific Foods and Disorders of Lipid Metabolism: Plant Sterols/Stanols. Available at: http://www.adaevidencelibrary.com/topic.cfm?cat=1059. Accessed August 25, 2006.

completion of the systematic review and after the completion of the Evidence-Based Guidelines for Nutrition Practice.

If the results are disseminated after the completion of the systematic review, the tables are often presented along with a description of the protocol used. Conclusion statements, evidence summaries, and tables are the results of a systematic review. The complete evidence analyses should be presented along with a description of the protocol used for the systematic review. Evidence tables may be included as attachments to evidence-based clinical practice guidelines or included as online-only appendixes to published articles, as was done for the Position of the ADA: Individual-, Family-, School-, and Community-Based Interventions for Pediatric Overweight (53). The value of this work requires dissemination to users, including practitioners, researchers, policy makers and payors, so that findings can be incorporated into practice and lead to more effective and higher quality care.

The following are important considerations or criteria that the ADA used when it selected EAL:

- Extent of access to dietetics practitioners, researchers, educators, and other target audiences at time of need

- Ability to continually update components of a review
- Ease of republishing an updated review
- Ability to share work between evidence analysis reports
- Ability to be transparent about the entire process and clearly link the research reviewed to the corresponding recommendations

STRENGTHS AND LIMITATIONS OF EVIDENCE-BASED MEDICINE

The systematic review process results in consideration of both the breadth and depth of the evidence. It also enables objective assessment of the levels of evidence and the strength of support for specific recommendations or intervention alternatives. EBDP promotes the use of effective interventions and the reduction of ineffective ones. It pushes the profession forward as practitioners make practice decisions that are supported by empirical data and recognize where uncertainties exist. When these uncertainties are formulated into answerable questions, available data

TABLE 12.2   Grading the Strength of the Evidence for a Conclusion Statement or Recommendation

Strength of Evidence Elements	Grades				
	I Good/Strong	**II** Fair	**III** Limited/Weak	**IV** Expert Opinion Only	**V** Grade Not Assignable
Quality Scientific rigor/validity. Considers design and execution.	Studies of strong design for question. Free from design flaws, bias and execution problems.	Studies of strong design for question with minor methodological concerns, OR only studies of weaker study design for question.	Studies of weak design for answering the question, OR inconclusive findings due to design flaws, bias, or execution problems.	No studies available. Conclusion based on usual practice, expert consensus, clinical experience, opinion, or extrapolation from basic research.	No evidence that pertains to question being addressed.
Consistency Of findings across studies.	Findings generally consistent in direction and size of effect or degree of association, and statistical significance with minor exceptions at most.	Inconsistency among results of studies with strong design, OR consistency with minor exceptions across studies of weaker design.	Unexplained inconsistency among results from different studies OR single study unconfirmed by other studies.	Conclusion supported solely by statements of informed nutrition or medical commentators.	NA
Quantity Number of studies. Number of subjects in studies	One to several good quality studies. Large number of subjects studied Studies with negative results have sufficiently large sample size for adequate statistical power	Several studies by independent investigators. Doubts about adequacy of sample size to avoid Type I and Type II error.	Limited number of studies. Low number of subjects studied and/or inadequate sample size within studies	Unsubstantiated by published research studies.	Relevant studies have not been done.

Source: Reprinted with permission from ADA Evidence Analysis Manual. Available at: http://www.adaevidencelibrary.com. Accessed February 10, 2007.

can be gathered and graded. When the level of evidence or the grade is low (III to V), additional studies are warranted. The identification of unanswered problems and uncertainties can stimulate research to fill gaps in important areas. The ADA EAL provides a search function that clearly identifies all questions where uncertainties exist, that is, those that are graded III, IV, or V (3).

The systematic reviews used in EBDP are subject to many of the same limitations as other types of research, including publication bias, delays between the gathering and publication of data, and methodological issues. Several limitations of systematic reviews are of particular concern: practitioner skill in conducting the search and evidence review, amount of time required to complete a thorough evidence review, lack of relevant research, and

applicability of RCT results to routine clinical settings (5,24–27,54). The methods used, and ways in which researchers and analysts are involved in completing the work of a systematic review, are extremely important in ensuring that the final results are valid and reproducible. Most groups that undertake a systematic review have several categories of people with various roles to ensure that the work completed is objective and there are checks and balances in the process.

If practitioners or institutions are expected to conduct evidence-based reviews, practitioners must have skills to precisely define a patient problem needing evidence to resolve, to conduct an efficient search of the literature, to select the best of the relevant studies, to apply rules of evidence to determine validity and reliability of individual

TABLE 12.3   Levels of Evidence and Grades of Recommendation

Grade of Recommendation	Level of Evidence	Therapy/Prevention, Etiology/Harm	Economic Analysis
A	1a	Systematic Review (SR) with homogeneity of Randomized Clinical Controlled Trials (RCTs)	Systematic Review (with homogeneity of Level 1 economic studies)
	1b	Individual RCT (with narrow Confidence Interval)	Analysis comparing (critically validated) alternate outcomes against appropriate cost measurement, and including a sensitivity variations in important variables
B	2a	SR (with homogeneity) of Cohort studies	SR (with homogeneity) of Level ≥ 2 studies
	2b	RCT; eg, < 80% follow-up (including low-quality individual cohort study)	Analysis comparing a limited number of alternative outcomes against appropriate cost measurement, and including a sensitivity analysis incorporating clinically sensible variations in important variables
	2c	"Outcomes Research"	
	3a	SR (with homogeneity) of case-control studies	
	3b	Individual case-control studies	Analysis without accurate cost measurement, but including a sensitivity analysis incorporating clinically sensible variations in important variables
C	4	Case-series (and poor-quality cohort and case-control studies)	Analysis with no sensitivity analysis
D	5	Expert opinion without explicit critical appraisal, or based on physiology, bench research or "first principles"	Expert opinion without explicit critical appraisal, or based on economic theory

Abbreviations: RCT, randomized clinical controlled trials; SR, systematic review.

Source: Adapted from Center for Evidence-based Medicine TOOL KIT. Available at: http://www.med.ualberta.ca/ebm/ebm.htm. Accessed August 6, 2006. Used with permission.

research reports, and to extract the clinical message and apply it to a patient problem. The rigor of the assessment of selected research is compromised if the practitioner lacks access to searching technology, knowledge of research principles, or experience in the topic being investigated. Institutions can plan and staff evidence analysis projects to overcome these limitations. However, most individual health care institutions have concluded that they lack the resources to conduct the types of systematic reviews necessary to develop evidence-based guidelines, and that this is more efficiently conducted by larger groups, the government, or professional associations.

A major barrier to the concept of EBDP is the time required for conducting a thorough systematic review when needed. To address this barrier, some institutions have created mechanisms for easy computer access to pre-processed reviews and guidelines (eg, terminals at the hospital unit or clinic and wireless PDAs). At some institutions, especially academic health centers, medical librarians are making rounds with the team so searches to resolve uncertainties can be quickly completed.

The primary use of systematic reviews of evidence is to provide the basis for clinical decision making, either through the development of profession-wide or institution-based clinical practice guidelines, MNT protocols, or clinical pathways to aid practitioner decision making for individual patients. Evidence summaries are often the basis behind policies regarding the types and amount of care that health plans will cover. Evidence summaries are also tremendously helpful in identifying gaps in research

TABLE 12.4   Summary of Descriptors of Strength of Evidence Supporting Recommendations

Users' Guide	CEBM	American Dietetic Association	American Diabetes Association	Chronic Kidney Disease	USPTF	NHLBI
A	**A**	**Strong**	**A**	**S**	**A**	**A**
Randomized trials Consistent results	Consistent level 1 studies	Benefits clearly exceed harms, excellent supporting evidence (Grade I or II)	Clear evidence	Analysis of data from single large, generalizable study of high quality	Strong	Randomized trials—rich body of data
B	**B**	**Fair**	**B**	**C**	**B**	**B**
Randomized trials Inconsistent or methodological weaknesses	Consistent level 2 or 3 studies or extrapolations from level 1 studies	Benefits exceed harms, supporting evidence is Grade II or III	Supportive evidence from well-conducted cohort studies	Compilation of original articles (tables of evidence)	Not strong, but sufficient	Randomized controlled trials—limited controls
C	**C**	**Weak**	**C**	**R**	**C**	**C**
Generalization from randomized trials or overwhelming observational studies	Level 4 studies or extrapolations from level 2 or 3 studies	Quality of evidence is low, or high-quality studies show little clear advantage for one vs another	Poorly controlled or non-controlled trials	Review of review & selected original articles	No recommendation for or against	Non-randomized studies, observational studies
C	**D**	**Consensus**	**E**	**O**	**D**	**D**
Other	Troubling inconsistent or inconclusive studies of any level	Expert opinion supports the recommendation even though evidence is not available	Expert consensus or clinical experience	Opinion	Recommends against	Panel consensus
		Insufficient Evidence			**I**	
		Both lack pertinent evidence and/or unclear balance between benefits and harms			Insufficient	

Source: Adapted from Myers EF. Systems for evaluating nutrition research for nutrition care guidelines: do they apply to population dietary guidelines? *J Am Diet Assoc.* 2003;103(12 suppl):S34–S41. Adapted with permission from the American Dietetic Association.

and focusing future research to answer important practice questions.

Another major limitation of EBDP is the premise that published research and evidence already have been, or can be, conducted to answer important clinical questions. It is virtually impossible to create or find research to answer all important clinical questions because of the high cost involved in research, the time required for research, and the difficulties inherent in conducting research (22). Furthermore, the gold standard for studies to determine whether a treatment is safe and effective is the RCT, which can be complex and costly to conduct. However, it is erroneous to conclude that a lack of research to answer a specific question is the same as evidence that a treatment is not warranted.

Further, there is debate about the applicability of RCT to patient populations (22,24–27,54). With tightly defined criteria for subject inclusion and the high commitment to compliance needed for valid clinical trials, the sample subjects studied in the trial may not reflect the

BOX 12.5   Sample Recommendation Summary Page:
RECOMMENDATION: 7. PLANT STANOLS AND STEROLS AND DISORDERS OF LIPID METABOLISM

Recommendation(s): (R7.1)

If consistent with patient preference and not contraindicated by risks or harms, then plant sterol and stanol ester enriched foods consumed two or three times per day, for a total consumption of two or three grams per day, may be used in addition to a cardioprotective diet to further lower TC by 4%–11% and LDL-C by 7%–15%. For maximal effectiveness, foods containing plant sterols and stanols (spreads, juices, yogurts) should be eaten with other foods. To prevent weight gain, isocalorically substitute stanol- and sterol-enriched foods for other foods. Plant stanols and sterols are effective in people taking statin drugs.

Strong

Conditional

Risks/Harms of Implementing this Recommendation

- Plant sterol/stanol products should not be used in individuals with sitosterolemia.
- Margarines are a common source of plant sterols/stanols, and can contain considerable calories. Caloric content should be considered and these foods should only be recommended when weight can be maintained.
- Consideration should be given to individuals with financial limitations, as these foods can be expensive.

Conditions of Application

None specified

Potential Costs Associated with Application

None specified

Recommendation Narrative

- Six high-quality RCTs of normocholesterolemic and seven high-quality RCTs of hypercholesterolemic individuals found sterol and stanol ester-enriched products lowered TC and LDL-C. Both sterols and stanols and the esterified and nonesterified forms were effective.
- Many studies provided sterols or stanols in foods other than margarines, such as low-fat yogurt, bakery products, and salad dressings, and beneficial effects still persisted.
- Beneficial effects were seen when phytosterols were given as part of a low-fat, low cholesterol diet in three high-quality RCTs.
- One study gave varying doses of plant stanols and found a dose response at lower levels, but increasing the dose from 2.4 to 3.2g/d did not provide further benefit.
- Two high-quality RCTs found that plant stanols are effective even when given with statin drugs.
- One RCT gave up to 9 g/day for eight weeks and found no evidence of adverse effects. This was confirmed by two other studies that gave lower does of plant sterol/stanols, but for longer periods of time.
- Three high-quality studies found no change in serum carotene levels after ingesting plant sterols/stanols, however several high-quality studies found that in general, alpha-tocopherol and alpha- and beta-carotene concentrations may be reduced with plant sterol/stanol consumption. To mitigate this effect, two studies found consuming foods rich in carotenoids and alpha-tocopherol with phytosterols maintained plasma levels.

Recommendation Strength Rationale

- Consistency of results among multiple high-quality RCTs.
- Although the ethnicity of study participants was not identified in all studies, few studies did report this information and studies included many populations such as Caucasians, blacks, Hispanics, and Asians; and men and women.
- A biological plausibility for mechanisms of action of plant stanol/sterol esters-containing foods exists.
- A dose-response relationship exists.
- Conclusions were Grade I, II, and III.

(Continued)

BOX 12.5   *(Continued)*

Areas of Uncertainty: To date, no clinical outcome studies have evaluated the effects of stanols and sterols on CHD events.

Supporting Evidence

The recommendations were created from the evidence analysis on the following questions. To see detail of the evidence analysis, see the following EA Questions:

- How are the effects of stanols and sterols on cholesterol levels altered when eaten as part of a cholesterol lowering diet?
- How do sterols and stanols compare in terms of their efficacy in lowering cholesterol?
- How do esterified and nonesterified forms of stanols and sterols compare in terms of their cholesterol lowering ability?
- Can plant stanols further reduce LDL cholesterol and total cholesterol even for people receiving statin therapy?
- Can statin dose be reduced through the use of stanols and sterols?
- What does the research indicate about the safety of stanol and sterol intake?
- Are there any unintended adverse effects when consuming stanols and sterols?
- How might the consumption of carotenoid-rich fruits or vegetables alter plasma carotenoid levels when also consuming sterols?
- What effect does the intake of plant sterols and stanols have on total cholesterol and LDL cholesterol?

Source: Reprinted with permission from American Dietetic Association Evidence Analysis Library. Specific Foods and Disorders of Lipid Metabolism: Plant Sterols/Stanols. Available at: http://www.adaevidencelibrary.com/topic.cfm?cat=1059. Accessed August 25, 2006.

range of patients that practitioners are likely to encounter in routine practice.

Reviews and the recommendations and guidelines developed from them can become obsolete as new research becomes available and new procedures and therapies are introduced. Splett developed a checklist to determine when it is necessary to update an evidence-based guide (51). In most areas of dietetics practice, updates of reviews should be considered in at least 2-year intervals (55). The Cochrane Collaboration also strives to update reviews every 2 years (36).

Although it is important to be included in peer-reviewed publications, peer-reviewed publications may not be as effective as other methods of disseminating systematic reviews in the long run. For example, after the systematic review is completed and published, key research may be completed that could change the findings; in cases like this, it is unlikely that a peer-reviewed publication will republish the updated review in a timely manner. Other methods are likely to be used in concert with peer-reviewed publications as we move to the concept of "living guidelines," in which guidelines are continuously reviewed for currency and updated on an ongoing annual basis vs at a set time period of 2 to 5 years.

ROLES OF PROFESSIONAL SOCIETIES

Criteria for Guidelines by Professional Societies

In 2000, Grilli et al developed minimum criteria for published guidelines prepared by professional societies: (a) description of the type of professionals involved in the guidelines development, (b) report of the strategy used to search for the primary evidence, and (c) use of explicit grading of recommendations according to the quality of supporting evidence (20). A total of 431 guidelines published from 1988 to 1998 were evaluated according to these criteria. Only 33% described the type of professionals involved in development, 13% reported search plan, and 18% used explicit criteria to grade the strength of the evidence to support their recommendations. Over half (54%) did not meet any of the three criteria, 34% met one criterion, and 7% met two of the three criteria. Forty-one percent of the guidelines were published from 1996 to 1998 (20). Clearly the rigor and description of guideline development have room for improvement.

TABLE 12.5   ADA Evidence-Based Guideline Recommendations: Definitions and Implications for Practice

Statement Rating	Definition	Implication for Practice
Strong	A **Strong** recommendation means that the workgroup believes that the benefits of the recommended approach clearly exceed the harms (or that the harms clearly exceed the benefits in the case of a strong negative recommendation) and that the quality of the supporting evidence is excellent (grade I or II).* In some clearly identified circumstances, strong recommendations may be made based on lesser evidence when high-quality evidence is impossible to obtain and the anticipated benefits strongly outweigh the harms.	Practitioners should follow a **Strong** recommendation unless a clear and compelling rationale for an alternative approach is present.
Fair	A **Fair** recommendation means that the workgroup believes that the benefits exceed the harms (or that the harms exceed the benefits in the case of a negative recommendation), but the quality of evidence is not as strong (grade II or III).* In some clearly identified circumstances, recommendations may be made based on lesser evidence when high-quality evidence is impossible to obtain and the anticipated benefits outweigh the harms.	Practitioners should generally follow a **Fair** recommendation but remain alert to new information and be sensitive to patient preferences.
Weak	A **Weak** recommendation means that the quality of evidence that exists is suspect or that well-done studies (grade I, II, or III)* show little clear advantage to one approach versus another.	Practitioners should be cautious in deciding whether to follow a recommendation classified as **Weak**, and should exercise judgment and be alert to emerging publications that report evidence. Patient preference should have a substantial influencing role.
Consensus	A **Consensus** recommendation means that Expert opinion (grade IV) supports the guideline recommendation even though the available scientific evidence did not present consistent results, or controlled trials were lacking.	Practitioners should be flexible in deciding whether to follow a recommendation classified as **Consensus**, although they may set boundaries on alternatives. Patient preference should have a substantial influencing role.
Insufficient Evidence	An **Insufficient Evidence** recommendation means that there is both a lack of pertinent evidence (grade V*) and/or an unclear balance between benefits and harms.	Practitioners should feel little constraint in deciding whether to follow a recommendation labeled as **Insufficient Evidence** and should exercise judgment and be alert to emerging publications that report evidence that clarifies the balance of benefit versus harm. Patient preference should have a substantial influencing role.

*Conclusion statements are assigned a grade based on the strength of the evidence. Grade I is good; grade II, fair; grade III, limited; grade IV signifies expert opinion only and grade V indicates that a grade is not assignable because there is no evidence to support or refute the conclusion. The evidence and these grades are considered when assigning a rating (Strong, Fair, Weak, Consensus, Insufficient Evidence—see chart above) to a recommendation.

Source: Reprinted with permission from American Dietetic Association Evidence Analysis Library. How Does ADA Develop Evidence-Based Nutrition Practice Guidelines. Available at: http://www.adaevidencelibrary.com/topic.cfm?cat=2690. Accessed February 10, 2007.

American Medical Association
Users' Guides to the Medical Literature

In the 1990s, the American Medical Association (AMA) published a series entitled *Users' Guides to the Medical Literature,* which have been a valuable foundation in the movement toward EBM (6,7,37,56–67). The first topic, in 1993, introduced the Evidence-Based Medicine Working Group members and provided the basics of evaluating literature to support medical practice (65). Users' guides

have included articles on how to use systematic reviews, decision analyses, practice guidelines, and economic analysis, along with articles that make treatment recommendations (6,7,37,56–57,67).

American Academy of Family Practice

The American Academy of Family Practice systematically reviews research journals to select articles focused on patient-oriented evidence that matters (POEM) (68). These selected articles address a clinical problem or clinical question that primary care physicians will encounter in their practice, use patient-oriented outcomes, and have the potential to change practice if the results are valid and applicable (69). These preprocessed evidence summaries are delivered via e-mail with approximately 30 to 35 research articles summarized on a monthly basis. A subscription on-line information search Web site (InfoRetriever) provides access to the best evidence available for a family practitioner through a sophisticated search engine that searches the various databases, including the Cochrane Library and Evidence-Based Guidelines as well as individual research articles.

American Dietetic Association

The ADA began the development of profession-wide protocols with the publication of the first edition of *Medical Nutrition Therapy Across the Continuum of Care* (1). The latest versions of the MNT protocols are called Evidence-Based Nutrition Practice Guidelines (EBGs) and are available in ADA Evidence Analysis Library. They are supported by evidence-based guide toolkits, available for purchase, which include implementation tools tailored for each EBG (70). Some ADA practice guides are supported by published validation studies, and studies are underway to validate other guides (71,72). The ADA's efforts to support and promote EBP led to the group being recognized as one of seven organizations that were leaders in EBM by the Joint Commission (formerly the Joint Commission on Accreditation of Healthcare Organizations) in 2002 (73).

ROLES OF GOVERNMENT AND OTHER ORGANIZATIONS

US Preventive Services Task Force

A series of articles describe the process developed and used by the 15-member US Preventive Services Task Force to evaluate the evidence for preventive services. Zaza and coworkers describe the lengthy data collection instrument for each research study included in the review (11).

Agency for Healthcare Research and Quality

AHRQ began funding comprehensive reviews of research in priority health conditions in the early 1990s (74). These reviews were initiated to define current practice and evidence

for the effectiveness of those practices. In its reviews, AHRQ recognized the role of experts, including researchers, experienced practitioners, and patients, as judges of clinical practices when research was lacking. AHRQ views research as the foundation for health care policies that affect clinical practice and, ultimately, health outcomes. AHRQ solicits input on the types of reviews to be conducted with federal funding through its 12 EPCs. A complete list of the EPC Evidence Review Reports is available on the Web site under the evidence-based practice section (75).

Institute for Clinical Systems Improvement

The ICSI developed a modified method of evaluating the evidence that attempts to address the limitations of the more restricted method employed by the public health community and national organizations (13). Its goal was to produce shorter, simpler guidelines that would be easily developed and employed by the practitioners who would use them (76).

Cochrane Collaboration Systematic Reviews

The Cochrane Collaboration, an international nonprofit and independent organization, produces and disseminates systematic reviews of health care interventions to address the effectiveness of these interventions. As part of their efforts, the group conducts paper and electronic literature searches for evidence in the form of clinical trials and other studies of interventions. The major product of the Cochrane Collaboration (40) is the Cochrane Database of Systematic Reviews, which is published quarterly as part of the Cochrane Library (41).

Systematic reviews of nutrition and dietetics topics are covered by several groups within the Cochrane Collaboration. To find systematic reviews on nutrition topics, search the Cochrane Library for the term *diet* or *nutrition*.

CONCLUSION

EBDP is the explicit linking of research to practice. It uses systematic reviews of the best currently available evidence, rather than a single study, to provide evidence for health care decisions. The final product of a systematic review is a summary document that can be used by others. Even with tables of evidence and resulting recommendations or guidelines, the dietetics practitioner must exercise clinical decision-making skills to determine if and how the results apply to individual clients or patients. EBDP requires expertise in knowing how to plan and conduct systematic reviews as well as how to use the summarized findings in practice. The process of evaluating or completing systematic reviews is another tool that dietitians must add to their repertoire of research skills.

REFERENCES

1. Myers EF, Pritchett E, Johnson E. Evidence-based practice guides vs. protocols: what's the difference? *J Am Diet Assoc.* 2001;101:1085–1090.
2. Scope of Dietetics Practice Framework. Section 4B, Definition of Terms. Available at: http://www.eatright.org/ ada/files/ Section4BTerms.pdf. Accessed August 25, 2006.
3. American Dietetic Association Evidence Analysis Library. ADA Evidence Analysis Manual. Available at: http://www.adaevidencelibrary.com/ tocip.cfm?cat=1155. Accessed August 26, 2007.
4. American Dietetic Association Evidence Analysis Library. How Does ADA Develop Evidence-Based Nutrition Practice Guidelines? Available at: http://www.adaevidencelibrary.com/ category.cfm?cid=16&cat=0. Accessed August 25, 2006.
5. Sackett DL, Straus SE, Richardson WS, Rosenberg W, Haynes RB. *Evidence-Based Medicine: How to Practice and Teach EBM.* St Louis, Mo: Churchill Livingstone; 2000.
6. Guyatt GH, Haynes RB, Jaeschke RZ, Cook DJ, Green L, Naylor CD, Wilson MC, Richardson WS. Users' Guides to the Medical Literature: XXV. Evidence-based medicine: principles for applying the Users' Guides to patient care. Evidence-Based Medicine Working Group. *JAMA.* 2000;284:1290–1296.
7. Guyatt GH. *Users' Guide to the Medical Literature: Essentials of Evidence-Based Clinical Practice.* Chicago, Ill: American Medical Association; 2002.
8. EBM tool kit—introduction to informatics. Available at: http://www. med.ualberta.ca/ebm/ebm.htm. Accessed February 13, 2007.
9. Resources for clinicians. Evidence-based medicine: finding the best clinical literature. Available at: http://www.uic.edu/depts/lib/lhs/resources/clinical. shtml Accessed August 25, 2006.
10. Carande-Kulis VG, Maciosek MV, Briss PA, Teutsch SM, Zaza S, Truman BI, Messonier ML, Pappaioanou M, Harris JR, Fielding J. Methods for systematic reviews of economic evaluations for the Guide to Community Preventive Services. Task Force on Community Preventive Services. *Am J Prev Med.* 2000;18(1 Suppl):75–91.
11. Zaza S, Wright-De Aguero LK, Briss PA, Truman BI, Hopkins DP, Hennessy MH, Sosin DM, Anderson L, Carande-Kulis VG, Teutsch SM, Pappaioanou M. Data collection instrument and procedure for systematic reviews in the Guide to Community Preventive Services. Task Force on Community Preventive Services. *Am J Prev Med.* 2000; 18(1 Suppl):44–74.
12. Briss PA, Zaza S, Pappaioanou M, Fielding J, et al. Developing an evidence-based Guide to Community Preventive Services—methods. The Task Force on Community Preventive Services. *Am J Prev Med.* 2000;18(1 Suppl):35–43.
13. Truman BI, Smith-Akin CK, Hinman AR, Gebbie KM, Brownson R, Novic LF, Lawrence RD, Pappaioanou M, Fielding J, Evans CA, Guerra FA, Vogel-Taylor M, Mahan CS, Fullilove M, Zaza S. Developing the Guide to Community Preventive Services—overview and rationale. The Task Force on Community Preventive Services. *Am J Prev Med.* 2000;18(1 Suppl):18–26.
14. Greer N, Mosser G, Logan G, Halaas GW. A practical approach to evidence grading. *Jt Comm J Qual Improv.* 2000;26:700–712.
15. Systems to Rate the Strength of Scientific Evidence. Evidence Report/Technology Assessment Number 47 of Agency for Healthcare Research and Quality. Available at: http://www.ahrq.gov. Accessed July 4, 2006.
16. Gyorkos TW, Tannenbaum TN, Abrahamowicz M, et al. An approach to the development of practice guidelines for community health interventions. *Can J Public Health.* 1994;85 Suppl 1:S8–13.
17. Clarke M, Oxman AD. *Cochrane Reviewer's Handbook 4.0.* Oxford, UK: Cochrane Collaboration; 1999.
18. NHS Research and Development Centre of Evidence-Based Medicine. Level of Evidence. Available at: http://cebm.jr2.ox.ac.uk. Accessed August 24, 2006.
19. US Surgeon General's Advisory Committee on Smoking and Health. *Smoking and Health: Report of the Advisory Committee to the Surgeon General of the Public Health Service.* Washington, DC: US Department of Health, Education and Welfare, Public Health Service; 1964.

20. Grilli R, Magrini N, Penna A, Mura G, Liberati A. Practice guidelines developed by specialty societies: the need for a critical appraisal. *Lancet.* 2000;355:103–106.

21. Shaughnessy AF, Slawson DC. POEMs: patient-oriented evidence that matters. *Ann Intern Med.* 1997;126:667.

22. Celermajer DS. Evidence-based medicine: how good is the evidence? *Med J Aust.* 2001;174:293–295.

23. Wolf FM, Shea JA, Albanese MA. Toward setting a research agenda for systematic reviews of evidence of the effects of medical education. *Teach Learn Med.* 2001;13:54–60.

24. Woolf SH, George JN. Evidence-based medicine. Interpreting studies and setting policy. *Hematol Oncol Clin North Am.* 2000;14:761–784.

25. AHRQ Center for Practice and Technology Assessment: Mission and Programs. Available at: http://www.ahrq.gov/about/cpta/cptafact.htm. Accessed May 18, 2006.

26. A Model for Establishing Upper Levels for Nutrients and Related Substances. Available at: http://www.who.int/ipcs/methods/ nra_final.pdf. Accessed July 4, 2006.

27. 2005 Dietary Guidelines Advisory Committee Report 2005. Available at: http://www.health.gov/ dietaryguidelines; dgs2005/report. Accessed July 4, 2006.

28. Critical Appraisal Skills Programme. Appraisal Tools. Oxford, UK. Available at: http://www.phru.nhs.uk/casp/reviews.pdf. Accessed August 25, 2006.

29. Bigby M. Challenges to the hierarchy of evidence: does the emperor have no clothes? *Arch Dermatol.* 2001;137:345–346.

30. Benson K, Hartz AJ. A comparison of observational studies and randomized, controlled trials. *N Engl J Med.* 2000;342: 1878–1886.

31. Concato J, Shah N, Horwitz RI. Randomized, controlled trials, observational studies, and the hierarchy of research designs. *N Engl J Med.* 2000;342:1887–1892.

32. Ernst E, Pittler MH. Systematic reviews neglect safety issues. *Arch Intern Med.* 2001; 161:125–126.

33. Grahame-Smith D. Evidence based medicine: Socratic dissent. *BMJ.* 1995;310:1126–1127.

34. Bannigan K, Droogan J, Entwistle V. Systematic reviews: what do they involve? *Nurs Times.* 1997;93:52–53.

35. Evans D. Systematic reviews of nursing research. *Intensive Crit Care Nurs.* 2001;17:51–57.

36. Cochrane Collaboration's Handbook of Systematic Reviews of Interventions. Available at: http://www.cochrane.dk/cochrane/ handbook/hbook.htm. Accessed August 23, 2006.

37. Craig JC, Irwig LM, Stockler MR. Evidence-based medicine: useful tools for decision making. *Med J Aust.* 2001;174:248–253.

38. Hopewell S, Clarke M, Lefebvre C, Scherer RW. Handsearching versus electronic searching to identify reports of randomized controlled trials. *Cochrane Database Methodol Rev.* 2002;(4). Available at: http://www.cochrane.org. Accessed April 9, 2007.

39. Avenell A, Handoll HH, Grant AM. Lessons for search strategies from a systematic review, in The Cochrane Library, of nutritional supplementation trials in patients after hip fracture. *Am J Clin Nutr.* 2001;73:505–510.

40. Scherer RW, Langenberg P, von Elm E. Full publication of results initially presented in abstracts. *Cochrane Database Methodol Rev.* 2005;(2). Article no. MR000005. Available at: http://www.cochrane.org. Accessed April 9, 2007.

41. The Cochrane Library. Available at: http:// www.The CochraneLibrary.com. Accessed August 15, 2006.

42. Goode CJ. What constitutes the "evidence" in evidence-based practice? *Appl Nurs Res.* 2000;13: 222–225.

43. Cooper MJ, Zlotkin SH. An evidence-based approach to the development of national dietary guidelines. *J Am Diet Assoc.* 2003;103(12 suppl): S28–S33.

44. Thompson RL, Summerbell CD, Hooper L, Higgins JPT, Little PS, Talbot D, Ebrahim S. Dietary advice given by a dietitian versus other health professional or self-help resources to reduce blood cholesterol. *Cochrane Database of Systematic Reviews.* 2003;(3). Article no. CD001366. DOI: 10.1002/14651858. CD001366.

45. Specific Foods and Disorders of Lipid Metabolism: Plan Sterols/stanols. Available at: http://www. adaevidencelibrary. com/topic.cfm?cat=1059. Accessed August 25, 2006.

46. QUOROM Checklist and Flowchart. Available at: http://www.consort-statement.org/Evidence/ evidence.html#quorom. Accessed August 25, 2006.

47. Altman DG, Schulz KF, Moher D, Egger M, Davidoff F, Elbourne D, Gøtzsche PD, Lang T, for the CONSORT Group. The Revised CONSORT Statement for Reporting Randomized Trials: Explanation and Elaboration. *Ann Intern Med.* 2001;134:663–694. Available at: http://www.consort-statement.org/ Explanation/ explanation.htm. Accessed August 25, 2006.

48. Strobe Statement: Strengthening the Reporting of Observational Studies in Epidemiology. Available at: http://www.strobe-statement.org/Checkliste.html. Accessed August 25, 2006.

49. The MOOSE Checklist. Available at: http:// www.consort-statement.org/Initiatives/ MOOSE/ Moosecheck.pdf. Accessed August 25, 2006.

50. The STARD Initiative—Towards Complete and Accurate Reporting of Studies on Diagnostic Accuracy. Available at: http://www. consort statement.org/Initiatives/newstard.htm. Accessed August 25, 2006.

51. Splett P. *Cost Outcomes of Nutrition Intervention: Part I Outcomes Research, Part II Measuring Effectiveness of Nutrition Interventions, Part III Economic and Cost Analysis.* Evansville, Ind: Mead Johnson; 1996.

52. Myers EF. Systems for evaluating nutrition research for nutrition care guidelines: do they apply to population dietary guidelines. *J Am Diet Assoc.* 2003;103(12 suppl):S34–S41.

53. Appendices A, B, and C to Position of the American Dietetic Association: Individual-, Family-, School-, and Community-Based Interventions for Pediatric Overweight. Available at: http://www.eatright.org/ ada/files/Appendices_A_B_C.pdf. Accessed August 15, 2006.

54. Rubin GL, Frommer MS. Evidence-based medicine—time for a reality check. *Med J Aust.* 2001;174:214–215.

55. Thomas L, Cullum N, McColl E, Rousseau N, Soutter J, Steen N. Guidelines in professions allied to medicine. Cochrane Database of Systematic Reviews Web site. Available at: http://www.mrw. interscience. wiley.com/cochrane/clsysrev/articles/CD000349/ frame.htm. Accessed August 25, 2006.

56. Archibald S, Bhandari M, Thoma A. Users' Guides to the Surgical Literature: how to use an article about a diagnostic test. Evidence-Based Medicine Working Group. *Can J Surg.* 2001;44: 17–23.

57. Dans AL, Dans LF, Guyatt GH, Richardson S. Users' Guides to the Medical Literature: XIV. How to decide on the applicability of clinical trial results to your patient. Evidence-Based Medicine Working Group. *JAMA.* 1998;279:545–549.

58. Guyatt GH, Sackett DL, Cook DJ. Users' Guides to the Medical Literature. II. How to use an article about therapy or prevention. A. Are the results of the study valid? Evidence-Based Medicine Working Group. *JAMA.* 1993;270:2598–2601.

59. Guyatt GH, Sackett DL, Cook DJ. Users' Guides to the Medical Literature. II. How to use an article about therapy or prevention. B. What were the results and will they help me in caring for my patients? Evidence-Based Medicine Working Group. *JAMA.* 1994;271:59–63.

60. Guyatt GH, Sackett DL, Sinclair JC, Hayward R, Cook DJ, Cook RJ. Users' Guides to the Medical Literature. IX. A method for grading health care recommendations. Evidence-Based Medicine Working Group. *JAMA.* 1995;274:1800–1804.

61. Hayward RS, Wilson MC, Tunis SR, Bass EB, Guyatt G. Users' Guides to the Medical Literature. VIII. How to use clinical practice guidelines. A. Are the recommendations valid? Evidence-Based Medicine Working Group. *JAMA.* 1995;274: 570–574.

62. Jaeschke R, Guyatt GH, Sackett DL. Users' Guides to the Medical Literature. III. How to use an article about a diagnostic test. B. What are the results and will they help me in caring for my patients? Evidence-Based Medicine Working Group. *JAMA.* 1994;271:703–707.

63. McAlister FA, Straus SE, Guyatt GH, Haynes RB. Users' Guides to the Medical Literature: XX. Integrating research evidence with the care of the individual patient. Evidence-Based Medicine Working Group. *JAMA.* 2000;283:2829–2836.

64. McGinn TG, Guyatt GH, Wyer PC, Naylor CD, Stiell IG, Richardson WS. Users' Guides to the Medical Literature: XXII. How to use articles about clinical decision rules. Evidence-Based Medicine Working Group. *JAMA.* 2000;284:79–84.

65. Oxman AD, Sackett DL, Guyatt GH. Users' Guides to the Medical Literature. I. How to get started. Evidence-Based Medicine Working Group. *JAMA.* 1993;270:2093–2095.

66. Randolph AG, Haynes RB, Wyatt JC, Cook DJ, Guyatt GH. Users' Guides to the Medical Literature: XVIII. How to use an article evaluating the clinical impact of a computer-based clinical decision support system. *JAMA.* 1999;282:67–74.

67. Wilson MC, Hayward RS, Tunis SR, Bass EB, Guyatt G. Users' Guides to the Medical Literature. VIII. How to use clinical practice guidelines. B. What are the recommendations and will they help you in caring for your patients? Evidence-Based Medicine Working Group. *JAMA.* 1995;274:1630–1632.

68. Shaughnessy AF, Slawson DC, Becker L. Clinical jazz: harmonizing clinical experience and evidence-based medicine. *J Fam Pract.* 1998;47:425–428.

69. Slawson DC, Shaughnessy AF, Ebell MH, Barry HC. Mastering medical information and the role of POEMs—patient-oriented evidence that matters. *J Fam Pract.* 1997;45:195–196.

70. Disorders of Lipid Metabolism Toolkit. Available at: https://www. adaevidencelibrary.com/store.cfm. Accessed August 25, 2006.

71. Kulkarni K, Castle G, Gregory R, Holmes A, Leontos C, Powers M, Snetselaar L, Splett P, Wylie-Rossett J. Nutrition Practice Guidelines for type 1 diabetes mellitus positively affect dietitian practices and patient outcomes. The Diabetes Care and Education Dietetic Practice Group. *J Am Diet Assoc.* 1998;98:62–70.

72. Franz M, Splett P, Monk A, Barry B, McCain K, Weaver T, Upham P, Bergenstal R, Mazze RS. Cost-effectiveness of medical nutrition therapy provided by dietitians for persons with non-insulin-dependent diabetes mellitus. *J Am Diet Assoc.* 1995;95: 1018–1024.

73. *Putting Evidence to Work: Tools and Resources.* Chicago, Ill: Joint Commission on Accreditation of Healthcare Organizations; 2002.

74. The outcome of outcomes research at AHCPR: final report. Available at: http:/www.ahcpr.org. Accessed August 25, 2006.

75. Agency for Healthcare Research and Quality. Evidence Based Practice. Available at: http://www.ahrq.gov/clinic/epcix.htm. Accessed August 25, 2006.

76. Institute for Clinical Systems Improvement. About ICSI. Available at: http://www.icsi.org/about/index.asp. Accessed August 25, 2006.

PART 6

Evaluation and Assessment Methods
in Research

13

Survey Research Planning and Questionnaire Design

Barbara E. Millen, DPH, RD, FADA, and Jacqueline A. Vernarelli, MS

Survey research is among the most important and frequently used approaches in human nutrition investigations at the individual, community, and population-based levels. It is central to the National Nutrition Monitoring and Related Research Program (NNMRRP)(1-3) and is broadly used in a wide variety of health-related research settings where links among nutrition, environmental factors, health characteristics, and outcomes are explored. Survey research is also used to evaluate many dimensions of the national food, nutrition, and agricultural systems in both the public and private sectors. These data extend our understanding of the nature and quality of the food supply; the production, distribution, and sales of agricultural commodities; and the features and impact of nutrition-related programs and services.

Given the importance, scope, and widespread application of survey research in nutrition and related domains and practice, it is essential that nutrition professionals develop relevant skills and expertise, particularly related to overall study design and questionnaire development. The following discussion describes the stages of survey research planning and implementation, with particular emphasis on the design of questionnaires and related protocols. Didactic components of the presentation are complemented by examples from the NHIS, NHANES, and CSFII surveys as well as from the authors' experiences in the Framingham Nutrition Studies (FNS) (4).

SURVEY RESEARCH APPLICATIONS

One of the primary applications of survey research methods is the NNMRRP, which includes the continuous National Health Interview Survey (NHIS) conducted by the Centers for Disease Control and Prevention (CDC) and state health departments (1), the US Department of Health and Human Services' ongoing National Health and Nutrition Examination Surveys (NHANES) (2), and the US Department of Agriculture (USDA) Continuing Survey of Family and Individual Intakes (CSFII) (3). (Refer to Chapter 10 for a detailed discussion of the NNMRRP.) The survey research elements of NNMRRP provide the chief mechanisms for assessing the health and nutritional status of the US population and for determining progress made toward national nutrition- and health-related policies and goals (eg, Healthy People 2010) (5). In this context, survey methods are used to evaluate the diet- and health-related knowledge, attitudes, and behaviors of individuals or households, and their environmental determinants. Nutrition survey data can be linked to individuals' biological risk factors or relevant health- or disease-related characteristics or outcomes (eg, nutrition-related acute, chronic, and infectious conditions and their comorbidities, complications, or consequences).

A second widespread application of survey methods in human nutrition research is in the field of nutrition epidemiology. This research domain has grown tremendously in the past decade as validated survey questionnaire methodologies (such as food frequency questionnaires and telephone-administered dietary assessment techniques) have emerged for use in population-based studies, and as advanced statistical techniques have been applied in innovative ways to large-scale nutrition data sets. Today, nutrition epidemiologists may test hypotheses relating to specific food or nutrient *exposures* to health outcomes of interest, and they may also assess relationships between health and exposure measures of *overall* dietary quality (6), such as the Healthy Eating Index and other Dietary Quality Indexes (7,8), male and female dietary patterns (6,9,10), or composite nutritional risk scores (6,10,11).

The domain of clinical nutrition research also often uses survey methods to assess the various dimensions of the individual's nutritional status (eg, retrospective and current dietary exposures, the key behavioral and ecological or environmental determinants of nutritional risk, and related health outcomes). Survey techniques are used to monitor controlled clinical trials. Information derived from these areas, often combined with findings from epidemiological investigations, has proven essential to evidence-based practice as well as for the design of effective preventive nutrition intervention strategies and medical nutrition therapies.

Survey research can extend to investigations of programs, communities, or entire systems. In the area of program or services evaluation research, survey methods may be used to assess the type, quality, impact, and efficacy of nutrition programs or interventions at the individual, community, or population levels. Alternatively, surveys may be designed to evaluate the characteristics of organizations, communities, or entire business frameworks (eg, availability of healthy food options, food retail stores, or farmers' markets) and their relation to population health.

In the agricultural sector, survey methods can be used to monitor the nature and quality of the US food supply and the nation's food production systems. This research provides information on commodities and the agricultural infrastructure, including domestic and international food production and distribution; food product imports and exports; and food processing practices (eg, pesticide and chemical use, animal feeds and treatment, acreage in organic farming). Survey research may also explore other wide-ranging dimensions of the food, foodservice, and nutriceutical industries.

SURVEY RESEARCH PLANNING

The goal of human nutrition survey research is to produce data on a sample of individuals drawn from a well-defined population of interest that relates to one or more of the following: nutrition-related beliefs, attitudes, and/or behaviors; their environmental influences, contexts, or determinants; and related health outcomes or consequences. Surveys may answer single or multiple research questions, test specific hypotheses, estimate population characteristics, formally model relationships between a set of nutritional characteristics and other variables, or accomplish other well-defined goals (12).

Critical to effective survey planning is a well-defined population of research interest (referent population) from which survey participants can be clearly identified and appropriately sampled. The term *population of interest* may include specific types of individuals, families, or households; consumer or professional subgroups; communities or populations with unique characteristics; or other key groups or entities with traits that may affect human nutrition. Unbiased, well-done investigations demand that the referent population's characteristics are carefully ascertained and that survey respondents are sampled with a known likelihood of participation; therefore, survey researchers typically use random or probability techniques rather than casual or convenience sampling (12–14).

Survey research protocols, including questionnaires, must be carefully constructed in order to establish that they will achieve the research's study goals and answer all research questions. Additionally, protocols must be designed to be well-suited to the research study subjects. It must be determined that the protocols can be understood and accurately completed by respondents with relative ease. These protocols must also conform to established research methods.

The survey research strategy also sets forth a coherent plan of operations for data collection, field operations (as appropriate), data set development, statistical analyses, and reporting. Survey research instruments and operating procedures are pretested and revised into final form to confirm that the array of survey methods is sufficient to achieve the established research goals and objectives and to answer all research questions. Quality control activities are performed throughout the research data collection activities as well as during research data coding and analysis. These procedures further confirm that high standards of research practice are achieved at all levels of survey operation.

An Ecological Framework for Nutrition Research Planning

At the outset of survey planning, you will carefully identify your research problem area and domains of research interest. You will specify the specific research questions; and the variables needed to achieve your study aims and answer all research questions. Nutrition and health experts have used the *ecological* framework to facilitate an understanding of relationships between potential domains of research investigations, including human behaviors (eg, diet), their environmental (ecological) determinants, and health-related outcomes.

The National Heart, Lung, and Blood Institute (NHLBI) recently used the ecological framework to inform its research planning processes for the examination of relationships among the environment, health-related behaviors including diet, and obesity-related health outcomes (15). A summary of an expert workshop on the topic can be found at the NHLBI Web site (16). Investigators from the Framingham Nutrition Studies added to the modeling by identifying methods for measuring overall diet behavior and quality. These included multivariable nutritional risk indexes as well as dietary patterns identified in the FNS populations of men and women (see Figure 13.1). Key considerations for applying the ecological model to survey research planning are summarized here.

The ecological framework identifies diet, including food and nutrient intake and composite measures of dietary quality (eg, dietary patterns and multiple-variable nutrient risk scores), as one of the primary modifiable human behaviors of research interest. The model acknowledges relationships between diet and other human behaviors, such as smoking and physical activity. It considers the complex array of environmental or ecological influences on these behaviors, including the following: characteristics of the individual (knowledge, attitudes, and other biological and demographic factors); the psychological, social or cultural, organizational, and physical environments in which the individual lives, functions, or is served or treated; and public and private policies, programs, and incentives that may influence diet and nutrition (such as Food Stamps or Medicare reimbursement of medical nutrition therapies). Any of these domains might become the focus of survey research. Therefore, during your initial survey planning and questionnaire design or protocol development activities, you should consider whether they are applicable to your research.

An important aspect of the ecological framework is the consideration of a wide range of nutrition- and health-related outcomes that may stem from dietary (or other lifestyle) behaviors, including biological risk factors and diseases or health conditions, as well as their comorbidities or consequences. The self-report of such health-related parameters may be of interest in your research and may be incorporated into your survey instrument or protocol development. Alternatively, relevant clinical data on nutrition-related health outcomes may be assessed independently (eg, plasma lipids or blood pressure) and linked analytically with survey research data. Such approaches enable the more thorough exploration of diet–disease risk relationships and may provide information and insights that are of use in the development of evidence-based interventions, therapies, and clinical practice guidelines.

The ecological framework can guide investigators in making careful decisions about broad domains or topics of research interest, focused research questions, and specific study variables. All of these considerations will be used in the survey planning process, particularly in the development of instruments and other research protocols. You may also be interested in exploring applications of the ecological model beyond survey research. Experts have used this approach extensively as a framework for intervention planning, and several key resources are available (17,18), including the National Cancer Institute's *Theory at a Glance: A Guide for Health Promotions Practice* (19).

Mapping the Survey Research Planning Process

Survey research is conducted in a series of complex stages (Box 13.1) that include the following: determining the research problem area and population of interest, creating a preliminary survey plan (including staff requirements, instruments and protocols), formulating the final survey plan and operating guidelines, implementing data collection (including quality control activities), and managing and analyzing data sets and reporting (12). Sound survey research employs a relatively systematic planning strategy, but experts acknowledge that the process unfolds dynamically during progressive stages of development and implementation. You can refer to a number of helpful full texts on survey research and Web-based resources for survey planning and instrument design (12–14,20–22).

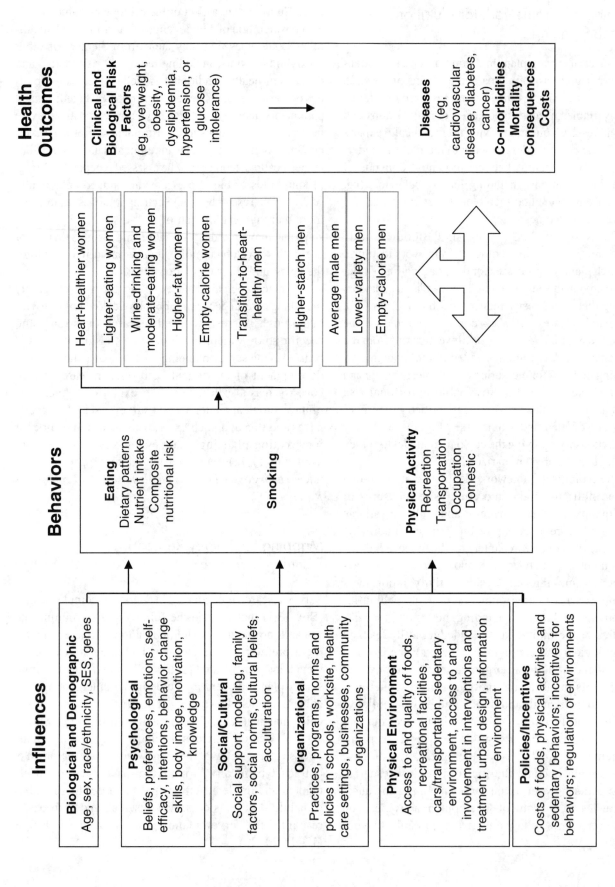

FIGURE 13.1   An ecological model of diet and health outcomes with dietary patterns. "SES" refers to socioeconomic status. "Heart-healthier women," "Average male men," and other similar terms refer to groups who meet specific eating patterns as determined by the Framingham dietary analysis.

BOX 13.1   Stages of Survey Research Planning

Step 1. Determine research problem area.
- Identify research aims, domains, and questions.
- Define population of interest.

Step 2. Create and pretest survey plan.
- Operationalize research questions.
- Create and pretest all survey protocols.
- Design plans for operations, analysis, and reporting.

Step 3. Finalize survey plan.
- Revise instruments and protocols.
- Hire and train personnel.

Step 4. Data collection.
- Select sample.
- Implement all survey protocols.
- Monitor quality control.

Step 5. Manage data analysis.
- Prepare and manage data sets.
- Conduct analyses and report findings.

At the outset of the survey planning process, you need to carefully state your overall goals and specify specific research aims and questions. You will closely identify the study population of interest and consider the resources and budget available to conduct the research. Most survey research is conducted on a fixed budget, so it is important that the planning process allocate resources, funding, and personnel to ensure that all research stages can be completed, including analysis and reporting. Research goals and questions, budget realities, and desired study population characteristics will guide the selection of the most appropriate and feasible survey methods. Your survey methods must be well defined and comprehensive and should include respondent sampling strategies, questionnaires/instrument design, data collection protocols, and plans for analysis and reporting. Regardless of the final research strategy, you should monitor all operations to ensure that quality control will be maintained throughout and that objective and ethical standards will be followed.

During the preliminary planning stages, you will typically review the existing literature to explore alternative approaches to your research design and data collection strategies. You will also identify the availability of established protocols for data collection, including validated survey questionnaires. As you begin to assemble your design elements and instruments, you should ask experts to review and comment on your approach. It is recommended that you conduct very preliminary pretests of survey protocols and specific questionnaire items. All research protocols, including subject sampling strategies, full questionnaires, and other data collection devices, should be as fully pretested as possible. It is optimal if multiple pretests can be accomplished and staged with one or more samples of suitable respondents whose profiles closely resemble the population of research interest. This enables you to fully understand the suitability of your methods and approaches vis-a-vis your subjects and research setting, and thorough pretesting may help prevent difficulties that could arise in actual survey operations.

Instrument and protocol pretesting often results in revisions of questionnaires and refinements to plans of research operation, including changes to one or more of the following: data collection methods, staff training, quality control procedures, and analytic plans. The pretesting stages will help you devise a survey management plan that will facilitate the smooth, objective, and ethical implementation of research and the successful achievement of research aims. Using an organized and tested plan, you will collect your data and compile them into one or more data sets. Your data sets must be carefully cleaned and edited before you undertake any statistical analyses. Then, you will summarize your findings in accordance with your research questions and produce reports or publications for various audiences.

It is important to consider each level of survey planning and operation in advance of data collection to ensure that your original goals are met, research quality is maintained, and resources are sufficient to implement and complete all stages of the research plan. In early planning stages, you should develop a clear understanding of the aims and scope of your study, fully characterize your study population, carefully define your research questions, and explore various methods for variable measurement and modes of data collection. It is particularly crucial to anticipate and outline your intended statistical analyses and reporting plans. You should recognize that all research surveys are subject to a variety of constraints (eg, budgetary constraints that may limit your sample size or the scope and methods of data collection). Understanding these potential limitations in the planning process will help you to optimize features of your study design. As appropriate, study limitations should be acknowledged in research reporting.

Survey research should be evidence-based, and new investigations should add to the body of evidence on a given topic or domain. Thus, peer-reviewed literature is used to inform as many of the research planning stages as possible, and insights from that literature are applied (as deemed feasible and appropriate) to each study. You will rely on available literature not only to carefully articulate your research questions but also to identify options for instruments and protocols, as well as data collection and statistical methods. The review of current literature and insights drawn from experts in the field of interest will also help you make informed decisions about study population characteristics, sampling strategies, methods to promote respondent participation and survey completion rates, and ways to enhance other features of the research.

Population Sampling

Your research aims and resources will affect your consideration of population sampling strategies. Choices include random, probability, or clustered sampling strategies, and your selection should be guided by published research and current state-of-the-art in the field. Advanced technologies are now available to facilitate random sampling and can be applied to telephone or Web-based surveys (eg, random-digit dialing and random e-mail access). Alternatively, increasingly complex probability or clustered sampling devices may be used to achieve efficiencies in research. These techniques will facilitate the selection and inclusion of respondents with specific characteristics (area/geography, age or racial/ethnic characteristics, and so on), and the data can be statistically modeled to allow your research results to more fully reflect your population of interest. You may want to refer to other resources and references on these topics (12–14,20–22).

Most of the previous discussion has pertained to single-population (sample) surveys. However, you may also be interested in comparing two or more populations (or subgroups) of research interest (eg, clinical cases vs control subjects, program/intervention participants compared with matched nonparticipants, or "majority" populations in contrast to underrepresented minorities). In these situations, you will carefully sample the various populations or subgroups of interest and make certain that you have sufficient numbers of subjects in each category to enable meaningful comparisons between groups of interest.

Estimating Statistical Power

When planning your study, you must determine the study's statistical power. Within available resources, you will need sufficient numbers of survey respondents (ie, adequate study power) to answer your research questions confidently. Depending on your stated research goals and aims, you need to be prepared to test your hypotheses, derive sound estimates of the characteristics or outcomes of interest, determine the effect of the treatments or interventions of interest, or explore relationships among research variables. To arrive at a sound survey design, you need to become accustomed early in the research planning process to thinking about your study power.

The existing literature provides important information for establishing a research study's power. You will need to review the research literature pertaining to your specific research problem area to identify what you might expect relating to each research question. For example, if you were interested in estimating a population's rate of a nutrition-related problem, you would review the available literature to assess what the expected rate(s) might be, including the confidence intervals around the estimates. To complete this task, you would examine the literature for the following: What proportion of the population of interest might be expected to have a specific nutrition problem (eg, overweight and obesity)? How do these rates vary in published population estimates?

In another study, you may be interested in examining the strength of association between a dietary exposure (eg, food or nutrient intake, level of dietary quality) and a potential set of behavioral determinants or certain health outcomes (eg, body weight or body mass index [BMI]). The researcher may pose additional questions about the observed relationship (eg, is a correlation between *trans* fat intake and overweight independent of intake levels for other key macro- or micronutrients or other characteristics of the individual?). In such cases, you would use the literature to quantify what you would expect to find (eg, How strong a correlation between the dietary factor and weight [or BMI] are you expecting? What are the confidence intervals around published estimates of these relationships?). To the extent possible, you will need to use published data relating to your research questions to make formal calculations of your research study's statistical power.

While you explore the published literature, you must also establish the tolerable levels of study error. Specifically, you will have to define the levels of α (type I) and β (type II) errors that you will accept in your research. Alpha (type I) error considers the following question: What is the risk of rejecting the null hypothesis if it is true? For example, what is the risk of concluding that a relationship exists between diet and a biological risk factor (such as low-density lipoprotein cholesterol levels), when it does not actually exist? Beta (type II error) considers the risk of accepting the null hypothesis when it is false. For example, what is the risk of concluding that diet is *unrelated* to the development of a disease when it actually is related? You can minimize α error by applying appropriate criteria in your statistical testing, and you can reduce β error by recruiting sufficient numbers of research subjects.

It may be suitable to rely on certain research conventions when you calculate a study's statistical power. For example, a typical approach sets the statistical α error limit at 5% or below (in this scenario, you will set significance levels for your statistical testing at $P < .05$). Using this criterion, the chance of rejecting the null hypothesis when it is true is 1 in 20 or lower. Another common convention to reduce β error is to set the power level at 15% or less. In this example, you will need to determine the numbers of subjects that are sufficient to answer your particular research question(s) with 85% or greater power. Here, there is a 15% or lower chance of accepting the null hypothesis when it is false (eg, concluding that diet is not associated with a health outcome when, in fact, it is related). Certainly, power calculations can be made with even stricter error criteria, but this will increase the number of study subjects needed for a given research investigation.

Statisticians can help you to estimate your study's statistical power. However, as the previous discussion and examples suggest, your expert consultants will expect you to provide the information needed to conduct the study's power calculations. You should become comfortable searching the literature for relevant data that can be used in power calculations as described earlier. Further discussions of study power calculations can be found in select key resources (14,23).

Personnel Planning Considerations

Final planning considerations include the recruitment, training, and monitoring of qualified survey research personnel. All staff need to be suitably experienced and fully trained in the protocols for which they are responsible. The requirements for staff training will be guided by your instrument and study protocol designs. Training should also focus on any problems or issues that are identified in the research pretesting process. You will need to apply quality control measures to all staff activities, including sampling, data collection, coding, statistical analyses, and reporting procedures. Quality control at all levels is essential to ensure that requisite research operational procedures are maintained and to achieve confidence in your research.

Survey Planning Examples

The following sections explore various survey planning activities as carried out in the NNMRRP and the Framingham Nutrition Studies. During this discussion, refer to the comparison of selected features of the national surveys that are summarized in Table 13.1. Information on survey questionnaire design is presented later in this chapter.

TABLE 13.1   Comparison of Three Federal Surveys

Survey Name	Year Begun	Current Sample Size	Goal	Methods Used	Domains
NHANES	1960	7,000/year	Continuous system of monitoring health, nutritional status and well-being in the United States	ACASI, CAPI, paper and pencil, MEC	Dietary intake; demographics; food security; health insurance; pesticide use; health behaviors; health status; drug use; full physical examinations; laboratory analysis of blood, tissue, and urine samples
CSFII	1985	33,000 noninstutionalized participants during a 2-year period	Determine and monitor the food consumption and nutrition knowledge in the United States	AMPM (dietary recall), CAPI, phone interview	Dietary intake, demographics, food source, water source, food program participation, food shopping practices, health status, dietary knowledge
NHIS	1957	106,000 noninstutionalized civilians/year	Monitor trends in health and health status	Paper and pencil, CAPI	Demographics, health behavior, health status, illness, disability status

Abbreviations: ACASI, audio computer assisted personal self interview; AMPM, automated multiple-pass method; CAPI, computer assisted personal interview; CSFII, Continuing Survey of Food Intakes by Individuals; MEC, mobile examination component; NHANES, National Health and Nutrition Examination Survey; NHIS, National Health Interview Survey.

National Health Interview Survey Planning

NHIS is a continuous cross-sectional survey of the US population that began in 1957. The instrument is updated every 10 to 15 years. As briefly explained in Chapter 10, NHIS was designed as a means of monitoring trends in the health and health status of Americans (including health behavior and outcomes such as illness and disability). The NHIS sample unit is the household unit, with one child and one adult randomly selected and interviewed from each household. Households are randomly selected by geographic probability sampling to ensure a nationally representative sample (24). The response rate for this survey is excellent, with annual completion rates in eligible households reaching more than 90% (24).

Starting in 1995, NHIS deliberately oversampled African-American (1.5:1) and Hispanic residents (2:1) to achieve a more nationally representative sample of respondents. The goal for the 1996 through 2004 surveys was to improve statistical reliability of the research findings for ethnic, racial, and regional subgroups of interest (24). Using such sampling strategies, the investigators also developed a more statistically powerful study design from which valid conclusions could be drawn on all selected subgroups.

Given the scope of the NHIS, the interviewers for this survey are drawn from the US Census Bureau staff, and they work in conjunction with the CDC. The approximately 400 interviewers used each year are thoroughly trained by the US Census Bureau regional offices (24).

Survey Planning for the Continuing Survey of Food Intakes by Individuals

CSFII began as a large, federally funded stand-alone study conducted by the USDA in 1985. It was designed to determine, at an individual level, "what we eat in America." CSFII's original goals were to identify the types and amounts of foods consumed by Americans and to assess the knowledge about diet and nutrition of a nationally representative sample of the US population. Between 1985 and 2002, there were six survey cycles, and details of the more recent examination of individual intake specifically (1994–1996) are discussed here. As noted in Chapter 10, CSFII was integrated into the NHANES survey beginning in 2002. However, the survey design and methods of earlier CSFII studies serve as a good example of national dietary study.

The study population for CSFII 1994–1996 was determined by the USDA. However, a private research firm conducted the specific sampling strategy, instrument design, promotional materials, pretesting, and implementation (3).

Population sampling and respondent selection involved a complex multistage probability sampling strategy. The entire United States was divided into population sampling units (PSUs) at the county level. Within the PSUs, individual dwelling units (DUs) were the household units sampled for the survey. Demographic breakdown of each PSU was obtained from US Census data to ensure a nationally representative sample, and sampling strategies included the oversampling of various racial and ethnic groups. A complete description of the sampling formulas and procedures for missed DUs can be found in the CSFII operations manual, which is available online (3).

The CSFII surveys were conducted by trained field and research personnel employed by the private research firm. These personnel included 80 English-speaking interviewers, 10 bilingual interviewers, 5 senior interviewers, 5 regional supervisors, and several data coders. Training materials for these staff members included an extensive manual, complete with examples, role-playing exercises, and coding instructions (3). Additionally, training sessions were conducted for several days depending on the position. In addition, USDA (Agricultural Research Service) staff members were extensively involved in oversight of the survey. A team of nutrition professionals, survey methodologists, statisticians, food specialists, and project managers was involved in planning and managing CSFII (3).

Planning for the National Health and Nutrition Examination Survey

NHANES is the largest federally conducted population study in the United States (25), with eight survey cycles conducted between 1971 and 2004. This population monitoring system was preceded by the National Health Examination Survey I–III (NHES), which was conducted in the 1960s (26). The goals of NHANES have been to determine the population prevalence of various diseases and biological risk factors (eg, dyslipidemia, hypertension, obesity), to monitor the trends in behavioral and environmental determinants of disease risk, to test hypotheses and model nutrition–disease risk relationships, and to explore a range of public health policy concerns (27). NHANES now serves as a continuous annual survey conducted for the purpose of monitoring the health and well-being of the US population. Survey response rates are close to 80% (25).

As is the case with any national study, the NHANES sample populations are selected using complex multistage probability sampling and weighting. A full description can be found on the NHANES portion of the CDC Web site (28), and is summarized in Chapter 10. The multiple survey sampling and data collection protocols and procedures for NHANES required careful recruitment of qualified staff and extensive training; this is an important consideration when designing multisite studies.

NHANES planning resulted in two primary modes of data collection; protocols are completed in mobile examination units and through in-home interviews. The mobile examination units allow NHANES to collect data on various domains of nutritional risk (eg, anthropometric, clinical, and biological samples from respondents) using standardized protocols. Home visits enable field staff to conduct in-person interviews and to carry materials to help facilitate data collection (eg, tools for food portion estimation and written directions). Staff in both field settings use laptop computers to conduct the mobile examination component (MEC) or computer-assisted personal interviews (CAPI). All staff are instructed to read introductory information, respondent instructions, and survey questionnaire items directly from their computer screens. This protocol standardizes questionnaire administration and is one of the field methods of research quality control.

Planning for the Framingham Nutrition Studies

The Framingham Study (originally known as Framingham Heart Study, or FHS) was initiated in 1948, and is one of the most important and longest-standing prospective epidemiological investigations ever conducted. This investigation was originally designed to study the natural history and determinants of cardiovascular disease (CVD) but has since been expanded substantially to examine a wide range of topics (eg, aging, other chronic disease endpoints, familial genetics).

The Framingham Study includes two major respondent cohorts: the original cohort of 5,209 men and women, ages 18 to 60 years (at baseline), who were initially recruited in the late 1940s; and the 5,135 Framingham offspring (of the original FHS cohort study participants) and their spouses, who were recruited in 1972 to comprise the Framingham Offspring Study (FOS) (29). Framingham, Massachusetts, was chosen as the study population of interest by the NHLBI of the National Institutes of Health (NIH) after a national investigation identified communities with population profiles that provided a suitable microcosm of the US population in the mid–20th century. Although the original Framingham cohort was considered a population representative of a typical American community, respondents were largely nonminority individuals (fewer than 2% of respondents were from minority populations). Framingham investigators point out this limitation with the original cohort and FOS studies; nonetheless, they also

emphasize that Framingham models of CVD and other disease risks have been confirmed and replicated in other, diverse populations worldwide. Detailed descriptions of the FHS and FOS methods have been previously published (29). In brief, the protocols include comprehensive behavioral and biological CVD risk factor assessments every 2 years (in the original cohort) and every 4 years (in the FOS), as well as confirmed appraisal of all health outcomes, including types and number of events and cause of mortality. Further details can be found on the study's Web site (30), which also provides a complete listing of Framingham publications, and a discussion of relatively new initiatives including the recruitment of a minority cohort, multigenerational studies, and other ancillary research.

The Framingham Nutrition Studies were initiated in 1984, after a more than decade-long hiatus in nutrition research at FHS. In the first 5 years, the FNS were funded as part of the FHS core contract with NIH. Since then, the FNS have been continuously funded with federal and private resources to investigate a wide range of nutrition topics and to examine diet–disease risk relationships in the FHS cohorts (4,9–11,16,31).

The motivation to develop the FNS was the increasing evidence of the importance of diet–disease relationships, in particular CVD outcomes. The FNS set forth to conduct a comprehensive assessment of dietary behaviors that were postulated to be of relevance to CVD morbidity and mortality, including established and emerging biological risk factors. The overall goals of the FNS were the following: to quantify trends in the Framingham population's food and nutrient intake; to develop traditional and innovative nutritional risk assessment methods; to examine the relationships between dietary behaviors, disease risk, and health outcomes; and to identify opportunities for preventive nutrition intervention strategies. FNS took particular interest in formal hypothesis testing and the statistical modeling of diet–disease risk and diet–disease outcome relationships; however, we were also keen to use this opportunity to develop nutrition-related epidemiological research methods and to conduct translational research on topics of relevance to evidence-based clinical practice and prevention nutrition interventions.

Given the fixed (existing) nature of the Framingham cohort populations, it was important to ascertain study power, particularly relating to the hypothesis testing and modeling of diet–disease relationships. The FNS team set its tolerable level of alpha error (in this case, the risk of finding an association between diet and disease risk when none exists) at less than 5% ($P < .05$). The investigators also had to examine β (type II) errors (ie, the risk of concluding that diet is *unrelated* to the development of CVD risk when it is actually related). To accomplish the power calculation, we examined the available published evidence on the strength of associations between diet, biological risk factors, and CVD outcomes. It was ascertained that many of the relationships of interest between diet and disease risk were likely to be clinically important but statistically relatively weak associations (correlations of $r \leq 0.2–0.4$). We used existing literature and available data to project the rate of development of all outcomes of research interest in both the men and women cohorts (at Framingham, disease-specific morbidity and mortality are confirmed with external clinical records and undergo complete internal expert panel review). This outcome evidence and projections are updated regularly and available for power calculations as well as research study statistical analyses.

Armed with available internal and published information, we were able a priori to conduct statistical power calculations. We ascertained that the original and FOS cohorts were of sufficient size to achieve a study power of 85% or greater (ie, the cohorts contained sufficient numbers of study respondents and numbers of projected outcomes). When carrying out formal multivariate statistical modeling of diet–disease risk relationships, it was thus determined that the risk of a beta error is 15% or less, giving us a high level of confidence in our findings of independent associations between diet and disease risk.

In addition to formal statistical power considerations, we regularly emphasize that errors inherent in all types of epidemiological research, but particularly in those relating to self-reported behaviors (eg, diet), may attenuate diet–disease relationships. We acknowledge these limitations in our reports, often noting that the relationships observed between diet and disease risk in our data analyses may actually *underestimate* the true diet–disease relationships. We also use advanced statistical modeling to attempt to correct for such self-report biases. See various reports of FNS findings for further discussion of the study (4,9–11,16,31–34). An excellent primer on statistical considerations in research planning is Ajetunmobi's text, *Making Sense of Critical Appraisal* (23).

METHODS OF SURVEY DATA COLLECTION AND QUESTIONNAIRE DESIGN

One of the most important stages of survey research is the selection of the mode(s) and method(s) of data collection, including the development of research questionnaires and other data collection protocols. The options for human survey data collection include self-administered (print or electronic) instruments and interviewer-administered questionnaires (using face-to-face or telephone formats). Data may be collected on one or more individuals in solo or group settings. In depth consideration of these topics is found in several classic and current texts (12–14,20) and Web-based resources (21). Selected key details of these processes are summarized here with applications to nutrition research.

The mode of data collection selected will depend on a variety of factors, including the ease of identifying suitable and available study subjects, the characteristics of respondents, the complexity and sensitivity of the desired survey data, the difficulty of reporting or data collection activities, the perceived optimal methods of data collection, staffing requirements, the project's budgetary and resource constraints, and so on (12–14). To make coherent decisions, you will consider each of these factors and select a mode or method that best suits your research interests and plan. Ideally, one or more of the selected strategies for data collection will allow you to collect a complex a set of desired data from a suitable sample of suitable respondents with the most efficient use of resources.

Early in the research planning process, you will consider whether your research questions demand that you assess one or more *domains* of an individual's nutritional risk or status, including dietary behavior, anthropometric indexes, clinical characteristics, biomarkers or biological risk factors, and diseases or other health outcomes. It is also important to assess whether information is needed on the environmental determinants of dietary behavior or nutritional risk or other outcomes (eg, hospital or long-term care admissions, costs of services). Once the domains of interest and specific research variables are articulated, you can better determine the ideal modes(s) and method(s) of data collection.

The design of the actual survey instrument will involve similar factors; you will weigh your options and arrive at a methodology that best suits your study goals and research questions, the characteristics of your subjects and the project staff, and the available financial and related resources. Early in the planning process, you will clearly define each research question and break it into its discrete component variables (12,14). Experts refer to this process as one of operationalizing your research questions and variables. Throughout this process, you seek to identify a final set of research domains and research questions and determine the comprehensive list of variables that are needed to answer all research questions. Each variable will then be linked to a method of measurement that will be incorporated into your data collection instrument(s) and protocol(s). In addition, you will consider how each variable measurement strategy relates to your data analysis plan.

There is a wide range of specific subject characteristics that may affect research protocols and methods of data collection. These include the respondents' location and your access to them; their primary language, literacy level, and levels of cognitive function and memory; their functional capacity or disability; and conditions or characteristics that may affect responses or behaviors, including willingness to participate in the research, likely compliance with protocols, and so on. If respondent characteristics pose serious limitations, research protocols will need to be adjusted. In some situations, proxy respondents may be used. Proxy respondents are suitable substitutes if they adequately represent the intended research subject and are able to answer a sufficient number of the research questionnaire items or complete the specified study protocols.

Your variable measurement strategies and research protocols will also affect your research staffing requirements. You will recruit and train personnel and implement quality control procedures that are appropriate to your data collection activities. You must consider these research dimensions prior to finalizing your data collection methods and in order to design and implement a coherent and suitable plan of research operation.

When you select data collection and measurement techniques, aim for an evidence-based study design that is feasible and appropriate to your research aims and questions, study population characteristics, and resources. You will always be faced with a wide range of issues and options to consider in setting your research plan and operations. As needed, you will weigh design complexity against what is suitable and manageable within resource constraints. During this process, data accuracy should not be sacrificed, as that will only undermine your confidence in the research plan and data. Refer to important references on this topic (12–14,21–23).

Data Collection Methods

Survey researchers employ a variety of data collection methods. The most common include qualitative or (semi)quantitative questionnaires that typically use one of the following approaches:

- **Self-administered:** mail or electronic (computer or Web-based) protocols
- **Interviewer-administered:** telephone or face-to-face (in-person) methodologies

Although interviews and questionnaires are often completed by self-report or with interviewer assistance in several formats, you may consider design modifications to increase response rates. For example, you may use a group format to complete self-administered questionnaires. Alternatively, you can use research staff to hand-deliver and/or pick up surveys. These data collection features may help to clarify questions or responses and enable interactions with survey participants that might increase their participation and completion of protocols.

Depending on the research questions of interest, survey instruments (questionnaires) may be qualitative, semiquantitative, or quantitative in nature. These methods are all broadly used in survey research. For example, nutrition epidemiologists may use qualitative questionnaires to assess dietary behaviors (eg, dietary supplement use, self-imposed or professionally recommended dieting) or environmental factors (eg, personal characteristics, cultural influences, involvement in private and public nutrition programs, interventions, or treatments) that may influence dietary exposures and their health-related outcomes. Semiquantitative questionnaires, such as certain food frequency instruments, can be used to characterize food intake behavior or estimate subjects' nutrient intake. Quantitative questionnaires can be used to determine an individual's level of food and nutrient intake or related characteristics and behaviors. The types of survey items and protocols need to be carefully considered because they will affect your mode of data collection and other dimensions of your research. Methods used to develop various types of questionnaires and specific survey items will be discussed in greater detail in the following chapter segment.

When selecting a mode of data collection, you also must consider types of research questions or variables. If the domains of research interest are quite sensitive, they may be better suited to self-administered methods of data collection that offer higher levels of potential anonymity (12,14). In contrast, biological, anthropometric, and clinical testing will rely on direct respondent contact unless an accurate alternative method of data collection can be identified (eg, mailed blood or urine samples for biological testing).

You will need to weigh additional advantages and disadvantages of each available mode of survey data collection. Interviewer-assisted methods have the advantages of providing a mechanism for personal contact, rapport building, review of survey questions and responses, and guidance of respondents through instruments and item sequences by trained staff. They also allow for clarification of instructions and questions and provide opportunities for the interviewer to probe respondent answers. The latter is particularly key if a questionnaire protocol includes items that are complex, such as a questionnaire with a large number of items, questions with numerous response categories, or questions that only certain respondents answer. In this situation, respondents may need instructions to successfully navigate the instrument (eg, directions to skip certain items) (12–14).

Self-administered questionnaires may ease respondent burden by giving participants the time to think through responses. Also, depending upon the location of administration, self-administered questionnaires may allow subjects to search for necessary data, complete diaries that may facilitate self-reporting, or check records for information that may influence responses. However, self-administered protocols may lack a level of quality control seen with other data collection modes. They may require higher literacy levels or cognitive functioning in respondents, and they do not enable investigators to control who actually completes the questionnaire. Computer technology may help investigators to maintain levels of quality control and check for consistency or erroneous responses.

CAPI and computer-assisted telephone interviews (CATI) may increase opportunities for research quality control. Interviewers can be guided by the system through the logic and detail of the interview questionnaire and can be prompted, as needed, if they make any mistakes. However, interviewer-administered surveys tend to be costly and time consuming, regardless of print or electronic administration (12–14). They may also pose field management difficulties if respondents are accessible only in dangerous or potentially hazardous settings. Under these circumstances, telephone interviewing may offer economies of time and cost efficiencies, and they may provide better population access and response rates than mail or electronic methods.

Mailed or Web-based, self-administered surveys are advantageous and particularly cost-efficient if respondents are not easily accessible; they also offer the aforementioned advantages of allowing respondents time to contemplate and complete instruments. However, these surveys do not provide an opportunity to personally guide respondents or offer clarification on items if needed. Furthermore, self-administered surveys may involve issues of (non)response bias, as noted earlier.

Another alternative to consider is the use of hand-delivered and picked up instruments. This approach enables survey staff to introduce the instrument, provide instructions, and clarify protocols, and it may provide opportunities to motivate respondents, increase response rates, and to check surveys for completeness at pick-up (12–14, 20).

You should carefully consider modes of data collection and select one or more methods that meet your research aims. The domains of research interest may also dictate that questionnaires be combined with the collection of biological, clinical, anthropometric, and potentially other types of data. As noted previously, the goal of the data collection methods, however simple or complex, is to achieve a strategy that accomplishes one's research aims with the highest level of accuracy possible, with the least respondent and staff burden, and with resource allocations that enable all stages of the research process to be accomplished, including analyses and reporting. Careful consideration also needs to be given to minimizing the potential for bias introduced by survey researchers or their staff or subjects. You should take care to maintain research objectivity and strict attention to protocols in conducting all levels of your research, including analyses and reporting. The potential influences of subject characteristics (eg, geographic inaccessibility or potential difficulties in completing research protocols) need to be assessed and addressed in all stages of survey planning. Once again, the literature and experts in the field can provide guidance on methods of minimizing research bias.

Questionnaire and Protocol Design

Having considered and selected one or more suitable modes of data collection, you need to construct your data collection instruments and research protocols, including survey questionnaires. The design of research instruments and protocols should follow a logical, systematic process that includes operationalizing your research questions and specifying all the information that is needed to achieve your research aims. Ideally, each question is translated into one or more specific research variables. Then, you can be more directed in your review of published literature and Web resources for suitable research protocols, instruments, or specific survey items and questions. Consider how your variable measurement strategies might influence research operations and staffing, and also dictate the data analysis plan. The final approaches to data collection will be those that you deem to be most suitable, accurate, and feasible within the project's aims, resources, and budget.

After selecting data collection methods, you will conduct one or more rounds of pretesting to evaluate your questionnaires, other study protocols (if used), and the overall plan of operations. You may need to revise instruments and protocols as you glean information from these activities.

During the instrument and protocol development process, it is important to clearly conceptualize what information is needed to answer each research question as completely as possible. Each research question needs to be formally operationalized (12,14) such that each of its components (ie, its attributes and characteristics) are clearly defined for measurement purposes. Investigators will recognize that variables can be assessed in a number of ways with techniques that may vary in complexity and accuracy (eg, self-report vs observed or measured dietary intake). Depending upon the complexity of the research variables, your mode of data collection (eg, staff measurement or interview or self-report) will be affected. Furthermore, investigators can use qualitative or (semi)quantitative strategies to perform variable measurement on various levels. These strategies may each vary in complexity (eg, type and format of questions, number of items). As data collection modes and techniques are considered, researchers will narrow their selection to those strategies that allow an optimal level and complexity of variable measurement. You should arrive at a set of instruments and protocols that enable you to answer your research questions as completely and accurately as possible with the highest likelihood of respondent participation and completion rates.

When constructing survey questionnaires, you should focus on a number of particularly key considerations. Each research variable is translated into one or more survey items, and each item should contain response categories that capture the variable meaningfully and completely. The items should also meet specific structural requirements; its response categories should be *mutually exclusive* and *exhaustive* (13,14). For each variable to have mutually exclusive responses, care should be taken to construct responses that can be classified in only one way. For example, gender is answered as "male" or "female," and employment status can be characterized as "employed" or "unemployed." Responses that are exhaustive will provide *all* suitable options (ie, every possible answer is mentioned). If needed, the "other" response category can be used as a convention to provide this dimension.

Appropriate variable measurement strategies also consider that the qualities and characteristics under investigation may have specific underlying attributes that determine their measurement and that will affect subsequent data analyses. Variables can be measured with nominal, ordinal, interval, or ratio scales. You should be aware that variable measurement terminology differs somewhat depending on the survey resources used. For example, variable measurement scales may also be described as discrete, categorical (binary or ranked), or continuous (normally distributed or skewed) (13,14,23). Relationships between the terms used in these different situations are integrated here.

Nominal variables are also discrete (binary or multiple categorical variables) and meet the aforementioned properties of being exhaustive and mutually exclusive. However, these variables are qualitative and do not have specified or implied quantitative relationships between responses. You can use nominal variable measurement techniques when evaluating a respondent's use of specific food items, types of diets, dietary supplements, or meals (eg, "Do you eat breakfast daily? Yes or No"). Response categories may also include lists of items for a respondent to consider ("Check all that apply"). You may use nominal measurement scales to assess the environmental characteristics that could influence a respondent's nutrition behavior or outcomes (eg, the individual's cultural background and characteristics, exposure to nutrition services, and family and household characteristics).

Ordinal (ranked, categorical) variables contain response categories that achieve the structure of being mutually exclusive and exhaustive, but responses are also logical and rank-ordered (eg, "Do you consider your current health to be: Excellent, Very Good, Good, Fair, or Poor?" or "How often do you consume breakfast? Rarely or Never, About Once a Month; Several Times a Month, Once a Week, Several Days a Week; or Daily"). Interval measurement of variables provides ordered *continuous* response categories with a unique distance between the responses. However, variable measurements of this sort contain an arbitrary "zero" point (eg, zero degrees on a temperature measurement scale is set arbitrarily).

Ratio measurement achieves all the characteristics of ordinal measurements, but here the distances between values on a scale are meaningful (eg, body weight is measured in pounds or kilograms; nutrient intake can be measured in grams or other established units). Many clinical or biological parameters of interest in nutrition research (eg, plasma lipid, glucose, or nutritional biomarker levels) also use ratio measurement scales. Be aware that ratio data can be continuous and normally distributed or skewed. It may require statistical adjustment (eg, log transformations) to handle such data correctly in your analyses.

For some research questions, nominal scales may be the only available variable measurement strategy, and this type of variable measurement can be used quite appropriately. However, if you have established the need for quantitative measurement of your research variables, appropriate interval or ratio (continuous) scales should be identified or developed to assess the relevant research variables. If the levels of desired variable measurement are not exactly clear at the outset, you would be advised to opt for higher levels of quantitative (continuous) measurement. This, of course, depends on whether suitable techniques are available or can be developed and tested within your research timetable (13,14).

The approaches to variable measurement outlined earlier have direct implications for the investigators' data analysis plan. A detailed discussion of this topic is beyond the scope of this chapter; for more information, consult Ajetunmobi's excellent primer (24).

A final consideration is the effects of variable measurement on respondents themselves, study personnel, and project implementation. Although you must design research questionnaires with sound and suitably complex methods to achieve study aims, the questionnaires must also be tailored to fit your resources and feasible and manageable for your personnel. Before finalizing your instruments and protocols, review and consider their impact on all persons involved in the conduct of your research, including intended respondents (and their proxies, as appropriate) and your research staff. Be certain that resources are adequate not only for data collection and management but also for your analyses and reporting activities. Develop training and quality control activities that ensure the successful completion of all data collection and maintain confidence in your analyses and reporting.

Formatting Questions and Surveys

Once the level and complexity of variable measurement level are established, questions can be carefully formatted and laid out in your survey instruments. Self-administered questionnaires often begin with the most interesting items to engage respondents. Interviewer-administered surveys may begin with the simplest items to build rapport. It is helpful to remember that the overall goal of the survey research is to use an appropriate array of statements, questions, and protocols to collect data in a manageable, defined manner from a carefully identified population. All of these elements of data collection are designed to achieve the intended level of research complexity, to accomplish your study aims, and to answer your research questions. A detailed discussion of these topics is found in key references and Web sites (12–14,21–22).

Instruments/questionnaires and protocols should contain suitable and unambiguous wording. Instructions, questions, and response categories should be clear and understood by staff and respondents. Avoid items that are likely to be misinterpreted. The terms and conditions used in specific questions need to be well-defined (eg, "Between midnight on [day/date] and 8 AM on [day/date], did you eat or drink anything other than water?"). Responses should have only single dimensions; double or multiple components (referred to as double-barreled items) should be avoided.

There are several other considerations related to the wording of your questionnaire items. You may use closed-ended questions (eg, "What is your gender? Male or Female") or open-ended items (eg, "Describe your usual weekday eating pattern."). You may incorporate certain qualifying statements to clarify items (eg, "Describe everything you ate or drank *since midnight*."). Qualifiers allow respondents to make a summary judgment (eg, "Considering all sources of influence on your eating behavior, what is most important?" or "Overall, would you say you are satisfied or not satisfied with your experience?"). Such items call for qualified adjectives (eg, "Identify your *most important* source of nutrition information."). As noted in the earlier discussion, items should include a set of responses (mutually exclusive and exhaustive). However, items may involve a long or complex list of choices for respondents to consider. Aim to make this task as easy for respondents as possible. Alternatively, open-ended responses allow respondents to provide information in their own forms. The process of formatting questionnaires is discussed in further detail in various resources and texts (12–14,20–22).

The physical design of Web-based surveys involves some considerations that are similar to issues encountered with printed surveys; however, factors unique to the Web need additional consideration. In both paper and Web surveys, an introductory statement that explains the survey itself (including the expected time for completion) and background on the importance of the survey may help increase response rates. All surveys should be attractive and easy to read (eg, printed in an appropriate text size, using readable fonts and colors), and they should not be difficult to complete. The layout and ordering of questions in a survey instrument is an essential consideration for all types of surveys.

For many surveys, using the Web is an attractive alternative to print because it offers options that may increase ease of administration (eg, pull-down menus, check boxes, motivating graphics). However, it is important to ensure that a Web-only survey does not introduce selection and response biases with regard to the target population. More importantly, a Web survey should only be used if it increases ease of response; using complex web surveys that slow down respondents may actually decrease response rates.

TABLE 13.2 Question Design of Web Based Surveys

Answer Format	Description	Used for
Pull-down menus	Click and hold to select and answer from a set list	One-line responses
Radio buttons	Open circles that are clicked to select the answer	Single- or multiple-answer questions
Check boxes	Clicking a box will insert a check mark, indicating the respondent's choice	Multiple-answer questions (eg, "Check all that apply")
Text boxes	Boxes where respondent can freely type in answers	Open-ended questions and free text

For the survey itself, there are a variety of questionnaire types that can be considered. Several examples of question formats are shown in Table 13.2.

There are some limitations to all of the question types identified in Table 13.2. Pull-down menus may save some space and may motivate the respondent, but they can also be difficult to use, resulting in incorrect or incomplete answers (21). Free-text boxes allow respondents to give both short and long answers, but the answers may be difficult to score.

Using a survey software package can reduce some of the problems with on-line surveys. The Survey System is an online resource for investigators that includes design tips and downloadable software packages that can target specific problems (eg, limiting e-mail responses to one per address). Web page design techniques can also aid in limiting inappropriate responses. You may want to require a survey Web site password or identifier (eg, an e-mail address or code) to restrict site access to only intended respondents. Resources on Web-based survey design (21) include the University of Maryland's on-line tools for beginning investigators to design Web-based surveys (22).

Once you have drafted your instruments and protocols, you will conduct one or more levels of pretesting to detect potential flaws or problems. You may wish to ask experts to assess item content, format, and overall layout of questionnaires or aspects of your research protocols. You can test your protocols in focus groups involving experts on the research topic or small sample of respondents (whose profile is similar to the study population of interest). You may also devise small-scale pretests to mimic your survey in operation. As the pretesting proceeds, you can revise research instruments and protocols. During this stage, you are likely to consult on a number of occasions with staff and respondents who are involved in the pretests. You may also want to observe staff and/or subject behavior during pretesting activities to observe and confirm that your research methods work in practice.

If you are developing new instruments or protocols, they must be formally tested for reliability and validity in advance of use. For more on these important tests, refer to texts that discuss them in detail (35,36).

Overall, the design of survey instruments should make their administration as easy as possible for respondents and staff. Self-administered surveys should be self-explanatory unless you intend for staff to interact with respondents. Questionnaire items should be clear, unambiguous, appropriate to the research, as short as possible, unbiased, and as positive in terminology as possible. Instruments should be clearly formatted and as short as possible. Related items should be clearly linked, with other items set apart. By embedding these features in the instruments and protocols, you will make the survey easier for your respondents and staff.

The following sections discuss the application of survey data collection and questionnaire design approaches in the NNMRRP and the FNS. (Refer also to Box 13.1.)

NHIS Instrument Considerations

The most recent NHIS instrument updates were introduced for the 1997 survey and will be described here. A complete description of the survey can be found on the CDC Web site (37). The 1997 revision restructured the survey to included three parts: the Basic module, the Periodic module, and the Topical module. The Basic module is itself broken down into three parts: the Family core, the Sample Adult core, and the Sample Child core. These cores include survey questions related to several broad variable domains associated with trends in health and health status of Americans, including health behavior and outcomes such as illness and disability.

CSFII Instrument Considerations

The survey examines a wide array of domains, including selected environmental determinants of dietary behavior, nutrition knowledge and attitudes, food and nutrient intake, and self-reported health parameters. During the sixth USDA CSFII cycle, several dietary survey instruments were completed; these used several modes of data collection, including an interviewer-administered personal interview, a self-administered paper questionnaire, and a telephone survey.

Dietary data were collected in person by using the 24-hour recall interview method. Two 24-hour dietary recall surveys were collected for two nonconsecutive days that were 3 to 10 days apart. Each 24-hour dietary recall was conducted by a trained registered dietitian (RD) in the homes of participants, with the RD using the automated multiple-pass method (AMPM), a computer-assisted interview that allows the interviewer to use the following five-step multiple-pass approach of obtaining the 24-hour recall so as to achieve the highest level of accurate response (3):

1. **Quick list**: Collect a list of foods and beverages consumed the previous day.
2. **Forgotten foods**: Probe for foods forgotten during the Quick List.
3. **Time and occasion**: Collect time and eating occasion for each food.
4. **Detail cycle**: For each food, collect detailed description, amount, and additions. Review 24-hour day.
5. **Final probe**: Final probe for anything else consumed.

During the 1994–1996 survey, food amounts were determined using various measuring cups (amount of vegetables), spoons (amount of oil), sticks (thickness of meat), and rulers (length of pizza, height of cake, and so on). The personal interviews were conducted in respondents' homes, and each respondent was permitted and encouraged to use personal serving materials to aid in the recall. In the 1998 survey, AMPM was used in conjunction with the *Food Model Booklet* (FMB), a booklet of visual aids to assist in determining portion sizes. The images in the booklet included both describable, measurable shapes (eg, thickness blocks to determine the amount and thickness of meat consumed) and computer-generated graphic images (eg, non-measurable images, such as amounts of cream cheese and other spreads).

Following the direct 24-hour dietary recall, the CSFII interview included a household questionnaire. The household portion of the survey included fewer nutrient-related food questions and more questions related to food consumption and preparation.

Food security is defined by the USDA as "access by all people at all times to enough nutritious food for an active, healthy life" (38). The CSFII contains four questions relating to food security. The following is an example of an item with mutually exclusive, exhaustive ordinal (categorical) responses (38): "Which of these statements best describes food eaten in your household in the last 3 months: enough of the kinds of food we want to eat; enough but not always the *kinds* of food we want to eat; sometimes not enough to eat; or often not enough to eat?"

The questions regarding food security deal not only with amount of food, but also types (kinds) of food. This aspect is an important variable in defining food security. Additional questions ask about the number of days or months that there was not enough food and the reasons why there was not enough food.

CSFII also includes other behavioral or health-related variables that may affect dietary intake, such as exercise. The survey uses common language to ask questions related to exercise, such as "exercise vigorously enough to work up a sweat" (28). The response options focus only on the number of occasions that the exercise occurred. Interestingly, the question does not ask about the duration of exercise, the type of exercise, or anything about the specific activity performed.

After the personal interview, the interviewer trained the participant how to fill out another 2-day dietary recall (a self-administered paper survey). Several weeks after the interview, one adult in the household was interviewed by telephone about knowledge of various dietary, health, and safety issues. This telephone survey, the Diet and Health Knowledge Survey Questionnaire (DHKS), was administered only to adults who had completed at least 1 day of dietary recall. DHKS was designed to test knowledge and health behavior of the respondents, and then examine how this knowledge shaped the individual's dietary habits. Between the 1989 and the 1994 CSFII surveys, the standardized Nutrition Facts food label was introduced. Several questions in the DHKS were designed to evaluate respondents' use and understanding of the new food labeling.

NHANES Instrument Considerations

The NHANES 2003–2004 survey marks the beginning of a new era of health monitoring; this survey is the first of a continuous monitoring of health and nutrition information, sampling approximately 7,000 individuals in 15 locations throughout the United States. The goal is to achieve a more longitudinal study, as opposed to a strictly cross-sectional study (26). One of the unique aspects of this study is the use of both the home interview and mobile examination units to conduct various aspects of the survey.

During the home interview, two types of information are collected:

• **Family or household information,** including information on respondent demographics, food security, health insurance, housing characteristics, income, pesticide use, and smoking habits

- **Individual information** regarding various medical conditions, diseases, weight, and vision

Following the initial home interview, the interviewer set up an appointment for each participant to take part in a full examination in the mobile examination unit (MEC). The rest of the survey takes place in the MEC, which has both interviewer-administered and self-administered survey components, including an audio computer-assisted personal self-interview (ACASI) questionnaire and a CAPI questionnaire. The ACASI covers survey components about behavioral risk factors that may involve legal, moral, or otherwise sensitive issues. It gives respondents complete privacy in reporting answers, which may increase the accuracy of the responses. Examples of all question types, as well as instructions for interviewers, can be found on the NHANES Web site (28). Protocols for these questions involve the following operational considerations:

- **Alcohol consumption:** Questions are asked of all participants older than 12 years. Behaviors of alcohol consumption are surveyed in two different ways. For minors, ages 12 to 19 years, questions regarding alcohol consumption are asked using the ACASI, because alcohol consumption at this age is illegal. For adults older than 20, questions regarding alcohol consumption are asked by a trained interviewer.
- **Mental/cognitive function (Youth Conduct Disorder):** The questions asked in this section examine potential illegal behavior conducted by minors ages 12 to 19 years.
- **Drug use:** Questions regarding drug use are administered to adolescents ages 12 to 19. The questions offered during the survey are based on answers to previous questions.
- **Sexual behavior:** Questions regarding sexual behavior are administered to participants ages 12 to 59 years via the ACASI. During this questioning process, the participant is reminded that his or her answers will be kept confidential.

The CAPI method is used to conduct a 24-hour dietary recall. The interviewer conducts the survey in a similar fashion to the CSFII survey, using both open- and closed-ended questions and relying on visual aids for measurement and quantity determinations. Interviews are conducted with all adults who were able to respond to the questionnaire; for all other participants (children, those with mental disabilities), a proxy responder is used. For example, caretakers of infants are asked specific questions regarding the intake of the infant, such as "In the past month did [name of infant] eat or drink any of these foods or beverages?" (28) followed by a list of various foods. Examples of questions, as well as interviewer instructions, can be found on the NHANES Web site (28).

The NHANES CAPI method is also used to determine levels of food security among participants. The questions related to food security are more in-depth in NHANES than in CSFII, and involve the emotions surrounding food security. Questions include wording such as, "(I/We) worried whether (my/our) family would run out of food before (I/we) got money to buy more." The questions also address the financial burden of purchasing specific types of foods (low-cost vs more expensive or better), which is an interesting difference between the two surveys.

Instrument Considerations for the Framingham Nutrition Studies

The FNS involve a complex array of qualitative and (semi)quantitative nutrition-related protocols for nutritional risk assessment. When initiating the FNS, the investigators considered these research goals and questions carefully, articulated the variables of interest, and explored alternative methods of data collection. The overall Framingham protocol enables access to information on respondent characteristics, including environmental factors (eg, personal, social, household), biological risk factors, clinical measurements, and disease or related health outcomes. FOS respondents undergo clinic-based examinations that include up to 4 hours of interviews, physical examinations, and diagnostic testing in a central clinical setting; these components are also supplemented with additional ancillary testing and supplementary self-administered questionnaires.

To maintain high levels of respondent participation and response rates, protocols have been honed to include only the most essential components. Response rates and protocol completions rates for the FNS protocols range from 70% to more than 95%, depending on the component. The FHS and FNS benefit from the strong commitment of both respondents and investigators, and from tremendous community and cohort rapport built during the many years of study operation.

When the FNS were initiated in 1984, only a few validated methods were available for application in large-scale, population-based nutrition epidemiology. The dietary history, 24-hour recall, and dietary record methods were the most widely available, validated techniques for quantitative estimates of food and nutrient intake. The dietary history was used alone in early studies of the original Framingham cohort but was not repeated in later research. The FNS team chose to include the validated dietary recall interview and 3-day dietary record methods. In addition, we introduced a validated telephone-administered dietary recall protocol that was administered in a random subsample of respondents. To estimate food portions, a validated two-dimensional visual with spoon sizes and a variety of shapes were used (4). RDs were employed in all interview-administered nutrition protocols. The FNS investigators also developed and validated the Framingham Food Frequency Questionnaire and a standardized Nutrition Behavior Questionnaire (4). Virtually all these methods used survey research techniques and were implemented according to strictly monitored protocols by trained staff. Details of the methods have been previously published (4,9,10,31,39) and are summarized throughout this chapter in relevant sections.

The 24-hour recall portion of the FNS allowed researchers to estimate population food and nutrient intake and compare that data with expert dietary recommendations. Unique to FNS was the development and validation of a two-dimensional food portion visual for estimating portion sizes. The recall technique was used in face-to-face and telephone interviews (in a random 10% sample of respondents only). In addition to recalls, subjects completed 3-day dietary record using standardized food record forms. RDs reviewed food records for completeness; if clarifications were needed, subjects were interviewed by telephone. FNS also developed and validated the semiquantitative Framingham Food Frequency Questionnaire to compare (rank) subjects' nutrient intake and to develop indexes of composite dietary quality, including dietary patterns and nutritional risk scores. Five unique and nonoverlapping dietary patterns of FOS men and women have been identified and validated (4,10,11,31). (See Figure 13.1.) FNS uses the patterns and nutrient risk scores to look at overall diet in relationship to health outcomes including obesity, CVD risk, and metabolic syndrome (10,31–34,39–42).

FNS also developed a Nutrition Behavior Questionnaire to assess detailed aspects of food and nutrient intake behaviors. The instrument included food preparation techniques, salt and visible fat usage, habitual meal patterns, self-reported height and weight at various ages, experiences with weight fluctuation, use of dietary supplements (including over-the-counter and prescribed vitamins and minerals or other products), use of physician-prescribed therapeutic diets, self-imposed dieting, perceptions concerning the importance of nutrition in health, and changes in dietary behavior for health-related reasons.

CONCLUSION

Evidence-based survey research entails careful systematic planning and adherence to valid, ethical, and strict protocols. Survey research planning is a complex process that needs to be carried out thoughtfully and thoroughly in order to ensure that your investigation adds meaningfully to the literature in a specified research domain and that your study questions are answered as completely as possible. You will consider many options for data collection and evaluate a wide array of factors before settling on the optimal study design, survey instruments, and research protocols.

This chapter has presented the basic concepts involved in survey planning and questionnaire design. From a research perspective, you should better appreciate the importance of a staged survey research planning process. You should also have an increased understanding of the methods of survey data collection and options for research variable measurement. It is hoped that you will be able to more critically evaluate the survey research literature and will find yourself increasingly comfortable in using it strategically to inform your own investigations. Among the literature's key uses are the identification of valid and suitable survey research techniques and protocols, and as the source of information needed to calculate your study's statistical power.

If the planning process is carefully accomplished, you should have confidence in your overall study design, including the respondent sampling procedures, methods of data collection, and other survey protocols and procedures. You will have laid out a sound plan of analysis and have resources allocated to complete all aspects of your work including research reporting. You will also comprehend the importance of conducting quality control of all survey activities, including staff training, and will recognize that research should be carried out according to established protocols and acceptable standards.

You have many opportunities to make professional contributions using survey research. The techniques have been applied to a wide range of nutrition-related areas. Among the most important are the assessment of a population's nutrition and health status and disease risk; the determination of progress toward achieving the nation's nutrition and health objectives; the development of new techniques of nutritional risk assessment; the establishment of relationships between dietary behavior and health outcomes; and the identification of effective and innovative nutrition services, programs, interventions, and medical nutrition therapies. Survey research methods are well-suited to investigations at the individual, community, and population levels. The techniques are also applicable to even broader realms that encompass the food, foodservice, pharmaceutical, and health-related industries. Given these widespread applications, RDs who develop sound survey research skills are positioned to make important contributions to the exciting and expanding field of nutrition.

REFERENCES

1. National Center for Health Statistics. National Health Interview Survey. Available at: http://www.cdc.gov/nchs/nhis.htm. Accessed May 2, 2006.

2. Centers for Disease Control and Prevention. National Center for Health Statistics. National Health and Nutrition Examination Survey Questionnaire. Hyattsville, Md: US Department of Health and Human Services, Centers for Disease Control and Prevention, 2003–2004. Available at: http://www.cdc.gov/nchs/about/major/nhanes/nhanes2003-2004/questexam03_04.htm. Accessed May 2, 2006.

3. Tippett K, Cypell Y, eds. *Design and Operation: The Continuing Survey of Food Intakes by Individuals and the Diet and Health Knowledge Survey, 1994–96.* Washington, DC: US Department of Agriculture; 1997. Available at: http://www.ars.usda.gov/SP2UserFiles/Place/12355000/pdf/Dor9496.pdf. Accessed May 2, 2006.

4. Millen BE, Quatromoni PA. Nutritional research within the Framingham Heart Study. *J Nutr Health Aging.* 2001;5:139–143.

5. US Department of Health and Human Services. *Healthy People 2010: Understanding and Improving Health.* 2nd ed. Washington, DC: US Government Printing Office; 2000.

6. Hu FB. Dietary pattern analysis: a new direction in nutritional epidemiology. *Curr Opin Lipidol.* 2002;13:3–9.

7. Kennedy ET, Ohls J, Carlson S, Fleming K. The Healthy Eating Index: design and applications. *J Am Diet Assoc.* 1995;95:1103–1108.

8. Haines PS, Siegra-Riz AM, Popkin BM. The Dietary Quality Index Revised: a measurement instrument for populations. *J Am Diet Assoc.* 1999;99:697–704.

9. Murabito JM, Garrison RJ, Millen BE. Lifestyle issues. In: *Fifty Years of Discovery: Medical Milestones from the National Heart, Lung and Blood Institute's Framingham Heart Study.* Hackensack, NJ: Center for Bio-Medical Communications; 1999:252–259.

10. Millen BE, Quatromoni PA, Copenhafer DL, Demissie S, O'Horo CE, D'Agostino RB. Validation of a dietary approach pattern for evaluating nutritional risk: the Framingham Nutrition Studies. *J Am Diet Assoc.* 2001;101:187–194.

11. Millen BE, Pencina MJ, Kimokoti RW, Meigs JB, Ordovas JM, D'Agostino RB. Nutritional risk and the metabolic syndrome in women: opportunities for preventive intervention from the Framingham Nutrition Studies. *Am J Clin Nutr.* 2006;84:434–441.

12. Czaja RF, Blair J. *Designing Surveys: A Guide to Decisions and Procedures.* 2nd ed. Thousand Oaks, Calif: Sage Publications; 2005.

13. Fowler FJ. *Survey Research Methods.* 3rd ed. London, UK: Sage Publications; 2002.

14. Babbie E. *The Practice of Social Research.* 6th ed. Belmont, Calif: Wadsworth Publishing; 1992.

15. Summary: Predictors of Obesity, Weight Gain, Diet, and Physical Activity Workshop; 2004. Available at: http://www.nhlbi.nih.gov/meetings/workshops/predictors/summary.htm. Accessed February 23, 2007.

16. Millen BE, Pencina MJ, Kimokoti RW, D'Agostino RB. The Framingham Nutrition Studies: insights into weight history, dietary patterns, obesity prevention, and risk reduction (abstract). Summary: Predictors of Obesity, Weight Gain, Diet, and Physical Activity Workshop; 2004. Available at: http://www.nhlbi.nih.gov/meetings/workshops/predictors/abstracts/millen.htm. Accessed May 2, 2006.

17. Green LW, Kreuter MW. *Health Promotion Planning. An Educational and Environmental Approach.* 2nd ed. Mountain View, Calif: Mayfield Publishing; 1991.

18. Glanz K, Lewis FM, Rimer BK, eds. *Health Behavior and Health Education. Theory, Research, and Practice.* San Francisco, Calif: Jossey-Bass Publishers; 1990.

19. Glanz K, Rimer B. *Theory at a Glance: A Guide to Health Promotion Practice.* Bethesda, Md: National Cancer Institute; 1997.

20. Fowler FJ, Mangione TW. *Standardized Survey Interviewing. Minimizing Interviewer-Related Error.* Newbury Park, Calif: Sage Publications; 1990.

21. The Survey System's Tutorial. Creative Research Systems. Available at: http://www.surveysystem.com. Accessed May 2, 2006.

22. University of Maryland. Online Survey Design Guide. Available at: http://lap.umd.edu/survey_design/index.html. Accessed May 15, 2006.

23. Ajetunmobi O. *Making Sense of Critical Appraisal.* London, UK: Hodder Headline Group; 2002.

24. Centers for Disease Control and Prevention. National Center for Health Statistics. NHIS Survey Description. Available at: http://www.cdc.gov/nchs/about/major/nhis/hisdesc.htm. Accessed January 11, 2007.

25. Centers for Disease Control and Prevention. National Center for Health Statistics. National Health and Nutrition Examination Survey Data. 2003–2004. Available at: http://www.cdc.gov/nchs/about/major/nhanes/nhanes2003-2004/nhanes03_04.htm. Accessed May 2, 2006.

26. Centers for Disease Control and Prevention. National Center for Health Statistics. National Health and Nutrition Examination Survey Questionnaire. 1959–1961. Available at: http://www.cdc.gov/nchs/about/major/nhanes/cyclei_iii.htm#Cycle1. Accessed May 3, 2006.

27. Centers for Disease Control and Prevention. National Center for Health Statistics. National Health and Nutrition Examination Survey Questionnaire. 2003–2004. Available at: http://www.cdc.gov/nchs/about/major/nhanes/nhanes2003-2004/questexam03_04.htm. Accessed May 2, 2006.

28. National Institutes for Health. NHANES Web site. Available at: http://www.cdc.gov/nchs/nhanes.htm. Accessed May 2, 2006.

29. Levy D, ed. *Fifty Years of Discovery: Medical Milestones from the National Heart, Lung and Blood Institute's Framingham Heart Study.* Hackensack, NJ: Center for Bio-Medical Communications; 1999.

30. Framingham Heart Study. 50 Years of Research Success. Available at: http://www.nhlbi.nih.gov/about/framingham/index.html. Accessed February 23, 2007.

31. Quatromoni PA, Copenhafer DL, D'Agostino RB, Millen BE. Dietary patterns predict the development of overweight in women: the Framingham Nutrition Studies. *J Am Diet Assoc.* 2002;102:1240–1246.

32. Millen BE, Quatromoni PA, Nam BH, O'Horo CE, Polak JF, D'Agostino RB. Dietary patterns and the odds of carotid atherosclerosis in women: the Framingham Nutrition Studies. *Prev Med.* 2002;35:540–547.

33. Millen BE, Quatromoni PA, Nam BH, O'Horo CE, Polak JF, Wolf PA, D'Agostino RB. Dietary patterns, smoking, and sub-clinical heart disease in women: opportunities for primary prevention from the Framingham Nutrition Studies. *J Am Diet Assoc.* 2004;104:208–214.

34. Sonnenberg LM, Pencina MJ, Kimokoti RW, Quatromoni PA, Nam BH, D'Agostino RB, Meigs JB, Ordovas JM, Cobain MR, Millen BE. Dietary patterns of women and the metabolic syndrome in obese and non-obese women: opportunities for preventive intervention on obesity from the Framingham Nutrition Studies. *Obes Res.* 2005;13:153–162.

35. Matthys C, Pynaert I, De Keyzer W, De Henauw S. Validity and reproducibility of an adolescent web-based food frequency questionnaire. *J Am Diet Assoc.* 2007;107:605–610.

36. Verkleij-Hagoort AC, de Vries JH, Stegers MP, Lindemans J, Ursem NT, Steegers-Theunissen RP. Validation of the assessment of folate and vitamin B(12) intake in women of reproductive age: the method of triads. *Eur J Clin Nutr.* 2007;61:610–615.

37. Centers for Disease Control and Prevention. National Center for Health Statistics. National Health Interview Survey. Available at: http://www.cdc.gov/nchs/nhis.htm. Accessed May 2, 2006.

38. US Department of Agriculture. Design and Operation of the CSFII/DHKS 1994–96. What We Eat in America 1994–1996 Day 1 Questionnaire. Available at: http://www.ars.usda.gov/SP2UserFiles/Place/12355000/pdf/day1.pdf. Accessed May 15, 2006.

39. Kimokoti R, Millen B, Pencina M, Meigs J, D'Agostino R. Dietary quality and the prospective development of the metabolic syndrome in women. The Framingham Nutrition Studies (abstract). *Obes Res.* 2005;13(suppl):A1–A270.

40. Kimokoti R, Millen B, Pencina M, D'Agostino R. Weight experience and nutrition risk in Framingham women. The Framingham Nutrition Studies (abstract). *Obes Res.* 2005;13(suppl):A1–A270.

41. Kimokoti RW, Pencina MJ, D'Agostino RB, Millen BE. Dietary quality and weight gain in women. The Framingham Nutrition Studies (abstract). *Circulation.* 2006;113:e301–e381.

42. Kimokoti RW, Millen BE, Pencina MJ, Zhu L, D'Agostino RB. Dietary quality, overweight and obesity in women. The Framingham Nutrition Studies (abstract). *FASEB J.* 2006;20:A818–A1474.

14

Dietary Assessment and Validation

Rachel K. Johnson, PhD, MPH, RD, Bethany A. Yon, MS, and
Jean H. Hankin, DrPH, RD

Diet is recognized as a primary determinant of health and disease at all ages. This chapter reviews methods appropriate for assessing individual or group intakes of nutrients, particular foods, or food groups, or individual or group dietary patterns. There is no single dietary method or "gold standard" that is applicable to all clinical, community, or research activities. Differences exist according to the purpose of the study, necessary precision, particular population, time period of interest, and available resources. Often, more than one method is used in a particular study; the methods should be tested for reproducibility, comparability, and validity of the reported dietary intake data. Thompson and Subar compiled descriptions of several existing methods and illustrations of questionnaires (1).

This chapter also discusses the validation of dietary intake methodology. Dietary assessment and validation of dietary intakes are increasingly incorporated into the design of national and international nutritional status and epidemiologic studies (1–7). Methods for estimating national food availability or disappearance data are described in other publications (8–12). Their major uses include measurement of the adequacy of the food supply and assessment of trends among and within countries. Nonetheless, Armstrong and Doll (11) correlated the per capita food and nutrient intakes from selected countries with incidence and mortality rates of cancer to illustrate associations of diet and disease, such as the hypothesized relationships between dietary fat and breast cancer and between meat intake and colon cancer. Such correlations provide leads for further research but cannot be used to demonstrate cause and effect

or true associations, as discussed by Willett (4). Chapter 10 of this book reviews the US Department of Agriculture (USDA) and US Department of Health and Human Services (HHS) National Nutrition Monitoring System used in the United States to identify dietary intakes of Americans.

24-HOUR DIETARY RECALL

In the 24-hour dietary recall method, the interviewer (usually a registered dietitian, nutritionist, or nonnutritionist trained in the use of the method) obtains information on all food items consumed during the past 24 hours, the previous day, or another defined 24-hour period. The information may be recorded and coded in the traditional way or may be recorded with the assistance of a computer (13). Interviewers should have knowledge of the foods available in the community, usual eating and cooking practices, and probing methods. Recalls may be administered face-to-face or by telephone with similar results (14–17). Visual aids, such as food models, geometric models, photographs, or household measuring utensils, may help subjects estimate quantities consumed (18).

It is important to have a quality control system in place to minimize errors and increase reliability of interviewing. Training and retraining sessions for interviewers (eg, via group meetings or periodic conference calls) are essential to discuss problems among interviewers. Some investigators tape telephone interviews (with the concurrence of the subjects). This technique has improved quality control in a large, multiethnic population study using 24-hour dietary recalls for calibration of a mailed quantitative food frequency questionnaire (FFQ) (19).

The major strength of the 24-hour dietary recall is that it facilitates comparisons of groups of people. For example, comparison of 24-hour recalls among men of Japanese ancestry living in San Francisco, Hawaii, and Japan demonstrated a stepwise increase in dietary fat intake and a similar decrease in carbohydrate intake from Japan to Hawaii to California, which paralleled the increase in coronary heart disease mortality rates among these populations (20). The USDA has shown that individual intakes, based on 2- or 3-day means, differ between blacks and whites, socioeconomic groups, geographic regions, and other demographic characteristics (21). These differences have been repeated in subsequent surveys. The National Health and Nutrition Examination Survey (NHANES) collects biological, anthropometric, and physiologic measurements on subjects. Hence, the data have been useful for examining group differences in diet in relation to various health and disease characteristics (22).

There are other advantages of the 24-hour dietary recall. It places little burden on the subjects. Also, if it is unannounced, it is unlikely to alter eating behavior. In addition, participants are generally willing to respond to the interviewer, and thus refusals are less likely to occur than in other, more demanding requests for dietary information. For group means, the method has been shown to be comparable to more cumbersome methods (23).

Data collection has been simplified by use of automated software for the direct coding of the foods reported during the interview; this software specifies the information needed for clarifying and coding each response (15,24). The software is being used in several studies in the United States; however, this procedure has the potential effect of losing the subject's verbal description, which would be available in the written recall conducted by an interviewer. The automated method may also be difficult to use if interviews are being conducted among heterogeneous ethnic populations who prepare and consume foods that are unfamiliar to the interviewer and are not included in the food composition database. The European Prospective Investigation into Cancer and Nutrition (EPIC) study developed a computer-assisted 24-hour dietary recall (EPIC-SOFT) as a means of collecting additional dietary intake data to calibrate the dietary assessments collected using different methods in each of the 11 study groups (25). A common food composition database, standardized for the European countries, was developed.

The USDA has used various dietary recall methods to survey the food intake of the American population. The most recent automated five-step multiple-pass 24-hour dietary recall has been used jointly since 2002 by the HHS, the National Center for Health Statistics, and the USDA for dietary data collection (7,26,27). These surveys are conducted on a continuous basis each year. The automated multiple-pass 24-hour dietary recall was designed specifically to limit the extent of underreporting of food intake in the USDA surveys. This method differs from the traditional 24-hour dietary recall because the interviewer uses computer-assisted interviewing instruments to conduct five distinct passes to gather information about a subject's food intake during the preceding 24 hours. These passes include the following:

- **First pass—quick list.** The respondent is asked to recall everything he or she ate the previous day using any recall strategy the respondent chooses without interruptions.
- **Second pass—forgotten foods.** The respondent is asked to clarify any foods mentioned in the quick list. For example, if the respondent reported that he or she ate breakfast cereal, the interviewer would then ask whether milk was consumed with the cereal and, if so, the type and amount.
- **Third pass—review.** The interviewer reviews the list of foods mentioned and probes for additional eating times and occasions (eg, "Did you eat anything after dinner, before bedtime?").
- **Fourth pass—detail cycle.** More difficult, detail-oriented questions are asked to elicit descriptions of foods and portion sizes.
- **Fifth pass—final probe review.** One last opportunity is provided to the respondent to remember any foods consumed.

One limitation of the 24-hour recall relates to the daily variation in food intakes of most people. Because of the large intraindividual variability in food and nutrient intakes of most people, a single 24-hour recall is not appropriate for estimating the usual intakes of one person (28). However, multiple 24-hour recalls obtained on random days during a 1-year interval may provide a satisfactory picture of the person's usual diet. When group assessment is the objective, the interviews should be scheduled on various days of the week to account for daily variation in food choices, particularly between weekdays and weekends, as well as between weeks and seasons of the year. As with all dietary intake methods, the 24-hour recall is subject to underreporting of energy, which is discussed in greater detail later in this chapter (29,30).

FOOD RECORDS OR DIARIES

Food records or diaries require participants to weigh, measure, or estimate and then record all foods consumed over a specified period of time, usually 3 to 7 consecutive days or multiple periods within a year. The method requires good instructions and demonstrations, and, ideally, some observations. Generally, persons who agree to participate are dedicated, highly motivated, literate subjects and thus may not be representative of the general population.

The most accurate food record method entails the weighing of all ingredients in recipes, the portion selected, and the plate waste. Because weighing foods may be difficult for some subjects, household measuring utensils, such as cups and spoons, have been used more frequently than scales in food record studies in the United States (1). However, weighed-food records are more common in the United Kingdom and Europe, where kitchen scales are commonly used (3,25). In both instances, directions should include methods of estimating and recording food items consumed away from home. Other methods of quantifying consumption have been reported. For instance, in a dietary cross-comparison study among multiethnic groups in Hawaii, Hankin and coworkers (31) gave subjects a book of photographs showing three different typical portions of various food groups for use in estimating amounts consumed. This method was appropriate for this population, many of whom were not familiar with household scales or even measuring utensils.

A major strength of food records is that they do not rely on memory. Because of the difficulty of assessing a person's true usual intake, investigators have used food records as a reference or standard for validating other dietary methods that are based on long-term recall (32). Although food records are not necessarily error-free, investigators have assumed that they approximated the truth with greater face validity than a diet history or FFQ. However, with the advent of biomarkers (indicators that measure body fluids or tissues and can independently reflect individual nutrient intakes), it is now known that none of the dietary intake methods (weighed-food records, 24-hour recalls, FFQs, or diet history questionnaires) give accurate estimates of the usual energy intakes of individuals (33).

Food records can provide helpful information for developing a structured FFQ for a particular population.

Food items that are important contributors to the intakes of particular dietary components (eg, macronutrients, micronutrients, and fiber) can be identified, along with the range of expected portion sizes for each item. In addition, records are often used to motivate participants in dietary intervention studies, which may encourage weight loss (34).

Along with its strengths, the use of food records has serious limitations. First, the selected time period for collecting and recording intakes may be atypical for the subject, possibly because of illness, business obligations, or travel. Also, this method may not be appropriate for people who consume most of their meals in restaurants. Second, as noted previously, persons who agree to keep detailed food records may not be representative of the general population in the study. Immigrants whose primary language is not English may find it difficult to keep a food record or diary. However, studies can be structured to reduce this problem. For example, Hankin and Huenemann (35) translated instructions for keeping 7-day food records into Japanese for first-generation immigrants in California and used trained bilingual persons to interpret and code the dietary intakes. Third, because of the labor-intensive methodology, food records are difficult to administer in large population studies and are costly in time and personnel. Fourth, food records provide data only on the current diet. If the investigator wishes to obtain dietary information on foods consumed 3 years in the past for an epidemiologic study, current intakes may be dissimilar. Fifth, food records covering a single series of 3 to 7 consecutive days most likely will not reflect the true variability in the diets of most individuals. Finally, the act of recording food intake may actually change people's dietary patterns. For example, people may choose to eat simpler meals or eliminate snacking to make record-keeping easier.

INTRAINDIVIDUAL VARIABILITY OF DIET

Both the single 24-hour dietary recall and the food record are limited by their short time coverage. For most people today, eating patterns are characterized by large variations from day to day, week to week, and often season to season. This is particularly true in developed countries, with their wide choice of available foods, and it is increasingly true in developing countries as well. Food intakes during the weekend usually differ considerably from meals consumed on weekdays, and dietary patterns are also likely to vary by season of the year. Furthermore, people are consuming more of their meals away from home. The large variation in daily and even weekly diets suggests that no single day or week can be representative of long-term usual intake.

Variability of diet within a population may be divided into within-person (or intraindividual) variation and between-person variation. It has been reported that within-person variation, which represents day-to-day differences in intake, is generally as large as or larger than between-person variation (23,28,36–39). Consequently, a longer time period is needed to characterize the usual diet of an individual than the usual diet of a group of persons. Several investigators have analyzed the variability in multiple 24-hour dietary recalls and food records and determined the number of days needed to achieve reliable estimates of mean nutrient intakes of individuals (23,28,38,40). For example, in a study of 29 adults who measured and recorded their food intakes for 1 year, Basiotis et al (28) found that 57 days were needed to estimate the individual total fat intakes within 10% of the true mean individual intakes for males with 95% confidence, whereas 71 days were needed for the same confidence level for females. To estimate vitamin A intake of individuals, 390 days were needed for males and 474 days for females. When the objective was to estimate mean intakes of the group with precision, a smaller number of days of food records was needed.

Other investigators have defined *precision* as an estimate within 20% of the true usual intake (41). With this increased latitude, considerably fewer days would be needed to estimate individual average intakes. These findings indicate that the use of a short recall or food record for diet and disease studies could lead to considerable error, with misclassification on the distribution of individual intakes occurring along a continuum (41).

FOOD FREQUENCY QUESTIONNAIRES

The first and classic diet history, conceived by Burke (42), was the forerunner of the more structured questionnaires used today. FFQs were developed for use in large epidemiologic studies on diet and coronary heart disease (and later cancer, osteoporosis, and other chronic diseases). The basic assumption of the FFQ is that the typical long-term diet, instead of dietary intakes during a few specific days, is the conceptually important exposure. With this method, precision is sacrificed. The method is simple to administer by a trained interviewer or by the respondent directly using a mailed questionnaire. The questionnaire can be computerized and optically scanned for analysis. The method is

objective because it is based on lists of selected foods and groups of items with similar nutrient values used interchangeably in the diet. In the past, food items were often selected to test particular hypotheses concerning diet and disease, such as a relationship between vitamin A or beta carotene intake and lung cancer risk (43–45). More recently, because of the uncertainty concerning the role of particular nutrients and other food components in the etiology of several chronic diseases, investigators have included a larger number and variety of foods in an attempt to assess the total diet. It is also valuable to examine interactions between dietary components and to have adequate data for analysis of particular foods, food groups, and eating patterns in relation to disease.

Selection of Food Items

It is preferable to select food items for the questionnaire based on the study population's eating patterns. General guidelines are to choose foods that are consumed by a sizable number of people, that vary in frequency and quantity of intake among the population, and that provide significant amounts of all dietary components. These food items may be selected using various methods. For example, Tucker et al (46) used 24-hour dietary recalls to describe the major food and nutrient contributors, as well as recipes and portion sizes commonly used, from a representative sample of the study population. Others have used population data, such as 24-hour recalls of adults participating in the NHANES II survey (47–49), for selecting particular food items for questionnaires. Some FFQs have been modified or expanded periodically to account for additional foods on the market or to test particular hypotheses (4).

Semiquantitative vs Quantitative Food Frequency Questionnaires

Some FFQs solicit frequency responses only (50–53), although a usual serving size may be listed with each item (50). These questionnaires are called *semiquantitative food frequency questionnaires*. The questionnaires developed for the Nurses' Health Study (50) and the Male Health Professionals Follow-up Study (54) illustrate this method. Frequencies are obtained by checking the appropriate column showing ranges per day, week, month, or year. The nutrient intakes are computed by multiplying the midpoint of the frequency interval by the nutrients in the specified portion of the food. This method may be satisfactory if all of the respondents generally consume similar amounts of the items (eg, 5 ounces of meat or a half-cup of vegetables) and if amounts are highly correlated with frequencies. A problem may occur if the usual portions of some subjects differ markedly from the portions specified and if the respondents do not adjust the frequencies accordingly. Marr (55), a distinguished pioneer in dietary methodology, indicated that a semiquantitative instrument could lead to a systematic bias toward either underestimates or overestimates of food and nutrient intakes. However, Willett et al (50) and Hunter et al (56) reported that specifications of quantities consumed provided little additional information to frequency data. These investigators concluded that the frequency of eating particular foods was a greater determinant of nutrient intakes than quantity, and that the use of a single serving size did not introduce a large error in the individual estimates.

The quantitative procedure assumes that amounts consumed are likely to vary among the population, and that more valid data will be obtained if subjects choose their own portion size according to their usual habits. Cummings and coworkers (57), Chu et al (58), and the multiethnic cohort study in Hawaii and Los Angeles (59) found that if a standard portion size is used, misclassification and inconsistent results may occur when compared with studies that allow subjects to choose their own serving size.

Various techniques have been employed to help subjects estimate amounts consumed. The directions for completing Block's questionnaire specify that a small portion is about one-half the specified medium serving size and a large portion is about one and one-half times as much the specified medium serving size (49). To assist subjects, several epidemiologists in Europe, such as Pietinen et al (60), have developed booklets that show different portion sizes of each item in the questionnaire. Canadian researchers used food portion photos on facing pages to help with portion size estimation (61). Others have used geometric models printed on a foldout that accompanies the questionnaire (15). The Hawaii group used color photographs of food items in three portion sizes in home interviews for several case-control studies (62–65).

FFQs may be processed in two ways. If the information is obtained by personal interview, the frequency interval may be precise (eg, "three times a month" or "four times a day"). However, FFQs are often self-administered. In this case, the respondent chooses the appropriate frequency interval from the listed series (eg, "one to three times a month") for each category of foods and the usual serving size. This format is designed for direct machine entry, such as optical scanning, and is generally preferable for the large population studies often administered by mail.

Some investigators (1,4) also include a few answers to be answered in writing. In this case, review of each questionnaire is needed before coding and processing.

Before using any dietary research instrument, it should be pretested extensively among representative samples of the population (66). When using a food frequency instrument, the pretesting should include a write-in section for recording other items usually eaten. This will help improve the questionnaire by yielding suggestions for the addition of particular foods or by highlighting a need for clarifying instructions. In addition, if the questionnaire will be self-administered by mail or completed by telephone interview, trial runs should be conducted among representative samples of the study population. In some geographic areas with large immigrant populations, it may be desirable to translate the instrument into other languages to ensure its comprehension. In some studies, participants may be videotaped to obtain an accurate estimate of individual intakes. Brown et al (67) tested this technique among elderly women living in a retirement home and showed that its accuracy was superior to that of the 24-hour dietary recall.

POTENTIAL ERRORS OF INDIVIDUAL DIETARY INTAKE METHODS

It is clear that none of the individual methods of dietary assessment are free from error. Witschi (34) classified errors into three categories: (a) respondent and recorder errors, (b) interviewer and reviewer errors (including all types of measurement errors, as described in Chapter 3), and (c) nutrient database errors. Briefly, in 24-hour dietary recalls and diet histories, subjects may fail to recall all foods and amounts consumed. Even for home-prepared meals, persons not involved in food preparation may not be aware of the components of mixed dishes. They may not know what kinds of fats and oils were used, or whether their portion of a mixed dish was 1 cup or 2 cups. Subjects may also want to please the interviewer, and they may be reluctant to admit consumption of alcoholic beverages or "sin foods," such as candy or desserts. Besides failure to recall all foods consumed (deletion errors), subjects may also report eating foods that were not actually consumed (addition errors), or they may substitute a different food for the one actually consumed (misclassification errors) (68). In addition, some persons may believe that certain foods are good or bad for health and may either exaggerate or underestimate their intakes of them. Some investigators have found that large intakes tend to be underestimated and small intakes overestimated (69,70).

The food composition databases are also not error-free. However, the values published by the USDA are carefully selected means from various sources and are reviewed and revised periodically (71). Although no longer available in a printed form, this online database is an appropriate primary resource for studies in the United States. However, it may need supplementation from other publications and sources, such as Pennington (72) and the Minnesota Nutrition Data System (73), as well as from commercial tables, and laboratory analyses of local foods. Food composition tables may include imputed values for some nutrients. There is divided opinion among researchers concerning the use of these imputed values, and it is likely that either inclusion or exclusion will result in some error in the estimated intakes. If used, food composition tables should be based on analyses of similar foods, and should be updated as new analytic information becomes available. Other potential unavoidable errors include changes in nutrient content occurring during food preparation or food storage, as well as in the bioavailability of some nutrients. Although differences exist between calculated and analyzed values of food intake data (32,55), these errors cannot be eliminated in large population studies.

The errors in dietary methodology, along with the large, random within-person variability, generally decrease the strength of the statistical association of diet with other variables, such as a biochemical measurement or disease status, provided that the errors are distributed randomly among the comparison groups. In contrast, if errors are biased and not random, as occurs with underreporting, this bias can obscure actual associations or create false ones (74).

Hence, failure to identify a relationship between a dietary variable and a disease does not necessarily mean the absence of an association. For example, there has been inconsistent evidence from epidemiologic studies on the relationship between dietary fat and breast cancer (75,76). This inconsistency may be due to the homogeneity of fat intakes within populations, substantial measurement error in dietary assessment (77–79), the large intraindividual variation in dietary fat intakes (80), or the selective under-reporting of high-fat foods (74).

Measurement error may be a substantial problem in large population or cohort studies that include subgroups for whom a single FFQ may perform differently; this fact complicates comparisons between the groups (19). To provide an unbiased estimate, data from the dietary questionnaire may be compared with dietary information from a second source, such as multiple 24-hour recalls from representative samples of the population groups. These data can then be used for correction of risk estimates obtained from analysis of nutritional factors and incidences of particular diseases among the groups. However, a number of biomarkers are now being used to both validate and calibrate dietary assessments instruments (3,5,81).

VALIDITY AND REPRODUCIBILITY OF DIETARY INTAKE DATA

To promote confidence in dietary data and diet-disease findings, the dietary method should be tested for both validity and reproducibility (ie, reliability) in a representative sample of the study population. Although it would be expedient to use a method evaluated in another population, the instrument is appropriate only if the eating patterns of the reference and study populations are similar. For example, a valid and reproducible questionnaire developed for nurses or health professionals in the United States would most likely not be appropriate for a multiethnic randomized population of Japanese Americans, Latinos, African Americans, native Hawaiians, and whites living in Hawaii and Los Angeles (59).

Several studies and reviews have evaluated particular dietary methods. A succinct and comprehensive review was written by Thompson and Subar (1). The National Cancer Institute also maintains a Web-based register of validation and calibration studies (82,83). This chapter includes only a brief review to illustrate the study objectives, general protocols, and relevant findings.

Dietary Validity or Comparability

Dietary validity is the ability of an instrument to measure what it purports to measure with regard to diet, such as the intake in a particular meal or day or the usual diet consumed during the past year. Validation requires that the truth be known, and the truth is difficult to obtain among free-living people for extended periods. This problem is particularly relevant today because of the large variability in people's eating patterns. However, dietary validity for short time intervals has been assessed by surreptitiously weighing foods of people eating in an institutional setting and then asking the subjects the following day to recall what they ate (69,70,84,85). In the past, FFQs were validated by measuring the relative validity of the new instrument in comparison to a method that had some evidence of greater accuracy (4,86). The choice was generally food records, in which food items were weighed, measured, or estimated, that were collected at multiple time periods during a year to reflect within-person variability among representative samples of the population. Some investigators have used 24-hour dietary recalls collected by trained interviewers of the same ethnic group as the respondents by personal interview or telephone (2,19) to obtain a second set of usual intakes for testing among the study population. Nonetheless, the reference data may underestimate the usual intakes of the people in the study. Investigators now use biomarkers as independent measures of dietary intake to validate food intake measurements (87,88).

FFQs are being used in several large cohort studies on diet and disease in the United States, Europe, and Asia (2,3,59,60,89). In these investigations, participants complete a dietary questionnaire at the start of the study. Several years later, the original dietary intakes are tested for associations with diseases that may have developed, such as cancer and heart disease. The aim is to identify dietary and other environmental or genetic factors that may be related to risk of disease. The findings, if confirmed among multiple populations and substantiated with biological research, may be used to identify potential risks and, it is hoped, to prevent these diseases. A major problem is that estimates of risk within cohorts can be substantially attenuated by measurement errors in assessing individual intakes (19). These problems are increased in cohort studies that include subgroups in which the questionnaire may perform differently. Consequently, the use of calibration substudies, in which data from the questionnaires are compared with data from a second source that is assumed to provide an unbiased estimate, allows for correction of the risk estimates for measurement error (19). In these studies, investigators begin by assuming that there is error in the FFQs. Thus, rather than trying to validate the frequency data, investigators use statistical methods, such as regression calibration and correlated measurement errors, to adjust the dietary intakes of each participant within the subgroup (90–93).

Use of Biomarkers to Validate Dietary Intake Methods

All the traditional dietary intake methods (24-hour dietary recalls, food records, diet histories, and FFQs) rely on information reported by the subjects themselves. It is now known that the assumption that this self-reported information is valid can be verified only by the use of external independent markers of intake (94). Hence, in recent years the search has begun for biomarkers that closely reflect dietary intake but do not rely on self-reports of food consumption (95).

Doubly Labeled Water

Doubly labeled water (DLW) is currently the most widely used and well-accepted biomarker. It is based on the principle that carbon dioxide production can be estimated by the difference in elimination rates of body hydrogen and oxygen. Through observations, Lifson and coworkers concluded that the oxygen in expired carbon dioxide was derived from total body water (96,97). This results from the equilibrium between the oxygen in body water and the oxygen in respiratory carbon dioxide (96). With this finding, the researchers predicted that carbon dioxide production could be indirectly measured by separately labeling both the hydrogen and oxygen pool of the body water with naturally occurring, stable isotopes. In 1982, Schoeller and van Santen first used this technique to measure total energy expenditure in free-living humans (98).

The DLW method provides an accurate measure of the total energy expenditure in free-living subjects. Hence, it is now well accepted as a gold standard to determine the validity of tools designed to measure energy intake (94). Its use as a validation tool is based on the principle of energy balance; that is, if a person is in energy balance, then his or her energy expenditure, as measured by DLW, must be equal to his or her energy intake (99,100). It is important to point out that DLW can determine the accuracy of a dietary intake method only with respect to energy. However, if a dietary assessment tool is accurate with respect to energy, there is a reasonable probability that it will also be accurate for specific macronutrients and micronutrients (101,102). In contrast, if a tool is not accurate with respect to energy, then it is not likely to provide an accurate measure of the absolute intake of other nutrients (101,102). Hence, it is accepted that when group estimates of energy intake are truly validated against a well-accepted criterion method (such as the DLW method), the coinciding estimates of macronutrient and micronutrient intakes can also be considered valid (103).

There are numerous advantages to the DLW technique, including the ease of administration and the ability of the subject to engage in free-living activities during the measurement period. This characteristic is extremely advantageous when the DLW method is used as an objective criterion measure to validate self-reported estimates of dietary intake, because the subject is not confined to a clinical research setting where usual activities are restricted.

Most important, the method is accurate and has a precision of between 2% and 8% (104).

Although there are many advantages to the DLW technique, there are also drawbacks—namely, the expense of the stable isotopes and the expertise required to operate the highly sophisticated and costly mass spectrometer for analysis of the isotopes. Thus, to date, the use of the DLW method has been confined to a few research laboratories around the world, and the method does not lend itself to routine use in large epidemiologic studies. It can be used, however, in a subsample from large cohort studies to validate energy intakes obtained from the dietary method of choice. This approach has been used by Bingham and colleagues in the EPIC study (105). DLW has also been used to compare self-reported dietary instruments in the Observing Protein and Energy Nutrition (OPEN) study (5). Currently, the USDA is conducting a DLW validation study with 400 volunteers to determine the accuracy of the automated five-step multiple-pass 24-hour dietary recall (7).

Other Biomarkers

Several other biomarkers that reflect nutrient intake have recently attracted considerable attention in nutrition epidemiology (106) and are being used to validate dietary assessment methods (5,107,108).

The pattern of fatty acids in the blood has been used as a biomarker of fatty acid intake (109). Andersen and colleagues demonstrated that intakes of eicosapentaenoic acid and docosahexaenoic acid, as well as of fish generally, were significantly related to concentrations of these fatty acids in plasma phospholipids (110). In this study, dietary intake data generated from a FFQ were validated when both dietary and biomarker data classified people into similar groupings of intake. This type of analysis can increase confidence that the estimated intake actually reflects the intake of a nutrient or a food containing that nutrient (111). For example, a biomarker confirming the quintile distributions of fat intake would have added substantially to the credibility of reports suggesting that a diet providing 30% of energy as fat was unlikely to result in a substantial reduction in the risk of breast cancer (112) or that total dietary fat was not associated with coronary heart disease in women (113).

Bingham and Cummings pioneered the use of urinary nitrogen measurement to validate protein intake. For people in energy and nitrogen balance, urinary nitrogen level, as assessed from 8 days of complete 24-hour urine collections, is an independent measure of protein intake (114). Bingham and colleagues have since used the 24-hour urinary nitrogen technique to validate reported protein intakes in 24-hour recalls, FFQs, and food records (95,105,115). Urinary potassium has recently been found to be as reliable as urinary nitrogen for use as a biomarker in dietary measurement studies (116).

Vegetables and fruits are the primary source of carotenoids in the diet (117), and circulating concentrations of carotenoids have been shown in feeding studies (118,119) to respond to dietary changes. Thus, serum carotenoid concentrations, as well as ascorbic acid levels, have been used as markers of fruit and vegetable consumption (108,120–123). Scott and colleagues examined the relationships between dietary intakes of lutein, lycopene, and beta carotene and their concentrations in blood and found that plasma carotenoid concentrations were indicative of dietary intake (122). Bingham used plasma carotenoids and vitamin C to validate dietary assessments for the EPIC study (105). Furthermore, British investigators determined that urinary fructose and sucrose can be used as markers to estimate total sugar and sucrose intake (124).

In the future, the collection of biological samples to validate estimates of dietary intake will become routine in nutrition epidemiology and surveillance (107). Researchers need to be aware of within-person variability in biomarkers. Block and colleagues recommend collecting at least two measurements per person to reduce attenuation (125). However, it is important to recognize that biomarkers cannot substitute for collecting estimates of dietary intake. As Conner states, "food intake is the bottom line as people eat food, not nutrients" (111).

UNDERREPORTING OF DIETARY INTAKE

Based on data collected from a variety of volunteers, it is now well accepted that underreporting of food intake is pervasive and increasing in prevalence (94,126). Underreporting occurs when people report food intakes so much lower than their measured total energy expenditure that the intakes are not biologically plausible. In other words, a person could not support fundamental physiological processes or survive over the long term on intakes so low.

Who Underreports?

Underreporters constitute anywhere from 10% to 45% of the total sample, depending on the age, gender, and body composition of the sample. In the past two decades, underreporting has been consistently shown to be more prevalent and more severe among obese in comparison with lean subjects (127–129). Underreporting is not confined to just obese people, however. In large nationwide surveys of both British and American adults, women were more likely than men to underreport (130–132). In addition, people of low socioeconomic status, characterized by low incomes and low education attainment, are more likely to report low-energy intakes (130–132).

Why Do People Underreport?

To fully understand the problem of underreporting, the reasons why people underreport their food intakes need to be known. Obesity does not cause people to underreport; instead, the psychological and behavioral characteristics associated with obesity probably lead people to underreport. Psychological characteristics associated with underreporting include a high need for social acceptance, high levels of body dissatisfaction, and a high level of dietary restraint among both men and women, obese and nonobese (133–136). Additionally, overweight people tend to consume larger meals. Their underestimation of food intake has been shown to be related to the meal size, as opposed to body size (137).

What Foods and Nutrients Are Prone to Underreporting?

If underreporting occurred simply across the board—that is, all foods and nutrients were underreported to the same degree—the solution to the problem of underreporting would be relatively simple. A correction factor could be added to the dietary intake data of underreporters, which would bring their intakes of all nutrients into line with those of the valid reporters. Unfortunately, the solution is not that simple because underreporters often fail to report those foods that have a "bad" or even "sinful" connotation (102).

In a large US nationwide survey, 1,224 out of 8,334 adults were found to be low-energy reporters. In comparing the low-energy reporters with those who were not low-energy reporters, the following were among the foods most likely to be underreported: cake and pie, savory snacks, cheese, white potatoes, meat mixtures, regular soft drinks, fat-type spreads, and condiments (138). British investigators found that underreporters reported consuming significantly less cake, sugar, fat, and breakfast cereal. However, the researchers found no discernible differences in reports of bread, potatoes, meat, or vegetable and fruit consumption between underreporters and other subjects (95).

At this time, there is no consensus as to whether or how much the macronutrients are differentially reported. Some research suggests that underreporters reported lower intakes of fat as a percentage of total energy, as well as higher intakes of protein and carbohydrate (132,139). However, other research suggests an underreporting bias toward not only fat but also carbohydrate and alcohol (5).

Effect of Underreporting on Conclusions about Diet and Health

In nutrition epidemiology, it is important to classify nutrient intakes correctly from low to high and then determine whether associations exist between nutrient intake and the occurrence of disease. As evidence of differential reporting of food and nutrients by underreporters accumulates, a real possibility of the misclassification of subjects' nutrient intakes in studies of diet and disease is highlighted.

This problem is exacerbated because the probability of underestimation of food intake, as well as of differential reporting of foods and nutrients, increases with other known factors of health risk, such as obesity and low socioeconomic status. For example, because obesity is a known risk factor for a number of chronic diseases, such as coronary heart disease, people at higher risk of these diseases are more likely to differentially report foods and macronutrients. Because bias in measuring dietary intake can both remove and create associations, it can generate seriously misleading conclusions about the impact of diet on disease (74,140–142).

Identifying Underreporters

Ideally, all dietary studies should incorporate independent biomarkers of energy intake as measures of validity. Unfortunately, no biomarkers are currently available that can be used in the field on a routine basis. However, researchers can apply the Goldberg cutoff, which has been extensively described by Goldberg and colleagues (143) and Black and colleagues (144). The Goldberg cutoff evaluates energy intake against estimated energy requirements and defines cutoff limits that identify the most obviously implausible intake values. A ratio of estimated energy intake (EI) to predicted BMR is calculated as EI/BMR. This ratio can then be compared with a study-specific cutoff value (using values suggested by Black et al [145]) that represents the lowest value of EI/BMR that could, within defined bounds of statistical probability (±2 standard deviations [SD]), reflect the habitual energy expenditure, given a sedentary lifestyle.

In the NHANES III, Briefel and colleagues used the Goldberg cutoff and classified 18% of the men and 28% of the women as underreporters (132). This illustrates how the Goldberg cutoff has been used to provide some indication of whether estimates of dietary intake are biased.

There are limitations to the Goldberg cutoff, however. It underestimates the incidence of underreporting because it assumes that all people have a sedentary physical activity level. For improved identification of individual underreporters, additional knowledge about lifestyle, occupation, and leisure physical activity is required to estimate subject-specific physical activity levels and calculate more subject-specific cutoffs (145,146).

McCrory and colleagues have developed an alternative method for identifying underreporters to compensate for some of these limitations (142). They found that using ±1 SD bounds, taking into account within-subject errors in the parameters of EI and predicted total energy expenditure may be more effective in identifying implausible dietary intakes.

Methods for Reducing Underreporting

Because underreporting is pervasive, it is increasingly important to identify means to improve validity of self-reports of food and energy intakes, so that researchers can make dietary recommendations to individuals and the population as a whole (147). Scagliusi and colleagues (148) developed a motivational training program that when combined with portion size aids and confrontation with dietary recalls showed some improvement in rates of underreporting. The use of technology (personal digital assistants) did not improve the validity of energy self-reports (149). Additional research is needed to investigate methods for increasing the validity of self-reported food and energy intakes.

Handling Underreporting in Dietary Intake Data

Researchers have not yet found good strategies for analyzing databases that contain large numbers of underreporters. One obvious technique is to exclude from analyses those people who report energy intakes that are biologically implausible. This technique is problematic, however, because underreporting is concentrated within specific subgroups of the population (130–132). Excluding these subjects would seriously alter the size and nature of the sample, eliminating people who might be of most concern in terms

of health risk (132). Their removal could mask or distort important diet-disease associations. Some investigators have analyzed their data using all observations and then reanalyzed the data with the underreporters removed, and have found significant improvements in the effect sizes of a number of dietary variables (150). If the findings remained consistent when reanalyzed in this manner, this procedure could improve confidence in the results and conclusions.

Upward adjustment of all nutrients equally to account for underreporting is another possible technique for handling underreporting, but it would be acceptable only if all nutrients are underreported, which is not the case. Underreporters tend to report diets that are micronutrient-rich in comparison with valid reporters (130). Adjusting all nutrients upward would create an artificial impression of the sample's nutritional status.

Epidemiologists recommend adjusting nutrient intakes for energy intake using the regression of nutrient vs energy (90). Again, this technique would be valid only when underreporting results from a systematic underestimation of portion sizes (across-the-board underestimation), but the actual foods are accurately reported. However, as stated earlier, it is likely that certain foods are underreported more than others (systematic omissions), so energy adjustment could make matters worse (151). For example, if foods containing fat are more likely to be underreported and foods containing vitamin A are less likely to be underreported, energy adjustment would provide a lower-than-actual measure of fat intake and a higher-than-actual measure of vitamin A intake. Researchers have acknowledged that energy adjustment cannot eliminate bias caused by selective underreporting of certain foods, which is further complicated by correlation of errors when estimating nutrient intake (130,152). Statistical adjustments have been further explored using data from the EPIC studies, and investigators have found that the effect of energy adjustment can vary widely when models of correlated measurement error are used (92,93).

CONCLUSION

No dietary intake assessment method can serve as a gold standard for all types of dietary research. The dietary assessment methods generally used include 24-hour dietary recalls, food records or diaries, diet histories, and FFQs. Researchers must determine which method is appropriate for their study based on the data being collected and the purpose of the research, as well as the strengths and weaknesses of the different methods. Once the method has been chosen, it should be tested for both reliability and validity in a representative sample of the study population.

The field of nutrition continues to advance substantially with the identification of a number of biomarkers that can be used to independently validate self-reports of dietary intake. These biomarkers have been used to identify the phenomenon of underreporting, and have furthered an understanding of who might underreport and what foods are more likely to be underreported. There is a pressing need for more research to identify novel methods of collecting dietary intake data. Ransley and colleagues (153,154) are currently exploring the use of supermarket receipts in estimating dietary intake. Additionally, there continues to be a need for further analytic approaches that can account for underreporting in dietary databases. In the meantime, researchers and practitioners must interpret dietary intake data with considerable skepticism; lack of skepticism would lead to the dissemination of misleading diet and health hypotheses and associations.

REFERENCES

1. Thompson FE, Subar AF. Dietary assessment methodology. In: Coulston AM, Rock CL, Monsen ER, eds. *Nutrition in the Prevention and Treatment of Disease.* San Diego, Calif: Academic Press; 2001:3–30.
2. Bingham SA, Riboli E. Diet and cancer—the European Prospective Investigation into Cancer and Nutrition. *Nature Rev.* 2004;4:206–215.
3. Bingham SA, Welch AA, McTaggart A, Mulligan AA, Runswick SA, Luben R, Oakes S, Khaw KT, Wareham N, Day NE. Nutritional methods in the European Prospective Investigation of Cancer in Norfolk. *Public Health Nutr.* 2001;4:847–858.
4. Willett W. *Nutritional Epidemiology.* 2nd ed. New York, NY: Oxford University Press; 1998.
5. Subar AF, Kipnis V, Troiano RP, Midthune D, Schoeller DA, Bingham S, Sharbaugh CO, Trabulsi J, Runswick S, Ballard-Barbash R, Sunshine J, Schatzkin A. Using intake biomarkers to evaluate the extent of dietary misreporting in a large sample of adults: the OPEN study. *Am J Epidemiol.* 2003;158:1–13.
6. Kipnis V, Subar AF, Midthune D, Freedman LS, Ballard-Barbash R, Troiano RP, Bingham S, Schoeller DA, Schatzkin A, Carroll RJ. Structure of dietary measurement error: results of the OPEN

biomarker study. *Am J Epidemiol.* 2003;158: 14–21.
7. Bliss RM. Researchers produce innovation in dietary recall. *Agric Res.* 2004;52:10–12.
8. Anderson SA, ed. *Guidelines for Use of Dietary Intake Data.* Washington, DC: US Food and Drug Administration; 1986.
9. Peterkin BP, Rizek RL, Tippett KS. Nationwide food consumption survey, 1987. *Nutr Today.* 1988;23:18–24.
10. Pao EM, Sykes KE, Cypel YS. *USDA Methodological Research for Large-Scale Dietary Intake Surveys, 1975–1988.* Washington, DC: US Department of Agriculture; 1989. Home Economics Research Report no. 49.
11. Armstrong B, Doll R. Environmental factors and cancer incidence and mortality in different countries, with special reference to dietary practices. *Int J Cancer.* 1975;15:617–631.
12. Jolliffe N, Archer M. Statistical associations between international coronary heart disease death rates and certain environmental factors. *J Chronic Dis.* 1959;9:636–652.
13. Mosfegh AF, Raper N, Ingerwesen I, Cleveland L, Anand J, Goldman J, LaComb R. An improved approach to 24-hour dietary recall methodology. *Ann Nutr Metab.* 2001;45(suppl 1): S156.
14. Galasso R, Panico S, Celentano E, Del Pezzo M. Relative validity of multiple telephone versus face-to-face 24-hour dietary recalls. *Ann Epidemiol.* 1994;4:332–336.
15. Morgan KJ, Johnson SR, Rizek RL, Reese R, Stampley GL. Collection of food intake data: an evaluation of methods. *J Am Diet Assoc.* 1987;87:888–896.
16. Lyu L-C, Hankin JH, Liu LQ, Wilkens LR, Lee JH, Goodman MT, Kolonel LM Telephone vs face-to-face interviews for quantitative food frequency assessment. *J Am Diet Assoc.* 1998;98:44–48.
17. Tran KM, Johnson RK, Soultanakis RP, Matthews DE. In-person versus telephone administered multiple-pass 24-hour recalls in women: validation with doubly labeled water. *J Am Diet Assoc.* 2000;100: 777–783.
18. Godwin SL, Chambers E, Cleveland L. Accuracy of reporting dietary intake using various portion-size aids in-person and via telephone. *J Am Diet Assoc.* 2004;104:585–594.
19. Stram DO, Hankin JH, Wilkens LR, Pike MC, Monroe KR, Park S, Henderson BE, Nomura AM,

Earle ME, Nagamine FS, Kolonel LM. Calibration of the dietary questionnaire for a multiethnic cohort in Hawaii and Los Angeles. *Am J Epidemiol.* 2000; 151:358–370.

20. Kagan A, Harris BR, Winkelstein W. *Epidemiologic Studies of Coronary Heart Disease and Stroke in Japanese Men Living in Japan, Hawaii, and California.* Hiroshima, Japan: Atomic Bomb Casualty Commission; 1972.

21. Human Nutrition Information Service, US Department of Agriculture. *Food Consumption: Households in the United States, Spring 1977.* Washington, DC: US Government Printing Office; 1982. Publication H-1.

22. Woteki C, Johnson C, Murphy R. Nutritional status of the US population: iron, vitamin C, and zinc. In: Food and Nutrition Board, National Research Council. *What Is America Eating?* Washington, DC: National Academies Press; 1986:21–39.

23. Beaton GH, Milner J, McGuire V, Feather TE, Little JA. Sources of variance in 24-hour dietary recall data: implications for nutrition study design and interpretation. Carbohydrate sources. Vitamins and minerals. *Am J Clin Nutr.* 1983;37:986–995.

24. Buzzard M. 24-hour dietary recall and food record methods. In: Willett W, ed. *Nutritional Epidemiology.* 2nd ed. New York, NY: Oxford University Press; 1998:50–73.

25. Riboli E, Hunt KJ, Slimani N, Ferrair P, Norat T, Fahey M, Charrondiere UR, Hemon B, Casagrande C, Vignat J, Overvad K, Tjonneland A, Clavel-Chapelon F, Thiebaut A, Wahrendorf J, Boeing H, Trichopoulos D, Trichopoulou A, Vineis P, Palli D, Bueno-de-Mesquita HB, Peeters PHM, Lund E, Engeset D, Gonzalez CA, Barricarte A, Berglund G, Hallmans G, Day NE, Key TJ, Kaaks R, Saracci R. European Prospective Investigation into Cancer and Nutrition (EPIC): study populations and data collection. *Public Health Nutr.* 2002;5: 1113–1124.

26. Moshfegh A, Borrud L, Perloff B, LaComb R. Improved method for the 24-hour dietary recall for use in national surveys. *FASEB.* 1999;13:A603.

27. Conway JM, Ingwersen LA, Vinyard BT, Moshfegh AJ. Effectiveness of the US Department of Agriculture 5-step multiple-pass method in assessing food intake in obese and nonobese women. *Am J Clin Nutr.* 2003;77:1171–1178.

28. Basiotis PP, Welsh SO, Cronin FJ, Kelsay JL, Mertz W. Number of days of food intake records

required to estimate individual and group nutrient intakes with defined confidence. *J Nutr.* 1987;117:1638–1641.

29. Black AE, Cole TJ. Biased over- or under-reporting is characteristic of individuals whether over time or by different assessment methods. *J Am Diet Assoc.* 2001;101:70–80.

30. Ferrari P, Slimani N, Ciampi A, Trichopoulou A, Naska A, Lauria C, Veglia F, Bueno-de-Mesquita HB, Ocke MC, Brustad M, Braaten T, Jose Tormo M, Amiano P, Mattisson I, Johansson G, Welch A, Davey G, Overvad K, Tjonneland A, Clavel-Chapelon F, Thiebaut A, Linseisen J, Boeing H, Hemon B, Riboli E. Evaluation of under- and over-reporting of energy intake in the 24-hour diet recalls in the European Prospective Investigation into Cancer and Nutrition (EPIC). *Public Health Nutr.* 2002;5:1329–1345.

31. Hankin JH, Wilkens LR, Kolonel LN, Yoshizawa CN. Validation of a quantitative diet history method in Hawaii. *Am J Epidemiol.* 1991;133:616–628.

32. Block G. A review of validations of dietary assessment methods. *Am J Epidemiol.* 1982;115: 492–505.

33. Sawaya AL, Tucker KT, Tsay R, Willett W, Salzman E, Dallal GE, Roberts SB. Evaluation of four methods for determining energy intake in young and older women: comparison with doubly labeled water measurements of total energy expenditure. *Am J Clin Nutr.* 1996;63:491–499.

34. Witschi JC. Short-term dietary recall and recording methods. In: Willett W, ed. *Nutritional Epidemiology.* 2nd ed. New York NY: Oxford University Press; 1990:52–68.

35. Hankin JH, Huenemann RL. A short dietary method for epidemiologic studies. I. Developing standard methods for interpreting seven-day measured food records. *J Am Diet Assoc.* 1967;50:487–492.

36. Hankin JH, Reynolds WE, Margen S. A short dietary method for epidemiologic studies. II. Variability of measured nutrient intakes. *Am J Clin Nutr.* 1967;20:935–945.

37. Marr JW, Heady JA. Within- and between-person variation in dietary surveys: number of days needed to classify individuals. *Hum Nutr Appl Nutr.* 1986;40:347–364.

38. Nelson M, Black AE, Morris JA, Cole TJ. Between-and within-subject variation in nutrient intake from infancy to old age: estimating the number of days required to rank dietary intake

with required precision. *Am J Clin Nutr.* 1989;50:156–167.

39. Sempos CT, Johnson NE, Smith EL, Gilligan C. Effects of intraindividual and interindividual variation in repeated dietary records. *Am J Epidemiol.* 1985;121:120–130.

40. Liu K, Stamler J, Dyer A, McKeever P. Statistical methods to assess and minimize the role of intraindividual variability in obscuring the relationship between dietary lipids and serum cholesterol. *J Chronic Dis.* 1978;31:399–418.

41. Block G, Hartman AM. Dietary assessment methods. In: Moon TE, Micozzi MS, eds. *Nutrition and Cancer Prevention. Investigating the Role of Micronutrients.* New York, NY: Marcel Dekker; 1989:159–180.

42. Burke BS. The dietary history as a tool in research. *J Am Diet Assoc.* 1947;23:1041–1046.

43. Samet JM, Skipper BJ, Humble CG, Pathak DR. Lung cancer risk and vitamin A consumption in New Mexico. *Am Rev Respir Dis.* 1985;131:198–202.

44. Ziegler RG, Mason TJ, Stemhagen A. Carotenoid intake, vegetables, and the risk of lung cancer among white men in New Jersey. *Am J Epidemiol.* 1986;123:1080–1093.

45. Hankin JH. Dietary methods for estimating vitamin A and carotene intakes in epidemiologic studies of cancer. *J Can Diet Assoc.* 1987;48:219–234.

46. Tucker KL, Maras J, Champagne C, Connell C, Goolsby S, Weber J, Zaghloul S, Carithers T, Bogle ML. A regional food-frequency questionnaire for the US Mississippi Delta. *Public Health Nutr.* 2005;8:87–96.

47. Block G, Dresser CM, Hartman AM, Carroll MD. Nutrient sources in the American diet: quantitative data from the NHANES II survey. I. Vitamins and minerals. *Am J Epidemiol.* 1985;122:13–26.

48. Block G, Dresser CM, Hartman AM, Carroll MD. Nutrient sources in the American diet: quantitative data from the NHANES II survey. II. Macronutrients and fats. *Am J Epidemiol.* 1985;122:27–40.

49. Block G, Hartman AM, Dresser CM, Carroll MD, Gannon J, Gardner L. A data-based approach to diet questionnaire design and testing. *Am J Epidemiol.* 1986;124:453–469.

50. Willett WC, Sampson L, Stampfer MJ, Rosner B, Bain C, Witschi J, Hennekens CH, Speizer FE. Reproducibility and validity of a semiquantitative food frequency questionnaire. *Am J Epidemiol.* 1985;122:51–65.

51. Stuff JE, Garza C, O'Brian Smith E, Nichols BL, Montandon CM. A comparison of dietary methods in nutritional studies. *Am J Clin Nutr.* 1983;37:300–306.

52. Gray GE, Paganini-Hill A, Ross RK, Henderson BE. Assessment of three brief methods of estimation of vitamin A and C intakes for a prospective study of cancer: comparison with dietary history. *Am J Epidemiol.* 1984;119:581–590.

53. Rohan TE, Potter JD. Retrospective assessment of dietary intake. *Am J Epidemiol.* 1984;120:876–887.

54. Rimm EB, Giovannucci EL, Stampfer MJ, Colditz GA, Litin LB, Willett WC. Reproducibility and validity of an expanded self-administered semiquantitative food frequency questionnaire among male health professionals. *Am J Epidemiol.* 1992;135:1114–1126.

55. Marr JW. Individual dietary surveys: purposes and methods. *World Rev Nutr Diet.* 1971;13:105–161.

56. Hunter DJ, Sampson L, Stampfer MJ, Colditz GA, Rosner B, Willett WC. Variability in portion sizes of commonly consumed foods among a population of women in the United States. *Am J Epidemiol.* 1988;127:1240–1249.

57. Cummings SR, Block G, McHenry K, Baron RB. Evaluation of two food frequency methods of measuring dietary calcium intake. *Am J Epidemiol.* 1987;126:796–802.

58. Chu SY, Kolonel LN, Hankin JH, Lee J. A comparison of frequency and quantitative dietary methods for epidemiologic studies of diet and disease. *Am J Epidemiol.* 1984;110:323–334.

59. Kolonel LN, Henderson BE, Hankin JH, Nomura AM, Wikens LR, Pike MC, Stram DO, Monroe KR, Earle ME, Nagamine FS A multiethnic cohort in Hawaii and Los Angeles: baseline characteristics. *Am J Epidemiol.* 2000;151:346–357.

60. Pietinen P, Hartman AM, Haapa E, Rasanen L, Haapakoski J, Palmgren J, Albanes D, Virtamo J, Huttunen JK. Reproducibility and validity of dietary assessment instruments. I. A self-administered food use questionnaire with a portion size picture booklet. *Am J Epidemiol.* 1988;128:655–666.

61. Shatenstein B, Nadon S, Godin C, Ferland G. Development and relative validity of a food frequency questionnaire in Montreal. *Can J Diet Pract Res.* 2005;66:67–75.

62. Kolonel LN, Yoshizawa CN, Hankin JH. Diet and prostate cancer: a case-control study in Hawaii. *Am J Epidemiol.* 1988;127:999–1012.

63. LeMarchand L, Yoshizawa CN, Kolonel LN, Hankin JH, Goodman MT. Vegetable consumption and lung cancer risk: a population-based case-control study in Hawaii. *J Natl Cancer Inst.* 1989;81:1158–1164.

64. LeMarchand L, Wilkens LR, Hankin JH, Kolonel LN, Lyu LC. A case-control study of diet and colorectal cancer in a multiethnic population in Hawaii (United States): lipids and foods of animal origin. *Cancer Causes Control.* 1997;8:637–648.

65. Goodman MT, Wilkens LR, Hankin JH, Lyu LC, Wu AH, Kolonel LN. Association of soy and fiber consumption with the risk of endometrial cancer. *Am J Epidemiol.* 1997;146:294–306.

66. Hankin JH. Development of a diet history questionnaire for studies of older persons. *Am J Clin Nutr.* 1989;50:1121–1127.

67. Brown JE, Tharp TM, Dahlberg-Luby EM. Videotape dietary assessment: validity, reliability, and comparison of results with 24-hour dietary recalls from elderly women in a retirement home. *J Am Diet Assoc.* 1990;90:1675–1679.

68. Rumpler WV, Kramer K, Rhodes DG, Moshfegh AJ, Paul DR. Identifying sources of reporting error using measured food intake. *Eur J Clin Nutr.* Advance online publication, 11 April 2007;doi: 10.1038.

69. Madden JP, Goodman SJ, Guthrie HA. Validity of the 24-hour recall. *J Am Diet Assoc.* 1976;68: 143–147.

70. Gersovitz M, Madden JP, Smickilas-Wright H. Validity of the dietary recall and seven-day record for group comparisons. *J Am Diet Assoc.* 1978;73:48–56.

71. US Department of Agriculture. *National Nutrient Data-base for Standard Reference, Release 18.* Available at: http://www.nal.usda.gov/fnic/foodcomp/search. Accessed June 18, 2006.

72. Pennington JAT, Douglass JS. *Bowes & Church's Food Values of Portions Commonly Used.* 18th ed. Philadelphia, Pa: Lippincott Williams and Wilkins; 2004.

73. Dixon LB. Minnesota Nutrition Data System (MNDS): food—a tool designed by researchers for researchers. Abstract presented at: Leadership through Diversity, 29th Annual Meeting of the Society for Nutrition Education, St Louis, Mo, July 20–24, 1996.

74. Johnson RK, Black AE, Cole TJ. Letter to the editor. *N Engl J Med.* 1998;338:917–919.

75. Willett WC, Reynolds RD, Cottrell-Hoehner S, Sampson L, Browne ML. Validation of a semiquantitative food frequency questionnaire: comparison with a l-year diet record. *J Am Diet Assoc.* 1987;87:43–47.

76. Hankin JH. Role of nutrition in women's health: diet and breast cancer. *J Am Diet Assoc.* 1993;93: 994–999.

77. Prentice RL, Pepe M, Self SG. Dietary fat and breast cancer: a quantitative assessment of the epidemiological literature and a discussion of methodological issues. *Cancer Res.* 1989;49: 3147–3156.

78. Bingham SA, Luben R, Welch A, Wareham N, Khaw K-T, Day N. Are imprecise methods obscuring a relation between fat and breast cancer? *Lancet.* 2003;362:212–214.

79. Freedman LS, Potischman N, Kipnis V, Midthune D, Schatzkin A, Thompson FE, Troiano RP, Prentice R, Patterson R, Carroll R, Subar AF. A comparison of two dietary instruments for evaluating the fat-breast cancer relationship. *Int J Epidemiol.* 2006;35:1011–1021.

80. Hegsted DM. Errors of measurement. *Nutr Cancer.* 1989;12: 105–107.

81. Johansson I, Hallmans G, Wikman A, Biessy C, Riboli E, Kaaks R. Validation and calibration of food-frequency questionnaire measurements in the Northern Sweden Health and Disease cohort. *Public Health Nutr.* 2002;5:487–496.

82. Thompson FE, Moler JE, Freedman LS, Clifford CK, Stables GJ, Willett WC. Register of dietary assessment calibration-validation studies: a status report. *Am J Clin Nutr.* 1997;65(suppl): 1142S–1147S.

83. Dietary Assessment Calibration/Validation Register: Studies and Their Associated Publications. National Cancer Institute. Available at: http://www.dacv.ims.nci.nih.gov. Accessed July 5, 2006.

84. Karvetti RL, Knuts LR. Validity of the estimated food diary: comparison of 2-day recorded and observed food and nutrient intakes. *J Am Diet Assoc.* 1992;92:580–584.

85. Linusson EEI, Sanjur D, Erickson EC. Validating the 24-hour recall method as a dietary survey tool. *Arch Latinoam Nutr.* 1974;24:277–294.

86. Subar AF, Thompson FE, Kipnis V, Midthune D, Hurwitz P, McNutt S, McIntosh A, Rosenfeld S. Comparative validation of the Block, Willett, and National Cancer Institute food frequency questionnaire. *Am J Epidemiol.* 2001;154:1089–1099.

87. Bogers RP, Dagnelie PC, Westerterp KR, Kester ADM, van Klaveren JD, Bast A, van den Brandt PA. Using a correction factor to correct for overreporting in a food frequency questionnaire does not improve biomarker-assessed validity of estimates for fruit and vegetable consumption. *J Nutr.* 2003;133:1213–1219.

88. Freedman LS, Midthune D, Carroll RJ, Krebs-Smith S, Subar AF, Troiano RP, Dodd K, Schatzkin A, Ferrari P, Kipnis V. Adjustments to improve the estimation of usual dietary intake distributions in the population. *J Nutr.* 2004;134:1836–1843.

89. Willett W. Dietary fat and breast cancer. In: Willett W, ed. *Nutritional Epidemiology.* 2nd ed. New York, NY: Oxford University Press; 1998: 377–413.

90. Willett WC, Howe GR, Kushi LH. Adjustment for total energy intake in epidemiologic studies. *Am J Clin Nutr.* 1997;65(suppl):1220S–1228S.

91. Fraser GE. A search for truth in dietary epidemiology. *Am J Clin Nutr.* 2003;78(suppl):521S–525S.

92. Michels KB, Bingham SA, Luben R, Welch AA, Day NE. The effect of correlated measurement error in multivariate models of diet. *Am J Epidemiol.* 2004;160:59–67.

93. Day NE, Wong MY, Bingham S, Khaw KT, Luben R, Michesl KB, Welch A, Wareham NJ. Correlated measurement error—implications for nutritional epidemiology. *Int J Epidemiol.* 2004;33: 1373–1381.

94. Black AE, Prentice AM, Goldberg GR, Jebb SA, Bingham SA, Livingstone MB, Coward WA. Measurements of total energy expenditure provide insights into the validity of dietary measurements of energy intake. *J Am Diet Assoc.* 1993;33: 572–579.

95. Bingham SA, Cassidy A, Cole TJ, Welch A, Runswick SA, Black AE, Thurnham D, Bates C, Khaw KT, Key TJ. Validation of weighed records and other methods of dietary assessment using the 24 h urine nitrogen technique and other biological markers. *Br J Nutr.* 1995;73:531–550.

96. Lifson N, Gordon GB, Visscher MB, Nier AO. The fate of utilized molecular oxygen and the source of heavy oxygen of respiratory carbon dioxide, studied with the aid of heavy oxygen. *J Biol Chem.* 1949;180:803–811.

97. Lifson N, Gordon GB, McClintock R. Measurement of total carbon dioxide production by means of D_2O^{18}. *J Appl Physiol.* 1955;7:704–710.

98. Schoeller DA, van Santen E. Measurement of energy expenditure in humans by the doubly labeled water method. *J Appl Physiol.* 1982;53: 955–995.

99. Poehlman ET. A review: exercise and its influence on resting energy metabolism in man. *Med Sci Sports Exerc.* 1989;21: 515–525.

100. Poehlman ET. Energy expenditure and requirements in aging humans. *J Nutr.* 1992;122:2957–2965.

101. Schoeller DA. How accurate is self-reported dietary energy intake? *Nutr Rev.* 1990;48:373–379.

102. Mertz W. Food intake measurements: is there a "gold standard"? *J Am Diet Assoc.* 1992;92:1463–1465.

103. Johnson RK, Driscoll P, Goran MI. Comparison of multiple-pass 24-hour recall estimates of energy intake with total energy expenditure determined by the doubly labeled water method in young children. *J Am Diet Assoc.* 1996;96:1140–1144.

104. Schoeller DA. Measurement of energy expenditure in free-living humans by using doubly-labeled water. *J Nutr.* 1988;118:1278–1289.

105. Bingham SA. Dietary assessments in the European Prospective Study of Diet and Cancer (EPIC). *Eur J Can Prev.* 1997;6:118–124.

106. Kok FJ, van't Veer P. *Biomarkers of Dietary Exposure: Proceedings of the 3rd Meeting on Nutritional Epidemiology.* London, UK: Smith-Gordon and Co; 1991.

107. Bingham S. Challenges in dietary approaches [abstract]. *Eur J Clin Nutr.* 1998;52(suppl):S4.

108. Bogers RP, van Assema P, Kester ADM, Westerterp KR, Dagnelie PC. Reproducibility, validity, and responsiveness to change of a short questionnaire for measuring fruit and vegetable intake. *Am J Epidemiol.* 2004;159:900–909.

109. Zock PL, Mensink RP, Harryvan J, de Vries JHM, Katan MB. Fatty acids in serum cholesterol esters as quantitative biomarkers of dietary intake in humans. *Am J Epidemiol.* 1997;145: 1114–1122.

110. Andersen LF, Solvoll K, Drevon DA. Very-long-chain n-3 fatty acids as biomarkers for intake of fish and n-3 fatty acid concentrates. *Am J Clin Nutr.* 1996;64:305–311.

111. Conner SL. Biomarkers and dietary intake data are mutually beneficial. *Am J Clin Nutr.* 1996;64: 379–380.

112. Willett WC, Stampfer MJ, Colditz GA, Rosner BA, Hennekens CH, Speizer FE. Dietary fat and the risk of breast cancer. *N Engl J Med.* 1987;316:22–28.

113. Hu FB, Stampfer MJ, Manson JE, Rimm E, Colditz GA, Rosner BA, Hennekens CH, Willett WC. Dietary fat intake and the risk of coronary heart disease in women. *N Engl J Med.* 1997;337:1491–1499.

114. Bingham SA, Cummings J. Urine nitrogen as an independent validatory measure of dietary intake: a study of nitrogen balance in individuals consuming their normal diet. *Am J Clin Nutr.* 1985;42:1276–1289.

115. Black AE. Under-reporting of energy intake at all levels of energy expenditure: evidence from doubly labeled water studies. *Proc Nutr Soc.* 1997;56:121A.

116. Tasevska N, Runswick SA, Bingham SA. Urinary potassium is as reliable as urinary nitrogen for use as a recovery biomarker in dietary studies of free living individuals. *J Nutr.* 2006;136:1334–1340.

117. Chug-Ahuja JK, Holden JM, Forman MR, Mangels AR, Beecher GR. The development and application of a carotenoid database for fruits, vegetables, and selected multicomponent foods. *J Am Diet Assoc.* 1993;93:318–323.

118. Yeum KJ, Booth SL, Sadowski JA, Liu C, Tang G. Human plasma carotenoid response to the ingestion of controlled diets high in fruits and vegetables. *Am J Clin Nutr.* 1996;64:5 94–602.

119. Martini MC, Campbell DR, Gross MD, Grandits GA, Potter JD. Plasma carotenoids as biomarkers of vegetable intake: the University of Minnesota Cancer Prevention Research Unit Feeding Studies. *Cancer Epidemiol Biomarkers Prev.* 1995;4:491–496.

120. Le Marchand L, Hankin JH, Carter FS, Essling C, Luffey D, Franke AA, Wilkens LR, Cooney RV, Kolonel LN. A pilot study on the use of plasma carotenoids and ascorbic acid as markers of compliance to a high fruit and vegetable dietary intervention. *Cancer Epidemiol Biomarkers Prev.* 1994;3:245–251.

121. Al-Delaimy WK, Ferrari P, Slimani N, Pala V, Johansson I, Nilsson S, Mattisson I, Wirfalt E, Galasso R, Palli D, Vineis P, Tumino R, Dorronsoro M, Pera G, Ocke MC, Bueno-de-Mesquite HB, Overvad K, Chirlaque MD, Trichopoulou A, Naska A, Tjonneland A, Olsen A, Lund E, Alsaker HER, Barricarte A, Kesse E, Boutron-Ruault M-C, Clavel-Chapelon F, Key TJ, Spencer E, Bingham S, Welch AA, Sanches-Perez M-J, Nagel G, Linseisen J, Quiros JR, Peeters PHM, van Gils CH, Boeing H, van Kappel AL, Steghens J-P, Riboli E. Plasma carotenoids as biomarkers of intake of fruits and vegetables: individual-level correlations in the European Prospective Investigation into Cancer and Nutrition (EPIC). *Eur J Clin Nutr.* 2005;59:1387–1396.

122. Scott KJ, Thurnham DI, Hart DJ, Bingham SA, Day K. The correlation between the intake of lutein, lycopene, and beta-carotene from vegetables and fruits, and blood plasma concentrations in a group of women aged 50-65 years in the UK. *Br J Nutr.* 1996;75:409–418.

123. Murphy SP, Bunch SJ, Kaiser LL, Joy AB. A food behavior checklist can measure changes resulting from a nutrition education intervention. Abstract presented at: Advancing Nutrition Education—Moving toward Healthful, Sustainable Diets, 31st Annual Meeting of the Society for Nutrition Education, Albuquerque, NM, July 18–22, 1998.

124. Tasevska N, Runswick SA, McTaggart A, Bingham SA. Urinary sucrose and fructose as biomarkers for sugar consumption. *Cancer Epidemiol Biomarkers Prev.* 2005;14:1287–1294.

125. Block G, Dietrick M, Norkus E, Jensen C, Benowitz NL, Morrow JD, Hudes M, Packer L. Intraindividual variability of plasma antioxidants, markers of oxidative stress, C-reactive protein, cotinine, and other biomarkers. *Epidemiology.* 2006;17:404–412.

126. Hirvonen T, Mannisto S, Roos E, Pietinen P. Increasing prevalence of underreporting does not necessarily distort dietary surveys. *Eur J Clin Nutr.* 1997;51:297–301.

127. Prentice AM, Black AE, Coward WA, Davies HL, Goldberg GR, Murgatroyd PR, Ashford J, Sawyer M, Whitehead RG. High levels of energy expenditure in obese women. *Br Med J.* 1986;292:983–987.

128. Lichtman SW, Pisarska K, Berman ER, Pestone M, Dowling H, Offenbacher E, Weisel H, Heshka S, Matthews DE, Heymsfield SB. Discrepancy between self-reported and actual caloric intake and exercise in obese subjects. *N Engl J Med.* 1992;327:1893–1898.

129. Bandini LG, Schoeller DA, Cyr HN, Dietz WH. Validity of reported energy intake in obese and nonobese adolescents. *Am J Clin Nutr.* 1990;52:421–425.

130. Price GM, Paul AA, Cole TJ, Wadsworth MEJ. Characteristics of the low-energy reporters in a longitudinal national dietary survey. *Br J Nutr.* 1997;77:833–851.

131. Pryer JA, Vrijheid M, Nichols R, Kiggins M, Elliot P. Who are the "low energy reporters" in the dietary and nutritional survey of British adults? *Int J Epidemiol.* 1997;26:146–154.

132. Briefel RR, Sempos CT, McDowell MA, Chien SCY, Alaimo K. Dietary methods research in the third national health and nutrition examination survey: underreporting of energy intake. *Am J Clin Nutr.* 1997;65(suppl):1203S–1209S.

133. Taren D, Tobar M, Hill A, Howell W, Shisslak C, Bell I, Ritenbaugh C. The association of energy intake bias with psychological scores of women. *Eur J Clin Nutr.* 1999;53:570–578.

134. Johnson RK, Friedman AB, Harvey-Berino J, Gold BC, McKenzie D. Participation in a behavioral weight-loss program worsens the prevalence and severity of underreporting among obese and overweight women. *J Am Diet Assoc.* 2005;105:1948–1951.

135. Novotny JA, Rumpler WV, Riddick H, Hebert JR, Rhodes D, Judd JT, Baer DM, McDowell M, Briefel R. Personality characteristics as predictors of underreporting of energy intake on 24-hour dietary recall interviews. *J Am Diet Assoc.* 2003;103:1146–1151.

136. Tooze JA, Subar AM, Thompson FE, Troiano R, Schatzkin A, Kipnis V. Psychosocial predictors of energy underreporting in a large doubly labeled water study. *Am J Clin Nutr.* 2004;79:795–804.

137. Wansink B and Chandon P. Meal size, not body size, explains errors in estimating the calorie content of meals. *Ann Intern Med.* 2006;145:326–332.

138. Krebs-Smith SM, Graubard BI, Kahle LL, Subar AF, Cleveland LF, Ballard-Barbash R. Low energy reporters vs others: a comparison of reported food intakes. *Eur J Clin Nutr.* 2000;54: 281–287.

139. Voss S, Kroke A, Lipstein-Grobusch K, Boeing H. Is macronutrient composition of dietary intake data affected by underreporting? Results from the EPIC-Potsdam study. *Eur J Clin Nutr.* 1998;52: 119–126.

140. Livingstone MB, Prentice AM, Strain JJ, Coward WA, Black AE, Barker ME, McKenna PG, Whitehead RG. Accuracy of weighed dietary records in studies of diet and health. *Br Med J.* 1990;300:708–712.

141. Hietmann BL, Lissner L. Can adverse effects of dietary fat intake be overestimated as a consequence of dietary fat underreporting? *Public Health Nutr.* 2005;8:1322–1327.

142. McCrory MA, Hajduk CL, Roberts SB. Procedures for screening out inaccurate reports of dietary energy intake. *Public Health Nutr.* 2002;5: 873–882.

143. Goldberg GR, Black AE, Jebb SA, Cole TJ, Murgatroyd PR, Coward WA, Prentice AM. Critical evaluation of energy intake data using fundamental principles of energy physiology: 1. Derivation of cut-off limits to identify under-recording. *Eur J Clin Nutr.* 1991;45: 569–581.

144. Black AE, Goldberg GR, Jebb SA, Livingstone MBE, Cole TJ, Prentice AM. Critical evaluation of energy intake data using fundamental principles of energy physiology: 2. Evaluating the results of published surveys. *Eur J Clin Nutr.* 1991;45: 583–599.

145. Black AE. Critical evaluation of energy intake using the Goldberg cut-off for energy intake:basal metabolic rate. A practical guide to its calculation, use and limitations. *Int J Obes.* 2000;24: 1119–1130.

146. Black AE. The sensitivity and specificity of the Goldberg cut-off for EI:BMR for identifying diet reports of poor validity. *Eur J Clin Nutr.* 2000;54: 395–404.

147. Blundell JE. What foods do people habitually eat? A dilemma for nutrition, an enigma for psychology. *Am J Clin Nutr.* 2000;71:3–5.

148. Scagliusi FB, Polacow VO, Artioli GG, Benatti FB, Lancha AH. Selective underreporting of energy intake in women: magnitude, determinants, and effect of training. *J Am Diet Assoc.* 2003;103:1306–1313.

149. Yon BA, Johnson RK, Harvey-Berino J, Gold BC. The use of a personal digital assistant for dietary self-monitoring does not improve the validity of self-reports of energy intake. *J Am Diet Assoc.* 2006;106:1256–1259.

150. Huang TTK, Roberts SB, Howarth NC, McCrory MA. Effect of screening out implausible energy intake reports on relationships between diet and BMI. *Obes Res.* 2005;13:1205–1217.

151. Carter LM, Whiting SJ. Underreporting of energy intake, socioeconomic status, and expression of nutrient intake. *Nutr Rev.* 1998;56:179–182.

152. Stallone DD, Brunner EJ, Bingham SA, Marmot MG. Dietary assessment in Whitehall II: the influence of reporting bias on apparent socioeconomic variation in nutrient intakes. *Eur J Clin Nutr.* 1997;51: 815–825.

153. Ransley JK, Donnelly JK, Khara TN, Botham H, Arnot H, Greenwood DC, Cade JE. The use of supermarket till receipts to determine the fat and energy intake in a UK population. *Public Health Nutr.* 2001;4:1279–1286.

154. Ransley JK, Donnelly JK, Botham H, Khara TN, Greenwood DC, Cade JE. Use of supermarket receipts to estimate energy and fat content of food purchased by lean and overweight families. *Appetite.* 2003;41:141–148.

15

Food Composition Data and Databases

Jean A.T. Pennington, PhD, RD

This chapter provides an overview of the features and uses of food composition databases and emphasizes the care that should be taken in using the data for various purposes. *Food composition data* refers to the levels of food components (nutrients, contaminants, and other constituents) per specified unit of foods (usually per 100 g or per specified serving size or portion). The data are the results of chemical analysis, calculations (eg, protein estimated from nitrogen or energy from calorie equivalents, or sums of values from recipe ingredients), imputations, or estimations. A *food composition database* refers to a collection of data on the levels of components in foods; usually the data are from various sources. Most food composition databases contain multiple foods and multiple food components; however, some databases, such as those for newly analyzed components or those for components that are not widespread in the food supply, may contain only one or only several food components.

AVAILABLE DATABASES

Major Databases

Many compilations of food composition data are available in the United States and in other countries (1,2). Most food composition databases are stored and maintained as computer files, and their availability to users may be as hard copies and/or electronic files. Many countries have a national or regional food composition database that reflects foods that are most commonly consumed by their populations (2). The national database for the United States is the Nutrient Database for Standard Reference (SR) developed by the Agricultural Research Service (ARS) of the US Department of Agriculture (USDA) (3). Release 19 of the SR (the most recent version as of this writing) contains 7,293 foods and data for up to 140 food components. It is routinely updated and serves as the foundation for many of the food composition databases that have been developed in US colleges, universities, hospitals, clinics, and private companies. Some of these US databases are listed in the *International Nutrient Databank Directory,* which was compiled by a committee of the National Nutrient Databank Conference (1). The SR also serves as the foundation for databases in several other countries where resources for analyzing local foods are limited or not available.

In addition to the SR, the ARS also maintains the Food and Nutrition Database for Dietary Surveys (FNDDS) (4), which is used to assess the food and nutrient intake of participants in the National Health and Nutrition Examination Survey (NHANES) conducted by the National Center for Health Statistics (NCHS) (5). The FNDDS includes about 7,000 foods and data for 62 food components. There are no missing values in this database; nutrient values that were not available from laboratory analysis or other sources were calculated from recipes or imputed by ARS. The foods in this database are generally in the "as-consumed" state, and the database is routinely updated to keep pace with trends and changes in American eating patterns.

Information about the development of food composition databases both in the United States and in other countries is available on the International Network of Food Data Systems (INFOODS) Web site (6). INFOODS was founded in 1984 to help improve the quality and quantity of food composition data and to facilitate data availability.

Features of food composition databases that may distinguish one database from another include the foods and food components contained, the form of the database (hard copy or electronic file), periodicity of update, format on the page or computer screen, intended uses (eg, reference, diet analyses, or product development), food and food component search capabilities, and associated software functions. Some databases are updated routinely as new data become available; others are updated at specific intervals, such as every year or every few years. Foods in databases may appear alphabetically or alphabetically by food group. One common format for listing foods and nutrients is to have the foods listed in the left-hand column with the nutrient values listed in columns across the page or screen. An alternative format is one food per page or screen, with the nutrients in the left-hand column and the values per 100 g and per serving portion in columns across the page or screen. The computer system for a database may allow the user to select several alternative formats for data display and presentation. Software features may allow for assessment of dietary intake, comparison of dietary intake with country standards, and calculation of the composition of recipe items from ingredients.

Special-Interest Databases

The ARS usually compiles data for newer food components in special-interest databases and then, when and if appropriate, incorporates the data into the SR. For example, the ARS special-interest database for carotenoids was merged into the SR (3). Currently ARS has special-interest databases for added sugars, choline, flavonoids, fluoride, isoflavones, oxalic acid, and proanthocyanidins (7). Because so few data are available for some food components, such as vitamins D and K, oxalic acid, chromium, and other trace minerals, these food components may be listed in separate tables in hard copy databases. In some cases the food component may occur in only a small number of foods (eg, vitamin D or vitamin K), or the cost or difficulty of analytic methods may limit the generation of data for many foods (eg, chromium).

Because of increasing interest in the relationships of carotenoids, flavonoids, polyphenols, and other measures of antioxidative capacity to measures of health and to diseases such as cancer, cardiovascular disease, and immune system diseases, scientific papers on the levels of these components (eg, references 8–32) are of great interest to database compilers. The carotenoids (beta carotene, alpha carotene, lutein, and lycopene) occur primarily in dark green, red, and yellow vegetables and in yellow and red fruits. There are about 5,000 flavonoid compounds; these substances are found primarily in vegetables, fruits, cereals, nuts, tea, coffee, and wine (33). Vegetables and fruits appear to be the major contributors to dietary intakes of polyphenols and other antioxidants (34). Data for these food components will continue to be developed and gathered in special-interest databases and/or incorporated into larger databases.

Dietary Supplement Databases

Databases on dietary supplements are essential to fully capture intakes of food components in nutrition surveys, in dietary research studies, and for patient care. Dietary supplements (capsules/pills, herbal preparations, and other dietary preparations) include thousands of different products with different brand names and potencies. There are also different potencies of the same compound with the same brand name. Data for dietary supplements are usually kept in separate databases rather than merged with food composition databases. A dietary supplement database was developed by NCHS for use with the NHANES dietary intake data (35,36). The Office of Dietary Supplement (ODS) at the National Institutes of Health (NIH) is currently working on a plan to develop a label-based dietary supplement database, and the ODS is also collaborating with the ARS to develop an analytic-based dietary supplement database (37–39). These and other databases for dietary supplements will likely evolve over the next decade as more research is conducted on the relationship of dietary supplements to health maintenance and disease prevention (40). (See Chapter 23 for more information about research on dietary supplements.)

Food Contaminant Databases

Data on the levels of contaminants in foods are usually not included in the databases that contain nutrient values. The development of food composition databases for food contaminants poses special challenges because average levels are not generally reported, and could be misleading if they were reported. The presence of pesticide residues, industrial chemicals, microbial toxins, toxic elements (eg, mercury, lead, arsenic, and cadmium), and other contaminants in foods is often a matter of chance. Experts in these areas speak of the number of *detections,* rather than average levels, and the residue levels are usually quite low compared with accepted standards. For example, an analysis of 200 samples of a food may reveal a pesticide residue in only 10 of the samples. The mean level for these 10 samples may be measurable; however, the mean for the 200 samples may be zero. In addition, levels of contaminants may be considerably reduced in foods during rinsing, peeling, and processing.

Although much work has been done to determine levels of pesticide residues and other contaminants in foods, it has been done to monitor the food supply (to assess safety by confirming that levels are below acceptable daily intakes), rather than to provide mean values for databases. It might be more informative for contaminant databases to provide a ratio of detected to nondetected contaminants and to provide reported values for the detected contaminants only, as well as for all samples analyzed. The databases for food contaminants are still being developed, and the accepted format and standards for these databases will likely evolve as the users and uses of these databases are made known.

In the United States, one of the primary sources of information on pesticide residues, industrial chemicals, radionuclides, toxic elements, and other contaminants in commonly consumed foods is the Food and Drug Administration (FDA) Total Diet Study (41). This study collects 280 foods four times per year from various US locations and ships them to the Total Diet Laboratory for analysis; the results of this study are posted on the FDA Web site (41). Another example of a contaminant database is that developed by Jakszyn et al (42) for assessing the relationship of cancer to dietary intake of nitrosamines, heterocyclic amines, and polycyclic aromatic hydrocarbons (43).

DATA USERS AND DATA USES

Food composition databases are used to assess the dietary status of patients, clients, and students; to assess dietary intakes of population groups with defined demographic characteristics; to plan and evaluate the dietary adequacy of meals and diets; and to discern relationships between diet, health, and disease from the results of national, clinical, and epidemiologic studies. Food composition databases may be used to assess the nutrient content of individual

foods or a group of similar foods for the purpose of developing food standards, formulating new food products, determining the potential use of foods in therapeutic diets, establishing definitions for dietary claims, or determining whether foods meet such claims. Databases are also used to develop nutrition education materials and programs for students, foodservice workers, caregivers, homemakers, and the general public.

Registered dietitians (RDs) and other nutrition professionals may have a specific need or range of needs for food composition data, depending on their place of employment and job responsibilities. RDs working in hospitals, schools, prisons, and other institutions and in private practice may use databases to plan and evaluate meals and daily diets, to develop therapeutic diets, and to educate patients or institutional residents. Within hospitals and clinics, databases may also be used to counsel patients and design diets for clinical trials. Academic nutrition professionals use databases for diet-disease epidemiologic research and for student education in nutrition, food science, and health courses. Government nutrition professionals at FDA, NIH, and USDA use databases to develop policies concerning nutrient fortification, food standards, and label claims; to assess the safety and adequacy of the food supply; to design and evaluate the results of epidemiologic studies and clinical trials; and to develop nutrition education materials for the general public and targeted population groups. Nutrition professionals who work in the food industry use databases for product development, nutrition labeling, and dietary claims. Grocery stores may use databases for shelf-labeling programs, and restaurants may use them to make nutrition claims about foods on their menus and to develop nutrition brochures for consumers.

FOOD ANALYSTS AND FOOD ANALYSIS

Food composition data originate from the work of chemists in government, industry, academic, and private laboratories who analyze individual or composite samples (mixtures of individual samples) of foods to determine the levels of food components. The procedures and accepted methods for collecting and analyzing foods for various food components are discussed in detail in *Food Composition Data: Production, Management, and Use* (44). It is important for analysts to document how the foods are sampled, selected, collected, prepared, and analyzed, as well as how the results are verified and evaluated. If calculations are required to determine nutrient levels (such as protein calculated from nitrogen content), these calculations should be explained and documented.

Each food that is analyzed requires a unique sampling design to ensure that the samples that are analyzed are representative of the foods typically consumed. The sampling design should include the variables that affect the composition of each food. Nationwide food sampling involves different variables than does local food sampling. The variables for raw fruits and vegetables may include season, geography, and cultivar (genetic strain or variety), whereas variables for processed foods may include the location of the processing plant and the market share of the brand-name products. If compositing methods are used, they should be appropriate for the intended purposes of the resulting data.

The Association of Official Analytical Chemists (45) provides information on the analytic methods and sample preparations that laboratories should use to determine the levels of each food component. Quality control procedures include duplicate analyses, recoveries of reference standards, recoveries of spiked/fortified samples, and the use of standard reference materials. Spiked/fortified samples contain a known added amount of the food component and are used to determine whether the analytic method accurately measures the amount present. Standard reference materials contain a government-certified amount of a component in a food and are purchased and analyzed by laboratories to ascertain the accuracy of their analytic methods.

When many samples of the same food are analyzed individually to determine the concentration of a food component, the distribution of those concentrations is rarely normal (Gaussian). Statistical treatment of analytic data typically includes the calculation of means, standard deviations, coefficients of variation, and medians. Means may be weighted by variety, cultivar, species, market share, or seasonal availability of the individual foods.

Much can be learned from evaluating the distribution of the analytic data points for each food component in a food. Outliers can be identified, and their treatment (ie, inclusion or omission from the evaluation) can be determined and documented. If bimodal or other modal distributions occur, it might be necessary to separate the samples into groups to obtain more useful data. For example, the distribution of the iron content of wheat-flake breakfast cereals might show a bimodal distribution reflecting two different levels of iron fortification (eg, 4.5 mg/oz and 18 mg/oz). The overall mean concentration of iron would be an intermediate value (between 4.5 and 18 mg/oz) that would not reflect either type of cereal. It would be best to list each type of cereal separately in a database, even if all the other nutrient values for the two types of cereal were similar.

DATA COMPILERS AND DATA COMPILATIONS

The data compiler gathers data from the available sources, organizes the food names into groups and subgroups, and evaluates and aggregates the data into a useful database (46). Compilers of food composition data may be employed by government agencies, food companies, academic institutions, hospitals, clinics, foodservice institutions, or private companies. They may be independent contractors hired by these organizations or be self-employed. Compilers should hold degrees in nutrition, dietetics, or food science and should be knowledgeable about food sampling, analysis, descriptions, and processing as well as about culinary terms and cuisines. Knowledge of computerized database systems and the retrieval of information from databases is also very important. It is best to have the compiler work directly with the person who designs the computer system so that the system performs the necessary operations accurately and efficiently.

Those who compile national databases usually have direct access to results from government or contract laboratories and supplement this with data from the scientific literature and from the food industry. Other database compilers gather data from national data sets (such as the SR and/or the FNDDS), scientific papers, food companies, the Internet, and other previous compilations. Data compilers in academia or clinical research might also obtain food component data directly from in-house or contract laboratories.

Compilers who use the SR or the FNDDS as the foundation for their databases select the foods and nutrients that they need from these sources and then add other foods and components that they obtain from the literature, food companies, restaurants, and other sources. Database compilers may fill in values that are missing in the SR by imputation or calculation, and they may add foods to the database that have nutrient values determined by imputation or calculation. Some compilers may include values from nutrition labels.

The data generated by food companies for the purpose of nutrition labeling is not of the same accuracy as data generated directly from food composition laboratories because the nutrition labeling data has been adjusted by the use of formulas and by rounding so that the resulting values are in compliance with FDA and USDA regulations. (The USDA regulates the nutrition labeling of meat and poultry and products containing meat and poultry; the FDA regulates the nutrition labeling of all other foods.) The information in Nutrition Facts panels on food labels are in grams and milligrams and/or percent Daily Values (DVs) for the food components. Vitamins A and C, calcium, and iron are provided only in percent DV. Therefore, the amounts of these four nutrients must be calculated based on their DVs.

The data from the various sources are collected by database compilers and incorporated into their files along with appropriate source documentation. Compilers cannot check the documentation for every food component value for every food with regard to sampling, number of samples, analytic method, and laboratory quality control. However, any data that appear to be clearly out of line should be questioned and either verified or omitted.

DATA AGGREGATION

Database compilers standardize food names and descriptions and aggregate the data for foods with the same name to prevent duplicate listings. Aggregation allows for summarizing the data for the same food (or very similar foods) and prevents repetition of the same food name in the database. Accurate aggregation requires that the data for foods that seem to have the same or similar name and descriptors be closely scrutinized to determine which foods and their corresponding nutrient values may be consolidated into a single food entry in the database. The compiler may also combine data for foods with similar descriptions that have identical (or nearly identical) composition data, such as different flavors for a brand name of reduced-fat yogurt or different cultivars of apples.

The aggregation of data from various sources has the potential benefit of enlarging or completing the nutrient profile for a food, because some sources may provide food components that are not provided by other sources. For example, one source might have extensive trace mineral values for a food, another source might provide individual carotenoid values for the same food, and another source may have the macronutrient content along with the levels of more common vitamins and minerals. Before combining data from different sources, it is important to be sure that the food names and descriptions indicate that the foods are the same and to check for comparability of common

data provided by the sources. Similarity of common nutrient values (eg, water, energy, protein, or fat) for information from several sources provides some basis for data aggregation. In addition, evaluation of major and minor nutrients might indicate that foods with slightly different names are basically the same food.

When data for the same food are aggregated from various sources, the challenge is usually to calculate representative values for the various food components using statistical models that weight the important factors contributing to variability. Data for aggregated foods may be averaged (ie, each data point carries the same value), or they may be weighted and averaged (eg, data for four brands of canned corn might be weighted and averaged by market share or averaged by the number of samples from each source to produce data for generic canned corn). The data sources and data manipulation should be documented, but it is not usually possible to provide this documentation within the database; this information usually remains in the files of the data compiler.

DATABASE FEATURES

Food Names and Descriptions

Database compilers must give accurate and appropriate names to each food and provide sufficiently descriptive terms to distinguish each food from all the other foods in the database. Foods that are vaguely named or that have inconsistent or ambiguous descriptive terms will cause confusion for the user and may lead to improper use of the data. Similarly, when food composition data are published in journals, the data should be accompanied by complete and accurate food descriptions.

Guidelines and methods for describing foods have been developed, and issues related to food descriptions and to the development of descriptive terms have been discussed (47–51). The luxuries of unlimited space for food names and open-ended food descriptors (as might be found in analytic reports or scientific papers) are not usually possible in databases available in hard copy or as electronic files, although the electronic files are more flexible with regard to space than are hard copy formats. Therefore, it is necessary to provide, within the allotted space, the food names and descriptive terms that will be most useful for the data user. The compiler should strive for uniformity in describing foods in a database by using a selected order of descriptors and standardized terms and abbreviations. For example, the

TABLE 15.1   Example of Order of Food Description Terms in a Database

Type of Term	Food with Descriptive Terms
Color	Apple, *red*, red delicious, with peel, without core, raw
Flavor	Pudding, *vanilla*, prepared from instant mix, Jell-O
Part of plant or animal	Beet, *greens and root*, diced, boiled
Accompaniments	Ice cream, vanilla *with chocolate syrup*
Preservation, treatment methods, and containers	Fruit cocktail *in light syrup, canned*, Del Monte
Preparation or cooking method	Frankfurter, beef and pork, *boiled*
Brand name	Peas, green, with cream sauce, frozen, *Birds Eye*

compiler might use the order of descriptors shown in Table 15.1.

Not all of the descriptors shown in Table 15.1 are applicable or useful for each food. The information for "part of plant or animal" would also indicate whether peel or seeds are present for fruits and vegetables, whether fat is present on meat cuts or has been trimmed away, whether rind is included or not for cheese, and so on. Redundant or commonly assumed information is not usually included (eg, that fruits and vegetables are rinsed before use, that ice cream is frozen, or that frozen or canned entrees are heated before serving). Footnotes might be added to provide ingredients for mixed dishes (eg, a footnote might say that a tuna-noodle-vegetable casserole contains tuna canned in water and drained, egg noodles, chopped frozen broccoli, and condensed mushroom soup), but footnotes are not usually necessary for well-known items with quality control (eg, a brand-name fast-food sandwich).

A thorough index with cross-references is useful for locating foods in a hard copy database because of the many synonyms for some foods (eg, green beans are also called snap beans and string beans; pancakes are also called hotcakes and flapjacks) and the many ways of describing and placing foods in alphabetical listings and within food groups (eg, corn may be either a vegetable or a cereal grain). Computerized systems usually have search functions that will bring up all foods with identified terms (eg, all foods called *sugar cookie* or all foods containing the words *soy* or *stir-fried*). These searches allow for very broad or narrow searching depending on the specificity of the terms and the number of terms used in the search. Some computerized systems also have built-in food name synonyms so that a search on a less-familiar term (eg, *aubergine, broad bean,* or *frankfurter*) would bring up the preferred terms in the database (eg, *eggplant, lima beans,* or *hot dog,* respectively).

When using the FNDDS (4) and other databases for assessing diets, the challenge is to appropriately match the foods described by study participants, students, patients, or clients to the foods listed in the databases (ie, to select the best fit). This challenge is one reason why food descriptions are so important. Because survey participants are not always able to provide accurate descriptions of the foods they eat, the FNDDS includes generic foods with the descriptor *not further specified* (NFS). The nutrient data for NFS foods are based on data for similar or representative foods. For example, *sandwich, NFS* might reflect the most commonly consumed sandwich in the survey (perhaps a cheese sandwich on white bread with mayonnaise), or it might be a composite sandwich with nutrient values calculated from weighted data from other sandwiches in the database.

Food Groupings

Database compilers often organize foods into groups based on food source (eg, grains, fruits, nuts, or vegetables) or food use (eg, beverages, breakfast cereals, condiments, desserts, entrees, or snacks). Food groups may then be further organized into subgroup hierarchies. Food groups and subgroups in databases help users locate items and prevent redundancy in terms, such as *ready-to-eat cereal* or *candy bar*. Food use groupings have cultural significance that might make a database useful in its country or region of origin but less useful internationally. Therefore, databases designed specifically for international use may need an alphabetical organizational structure or food groups that are based on food source rather than food use.

Because there are many potential hierarchies for food subgroups, thought must go into constructing them so that they will be most useful. A consideration of the potential subgroups and hierarchical structure for pizza (Figure 15.1) shows subgroups according to crust (deep-dish, regular, thick, or thin), topping (cheese, mushroom, pepperoni, or sausage), source (frozen, carryout, homemade, or restaurant chain), or brand name. The resulting hierarchies are affected by the order in which the variables are selected. Likewise, cakes may be subgrouped by flavor (chocolate, cherry, pound, or yellow) or by source (bakery, homemade, box mix, or frozen). Ready-to-eat cereals may be grouped

Crust (level 1)	Topping (level 2)	Location of Preparation (level 3)
Deep-dish	Cheese	Carryout
Regular	Mushroom	Frozen
Thick	Pepperoni	Homemade
Thin	Sausage	Restaurant

Pizza Hierarchy Example

Level 1   Deep-dish
  Level 2   Cheese
    Level 3   Carryout
    Level 3   Frozen
    Level 3   Homemade
    Level 3   Restaurant
  Level 2   Mushroom
    Level 3   Carryout
    Level 3   Frozen
    Level 3   Homemade
    Level 3   Restaurant
  Level 2   Pepperoni
    Level 3   Carryout
    Level 3   Frozen
    Level 3   Homemade
    Level 3   Restaurant
  Level 2   Sausage
    Level 3   Carryout
    Level 3   Frozen
    Level 3   Homemade
    Level 3   Restaurant

Level 1   Regular crust
  Repeat above for levels 2 and 3.
Level 1   Thick crust
  Repeat above for levels 2 and 3.
Level 1   Thin crust
  Repeat above for levels 2 and 3.

FIGURE 15.1   Example of a subgroup hierarchy for pizza. This example uses only four descriptive terms from each of the three subgroups and shows only part of one hierarchical arrangement (crust first, topping second, and location of preparation third). Fifteen other hierarchical arrangements are possible with these three subgroups.

by grain type (corn, oat, rice, or wheat), listed alphabetically by cereal brand name (Trix, Froot Loops, or Shredded Wheat), or subgrouped according to the manufacturer's name (General Mills, Kellogg's, or Post). The decisions for grouping and subgrouping are made by the compiler and often depend on how many items are available under each subgrouping. The group and subgroup designations affect the usefulness of the compilation, so the compiler must make these decisions with care.

Basis of Data

Data for foods in databases are presented on a wet-weight (ie, as-consumed) basis, so data reported on a dry-weight basis (as may be done for literature papers on trace elements or contaminants) should be converted to wet weight before being added to a database. (Dry-weight basis means that all the water in the food has been removed by a dehydration process and that the food is in a powdered state.) Dry-weight data should not be included in a food composition database unless the product is available as a powder. It is important for analysts to include the percent water content with the other food components for each food when they publish data in the scientific literature to allow food component values to be converted from a dry-weight to a wet-weight basis.

It should be clear in the database whether the data are presented *as purchased* (ie, with waste or refuse) or as *edible portion,* and whether the weight of the food includes or excludes possible waste or refuse (ie, bone, peel, core, husk, or shell). For example, the data for an apple presented on a 100-g basis may or may not include the weight of the core and the peel, or the data for a baked chicken breast may or may not include the weight of the bones and skin. The database should indicate whether the foods are raw, cooked, or processed; the specific methods of cooking and processing; and if ingredients are added during cooking or processing (eg, a fried chicken leg may have been battered and salted).

RDs are most likely to need nutrient values per weight of edible portion of foods as consumed (eg, cooked meat without bones, popped popcorn, or apples without cores). The food weight in the database may be per typical serving portion or per 100 g. If a serving portion is given, it should be unambiguously described and a corresponding gram weight for the serving size should be included. Consistency in listing serving portions within each food group of a database is useful for comparative purposes so that users can compare nutrient values for similar quantities of foods (eg, 8 fl oz of milks, 1 oz of ready-to-eat cereals, 1 cup of cooked vegetables, 1 oz of nuts or seeds, and 1 oz of cheeses).

Aggregation of nutrient data for the same food from various sources requires that food components have the same specificity and units for measurements. For example, two different sources of vitamin E for the same food may include one expressed in International Units and one expressed in milligrams of individual tocopherols.

Missing Values

When data are missing from a database, it is usually because the analyses have not been performed or because the manufacturers are unable to release the data. Currently, data for many multi-ingredient foods are not available for inclusion in food composition databases. This is especially common for some homemade, frozen, and shelf-stable entrees and desserts; fast foods and carryout foods; other restaurant foods; and ethnic foods. Unfortunately, a common mistake made by database users is to assume that missing values are zeros. This can lead to underestimation of daily food component intakes and/or to inappropriate foods being allowed on restricted diets. True zeros in a database are indicated with zeros.

Reference databases contain data gathered from available sources and generally do not contain imputed or calculated data for missing values, whereas databases used to analyze dietary information from food consumption surveys and studies (such as the FNDDS) should have as few missing values as possible.

Procedures used to impute food composition values are found in Chapter 5 of *Guidelines for Compiling Data for Food Composition Databases* (46). Some blanks may be filled in with zeros (eg, cholesterol and vitamin B-12 for plant materials or dietary fiber for animal-based foods). Other data may be imputed from a different form of the same food (eg, some data for canned corn might be used for frozen corn [except for the sodium content]) or from similar foods (eg, data for pinto beans might be used for navy beans). Missing values for multi-ingredient foods may be filled in with data calculated from recipes. These calculations usually require corrections for refuse (eg, bone, shell, peel, or trimmed fat), loss or gain of moisture or fat during cooking, and nutrient loss or retention during cooking. Chapter 6 of *Guidelines for Compiling Data for Food Composition Databases* (46) provides information on how to estimate nutrients for multi-ingredient foods. Imputed or calculated values in databases should be identified as such, and the process used for imputation should be documented.

Database Checks

Computerized tools are available to help the compiler assess the validity and integrity of the compiled database (52). These tools include checks for weights of major nutrients compared with the total weight of the food, caloric sums of energy-yielding nutrients compared with the total caloric value of the food, and limits of nutrient concentrations in various food groups. For example, 1 cup of boiled mashed pumpkin weighs 245 g (3), and the sum of the weights of the component values for water (229.54 g), protein (1.76 g), fat (0.17 g), and carbohydrate (12.01 g) is 243.48 g, which rounds to 243 g. The energy value of this food is 49 kcal per cup (3), and the sum of the energy equivalents of the protein (7.04 kcal), fat (1.53 kcal), and carbohydrate (with a correction for 2.7 g of dietary fiber) (37.24 kcal) content is 45.81 kcal, which rounds to 46 kcal. These checks indicate data comparability (ie, 243 g is close enough to 245 g, and 46 kcal is close enough to 49 kcal). The computer system can identify foods and nutrients with potential problems to allow the database compiler to evaluate them. Foods with missing values will generally be flagged by the database checks unless the system is designed to exclude them from this process. Computer systems can also check for outliers by listing the 10 highest and lowest values for each food component or by setting high and low threshold values for each food component and flagging foods that are above or below these thresholds.

Food Component Variability

Except perhaps for carefully formulated products (eg, medical formulas and infant formulas), the food component levels in databases should be expected to have inherent and acquired variability. For example, the mean vitamin C content of a 131-g orange ($2^5/_8$-inch diameter) as listed in the SR is 69.7 mg (3), but the actual vitamin C content of an orange depends on factors such as season, sunlight exposure, cultivar, species, variety, time of day of harvest, length of storage time, storage temperature, and ripeness at harvest. Mean values for individual food components may have large standard deviations. It is useful if the food composition database is able to provide standard deviations and the number of samples analyzed so that users get a better feel for the basis for the data.

The many causes of food component variation are compounded in food composition databases because the data are aggregated from various sources. Variables within any one food include genetics; environmental conditions (climate, temperature, and soil); and methods of preservation, processing, and preparation. Because multi-ingredient foods are made from mixtures of different foods, they have mixtures of these variables. Contributing further to nutrient variation are different analytic methods and techniques, use of different recipes to calculate nutrient values for a mixed dish, and the compiler's unique methods of aggregating foods and nutrient values.

Recent literature on food component variation includes the evaluation of such variables as time of day of collecting breastmilk (53); variety/cultivar (13,19,25,54,55); cultivation/growing conditions (20,56,57); geography (58); fertilization (14,20); season (15,16); crop yield (59); germination (30); feed composition (60); food cooking, processing, and storage (8,22,23,29,31,61); brewing techniques (for tea) (32); brand names (11,62); and analytic and calculation issues (57,63,64). Leskova et al have provided an extensive review of the retention of vitamins in foods after heat treatment (65).

Considering the extent of food component variation, diet recommendations for patients and clients should not be rigid. One food should not be recommended over another as a better or lesser source of a food component unless the difference between the foods will be of practical importance for the patient or client. Small differences in average values for nutrients should not be used to make comparative selections for foods. Rigid dietary recommendations by RDs may override the dietary variety that is necessary to ensure adequate nutrient intake.

Database Inconsistencies

Some inconsistencies in food component values may be identified during database checks and may then be verified or corrected. Other inconsistencies may become apparent only when one compares nutrient values for foods with those of a group or subgroup. For example, one might expect higher values for a raw fruit than for the canned or frozen fruit, but the aggregated data from different varieties, regions, and seasons may show somewhat higher mean levels in the canned or frozen product. Such apparent inconsistencies might reflect the fact that the data for the raw and processed foods came from different sources or might be the result of differences in food storage and sampling or differences in laboratory analytic methods and techniques.

One example of an apparent inconsistency is that the cholesterol content of tuna canned in vegetable oil (15 mg cholesterol per 3-oz drained tuna) is less than that for tuna canned in water (26 mg cholesterol per 3-oz drained tuna) (3). Because cholesterol is lipid-soluble, some of it dissolves into the vegetable oil and thereby reduces the amount of cholesterol in the drained tuna. Tuna in vegetable oil therefore might appear to be a better choice for cholesterol-conscious individuals; however, the cholesterol difference

(9 mg per 3 oz of tuna) is not of practical significance. Tuna canned in water is still a better choice for people following diets low in total fat and energy because it contains 99 kcal and 0.7 g fat per 3 oz, whereas tuna canned in oil contains 168 kcal and 7.0 g fat per 3 oz (3).

IMPLICATIONS FOR REGISTERED DIETITIANS

Some basic tips to help RDs use databases are listed here:

- Be diligent in searching for the best match between the food of interest and the foods listed in the database. Consider food name synonyms and appropriate descriptive terms.
- Do not assume that missing values are zeros. (If a food component value is missing, look for the level of that component in a similar food to get some idea of what the value might be.)
- Adjust the serving portion to what was or will be consumed (ie, do not assume that the serving portion listed in the database is the amount that should be used).

Try not to extend the uses of food composition databases beyond their limitations. Databases may be used for multiday individual dietary assessments or 1-day group dietary assessments. However, because of intraindividual variation, they probably should not be used to assess the dietary adequacy or deficiency of 1-day diets of individuals. Databases are not accurate enough to use for planning or assessing diets for metabolic research or balance studies, nor are they accurate enough to plan diets for patients on very restricted diets. Specific information from food manufacturers about the composition of some foods might be used in research studies or for planning restricted diets. If physiologic measures of body fluids are to be made after specific foods are consumed (eg, serum carotenoids measured after eating tomatoes), then samples of the consumed foods need to be analyzed and the exact portions consumed by the subjects need to be measured.

Use databases knowledgeably and do not become unduly alarmed about uneven quality (eg, more detailed descriptions and nutrient data for some foods than others) or inconsistencies. However, you should not accept unreasonable data; try to determine the reasons for values that appear to be out of line with values for similar foods. Several sources are available to address concerns or questions about the food component content of foods in databases. The ARS and food trade associations are good sources of information regarding the composition of basic and traditional foods. The ARS should be contacted for concerns about data in the SR and the FNDDS (3). Food companies can be contacted regarding data for brand-name products.

The selection of a nutrient database or database system for use in a dietary department, educational facility, or research clinic requires consideration of the specific needs of the users and the features and limitations of the various database systems (66–68). Consider factors such as the number and types of foods included, the food components included and their units of measure, the sources of the data, the quality of the data, availability and frequency of data updates, food search capabilities, and the desired software features, along with considerations for such items as initial cost, maintenance costs, and hardware concerns. Talk with individuals who use different database systems and to ask specific questions of the database system developers. Experimentation with database systems at conference exhibits also may be helpful.

OUTLOOK FOR FOOD COMPOSITION DATABASES

Food composition databases will continue to become more accurate over time as work continues to improve and develop new analytic methods, quality assurance techniques, and statistical analysis of results. Needs for current databases are to fill in the missing or imputed values for food components with analytic values and to analyze foods for which data are most needed. Several publications (69–71) indicate that when databases are updated, changes in dietary intake of nutrients are observed (ie, changes to the database affect the results from food consumption surveys). Thus, maintaining and improving food composition data is important to obtain reliable information about dietary status and diet-health relationships.

Improvements in food composition data quality do not result in decreased data variability because food component variability is inherent in the food materials. However, improved data quality does allow variability to be more readily measured. As more data become available for the same food, outlying values are more clearly identified and can be omitted when averages are determined. For the future, better ways of determining and expressing nutrient variability and validating nutrient data in compiled databases should be found so that RDs can more easily

evaluate the results of their nutrition surveys and studies, help patients and clients with dietary instruction, and educate students about the composition of foods.

Activities are underway to continue to enhance the quality and quantity of food composition data. The NIH and the ARS are collaborating on the National Food and Nutrient Analysis Program (NFNAP), which allows support money from the NIH and other agencies within the US Department of Health and Human Services to be transferred to the ARS for the analysis of foods (72). The *Journal of Food Composition and Analysis* (73) is devoted specifically to the publication of articles dealing with the composition of foods and allows a venue for sharing data. The US National Nutrient Databank Conference continues to meet on a yearly basis, providing a forum for oral and poster presentations relating to food composition (74), and the International Food Data Conference (75) meets every other year to share information and data on foods on an international basis.

REFERENCES

1. National Nutrient Databank Conference (NNDB). International Nutrient Databank Directory. Available at: http://www.nal.usda.gov/fnic/foodcomp/conf/index.html. (Follow link for PDF file.) Accessed April 11, 2006.
2. International Network of Food Data Systems. International Food Composition Tables Directory. Available at: http://www.fao.org/infoods/directory_en.stm. Accessed April 11, 2006.
3. US Department of Agriculture, Agriculture Research Service. Nutrient Data Laboratory. Available at: http://www.nal.usda.gov/fnic/foodcomp/search. (Search the USDA National Nutrient Database for Standard Reference Release 19.) Accessed April 18, 2007.
4. US Department of Agriculture, Agriculture Research Service. USDA Food and Nutrient Database for Dietary Studies (FNDDS). Available at: http://www.ars.usda.gov/Services/docs.htm?docid=7673. Accessed April 11, 2006.
5. Centers for Disease Control and Prevention, National Center for Health Statistics. National Health and Nutrition Examination Survey. Available at: http://www.cdc.gov/nchs/nhanes.htm. Accessed April 11, 2006.
6. International Network of Food Data Systems. Background to INFOODS. Available at:

http://www.fao.org/infoods/index_en.stm. Accessed April 11, 2006.

7. US Department of Agriculture, Agriculture Research Service. Products & Services, Data Sets Prepared by USDA-ARS's Nutrient Data Laboratory. Available at: http://www.ars.usda.gov/Services/docs.htm?docid=5121. Accessed April 11, 2006.

8. Xianquan S, Shi J, Kakuda Y, Yueming J. Stability of lycopene during food processing and storage. *J Med Food.* 2005;8:413–422.

9. Hulshof PJM, van Roekel-Jansen T, van de Bovenkamp P, West CE. Variation in retinol and carotenoid content of milk and milk products in the Netherlands. *J Food Comp Anal.* 2006;19:67–75.

10. Lisiewska Z, Kmiecik W, Korus A. Content of vitamin C, carotenoids, chlorophylls and polyphenols in green parts of dill (*Anethum graveolens L.*) depending on plant height. *J Food Comp Anal.* 2006; 19:134–140.

11. Vanamala J, Reddivari L, Yoo KS, Pike LM, Patil BS. Variation in the content of bioactive flavonoids in different brands of orange and grapefruit juices. *J Food Comp Anal.* 2006;19:157–166.

12. Nardini M, Natella F, Scaccini C. Phenolic acids from beer are absorbed and extensively metabolized in humans. *J Nutr Biochem.* 2006;17:14–22.

13. Luthria DL, Pastor-Corrales MA. Phenolic acids content of fifteen dry edible bean (*Phaseolus vulgaris L.*) varieties. *J Food Comp Anal.* 2006;19:205–211.

14. Toor RK, Savage GP, Heeb A. Influence of different types of fertilizers on the major antioxidant components of tomatoes. *J Food Comp Anal.* 2006;19:20–27.

15. Raffo A, La Malfa G, Fogliano V, Maiani, G, Quaaglia G. Seasonal variations in antioxidant components of cherry tomatoes (*Lycopersicon esculentum* cv. Naomi F1). *J Food Comp Anal.* 2006;19:11–19.

16. Toor RK, Savage GP, Lister CE. Seasonal variations in the antioxidant composition of greenhouse grown tomatoes. *J Food Comp Anal.* 2006;19:1–10.

17. Yilmaz Y, Toledo RT. Oxygen radical absorbance capacities of grape/wine industry byproducts and effect of solvent types on extraction of grape seed polyphenols. *J Food Comp Anal.* 2006;19:41–48.

18. Iwalewa EO, Adewunmi CO, Omisore NOA, Adebanji OA, Azike CK, Adigun AO, Adesina OA, Olowoyo OG. Pro- and antioxidant effects and cytoprotective potentials of nine edible vegetables in Southwest Nigeria. *J Med Food.* 2005;8:539–544.

19. Cantos E, Carlos Espin C, Tomas-Barberan FA. Varietal differences among the polyphenol profiles of seven table grape cultivars studied by LC-DAD-MS-MS. *J Agric Food Chem.* 2002;50: 5691–5696.

20. Robbins RJ, Keck AS, Banuelos G, Finley JW. Cultivation conditions and selenium fertilization alter the phenolic profile, glucosinolate, and sulforaphane content of broccoli. *J Med Food.* 2005;8:204–214.

21. Soong YY, Barlow PJ. Antioxidant activity and phenolic content of selected fruit seeds. *Food Chem.* 2004;88:411–417.

22. Ninfali P, Bacchiocca M. Polyphenols and antioxidant capacity of vegetables under fresh and frozen conditions. *J Agric Food Chem.* 2003;51:2222–2226.

23. Zhang D, Hamauzu Y. Phenolics, ascorbic acid, carotenoids and antioxidant activity of broccoli and their changes during conventional and microwave heating. *Food Chem.* 2004;88:503–509.

24. Sellapan S, Akoh CC. Flavonoids and antioxidant capacity of Georgia-grown Vidalia onions. *J Agric Food Chem.* 2002;50: 5338–5342.

25. Lachman K, Pronek D, Hejtmankova A, Dudjak J, Pivec V, Faitova K. Total polyphenol and main flavonoid antioxidants in different onion (*Allium cepa L.*) varieties. *Hort Sci.* 2003;30: 142–147.

26. Xu X, Gu L, Holden J, Haytowitz DB, Gebhardt SE, Beecher G, Prior RL. Development of a database for total antioxidant capacity in foods: a preliminary study. *J Food Comp Anal.* 2004;17:407–422.

27. Peterson JJ, Dwyer JT, Beecher GR, Bhagwat SA, Gebhardt SE, Haytowitz DB, Holden JM. Flavanones in orange, tangerines (mandarins), tangors, and tangelos: a compilation and review of the data from the analytical literature. *J Food Comp Anal.* 2006;19:S66–S73.

28. Peterson J, Beecher GR, Bhagwat SA, Dwyer JT, Gebhardt SE, Haytowitz DB, Holden JM. Flavanones in grapefruit, lemons, and limes: a compilation and review of the data from the analytical literature. *J Food Comp Anal.* 2006;19:S74–S80.

29. Choi MS, Rhee KC. Production and processing of soybeans and nutrition and safety of isoflavone and other soy products for human health. *J Med Food.* 2006;9:1–10.

30. Lopez-Amoros ML, Hernandez T, Estrella I. Effect of germination on legume phenolic compounds and their antioxidant activity. *J Food Comp Anal.* 2006;19:277–283.

31. van Jaarsvela PH, Marais DW, Harmse E, Nestel P, Rodriguez-Amaya DB. Retention of beta-carotene in boiled, mashed orange-fleshed sweet potato. *J Food Comp Anal.* 2006;19:321–329.

32. Su X, Duan J, Jiang Y, Shi J, Kakuda Y. Effects of soaking conditions on the antioxidant potentials of oolong tea. *J Food Comp Anal.* 2006;19:348–353.

33. Bravo L. Polyphenols: chemistry, dietary sources, metabolism, and nutritional significance. *Nutr Rev.* 1998;56:317–333.

34. Pennington JAT. Food composition databases for bioactive food components. *J Food Comp Anal.* 2002;15:419–434.

35. Ervin RB, Wright JD, Kennedy-Stephenson J. Use of dietary supplements in the United States, 1988–94. *Vital Health Stat.* 1999;11(244).

36. Dwyer JT, Picciano MF, Raiten DJ. Food and dietary supplement databases for What We Eat in America-NHANES. *J Nutr.* 2003;133:624S–634S.

37. Dwyer JT, Picciano MF, Betz JM, Coates PM. Mission and activities of the NIH Office of Dietary Supplements. *J Food Comp Anal.* 2004;17:493–500.

38. Dwyer JT, Picciano MF, Betz JM, Fisher KD, Saldanha LG, Yetley EA, Coates PM, Radimer K, Bindewald B, Sharpless KE, Holden J, Andrews K, Zhao C, Harnly J, Wolf WR, Perry CR. Progress in development of an integrated dietary supplement ingredient database at the NIH Office of Dietary supplements. *J Food Comp Anal.* 2006;19: S108–S114.

39. Office of Dietary Supplements. Dietary Supplement Ingredient and Labeling Databases. Available at: http://dietary-supplements.info.nih.gov/ Health_Information/Dietary_Supplement_Ingredient_ and_Labeling_Databases.aspx. Accessed April 11, 2006.

40. Costello RB, Saldanha LG. *Annual Bibliography of Significant Advances in Dietary Supplement Research 1999.* Bethesda, Md: NIH Office of Dietary Supplements; 1999. Available at: http:// dietary-supplements.info.nih.gov/publications/ publications.html.

41. Food and Drug Administration. Total Diet Study. Available at: http://www.cfsan.fda.gov/~comm/ tds-toc.html. Accessed April 11, 2006.

42. Jakszyn P, Ibanez R, Pera G, Garcia-Closas R, Agudo A, Amiano P, Gonzalez CA. *Food Content of Potential Carcinogens.* Barcelona, Spain: Catalan Institute of Oncology; 2004. Available at: http:// epic-spain.com/libro.html. Accessed March 1, 2007.

43. Jakszyn P, Agudo A, Ibanez R, Garcia-Closas R, Pera G, Amiano P, Gonzalez CA. Development of a food database of nitrosamines, heterocyclic amines, and polycyclic aromatic hydrocarbons. *J Nutr.* 2004;134:2011–2014.

44. Greenfield H, Southgate DAT. *Food Composition Data: Production, Management, and Use.* London, UK: Elsevier Applied Science; 1992.

45. *Official Methods of Analysis of AOAC International.* 18th ed. Gaithersburg, Md: Association of Official Analytical Chemists; 2005.

46. Rand WM, Pennington JAT, Murphy SP, Klensin JC. *Guidelines for Compiling Data for Food Composition Databases.* Hong Kong: UNU Press; 1991.

47. Truswell AS, Bateson DJ, Madafiglio KC, Pennington JAT, Rand WM, Klensin JC. INFOODS guidelines for describing foods: a systematic approach to facilitate international exchange of food composition data. *J Food Comp Anal.* 1991;4:18–38.

48. McCann A, Pennington JAT, Smith EC, Holden JM, Soergel D, Wiley RD. FDA's Factored Food Vocabulary for food product description. *J Am Diet Assoc.* 1988;88:336–342.

49. Pennington JAT, Smith EC, Chatfield MR, Hendricks TC. LANGUAL: a food description language. *Terminology.* 1995;1:277–289.

50. Pennington JAT. Issues of food description. *Food Chem.* 1996;57:145–148.

51. Pennington JAT. Cuisine: a descriptive factor for foods. *Terminology.* 1996;3:155–169.

52. Murphy SP. Integrity checks for nutrient databases. In: Stumbo PJ, ed. *Proceedings of the Fourteenth National Nutrient Databank Conference.* Ithaca, NY: CBORO Group; 1990:89–91.

53. Lubertzky R, Littner Y, Mimouni FB, Dollberg S, Mandel D. Circadian variations in fat content of expressed breast milk from mothers of preterm infants. *J Am Coll Nutr.* 2006;25: 151–154.

54. Skupien K, Oszmian J. Comparison of six cultivars of strawberries (Fragaria x ananassa Duch.) grown in northwest Poland. *Eur Food Res Technol.* 2004;219: 66–70.

55. Peterson J, Dwyer J, Jacques P, Rand W, Prior R, Chui K. Tea variety and brewing techniques influence flavonoid content of black tea. *J Food Comp Anal.* 2004;17:397–406.

56. Kuman V, Rani A, Solanki S, Hussain SM. Influence of growing environment on the biochemical composition and physical characteristics of soybean seed. *J Food Comp Anal.* 2006;19: 188–195.

57. Kim HK, Ye SH, Lim TS, Ha TY, Kwon JH. Physiological activities of garlic extracts as affected by habitat and solvents. *J Med Food.* 2005;8:476–481.

58. Nikkarinen M, Mertanen E. Impact of geological origin on trace element composition of edible mushrooms. *J Food Comp Anal.* 2004;17:301–310.

59. Davis DR, Epp M, Riordan H. Changes in USDA food composition data for 43 garden crops, 1950 to 1999. *J Am Coll Nutr.* 2004;23:669–682.

60. Milinsh MC, das Gracas Padre R, Hayashi C, de Oliveira CC, Visentainer JV, de Souza NE, Matsushita M. Effects of feed protein and lipid contents on fatty acid profile of snail (*Helix aspersa maxima*) meat. *J Food Comp Anal.* 2006;19:212–216.

61. Judprasong K, Charoenkiatkul S, Sungpuag P, Vasanachitt K, Nakjamanong Y. Total and soluble oxalate contents in Thai vegetables, cereal grains and legume seeds and their changes after cooking. *J Food Comp Anal.* 2006;19:340–347.

62. Gallaher RN, Gallaher K, Marshall AJ, Marshall AC. Mineral analysis of ten types of commercially available tea. *J Food Comp Anal.* 2006;19:S53–S57.

63. Menezes EW, de Melo AT, Lima GH, Lajolo FM. Measurement of carbohydrate components and their impact on energy value of foods. *J Food Comp Anal.* 2004;17:331–338.

64. Smit LE, Schofeldt HC, de Beer WHJ. Comparison of the energy values of different dairy products obtained by various methods. *J Food Comp Anal.* 2004;17:361–370.

65. Leskova E, Jubikova J, Kovacikova E, Kosicka M, Porubska J, Holcikova K. Vitamin losses: retention during heat treatment and continual changes expressed by mathematical models. *J Food Comp Anal.* 2006;19:252–276.

66. Buzzard IM, Price KS, Warren RA. Considerations for selecting nutrient-calculation software: evaluation of the nutrient database. *Am J Clin Nutr.* 1991; 54:7–9.

67. Stumbo P. Considerations for selecting a dietary assessment system. *J Food Comp Anal* (in press).

68. Probst YC, Tapsell LC. Overview of computerized dietary assessment programs for research and practice in nutrition education. *J Nutr Educ Behav.* 2005;37:20–26.

69. Guenther PM, Perloff BP, Vizioli TL Jr. Separating fact from artifact in changes in nutrient intake over time. *J Am Diet Assoc.* 1994;94:270–275.

70. Guilland JC, Aubert R, Lhuissier M, Peres G, Montagnon B, Fuchs F, Merlet N, Astorg PO. Computerized analysis of food records: role of coding and food composition database. *Eur J Clin Nutr.* 1993;47:445–453.

71. Ahuja J, Goldman JD, Perloff BP. The effect of improved food composition data on intake estimates in the United States of America. *J Food Comp Anal.* 2006;19:S7–S13.

72. Agricultural Research Service, USDA. National Food and Nutrient Analysis Program (NFNAP). Available at: http://www.ars.usda.gov/Services/docs.htm?docid=9446. Accessed April 11, 2006.

73. Journal of Food Composition and Analysis. Available at: http://www.elsevier.com/wps/find/journaldescription.cws_home/622878/description. Accessed April 11, 2006.

74. National Nutrient Databank Conference. Available at: http://www.nal.usda.gov/fnic/ foodcomp/conf/index.html. Accessed April 11, 2006.

75. International Food Data Conference. Available at: http://www.fao.org/infoods/food_data_conf_en.stm. Accessed January 3, 2007.

16

Using the Dietary Reference Intakes to Assess Intakes

Suzanne P. Murphy, PhD, RD, Susan I. Barr, PhD, RD, and Alicia L. Carriquiry, PhD

In the past, nutrient standards for the United States were the Recommended Dietary Allowances (RDAs) and those for Canada were the Recommended Nutrient Intakes (RNIs). A single standard (either the RDA or the RNI) was typically specified for each nutrient. However, new nutrient standards have now been set for the two countries, using a paradigm that considers the distribution of nutrient requirements as well as the possibility of nutrient excess. As a result, it is possible to set multiple standards for each nutrient. This collection of nutrient standards is called the Dietary Reference Intakes (DRIs). Box 16.1 gives the definitions for each of the DRIs (1–9). The first section of this chapter discusses each of the DRIs, how they were set, and how they may be used. Methods for using the DRIs to assess intakes for individuals are presented in the next section, and the final section covers methods for using the DRIs to assess intakes of population groups.

THE DIETARY REFERENCE INTAKES: A NEW PARADIGM

The DRIs were set by several expert panels that were convened by the Food and Nutrition Board of the Institute of Medicine. Six reports on the DRIs for groups of nutrients were published between 1997 and 2005 (1–6). In addition, two reports on the applications of the DRIs were published, one on using the DRIs to assess dietary intakes (7) and the other on using the DRIs to plan diets (8). A summary report covering all eight of the previous DRI reports

has recently been published (9). A complete set of the DRI values is available at the Institute of Medicine's Web site (http://www.iom.edu/?id=21377).

Estimated Average Requirement and the RDA

Whenever possible, an average requirement was determined for a nutrient and designated as the Estimated Average Requirement (EAR). For each nutrient with an EAR, an indicator or criterion of adequacy was specified. Because the EAR is the level of usual intake that would be adequate for half of the people, the risk of inadequacy would be 0.5 (or 50%) if a person's usual intake is equal to the EAR. The usual intake of an individual is typically defined as the long-term average or habitual nutrient intake. Among a group of people with intakes exactly equal to the EAR, we would expect 50% of them to have intakes that are inadequate for the criterion that was chosen. For example, the EAR for vitamin C for men is 75 mg/d, and the criterion for adequacy is near-maximal maintenance of neutrophil vitamin C concentrations with minimal urinary loss. With an intake of 75 mg/d, a man would have a 50% chance of being unable to maintain near-maximal concentrations in his neutrophils. EARs can differ across 22 life stage categories: two for infants, two for young children, six for boys and men, six for girls and nonpregnant, nonlactating women, three for pregnant women (depending on age group), and three for lactating women (also depending on age group).

BOX 16.1   Dietary Reference Intake (DRI) Definitions

Estimated Average Requirement (EAR): The average daily nutrient intake that is estimated to meet the requirement of half the healthy individuals in a particular life stage and gender group.
Recommended Dietary Allowance (RDA): The average daily dietary nutrient intake that is sufficient to meet the nutrient requirements of nearly all (97% to 98%) healthy individuals in a particular life stage and gender group.
Adequate Intake (AI): The recommended average daily intake level based on observed or experimentally determined approximations or estimates of nutrient intake by a group (or groups) of apparently healthy people that are assumed to be adequate—used when an RDA cannot be determined.
Tolerable Upper Intake Level (UL): The highest average daily nutrient intake level that is likely to pose no risk of adverse health effects to almost all individuals in the general population. As intake increases above the UL, the risk of adverse effects may increase.

Source: Data are from references 1–9.

After deciding on the mean (or median) requirement for a nutrient, the panel members were asked to estimate the distribution of requirements. For all nutrients except iron, the distribution was assumed to be normal (or, in the case of protein, the logarithms of the requirements were distributed normally). Because the data are sparse on the standard deviation (SD) of requirements, a coefficient of variation (CV) of 10% was assumed for most nutrients [CV = (SD/Mean) × 100]. Other estimates of the CV were used for protein (12.5%), niacin (15%), and vitamin A (20%). Because the distribution of iron requirements is skewed, especially for menstruating women, the components of iron requirements were modeled to determine the risk of inadequacy at various levels of intake.

Figure 16.1 shows a graph of the risk (or probability) of inadequacy as intake increases for a hypothetical nutrient. When intake is zero, the risk of inadequacy is 1.0 (or 100%). As intake increases, the risk of inadequacy decreases until it is essentially zero. In Figure 16.1 (9), the EAR is the point on the curve where the risk of inadequacy is 50%. A second point on the curve is labeled the RDA. When intake is equal to the RDA, the risk of inadequacy is low, about 2.5%. The RDA is 2 SD above the EAR, and thus can be calculated if the mean (EAR) and SD are known. For nutrients with a CV of 10% of the requirement, the RDA is 20% above the EAR (ie, RDA = EAR × 1.2). Continuing with the

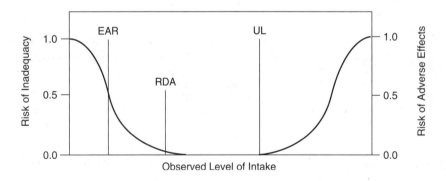

FIGURE 16.1   Relationship among Dietary Reference Intakes. This figure shows that the Estimated Average Requirement (EAR) is the intake at which the risk of inadequacy is 0.5 (50%) to an individual. The Recommended Dietary Allowance (RDA) is the intake at which the risk of inadequacy is very small—only 0.02 to 0.03 (2% to 3%). The Adequate Intake (AI) does not bear a consistent relationship to the EAR or the RDA because it is set without estimation of the requirement. At intakes between the RDA and the Tolerable Upper Intake Level (UL), the risks of inadequacy and of excess are both close to zero. At intakes above the UL, the risk of adverse effects may increase. Reprinted from Institute of Medicine. *Dietary Reference Intakes: The Essential Guide to Nutrient Requirements.* Washington, DC: National Academies Press; 2006:12. Used with permission of the National Academies Press.

vitamin C example for men, the EAR is 75 mg/d and the SD is 7.5 mg/d (a CV of 10%). Thus, the RDA for men for vitamin C is $75 \times 1.2 = 90$ mg/d. The RDA is often used to plan diets for individuals, because intake at the RDA for a nutrient has a low risk of being inadequate.

Although the new RDAs are conceptually similar to the RDAs that were used as nutrient standards in the United States in the past, they differ in the way they are determined. Because the new RDAs are specifically derived from EARs, it is possible to calculate other nutrient standards that may be used instead of the RDA. For example, if a 15% probability of inadequacy were considered acceptable for an individual (instead of the 2% to 3% inherent in the RDA), a number lower than the RDA could be used as a target (approximately the EAR plus 1 SD, rather than the EAR plus 2 SD).

The Adequate Intake (AI)

When the data are insufficient to set an EAR, and therefore an RDA, an Adequate Intake (AI) is set. An AI is ideally the mean intake of a healthy population (ie, one with a low prevalence of inadequacy based on the defined criterion). However, other methods have been used to derive an AI, such as experimentally determined intake. An AI is used as the nutrient standard for almost all nutrients for infants and is based on the mean intake supplied by human milk for healthy, exclusively breastfed infants.

An AI is expected to exceed the RDA for a nutrient, if an RDA could be determined, because the mean intake of a healthy population could be well above the RDA. If the mean intake were below the RDA, you would expect to see some evidence of inadequacy within the population, and thus it would not be considered healthy.

As an example, calcium currently has an AI as the nutrient standard for adequacy. Because the AI is a single number (ie, 1,000 mg/d for men and women ages 19 to 50 years), it is not possible to construct a risk curve like the one shown in Figure 16.1. If an intake is below 1,000 mg/d, it is not possible to estimate the risk of inadequacy, because no information on the distribution of requirements is available. An intake below 1,000 mg/d may still have a low risk of inadequacy.

The Tolerable Upper Intake Level

Although intakes at or above the RDA have a very low risk of inadequacy, at some point intake can become high enough to increase the risk of consuming an excessive amount of the nutrient. As illustrated in Figure 16.1, the risk of an intake being excessive begins to increase at levels above the Tolerable Upper Intake Level (UL). For each nutrient with a UL, a specific adverse effect was identified. The goal was to select the adverse effect that would first appear as intake became excessive, so the initial adverse effect might be relatively mild. For example, the adverse effects for excessive vitamin C intake are osmotic diarrhea and related gastrointestinal disturbances. The vitamin C UL for adults is 2,000 mg/d. If usual intake exceeds this level, the risk of diarrhea is increased. At even higher levels, other adverse effects might occur, but multiple ULs are not set for a nutrient. For many nutrients, the data were insufficient to set a UL. The lack of a UL does not mean that intake at any level is considered safe, only that data were lacking.

Nutrient Standards for Energy and Macronutrients

The nutrient standard for energy intake is the Estimated Energy Requirement (EER). It is the average energy intake that is needed to maintain energy balance in an adult. For children, the EER also includes the energy needed for growth; for pregnant women, it includes the energy for growth of fetal and maternal tissues; and for lactating women, it includes the energy for the secretion of milk. For adults, the EER is calculated using equations that consider the person's age, weight, height, and level of physical activity.

For macronutrients, the standard is the Acceptable Macronutrient Distribution Range (AMDR), which is expressed as a percent of energy intake from five macronutrients: total fat, n-6 polyunsaturated fatty acids (linoleic acid), n-3 polyunsaturated fatty acids (alpha-linolenic acid), carbohydrate, and protein. The AMDRs represent intakes that minimize the risk of chronic disease and permit an adequate intake of essential nutrients. Protein and carbohydrate also have EARs and RDAs, which are expressed as grams per day.

Food Composition Tables and the Nutrient Forms Used for the DRIs

Some of the new DRIs are expressed in forms and units of nutrients that are not traditionally included in food composition tables (10,11). As a result, it can be challenging to evaluate nutrient intakes by comparing them to the DRIs.

This has been a particular problem for the following three nutrients:

- **Vitamin E**—EAR and RDA of vitamin E are expressed in milligrams of alpha-tocopherol, rather than in milligrams of alpha-tocopherol equivalents. Tocopherols other than alpha-tocopherol are assumed to have no vitamin E activity.
- **Vitamin A**—EAR and RDA of vitamin A are expressed in micrograms of retinol activity equivalents (RAE) rather than in micrograms of retinol equivalents (RE). The difference is the conversion factors that are used for carotenoids: to calculate RE, the micrograms of beta carotene are divided by 6 and the micrograms of the other provitamin A carotenoids are divided by 12. However, the calculation for RAE assumes a 50% lower conversion of carotenoids to vitamin A, and factors of 12 and 24 are used.
- **Folate**—EAR and RDA of folate are expressed in micrograms of dietary folate equivalents (DFE) rather than in micrograms of folate (or folacin). One microgram of folate naturally occurring in food is equal to 1 DFE, but 1 µg of synthetic folate (added to foods or in dietary supplements) is equal to 1.67 DFE.

Furthermore, for some nutrients, the UL is applied to a different form of the nutrient than was used for the EAR and RDA. For example, the ULs for folate, vitamin E, and niacin apply only to synthetic forms of these nutrients, such as those added as fortificants or in dietary supplements. The UL for vitamin A is only for the preformed vitamin (retinol). For magnesium, the UL applies only to magnesium salts in supplements. Thus, to compare intakes to these ULs, it is necessary to separately calculate intakes from these specific forms of each nutrient. Unless the food composition table disaggregates the sources of these vitamins, it is not possible to make such comparisons.

Fortunately, the primary databases used in the United States and Canada have been updated to allow most of the desirable comparisons to the new DRI units and forms. For more on food composition tables, refer to Chapter 15.

ASSESSING INTAKES OF INDIVIDUALS

Does an individual's diet meet his or her nutrient requirements? Is he or she at risk of adverse effects from excessive intakes? The way in which these seemingly simple questions are addressed may vary considerably between what is practical and feasible in the practice setting and what is appropriate in a research context. In the practice setting, registered dietitians (RDs) may use relatively informal methods to assess their clients' nutrient intakes. For example, an RD might compare a client's intake on a "typical day" to serving recommendations from MyPyramid (12). Inferences about nutrients for which intakes could be low are often made on this basis (eg, it might be inferred that calcium intake was low if few servings of dairy products were consumed).

In contrast, in a research setting it may be important to obtain a quantitative assessment of the adequacy of an individual's usual nutrient intake—in other words, to determine whether the individual's usual intake meets his or her requirements. It is not easy to do this with accuracy because a given individual's actual requirement is almost never known. In addition, measuring an individual's long-term usual intake of the nutrient is difficult, due to day-to-day variation in intake. Because access to food intake data is typically limited to intake on a single day or small number of days, this observed or reported intake rarely represents the individual's usual intake (7). For these reasons, it is not possible to state with complete certainty whether an individual's intake of a nutrient meets his or her requirement.

However, a statistical approach has been developed that provides an estimate of the *level of confidence* that an individual's usual intake meets his or her requirement (7). This approach first considers the probability that the individual's intake meets his or her requirement, assuming that the intake quantified by the food records or 24-hour dietary recalls represents his or her true usual intake. Next, the impact of inferring usual intake from observed intake is considered. The remainder of this section describes how this approach is executed. In all cases, it is essential to begin with accurately measured food intake data, avoiding intakes that are either overestimated or underestimated (13).

Nutrients with an EAR

Probability of Adequacy

Although an individual's requirement for a nutrient is generally not known, knowledge of the EAR and CV of the requirement distribution provides information on the range within which the requirement likely falls. As described earlier, the requirement distribution for most nutrients is assumed to be normal, with a mean at the EAR and a CV of 10%. Figure 16.2 shows an example of a requirement distribution, in this case magnesium, for women ages 19 to 30 years. The EAR is 255 mg/d, and the SD is 25.5 mg/d

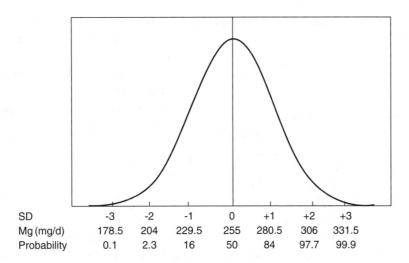

SD	-3	-2	-1	0	+1	+2	+3
Mg (mg/d)	178.5	204	229.5	255	280.5	306	331.5
Probability	0.1	2.3	16	50	84	97.7	99.9

FIGURE 16.2   Example of a requirement distribution: magnesium requirements for women aged 19 to 30 years. *Note*: The requirement distribution for magnesium for women aged 19 to 30 years is shown. The Estimated Average Requirement (EAR) is 255 mg/d, and the standard deviation (SD) is 25.5 mg/d (based on an assumed coefficient of variation [CV] of 10%). Also shown are the probabilities of adequacy for usual intakes at the EAR, and 1, 2, or 3 SD above or below the EAR.

(based on an assumed CV of 10%). It can be seen that most individuals have requirements that are relatively close to the EAR, whereas smaller proportions have requirements that are considerably higher or lower.

Figure 16.2 also shows the probability that a given usual intake is adequate. Based on characteristics of the normal curve, the probability ranges from near zero (at intakes more than 2 SD below the EAR) to nearly 100% (at intakes more than 2 SD above the EAR). The probability is calculated by subtracting the EAR from the usual intake and dividing by the SD of the requirement distribution to yield a z score (a difference divided by its SD) and then consulting a table of z scores to determine the associated probability. For example, the probability that a usual magnesium intake of 280 mg/d is adequate would be estimated as follows: $z = (\text{Intake} - \text{EAR})/\text{SD} = (280 - 255)/25.5 = 0.98$. A z score of 0.98 (about 1.0) is associated with a probability of about 84%. In other words, a usual intake of 280 mg/d meets or exceeds the magnesium requirements of about 84 of 100 women ages 19 to 30 years.

Uncertainty of Estimating an Individual's Usual Intake

The preceding discussion of the probability of adequacy is based on the individual's true long-term usual intake. As alluded to previously, because of day-to-day (within-person) variability, in most cases intake recorded on one day or even many days does not accurately reflect the individual's true long-term usual intake. The extent of uncertainty about an individual's true usual intake is a function of both the

number of days for which records or recalls are kept (collecting intake data over a larger number of days leads to less uncertainty) and the specific nutrient being assessed. There is much more day-to-day or within-person variability (and therefore uncertainty) in intakes of nutrients found in high concentrations in a small number of foods compared with those nutrients widely distributed throughout the food supply. Estimates of within-person variability for many nutrients have been computed from nationwide food consumption surveys (7). For example, for women ages 19 to 50 years, the within-person or day-to-day variability in magnesium intake is 86 mg (a within-person CV of 38%).

A method of combining the uncertainty about the individual's requirement and that regarding his or her usual intake has been proposed. This method also results in the calculation of a z score, which can then be used to estimate the level of confidence that an individual's usual intake is adequate. The procedures for these calculations are described in detail in *Dietary Reference Intakes: Applications in Dietary Assessment* (7). Consider the example of magnesium provided earlier, in which the probability that a usual intake of 280 mg/d was adequate was determined to be 84%. If a woman's usual intake was estimated from 4 days of food records, you could calculate the level of confidence that her usual intake was adequate to be 69%. Therefore, the level of confidence that her intake was adequate is less when you consider the uncertainty associated with estimating her usual intake from 4 days of records.

These methods cannot be used when the within-person variability exceeds 60% to 70%. In general, they are not appropriate for vitamin A, carotene, vitamin C, and vitamin B-12.

Nutrients with an AI

By definition, the EAR is unknown for nutrients that have an AI, and the approach described earlier to estimate the degree of confidence that the individual's intake exceeds his or her requirement cannot be used for nutrients with an AI. However, a statistically based hypothesis testing procedure can be used to compare intake to the AI. This equation accounts for the uncertainty in the reported nutrient intake, as it includes the day-to-day (within-person) variation of nutrient intake. If there is a high degree of confidence that an individual's usual intake equals or exceeds the AI after applying this statistical test, it can be concluded that the diet is almost certainly adequate, as the AI is thought to exceed the requirements of almost everyone. If, however, intake falls below the AI, no quantitative (or qualitative) estimate can be made of the probability of nutrient inadequacy, because the requirement is not known and cannot be estimated from the AI. Nutrition professionals should use their judgment, after considering additional types of information about the individual, when interpreting intakes below the AI. For example, it is not possible to determine whether an adolescent female with a calcium intake of 900 mg/d (where the AI is 1,300 mg/d) is obtaining enough calcium to support optimal rates of bone mineral deposition, and it would be inappropriate to state that she was "deficient" in calcium intake. Nevertheless, it is likely that an RD would recommend that she increase her intake to meet the AI so that adequacy could be ensured.

Nutrients with a UL

The UL may be used to assess whether an individual's usual nutrient intake is so high that it poses a potential risk of adverse health effects. A statistical test similar to the one proposed for the AI can be used to determine the level of confidence that usual intake is below the UL. For some nutrients, the UL applies only to intake from supplements, fortificants, or medications, whereas for other nutrients, total intake from all sources is considered.

Macronutrients with an AMDR

Because the AMDRs have both lower and upper boundaries, one would need to conduct two sets of assessments to determine the level of confidence that an individual's usual intake fell within the AMDR. The equation developed for use with the AI could be adapted to assess the level of confidence that usual intake was above the lower boundary, and the equation developed for use with the UL could be adapted to assess the level of confidence that usual intake was below the upper boundary. Intake data would be expressed as a percentage of total energy, and the standard deviations of within-person variability for percentage energy from carbohydrate, protein, fat, n-3 fatty acids, and n-6 fatty acids would need to be generated from large data sets.

Evaluating Energy Intake Using the EER

In most cases, it is not appropriate to use the EER to evaluate the adequacy of an individual's energy intake—an EER that has a high probability of being "adequate" for an individual (eg, an intake 2 SD above the mean) would have an equally high probability of leading to weight gain. Furthermore, energy intake is subject to underreporting (13,14). Unlike for other nutrients, for energy there is a valid, reliable, and accessible indicator of whether energy requirements are being met: stability or change in body weight.

Assessing Individual Diets Using the DRIs: An Example

A hypothetical example of a dietary assessment for a 74-year-old man is shown in Table 16.1. This individual reported 3 days of dietary data, and nutrient intake has been calculated for four nutrients (riboflavin, folate, calcium, and zinc). The appropriate statistical equations were used to determine the level of confidence that his usual intake meets his requirement (for nutrients with an EAR) or exceeds the AI, and is below the UL. Several points are apparent from this example:

- Although riboflavin intake was well above the EAR, and even above the RDA of 1.3 mg/d, because of day-to-day variation in intake, the level of confidence that his usual intake is adequate is less than 100%. A similar situation exists for zinc, where his intake equals the RDA of 11 mg.
- Folate intake is well below the EAR, and the confidence of adequacy is only 10%.
- Calcium does not have an EAR or RDA, but only an AI of 1,200 mg/d. The man's intake was 1,250 mg/d, above the AI, and therefore adequate if true long-term intake was accurately captured. However, because of the day-to-day variation in calcium intake, the confidence that intake is above the AI is about 60%.

TABLE 16.1   Evaluation of a 74-Year-Old Man's Diet Based on 3 Days of Intake

Nutrient	Mean Intake	EAR or AI	UL	Confidence That Intake Is Adequate (or > AI)	Confidence That Intake Is < UL
Riboflavin, mg	1.5	1.1 (EAR)	Not established	~80%	No UL
Folate, µg DFE	200	320 (EAR)	1,000 (synthetic folate only)	~10%	He does not use supplements and has little intake from fortified foods; confidence would be very high (> 98%).
Calcium, mg	1,250	1,200 (AI)	2,500	60% (reflects confidence that intake > AI, not confidence of adequacy)	Very high (> 98%)
Zinc, mg	11	9.4 (EAR)	40	63%	Very high (> 98%)

Abbreviations: AI, Adequate Intake; DFE, dietary folate equivalent; EAR, Estimated Average Requirement; UL, Tolerable Upper Intake Level.

A similar approach would be used to determine whether this man's intakes are below the UL. Of the nutrients in the illustration, ULs have been set for three: folate (from supplements and fortificants only), calcium, and zinc. Because none of his intakes is close to the corresponding UL, excessive intake is not a concern.

ASSESSING INTAKES OF POPULATIONS

When using the DRIs to assess the nutrient intakes of population groups, the goal is to estimate the *prevalence of inadequate intakes* (ie, the percentage of the group that has usual intakes that do not meet their requirements). Although it is seldom feasible to collect many days of dietary data for each individual within the group, it is still possible to estimate the distribution of usual intakes using a statistical adjustment. Once this distribution is obtained, the prevalence of inadequacy can often be calculated as the percentage of the group with intakes below the EAR. Thus, the EAR, rather than the RDA, is the DRI that is used in assessing the intakes of populations. The following sections of this chapter give the theoretical basis and the details of the appropriate calculations when assessing the intakes of groups.

Differences between Individuals and Groups: Adjusting Intake Distributions

The first step in assessing the intakes of a group is to obtain the distribution of usual intakes. However, the distribution of 1-day intakes is not the same as the distribution of usual intakes because the former includes both between-person variability (some people habitually have higher nutrient intakes than others) and within-person variability (on the day of the recall, a given person's intake might be much higher or much lower than his or her usual intake). As shown in Figure 16.3, the variance (or spread) of nutrient intakes in the distribution of 1-day intakes is much greater than the variance in a distribution of usual intakes that reflects only between-person variability. Such differences would usually be seen even if multiple days of intake data were available for each person. Because the prevalence of nutrient inadequacy in a group can often be estimated from the proportion of individuals in the group with intakes below the EAR for the nutrient, it is important to estimate the distribution correctly. As seen in Figure 16.3, the prevalence of inadequacy of vitamin C intakes (those below the EAR of 56 mg/d) for this group of women would be substantially overestimated if the distribution of one-day intakes was used.

Several approaches have been proposed to adjust daily intake distributions so that the estimated usual intake distributions reflect between-person variability and therefore have the correct variance. Three of the approaches are described here; all require at least 2 days of intake data for at least a representative subsample of the population group of interest so that the day-to-day variation in intakes can be calculated. Although it is possible to use estimates of day-to-day variation from a different, but similar, group, it is preferable to calculate this variability directly from the group being evaluated.

None of the methods can correct for under- or over-reporting of different foods (ie, for biases in the intake data). It is known that individuals tend to underreport energy and protein, although little is known about how precisely they report other nutrients (14). If daily intake of the nutrient, as measured by 24-hour recalls, is underreported, the estimated usual intake distributions obtained by any of the three

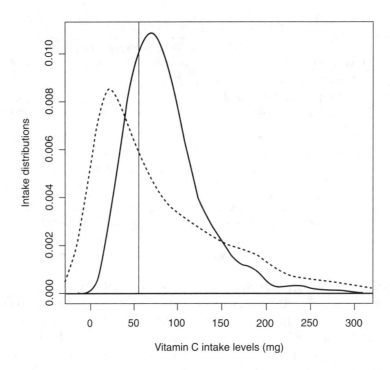

FIGURE 16.3 Estimated usual intake distribution for vitamin C for nonpregnant, nonlactating, nonsmoking women aged 19 to 30 years in the 1994–1996 Continuing Survey of Food Intakes by Individuals. The dashed curve represents 1 day of intake data; the solid curve uses the Iowa State University method. The vertical line denotes the EAR, which is 56 mg/day. The prevalence of inadequacy is estimated as the proportion of the population with intakes below the EAR.

methods described here will have the correct shape but will be shifted to the left by an amount that is roughly proportional to the underreporting (14).

Adjusting Intake Distributions with the National Research Council Method

The National Research Council (NRC) was the first to propose an approach to estimating usual intake distributions (15). The method proposed by the NRC consists of the following steps.

First, daily intakes are transformed by applying a transformation such as a square root or a logarithmic transformation to them. This is done so that in the transformed scale, daily intakes of a nutrient can be assumed to be normally distributed.

In the normal scale, you then obtain an estimate of the within-person variance and an estimate of the between-person variance. Formulas to compute the within- and the between-person variances have been published (16).

Once these variances have been determined, it is possible to calculate an adjustment factor that considers the relative size of the two types of variance and the number of days of intake available for each individual. The factor is then used to adjust the intake of the nutrient for each person in the group based on the difference between the person's mean intake and the group's mean intake. Thus, individual intakes that are farther from the group's mean will be adjusted more than those that are close to the mean, and the resulting adjusted intake distribution will be narrower, and will better approximate a distribution of usual intakes.

The last step in the method proposed by the NRC (15) consists of back-transforming the estimated usual intakes for each person to the original scale. For example, if the transformation into the normal scale was the square root of daily intake, the inverse or back-transformation to obtain usual intakes is the square. Further details on these calculations, and a sample SAS program, are found in Appendix E of *Dietary Reference Intakes: Applications in Dietary Planning* (8).

The NRC method requires that individual usual intakes be first estimated, and the distribution of usual nutrient intake is then obtained from these individual estimates. That means that when the group size is small (eg, fewer than 50 persons), individual percentiles of the usual nutrient intake distribution may be estimated with some inaccuracy.

Adjusting Intake Distributions with the Iowa State University Method and PC-SIDE

The second method described was proposed by Nusser et al (17) and is known as the Iowa State University (ISU) method. It was developed to overcome some of the limitations of the adjustment procedure that had been proposed by the NRC (15) and consists of almost the same steps. The differences are noted here, but the technical underpinnings of the ISU method are not described in detail. For the technical details, the reader is referred to references 16 and 17.

Perhaps the biggest difference between the NRC method and the ISU method resides in the transformation step into the normal scale. The comprehensive approach proposed by Nusser et al (17) to transform daily intakes is incorporated. Also, the ISU method does not require that individual usual intakes be estimated in order to calculate the usual nutrient intake distribution. The back-transformation proposed by Nusser et al (17) consists of the naive inverse transformation employed by the NRC method plus an adjustment factor. This additional adjustment factor decreases the bias that is inevitably introduced by the naive back-transformation step.

The ISU method can be implemented using either C-SIDE (18) or PC-SIDE, two programs available from ISU. C-SIDE was designed to run on Unix platforms, whereas PC-SIDE is a Windows-based program. Before implementing the steps in the ISU method, both programs permit preliminary adjustments of daily intakes to remove effects of day of week, survey method, survey sequence, and other similar effects chosen by the user. These adjusted intakes are then used to estimate usual intake distributions as described earlier. The output from the programs includes the mean, SD, skewness, and other attributes of the usual intake distribution in the group together with any percentiles requested by the user. By default, the programs produce a set of percentiles from the 1st to the 99th, together with their standard errors. The programs also provide the proportion of individuals in the group with usual intakes below a set of cutoffs provided by the user, and the corresponding standard errors. It is important to note that if survey weights are available for individuals in the group, both C-SIDE and PC-SIDE compute the correct, survey design–adjusted standard errors so resulting estimates are generalizable to the population from which the sample of individuals was drawn. Enhancements included in the newer PC-SIDE include graphing capabilities, the possibility of easily incorporating variance estimates obtained from an external data set (which permit, for example, adjusting distributions even when there is only 1 day of daily intake information available on each person in the group), the chance to compute individual estimated usual intakes, and a way to generate a sample of usual intakes of any size from the usual intake distribution.

Adjusting Intake Distributions with the Bias-Corrected NRC Method

A third approach for estimating usual nutrient intake distributions incorporates some of the features of the ISU method but retains the ease of implementation of the NRC method. This approach, called the bias-corrected NRC (BC-NRC) method, is essentially the same as the NRC method up to the back-transformation step. However, the back-transformation step is improved so that the resulting estimated usual nutrient intake distribution closely approaches the distribution that results from applying the ISU method. The adjustment to the naive back-transformation depends both on the power that was used to transform daily intakes into the normal scale and on the size of the day-to-day variance in intakes in the normal scale. The general methodology, including its theoretical justification, has been published (19).

Calculating the Prevalence of Adequacy/Inadequacy

Researchers and public health officials are often interested in estimating the prevalence of nutrient inadequacy in a group. This information may be required for a variety of reasons, including monitoring the health status of the group or designing interventions to improve intakes for a given group.

A person does not consume an adequate amount of a nutrient when his or her usual intake of the nutrient does not meet his or her requirement for the nutrient. Similarly, the proportion of persons in a group with inadequate intakes is given by the proportion whose intakes do not meet their requirements. In principle, therefore, it would seem that in order to estimate the prevalence of nutrient inadequacy in a group, you would need to know, for each person in the group, both his or her usual intake of the nutrient and his or her requirement for the nutrient. Because you never know each person's requirement for a nutrient, and because you can only estimate each person's usual intake, estimating prevalence seems, at first glance, to be an impossible task.

However, under some assumptions, and with knowledge about the distribution of requirements in the group and the distribution of usual intakes in the same group, it is possible to obtain an estimate of the prevalence of inadequacy. Two approaches that have been proposed to do so are called the *probability approach* and the *EAR cut-point method*.

The Probability Approach

The probability approach for estimating the prevalence of nutrient inadequacy was first proposed by the NRC (15). The idea is straightforward: Using the distribution of requirements in a group, first compute the risk curve, which indicates the risk of inadequacy at each usual intake level. For example, if the distribution of requirements in a group is normal with an EAR (mean) equal to 100 units of the nutrient and an SD equal to 10 units, then from a normal probability table we can read off the risks associated with any level of intake directly. Figure 16.2 shows that the risk associated with any level of usual intake depends on how far the intake is from the mean (ie, the number of SDs between the intake and the mean).

If estimates of usual intake for each person in the group have been obtained (eg, if the NRC method or the BC-NRC method has been used to estimate the usual intake distribution, or if the option of producing individual-level estimates was used with PC-SIDE), risk of inadequacy can be computed for each person in the group. The risks associated with each intake (illustrated in Figure 16.2) can be calculated using statistical software, such as the PROBNORM function in SAS. Using the mean (EAR) and the SD of the requirement, the program will calculate the probability (risk) of inadequacy for each person. The prevalence of inadequacy would then be computed as the simple average of the individual-level risks.

The probability approach for estimating the prevalence of inadequacy relies on few assumptions. The distribution of requirements does not need to be normal or symmetric. Usual intake distributions can have any shape, and in particular can be skewed. The method cannot be applied, however, when intakes and requirements are not independent, as is the case with energy. Finally, it is not possible to apply the probability approach for estimating prevalence of inadequacy unless the requirements distribution is known. By this we mean that you must at least know the mean and SD (or the CV) of requirements in the group and be willing to make some assumption regarding the shape of the distribution of requirements before you can

implement this method. Thus, the probability approach cannot be applied to nutrients for which an AI, but not an EAR, has been established.

The Cut-Point Approach

Beaton (20) and later Carriquiry (21) proposed a shortcut to the probability approach for estimating the prevalence of nutrient inadequacy in a group that is known as the EAR cut-point method. The method is simple to implement if an estimate of the usual intake distribution in the group is available.

Essentially, the EAR cut-point method consists of estimating the prevalence of nutrient inadequacy as the proportion of persons in a group whose usual intakes of the nutrient are below the EAR for the nutrient. The theoretical underpinnings of the EAR cut-point method can be found in Carriquiry (21), whereas *Dietary Reference Intakes: Applications in Dietary Assessment* (7) provides an extensive discussion of the approach, including a derivation of the method. It is crucial that intake distributions be adjusted to reflect usual intake before using the EAR cut-point method. For example, the prevalence of inadequacy of vitamin B-6 intakes for women was examined before and after adjustment (7). The prevalence estimate based on 1 day of intake was approximately 32%, whereas the prevalence computed using the adjusted distribution is approximately 18%. This example illustrates the importance of properly adjusting daily intakes for within-person variance.

The EAR cut-point method can be implemented in PC-SIDE or in C-SIDE by supplying the EAR as a cut-off value to the programs. The programs will then output the proportion of persons in the group with usual intakes below the cutoff value (the EAR), and will also produce a standard error for the proportion. If the NRC or the BC-NRC method is used to estimate the usual intake distribution in the group, an estimate of prevalence can be obtained by counting the number of persons with estimated usual intakes below the EAR and then dividing the resulting number by the total number of persons in the group.

Although the EAR cut-point method is relatively simple to implement, it relies on more assumptions than the probability approach does, and thus cannot be applied as widely. As in the case of the probability approach, the EAR cut-point method works well only when intakes and requirements can be assumed to be independent. Therefore, the EAR cut-point method cannot be used with energy. Further, the EAR cut-point method requires that the distribution of requirements be normal or at least symmetric around the EAR. As a consequence, it cannot be used to estimate the prevalence of iron inadequacy in a group (the probability approach, however, can be applied to iron intake). In addition, the EAR cut-point method works well when the variance of requirements is less than the variance of usual intakes, an assumption that is likely to hold for most nutrients, at least in free-living populations. On the positive side, it is not necessary to know the exact SD of the requirement (ie, the variance of the requirement) when applying the EAR cut-point method, as long as this variance is relatively small compared with the variance of intakes.

The EAR cut-point method provides a closer approximation to the prevalence than that estimated by the probability approach when the true prevalence of inadequacy in the population is neither too low nor too high. Clearly, as is the case with the probability approach, the method cannot be applied when an EAR for the nutrient has not been established.

Iron as a Special Case

The probability approach (rather than the EAR cut-point method) must be used for iron because the requirement distribution is known to be skewed. Percentiles of the requirement distributions for iron are available by age and sex group in *Dietary Reference Intakes for Vitamin A, Vitamin K, Arsenic, Boron, Chromium, Copper, Iodine, Iron, Manganese, Molybdenum, Nickel, Silicon, Vanadium, and Zinc*, Appendix Tables I-3 and I-4 (4).

Limitations of AIs

The approaches addressed thus far cannot be used for nutrients with an AI because the requirement distribution is not known for these nutrients. For this reason, the AI is of limited use in assessing the adequacy of nutrient intake for groups. Nevertheless, the following statements can be made:

- If a group has a mean or median intake at or above the AI, it is likely that there is a low prevalence of inadequate intakes. However, because the AIs are set using different criteria, one's confidence in this assessment varies and is high only if the AI represents the mean or median intake of an apparently healthy group of people. The derivation of each AI is described in the individual DRI reports (1–6).
- It is not possible to make any assumptions about the prevalence of inadequacy when the mean intake of

a group is below the AI: it is possible that the prevalence of inadequate intake could be extremely low. For example, pantothenic acid deficiency is virtually unknown in North America, so even among a group with a mean intake below the AI, it is probable that pantothenic acid status would be satisfactory.
- Although the percentage of individuals with usual intakes less than the AI can be estimated, this proportion *cannot* be interpreted as having "inadequate" intakes.

Calculating the Prevalence of Potentially Excessive Intakes

The prevalence of potentially excessive intakes is estimated by determining the proportion of the usual intake distribution that falls above the UL for the age and sex group. It is important to ensure that usual intakes of the appropriate form of the nutrient are being assessed. For example, for vitamin A, one would determine the prevalence of usual intake of preformed retinol above the UL, rather than of the total vitamin A intake from both retinol and carotenoids.

Assessing Energy and Macronutrients with the EER and AMDR

Energy

The mean energy intake of a group that is weight-stable (or, in the case of children or pregnant women, gaining weight at an appropriate rate) should be equal to the group's mean energy requirement. This means that the adequacy of a group's energy intake could theoretically be assessed by comparing the mean energy intake to the mean predicted EER for the group: a mean intake approximating the EER would reflect an adequate energy intake, whereas a mean intake below or above the mean EER would reflect an inadequate or excessive intake, respectively. However, as was also the case for individuals, it is more appropriate to assess the adequacy of a group's energy intake by assessing group members' relative weights, most commonly using body mass index.

Macronutrients

For each macronutrient with an AMDR, the proportion of the usual (adjusted) intake distribution that falls within the AMDR would be assessed as having intakes consistent with minimizing the risk of chronic disease and permitting adequate intakes of essential nutrients.

What to Do with Small Groups

A question that is often asked by practitioners is how many individuals constitute a "group." The answer, unfortunately, is not always 30 or 50 or 100. Rather, whether persons are just individuals or form a group depends in great measure on the objectives of the investigation. If the final objective is to provide nutrition counseling to each person, then even a sample of 1,000 persons should be treated as 1,000 individuals, and their nutrient intakes should be assessed as described in the section in this chapter on assessing intakes of individuals. If, however, the goal of the study is to characterize the intake distribution in a population or perhaps to estimate the prevalence of inadequate intakes of a nutrient, those persons should be treated as a group. However, it is still difficult to give a specific number because the appropriate sample size depends on several factors.

One important consideration is the number of persons in the group with at least one replicate observation. It may be better to have 100 individuals in the group when 2 days of daily intakes have been collected on each than to have a sample of 500 individuals for whom a replicate observation is available on only 25.

The size of the group will determine the precision with which percentiles of the usual nutrient intake distribution can be estimated. If only a rough estimate of the usual intake distribution is required, then a small group with 30 or 40 individuals might suffice. In this case, the practitioner might be able to reliably estimate the mean, variance, and skewness of the usual intake distribution, but will be surrendering the capability of estimating percentiles at the tails with any degree of accuracy.

Finally, those nutrients with large (and perhaps heterogeneous) day-to-day variance in intake require larger sample sizes for reliable estimation. It is "easier" (in terms of group size) to estimate the usual intake distribution of, for example, protein than to estimate the usual intake distribution of, for example, vitamin A.

A group of size 100, in which at least half of the individuals have a replicate observation, is probably almost always large enough to implement any of the three methods described earlier to estimate usual nutrient intake distributions. At the other end, a group with 30 or fewer individuals, even if all have a replicate intake observation, is probably too small to implement any of the three approaches.

Statistical Tests of Differences between Groups

Nutrition researchers often want to know whether the difference in nutrient intakes between two groups is significant. A relevant question that can be addressed using the DRIs is, do the two groups differ in the prevalence of dietary nutrient inadequacy (or adequacy)?

Without Adjustment for Covariates

The dietary adequacy of two groups can be compared with relatively simple statistical tests. For example, suppose the adequacy of intakes of vitamin C of adolescent boys is to be compared with that for adolescent girls. The first step would be to determine the prevalence of adequate vitamin C intakes for each group, after appropriately adjusting the intake distributions for the effect of day-to-day variation (as described earlier). Then, the prevalence of adequate intakes for each group would be estimated as the percentage of the group with intakes above the EAR. Finally, a statistical test, such as a t-test, can be used to determine whether the prevalence for boys is statistically different from that for girls.

With Adjustment for Covariates

When comparing the nutrient adequacy of two groups, it is often desirable to consider covariates, such as age, income, and education level that might affect nutrient intakes. For example, when comparing adolescent boys and girls, one might wish to adjust for their ages. One possible approach is to remove the effect of potentially confounding covariates from the intake observations before estimating prevalence. In this example, you would adjust daily intakes of boys and girls for age, and then estimate prevalence in the two sex groups. Nusser et al (17) and Dodd (18) have described examples of this type of adjustment.

In some circumstances, it may be of interest to estimate the association between a person-level covariate and adequacy. For example, you might be interested in comparing different food assistance packages by testing whether persons enrolled in the different programs have different probabilities of inadequacy. There are many possible approaches to carrying out this type of analysis. An approach relying on multivariate analysis has been proposed (7) but has not been widely used to date.

Heterogeneous Groups: Assessment Using the Ratio of Intake to EAR

In some cases, it might be of interest to estimate the prevalence of nutrient inadequacy in a group of persons whose ages and perhaps gender do not coincide with the groupings that were used to define the DRIs. For example, suppose that the group of interest consists of boys ages 7 years to 16 years and that we are interested in assessing prevalence of magnesium inadequacy in that group of boys. The EAR for boys ages 4 to 8 years has been set at 110 mg/d, the EAR for boys ages 9 to 13 years is 200 mg/d, and the EAR for boys ages 14 to 18 years is 340 mg/d. The easiest approach to estimating the prevalence of inadequacy in such groups is to "normalize" daily intakes to a common EAR, as follows:

1. Divide each daily intake of a person by the appropriate EAR for that person's group. In the preceding example, you would divide the intakes of each boy ages 7 or 8 years by 110, the daily intakes of the boys ages 9 to 13 years by 200, and the daily intakes of the boys ages 14, 15, or 16 years by 340.
2. Estimate the distribution of "normalized" usual intakes, using the daily intakes divided by the corresponding EARs.
3. Estimate the prevalence of nutrient inadequacy as the proportion of individuals in the group with "normalized" usual intakes below 1.0.

This approach was first proposed by Devaney et al (22) and is identical to the EAR cut-point method described earlier ("The Cut-Point Approach"), except that the cut-point here is not the EAR but the number 1.0.

Examples of Applications for Groups

Two recent large studies have utilized the foregoing approaches to evaluate the prevalence of inadequate intakes for large population groups (23,24). One is the description of the results of the dietary portion of the National Health and Nutrition Examination Survey 2001–2002 (23). The Food Surveys Research Group of the US Department of Agriculture has published a report that not only gives the means, standard errors, and percentiles of intake for 60 nutrients but also gives the prevalence of inadequacy (from food sources alone—ie, the contributions of supplements were not considered) for nutrients with an EAR. The prevalence of intakes above the UL is also reported. The intake distributions were adjusted using the C-SIDE program.

A second report was published by the Institute of Medicine as part of an evaluation for the food packages for the Special Supplemental Nutrition Program for Women, Infants and Children (WIC) (24). Usual intakes for age groups eligible for WIC were evaluated to determine the prevalences of inadequacy, and prevalences of potentially excessive intakes, for a variety of nutrients. Those nutrients for which intakes were particularly low (or high) were then targeted for change when revisions to the WIC food packages were recommended. The data were from the Continuing Survey of Food Intakes by Individuals, conducted in 1994–1996 and 1998, and the distributions were adjusted using the C-SIDE program.

REFERENCES

1. Institute of Medicine. *Dietary Reference Intakes for Calcium, Phosphorus, Magnesium, Vitamin D and Fluoride.* Washington, DC: National Academies Press; 1997.
2. Institute of Medicine. *Dietary Reference Intakes for Thiamin, Riboflavin, Niacin, Vitamin B6, Folate, Vitamin B12, Pantothenic Acid, Biotin, and Choline.* Washington, DC, National Academies Press; 1998
3. Institute of Medicine. *Dietary Reference Intakes for Vitamin C, Vitamin E, Selenium and Carotenoids.* Washington, DC: National Academies Press; 2000.
4. Institute of Medicine. *Dietary Reference Intakes for Vitamin A, Vitamin K, Arsenic, Boron, Chromium, Copper, Iodine, Iron, Manganese, Molybdenum, Nickel, Silicon, Vanadium, and Zinc.* Washington, DC: National Academies Press; 2000.
5. Institute of Medicine. *Dietary Reference Intakes for Water, Potassium, Sodium, Chloride, and Sulfate.* Washington, DC: National Academies Press; 2004.
6. Institute of Medicine. *Dietary Reference Intakes for Energy, Carbohydrate, Fiber, Fat, Fatty Acids, Cholesterol, Protein, and Amino Acids (Macronutrients).* Washington, DC: National Academies Press; 2002/2005.
7. Institute of Medicine. *Dietary Reference Intakes: Applications in Dietary Assessment.* Washington, DC: National Academies Press; 2000.
8. Institute of Medicine. *Dietary Reference Intakes: Applications in Dietary Planning.* Washington, DC: National Academies Press; 2003.

9. Institute of Medicine. *Dietary Reference Intakes: The Essential Guide to Nutrient Requirements.* Washington, DC: National Academies Press; 2006.

10. Murphy SP. Changes in dietary guidance: implications for food and nutrient databases. *J Food Comp Anal.* 2001;14:269–278.

11. Murphy SP. Dietary reference intakes for the U.S. and Canada: update on implications for nutrient databases. *J Food Comp Anal.* 2002;15:411–417.

12. US Department of Agriculture. *MyPyramid. Steps to a Healthier You.* Available at: http://www. MyPyramid.gov. Accessed December 28, 2006.

13. Black AE, Cole TJ. Biased over- or under-reporting is characteristic of individuals whether over time or by different assessment methods. *J Am Diet Assoc.* 2001;101:70–80.

14. Subar AF, Kipnis V, Troiano RP, Midthune D, Schoeller DA, Bingham S, Sharbaugh CO, Trabulsi J, Runswick S, Ballard-Barbash R, Sunshine J, Schatzkin A. Using intake biomarkers to evaluate the extent of dietary misreporting in a large sample of adults: the OPEN study. *Am J Epidemiol.* 2003;158:1–13.

15. National Research Council. *Nutrient Adequacy. Assessment Using Food Consumption Surveys.* Washington, DC: National Academies Press; 1986.

16. Carriquiry AL. Estimating the usual intake distributions of nutrients and foods. *J Nutr.* 2003; 133:601–608.

17. Nusser SM, Carriquiry AL, Dodd KW, Fuller WA. A semiparametric approach to estimating usual nutrient intake distributions. *J Am Stat Assoc.* 1996;91: 1440–1449.

18. Dodd KW. *A Technical Guide to C-SIDE (Software for Intake Distribution Estimation).* Technical Report 96-TR 32. Dietary Assessment Series Report 9. Ames, Iowa: Department of Statistics and Center for Agricultural and Rural Development, Iowa State University; 1996.

19. Dodd KW, Guenther PM, Freedman LS, Subar AF, Kipnis V, Midthune D, Tooze JA, Krebs-Smith SM. Statistical methods for estimating usual intake of nutrients and foods: a review of the theory. *J Am Diet Assoc.* 2006;106:1640–1650.

20. Beaton GH. Criteria of an adequate diet. In: Shils ME, Olson JA, Shike M, eds. *Modern Nutrition in Health and Disease.* 8th ed. Philadelphia, Pa: Lea and Febiger; 1994:1491–1505.

21. Carriquiry AL. Assessing the prevalence of nutrient inadequacy. *Public Health Nutr.* 1999;2:23–33.

22. Devaney B, Carriquiry AL, Camano G, Kim M. *Assessing the Nutrient Intakes of High-Risk Subgroups.* Princeton, NJ: Mathematica Policy Research Report; 2002. MPR # 8935-200.

23. Moshfegh A, Goldman J, Cleveland L. *What We Eat in America, NHANES 2001–2002: Usual Nutrient Intakes from Food Compared to Dietary Reference Intakes.* Washington, DC: Agricultural Research Service, US Department of Agriculture; 2006. Available at: http://www.ars.usda.gov/foodsurvey. Accessed December 28, 2006.

24. Institute of Medicine. *WIC Food Packages. Time for a Change.* Washington, DC: National Academies Press; 2006.

17

—⚉—

Biomarkers in Nutrition Research

Cheryl L. Rock, PhD, RD, and Johanna W. Lampe, PhD, RD

A *biomarker* is most simply defined as a biological marker or indicator. This term encompasses diverse biological markers that differ in conceptual basis, interpretation, and use. Some biomarkers of particular interest in nutrition research are biological markers or indicators of dietary intake, which are useful in the validation of dietary intake measures or as a way of quantifying exposure to various foods or dietary factors (1,2). Another type of biomarker reflects the biological or cellular activity of dietary constituents (or pharmacological agents), although the activity may not be the primary mechanism by which the constituent or agent affects the disease process (3). Finally, certain biological markers are useful in nutrition research as surrogate end point biomarkers: the molecular or cellular markers that reliably predict disease risk (4), typically reflecting a specific molecular mechanism that appears to play a role in the promotion or inhibition of the disease process. These biomarkers are cellular, biochemical, molecular, or genetic alterations by which a normal or abnormal biological process can be identified or monitored, and they are measurable in tissues, cells, or body fluids. As disease precursors, these alterations reflect inherited or acquired genetic susceptibility, metabolism of carcinogens, damage or repair of genetic material, abnormal cellular proliferation, or another aspect of the pathophysiological process of disease. In nutrition research on diseases that are preceded by a defined pathological lesion or morphological tissue changes, cytological or histological characteristics of tissues can also be used as biomarkers.

Using biomarkers in nutrition research involves measuring biological materials, such as blood or urine samples, surgical specimens, or tissue biopsies. Blood collection enables the measurement of several different components or circulating pools, such as serum (the fluid portion remaining when blood has been allowed to clot and the clotted material has been discarded), plasma (the fluid portion remaining when clotting has been inhibited and the formed elements, red and white blood cells, have been removed), and red and white blood cell fractions. Although blood and the various components of blood are liquid at ambient temperature, blood should be considered and described as tissue, as one would consider and describe peripheral or solid tissue, such as cervix or skin. The collection of urine allows the measurement of excretory products and urinary metabolites that may reflect dietary intake or be responsive to interventions. Urine collections used in nutrition research are typically timed collections (eg, urine collected over a 24-hour period).

Biological samples are considered biohazardous materials because exposure to microorganisms during the collection and processing of these samples presents a potential health risk. Health care facilities and research units or institutions at which biological materials are collected, handled, or measured must adhere to strict guidelines for the handling of the samples, and careful monitoring and documentation of these procedures is necessary. Universal precautions that must be employed to safely handle biological materials are described in detail elsewhere (5).

The factors being measured in biological samples are likely to be present in small concentrations and are usually vulnerable to degradation once outside their normal environment, the biological system. Thus, scrupulous collection and handling procedures are necessary to obtain quality data on biomarkers. Collection and processing procedures are nearly always specific to the biomarker of interest. Therefore, one should determine the measurements desired before sample collection and processing begins.

This chapter presents the basic concepts and key issues involved in the use of biomarkers in nutrition research. It addresses some areas of current interest, with an emphasis on clinical and community-based research applications. Most of the examples presented relate to cancer research; however, the basic principles and key issues are uniformly applicable to any aspect of nutrition research in which biomarkers enhance the ability to answer a research question.

BIOMARKERS: NUTRITION ASSESSMENT AND DIETARY INDICATORS

Biomarkers are used in nutrition assessment for several reasons. One basic reason is to provide biochemical data on nutritional status by generating objective evidence that enables the evaluation of dietary adequacy or the ranking of individuals on exposure to particular nutrients or dietary constituents. Biochemical or biological measurements may also be collected to provide objective evidence of a dietary pattern, such as overall fruit and vegetable consumption, or to validate dietary assessment instruments or self-reported dietary data. Another possible purpose for obtaining these biological measures is to establish the biological link between a nutritional factor and a physiological or biochemical process.

Biological Measures in Nutrition Assessment

Because of the well-known limitations in the use of self-reported dietary intake data, the development and increased availability of dietary biomarkers is of critical importance in research on nutrition and disease risk (6). Biochemical measures of nutrients or other dietary constituents can be a valuable component of nutrition assessment and monitoring. Overall, the usefulness of biochemical indicators of nutritional status or exposure is based on knowledge of the physiological and other determinants of the measure. For several micronutrients, the concentration of the nutrient in the circulating body pool (eg, serum) seems to be a reasonably accurate reflection of a nutrient's overall status. In contrast, the amounts of some micronutrients in the circulating pool may be homeostatically regulated when the storage pool is adequate, or they may be unrelated to intake and thus have little relationship to total body reserves or overall status. Figure 17.1 illustrates the relationships between various compartments or body pools that may be sampled in the measurement of biological indicators.

Knowledge of the influential nondietary factors is particularly important for accurate interpretation of the nutrient concentration in tissues. For example, tocopherols and carotenoids are transported in the circulation nonspecifically by the cholesterol-rich lipoproteins (7); therefore, higher concentrations of these lipoproteins are predictive of higher concentrations of the associated micronutrients in the circulation, independent of dietary intake or total body pool. Smoking and alcohol consumption need to be considered in the interpretation of serum and other tissue concentrations of several micronutrients, particularly compounds that may be subject to oxidation (eg, vitamin C, tocopherols, carotenoids, folate). Knowledge of the relationship between the indicator and the risk of nutrient depletion, in addition to knowledge of the responsiveness of the indicator to interventions or change, is also necessary (8). For some nutrients, such as calcium and zinc, specific sensitive biomarkers of diet or biochemical status have not yet been identified.

Practical considerations in the use of a biochemical measure of status include the ability to conveniently access the body compartment for measurement, the procedures necessary for collecting and processing the sample, subject burden, and the resources for laboratory analysis. For example, accurate quantification of vitamin C or folate in a circulating body pool requires processing steps that must be conducted immediately after blood collection to preserve the sample appropriately and prevent degradation that would result in an inaccurate measurement. These extra steps can add time and effort to the labor of blood processing, making these measurements more difficult to obtain in a large study in which resources are limited.

Technological challenges (and capabilities) are also often linked with biochemical measurement capabilities. For example, the development of high-performance liquid chromatography (HPLC) in the 1970s and improved detection technologies that are currently emerging allow the separation and quantification of many micronutrients and other dietary constituents that are present in very low concentrations in biological samples. The development of specialized cell separation tubes for blood collection now permits easier separation of the leukocyte pool, allowing

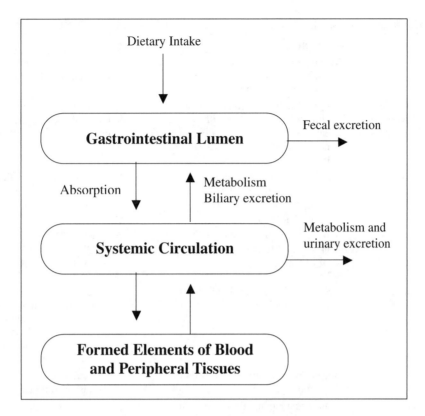

FIGURE 17.1   Relationships between compartments or body pools sampled in the measurement of biological indicators of nutritional status of exposure.

much easier measurement of micronutrients such as vitamin C and zinc in this pool.

Table 17.1 lists biochemical measures of micronutrients that may be useful in nutrition assessment or dietary intake monitoring. An important concept is that a static measurement (eg, a tissue concentration) is typically not as sensitive as a functional marker in the assessment of status. Also, a functional measure, such as the in vitro activity of an erythrocyte-derived enzyme with and without the micronutrient cofactor, will more directly reflect the body function. However, good functional measures are still lacking in many instances, and in some cases the extra labor involved in the procedures limits the ability to use the functional measures in large-scale studies. In-depth reviews of biological status indicators for the various micronutrients give more details (9–15).

Biomarkers as General Dietary Indicators

Monitoring overall dietary patterns or changes in patterns in response to dietary interventions presents additional challenges. The goal is to assess and monitor the intake of certain types of foods or food groups, rather than specific nutrients; therefore, these dietary indicators ideally should be distributed generally within certain types of foods.

Plasma carotenoids provide a good example of the use of biomarkers as a dietary indicator when the goal is to assess and monitor dietary patterns. Vegetables and fruits contribute the vast majority of carotenoids in the diet, and plasma carotenoid concentrations have been shown to be useful biomarkers of vegetable and fruit intakes in cross-sectional descriptive studies, controlled feeding studies, and clinical trials (16–18). The consistency of this relationship across diverse groups and various concurrent diet manipulations (with differences in amounts of dietary factors that could alter carotenoid bioavailability) is notable, although considerable interindividual variation in the degree of response is typically observed. Also, nondietary factors that are determinants of plasma carotenoid concentrations (eg, body mass, plasma cholesterol concentration) will influence the absolute concentration that is observed in response to dietary intake.

TABLE 17.1   Biological Indicators Useful in Nutrition Assessment or Dietary Intake Monitoring*

Nutrient	Characteristics	Comments†
Tocopherols, plasma or serum	Vary directly with vitamin E (tocopherol) intake; slow tissue turnover and relatively large body pool	Influenced by cholesterol-carrying lipoprotein levels and smoking status
Carotenoids, plasma or serum (beta carotene, alpha carotene, lycopene, lutein, β-cryptoxanthin, zeaxanthin)	Vary directly with carotenoid intakes, although relationship with specific calculated intakes is usually modest; generally reflects total vegetable and fruit intake	Influenced by cholesterol-carrying lipoprotein levels, smoking status, body mass, and alcohol intake
25-Hydroxyvitamin D, plasma or serum	Good biochemical indicator of overall vitamin D status (intake plus endogenously synthesized in response to sun exposure)	Effect of skin pigmentation can be great and should should be considered in interpretation of results; seasonal changes can also be notable
Vitamin C, plasma or serum	Varies directly with vitamin C intake only up to a threshold level	A preservative must be incorporated into the sample immediately after blood collection and separation, prior to preparing aliquots and freezing; influenced by smoking status
Folate, whole blood or erythrocyte	Acceptable biochemical indicator of long-term folate status	A preservative must be incorporated into the sample immediately after blood collection, prior to freezing; influenced by smoking status; hemoglobin measurement (which must be conducted with fresh blood) necessary for interpretation of results
Pyridoxal-5-phosphate, plasma	Acceptable biochemical indicator of vitamin B-6 status	Influenced by circulating albumin concentration, exercise, and protein and carbohydrate intakes
Vitamin B-12, plasma or serum	Not the first biochemical change that occurs in response to dietary vitamin B-12 deficiency, but a definitive indicator of prolonged vitamin B-12 inadequacy	Low concentrations can result from several physiological abnormalities (eg, pernicious anemia, atrophic gastritis, hypochlorhydria, and gastric surgery), in addition to dietary inadequacy
Ferritin, serum	Considered the most sensitive and specific indicator of overall iron status; increased concentration in response to excess iron uptake and body stores	Reference (normal) ranges vary depending on method used; increased in several physiological abnormalities in which normal uptake regulation is overridden (eg, hereditary hemochromatosis), resulting in excessive accumulation of iron
Fatty acids, serum phospholipid or plasma	Modified in response to inadequate fat intake and also in response to substantial changes in n-6 and n-3 fatty acid ingestion	Used as a biomarker of compliance with supplementation in fish oil supplement studies

*Good or acceptable biochemical indicators of status have been established for several nutrients not on this list, but the effort involved in the analytic procedures precludes their usefulness in large clinical or community-based nutrition research studies. Also not listed are several nutrients (eg, zinc, copper, and calcium) for which serum or plasma concentrations are easily measured and may contribute to the evaluation of status, but the values produced need substantial additional information for accurate interpretation.

†Includes additional measures that must be obtained concurrently for interpretation, as well as other factors crucial to the usefulness of values obtained. Notably, demographic characteristics (eg, age, gender, and racial/ethnic group) are also useful in the interpretation of all of these measures.

Source: Data are from Institute of Medicine, 1998, 2000, and 2002 (12–15).

Although vitamin C also is provided predominantly by fruits and vegetables in the diet, this measure is much less useful as a biomarker of this dietary pattern because the relationship between vitamin C intake and plasma concentration is linear only up to a certain threshold (14). The use of vitamin C supplements (which is common) often increases the intake level beyond the range in which linearity between intake and plasma concentration occurs, and it also obscures the relationship between food choices and tissue concentrations.

Lignans are a group of compounds that are present in high-fiber foods, particularly cereals and fruits (19). These compounds are not found in animal products and, like carotenoids, are useful markers of a plant-based diet (20).

Lignans exemplify how using dietary constituents as biomarkers requires an understanding of the metabolism of the compounds. Lignans in plant foods are altered by intestinal microflora; therefore, the specific compounds monitored in plasma or urine are actually bacterial metabolites. Generally, enterolactone and enterodiol are measured. Because of this bacterial conversion, lignan concentrations in urine or plasma in response to a similar dietary dose will vary significantly among individuals. In addition, nondietary factors (eg, orally administered antibiotics) will reduce enterolactone and enterodiol production (21).

As another example, the fatty acid composition of membrane phospholipids is in part determined by the n-6 and n-3 fatty acid composition of the diet. Thus, the fatty acid pattern of serum phospholipids or plasma aliquots has been used as a biomarker of compliance with n-3 fatty acid supplementation in clinical trials (22,23). Although enzyme selectivities and other physiological factors are also important determinants of the fatty acid composition of phospholipids, a diet high in n-3 polyunsaturated fats will result in increased amounts of eicosapentaeneoic and docosahexaenoic acids in circulating tissue pools.

Specific fatty acids can be associated with certain types of foods. Pentadecanoic acid (15:0) and heptadecanoic acid (17:0) are fatty acids produced by bacteria in the rumen of ruminants. These fatty acids are not synthesized by humans; therefore, their presence in human biological samples can be indicative of dietary exposure to milk fat. Proportions of 15:0 and 17:0 in adipose tissue and concentrations of 15:0 in serum have been found to correlate with milk fat intake in men and women (24,25).

Biomarkers of Phytochemical Intakes

Although not recognized as essential for life, numerous dietary components—particularly of plant origin—have demonstrated biological activity and are thought to play an important role in the prevention of chronic disease. These phytochemicals are absorbed, often metabolized in the intestinal epithelium and liver, and excreted; thus, the metabolites can be monitored in urine, serum, or plasma.

Dietary exposure to flavonoids and other polyphenols can be monitored in urine or plasma (26). The isoflavones daidzein and genistein are highly concentrated in soybeans and soy products. Much remains to be learned about their metabolism in human beings (27,28). These compounds can be measured in urine and plasma by immunoassay or HPLC with diode array, coulometric array detection, or mass spectrometry. Urinary isoflavone excretion is associated strongly and directly with soy protein intake under controlled dietary conditions (29). In observational studies of populations that generally consume soy, soy food intake and urinary isoflavonoid excretion also are positively correlated (30–32). Because the plasma half-lives of the isoflavones genistein and daidzein are short (6 to 8 hours) (33), intermittent soy consumption may be severely underestimated or overestimated if isoflavone exposure is monitored in plasma or spot urine specimens. The metabolism of isoflavones is also inextricably linked to the health of colonic bacterial populations, and plasma and urinary levels may be influenced by the effects of diet and drugs on the colonic environment.

Other compounds that have been used as biomarkers of dietary intake, such as sulforaphane and other isothiocyanates in cruciferous vegetables, have been of interest because of putative chemopreventive effects. Dithiocarbamates (metabolites of isothiocyanates) can be quantified in urine, following extraction and measurement by HPLC, and provide an estimate of cruciferous vegetable exposure (34).

Biomarkers of Energy Intake

To date, there are few biological measures that objectively monitor energy intake, and collecting those measures that are available is either cumbersome in free-living populations, expensive, or both. Under steady-state conditions, indirect calorimetry provides an estimate of energy expenditure and some insight about intake. Indirect calorimetry estimates the rate of oxidation or energy expenditure from the rate of oxygen consumption (Vo_2) and the rate of carbon dioxide production (Vco_2). This technique is relatively inexpensive and portable, although some subject effort is required. These traits lend the technique to clinical applications (35).

The chief premise behind indirect calorimetry is that Vo_2 and energy metabolism are proportional. All energy-dependent metabolic processes depend on energy liberated from adenosine triphosphate (ATP) hydrolysis. The ATP utilization rate dictates substrate oxidation (36). Total body oxygen storage is very low compared with oxygen consumption. Given the first law of thermodynamics, energy from oxidative metabolism is converted to heat and work. If the subject is resting in a thermoneutral environment, heat released by oxidation and measurable by indirect calorimetry is equal to heat lost to the environment and measurable by direct calorimetry.

Indirect calorimetry produces two types of information: resting energy expenditure (REE) and the respiratory quotient (RQ). The REE estimates fasting energy expenditure in an awake, resting person and is approximately 10% greater than basal energy requirements. The REE correlates with lean body mass (37). The RQ is the ratio of carbon dioxide produced to oxygen consumed (V_{CO_2}/V_{O_2}) and indicates contributions from each substrate. An RQ of 1.0 suggests 100% glucose utilization, whereas an RQ of 0.7 corresponds to oxidation of 100% fat. Protein utilization results in an RQ near 0.8. However, urinary nitrogen excretion is used to determine what portions of the V_{CO_2} and V_{O_2} are contributed by protein utilization. Exclusion of the effects of protein produces the nonprotein respiratory quotient (NPRQ). Thus, for NPRQs between 0.7 and 1.0, proportions of fat and carbohydrate oxidation can be identified (38,39). Note that the RQ represents substrate oxidation, which may or may not equal exogenous macronutrient intake. In using the RQ to determine substrate oxidation, two assumptions are made: (a) the participant is in a metabolically steady-state condition, and (b) all expired carbon dioxide measured represents substrate oxidation (35).

Various types of equipment are used in indirect calorimetry, with both open- and closed-circuit systems available. The closed-circuit system allows the participant to breathe from a pure-oxygen reservoir and calculates oxygen consumption from disappearance data. The more sophisticated open-circuit system, in which subjects breathe room air and detectors calculate the difference between gases inhaled and those exhaled, is more widely available in the United States. The apparatus used to collect respiratory gases may take the form of a tentlike canopy, a fitted face mask, or a mouthpiece with nose clips that directs all inhalation and expiration through the mouth. The canopy system may be best suited to clinical and research applications because it is comfortable and requires no fitting (40), whereas the face mask system has been tested in healthy adults restricted to bed (41). Despite validation in healthy participants, indirect calorimetry is generally applied to critically ill individuals, due to the availability of instruments and its greater precision for prescribing nutrition support in those instances.

The limitations of indirect calorimetry in the community-based setting are substantial. If the REE is measured, participants must provide accurate typical-activity records for adjustment of the results to total energy expenditure. Such records introduce reporting bias and general inaccuracy. Indirect calorimetry can be used to measure total energy expenditure, but long data collection periods are necessary to control error associated with extrapolation, and it is likely that a participant's usual activity would be hindered by even the most mobile system. Even measuring energy expenditure for a full day would leave day-to-day variability unacknowledged (42).

Energy expenditure can also be measured using a doubly labeled water (DLW) technique (43). This method uses nonradioactive isotopes of hydrogen (^2H) and oxygen (^{18}O) to measure free-living total energy expenditure by monitoring urinary isotope excretion. Within the calorimeter environment, energy expenditures determined by room calorimetry, indirect calorimetry, and DLW are not significantly different; however, in free-living subjects, DLW energy expenditures are found to be 13% to 15% higher than energy expenditures from other methods (42). The DLW method has the distinct advantage of allowing subjects to go about their usual activities, with energy expenditure calculated after a study period of 7 to 14 days. Unfortunately, the ^{18}O isotope required to conduct DLW studies is expensive and often in short supply. Although DLW studies are suited to nutrition research aimed at quantifying total energy expenditure for specific groups, the cost for large samples limits their broad use.

One of the most important and relevant uses of DLW methodology in community-based nutrition research has been to produce an estimate of energy requirements, which can then be compared with the reported energy intakes obtained from various dietary assessment methodologies (44). Underreporting is a recognized problem in dietary assessment (see Chapter 14), and DLW may be used to validate (or calibrate) assessment methods such as dietary recalls and food frequency questionnaires. Although the data produced are objective and the approach is less disruptive to normal life activities than indirect calorimetry, measurement error does occur and can be compounded by estimates of various physiological factors and assumptions that are used in the calculations. Furthermore, one of the most notable findings from the use of DLW methodology is that total daily energy expenditure varies dramatically among healthy, free-living human beings (45).

BIOMARKERS OF BIOCHEMICAL ACTIVITY AND SURROGATE END POINT BIOMARKERS

If a nutritional factor or dietary constituent has a known biochemical activity, measuring markers of that activity can be useful. One purpose is to identify the dosage or concentration necessary to achieve a clinically meaningful effect. Often, a biochemical activity may have been linked to the pathogenesis of disease, but the biomarker cannot be considered a surrogate end point biomarker unless its modulation has been shown to be indicative of progression or reversal of the disease process. In an intervention trial, the use of surrogate end point biomarkers (rather than the diagnosis of disease) requires substantially less time and fewer resources in the evaluation of efforts aimed at reducing risk for chronic diseases such as cancer, cardiovascular disease, and osteoporosis. To date, few markers have been established as true surrogate end point biomarkers.

Biomarkers of Oxidative Stress

Biochemical indicators of oxidative stress illustrate a type of biomarker that reflects a biological activity. Oxidative stress has been suggested to play a role in the pathophysiological disease process in cancer, atherosclerotic cardiovascular disease, and many other acute and chronic conditions (46), although the specific relationship with the disease process remains to be established in most instances. Cellular damage caused by reactive oxygen species—which are generated from cellular respiration, co-oxidation during metabolism, and the activity of phagocytic cells of the immune system—is controlled by antioxidant defense mechanisms that involve several micronutrients. Oxidative stress describes the condition of oxidative damage that results when the balance between free-radical generation and antioxidant defenses is unfavorable. Direct measurement of active oxygen and related species in biological samples is very challenging, mainly because these compounds have very short half-lives. Thus, the oxidative stress biomarkers used in studies of human beings are typically adducts or end products reflecting reactions that have occurred between free radicals and compounds such as lipids, proteins, carbohydrates, DNA, and other molecules that are potential targets (47).

One frequently described assay used as an oxidative stress biomarker is the thiobarbituric acid reactive substances assay. This assay basically quantifies a product of malondialdehyde, which presumably reflects lipid hydroperoxides in the sample. However, this assay has some serious limitations in specificity, and the product measured cannot be interpreted as directly reflecting lipid peroxidation in vivo (47). Direct measurement of malondialdehyde in biological samples using HPLC has also been examined as an alternative approach, although the specificity of the more direct HPLC measurement has also not been established to the level desired.

Breath pentane is another biomarker of oxidative stress that has been used in studies of human beings (48).

The approach basically involves collecting exhaled air for the measurement of the products of peroxidation of unsaturated fatty acids, a portion of which are volatile and released in the breath, using gas chromatography (GC) methods. However, the measurement methodologies vary and are not always reliable; standardization of the procedure and knowledge of various influencing factors are needed to improve the usefulness of this approach (47).

Another biomarker of oxidative stress involves the measurement of urinary 8-hydroxydeoxyguanosine (8OHdG) using HPLC and electrochemical detection (3,49). The 8-hydroxylation of the guanine base is a frequent type of oxidative DNA damage, and 8OHdG is subsequently excreted without further metabolism in the urine after repair in vivo by exonucleases. In previous studies, certain demographic factors and physiological characteristics, such as gender and body mass (50), have been observed to influence urinary 8OHdG concentration, so these factors may need to be considered in interpretation. Urinary 8OHdG is increased in association with conditions known to be characterized by increased oxidative stress, such as smoking, whole body irradiation, and cytotoxic chemotherapy (49–51). Prostaglandin-like compounds produced by nonenzymatic free radical–catalyzed peroxidation of arachidonic acid, termed F_2-isoprostanes, are currently of great interest as useful biomarkers of oxidative damage. Specific gas chromatography–mass spectrometry (GC-MS) assays for the measurement of some of these compounds, such as $iPF_2\alpha$-III (also called 8-iso-$PGPF_2\alpha$) and $iPF_2\alpha$-VI, have been developed and used to quantify them in urine and blood samples. These biomarkers have been shown to be less variable than 8OHdG (52), and elevated levels have been observed in plasma and urine samples from subjects under a wide variety of conditions of enhanced oxidative stress (53–55).

Another approach to measuring DNA oxidative damage that appears to be useful in human nutrition research is the measurement of 5-hydroxymethyluracil levels in DNA in blood. 5-Hydroxymethyluracil, produced when DNA is exposed to oxidants, is relatively stable compared with other oxidation products and can be quantified with GC-MS (56). In a small cross-sectional study, 5-hydroxymethyluracil concentration was observed to be inversely associated with cooked vegetable intakes and directly related to beef and pork intakes in the diets of women enrolled in a low-fat diet intervention trial (57).

Oxidative damage to low-density lipoproteins (LDL) has been specifically linked to atherogenesis, and in an application of this biological activity, LDL oxidation measured ex vivo has been used in clinical studies as a biomarker of oxidative stress (58). Basically, this process involves isolating the LDL fraction from a blood sample, exposing this fraction to oxidants such as Cu^{2+}, and measuring the lag time before oxidation. Although this biomarker might appear to be specific to cardiovascular disease risk, results from this assay have not yet been specifically linked with risk for disease, so results should be interpreted as simply another approach to the assessment of oxidative stress (47). Also, a variety of specific methodologies are used across laboratories, and the lack of standardization in the approaches in use constrains the ability to make comparisons across studies.

Several other approaches to measuring biomarkers of oxidative stress have been proposed and are under study. Handelman and Pryor provide a useful review of this topic (47).

Biomarkers of Metabolizing Enzyme Activity

Understanding how diet influences enzyme systems is important in developing strategies for disease prevention and treatment. For example, dietary modulation of enzymes involved in carcinogen metabolism may be important in reducing cancer risk. Dietary intervention that reduces the expression of rate-limiting enzymes in cholesterol synthesis may alter cardiovascular disease risk. Direct measurement of enzyme expression or activity in human studies is a challenge, however. Often the enzymes of interest are located primarily in tissues that are not readily accessible (eg, liver, intestine, lung).

One approach to meeting this challenge is to measure the enzymes in more accessible tissue; for example, enzymes that are present in high levels in the liver can often be measured in plasma or serum as a result of normal hepatocyte turnover. Enzyme activity of glutathione-S-transferase (GST), a biotransformation enzyme important in carcinogen detoxification, can be measured spectrophotometrically in serum (59), or concentrations of the enzyme itself can be determined in serum by immunoassay (60). Serum concentration of the GST isoenzyme GST-α has been shown to increase when cruciferous vegetables are added to the diet (60). A limitation of using serum measures of a hepatic enzyme is that the liver function is assumed to be normal. Thus, it is important to include other measures of liver function in the data collection to verify that there is no underlying hepatic disease that could result in spurious GST values. Additionally, some enzymes are present in isoforms in various tissues. GST-μ, another GST isoenzyme, is present in lymphocytes as well as in liver; therefore, for this isoenzyme, GST activity or protein concentration can be measured in cells extracted from blood samples.

In another approach, enzyme activity can be measured using a drug probe. Many of the same xenobiotic enzymes that metabolize carcinogens also are induced by, and metabolize, commonly used drugs. The metabolites of these drugs can be monitored in serum, plasma, or urine and used to determine enzyme activities. Caffeine metabolites measured in urine samples collected 4 hours after consumption of 500 mg of caffeine allow determination of cytochrome P-450 1A2, N-acetyltransferase, and xanthine oxidase activities (61). Similarly, acetaminophen (paracetamol) is used to measure UDP-glucuronosyltransferase and sulfotransferase activities (62). Drugs can be administered as probes following a nutrition intervention to determine the degree of change in enzyme activity in response to diet (63,64).

Biomarkers Reflecting Other Biochemical Activities

The specificity of the biochemical activities of the dietary constituent of interest means that a wide variety of markers that are indicators of biological activity may be useful in nutrition research. For example, folate is an essential micronutrient in DNA methylation. The degree of methylation in DNA extracted from tissue samples has been used in human studies as a biomarker of folate function (65). A possible link to disease process is that DNA hypomethylation is known to be an early step in colon carcinogenesis (66). However, it is possible that the effect of dietary folate is modified by other, influencing factors, such as dietary methyl donors and certain genetic polymorphisms (67), and specific areas of hypermethylation of genes have also been identified in colon carcinogenesis (66). Thus, the degree of DNA methylation has been examined as a possible biomarker of folate biochemical activity, but direct links between dietary folate, methylation abnormalities, and human colon carcinogenesis have not yet been established.

Measurement of arachidonic acid metabolism, which involves measuring the concentration of prostaglandins, leukotrienes (metabolic products), or enzymes in the eicosanoid metabolic pathway (cyclooxygenase), provides another example. Altered arachidonic acid metabolism is among the biochemical activities of nonsteroidal anti-inflammatory agents and may also be influenced by antioxidant micronutrients, such as vitamin E (68), and quantitative changes in these products or enzymes in tissues serve as biomarkers of this activity (69). As with the link between disease process and DNA hypomethylation, a reasonable amount of biological evidence suggests some role for this enzymatic pathway in colon carcinogenesis (70); however, the overall relationship with the disease process is still under investigation.

Cellular Biomarkers

Cellular markers of proliferation, differentiation, and apoptosis (programmed cell death) can be useful as biomarkers in research focused on nutritional factors and cancer, although the measured effect is more of a general indicator of an altered cell growth regulation effect than a measure of specific biochemical activity.

As a general rule, increased proliferation of undifferentiated cells is one aspect or characteristic of carcinogenesis, and in colon cancer this relationship has been well established. For example, cell proliferation occurs at the base of the colonic crypts, and as cells migrate from the crypts to the luminal surface, they become increasingly differentiated and mature and lose their proliferative capabilities (71). The shift in which the proliferative zone extends to the surface, so that cells on the luminal surface retain proliferative capabilities and are immature and underdifferentiated, may be considered a field defect that sets the stage for current and future neoplastic changes (72–74). With increased sensitivity in immunohistochemical techniques, proteins present in proliferating cells (eg, proliferating cell nuclear antigen [PCNA] and Ki67) now are used to quantify proliferative activity in tissue specimens. Labeling indexes have been used to quantify the proliferative activity in colonic mucosal samples from human subjects (73) and have been used successfully as end points in several nutrition intervention studies to prevent colon cancer (74). These indexes are being further refined by staining for proteins present during apoptosis (eg, Bax, Bcl-2) and in differentiated cells to provide a more complete picture of cell dynamics.

In cases where specific genetic mutations may be indicative of disease risk or progression, or may be modified by nutritional factors, genetic markers can also be useful biomarkers. Various molecular techniques have been developed to help characterize genetic variation. Genetic factors are important considerations in nutrition research for several reasons. First, it is increasingly evident that genetic polymorphisms (ie, variations in DNA coding sequences of genes) may contribute substantially to differences in the response to environmental and dietary exposures (75), and analysis by subgroup according to differences in genetic susceptibility permits a more refined

evaluation and interpretation of the observed effect of nutrition interventions and associations. For example, genetic variations in the expression of the xenobiotic metabolizing enzymes may mediate the potentially carcinogenic effect of heterocyclic amines (obtained from meat cooked at high temperatures) (76). Also, results from laboratory animal studies suggest that dietary modifications can cause noncoding alterations in DNA that affect DNA stability and gene expression (77). Thus, measuring genetic variation and change may be considered an approach to demonstrating a biological link between dietary factors and disease risk.

With the development of more sensitive, high-throughput analytic laboratory instruments and greater computing capacity, diet effects can now be measured using biomarker profiling techniques that rely on monitoring thousands of components simultaneously, rather than focusing on one or two measures. Expression of tens of thousands of genes can be monitored in a single tissue sample using high-throughput technologies such as cDNA microarrays. Similarly, in the areas of proteomics and metabolomics, the quantity and types of multiple proteins and other, smaller-molecular-weight compounds in biological samples and tissues are measured to provide a profile or fingerprint (78,79). These types of markers are currently under study because they could illuminate the effects of dietary intakes on metabolic processes that relate to disease risk and progression (78).

These molecular approaches show increasing potential and usefulness in clinical and community-based nutrition research because of improved molecular methodologies, and they are feasible if appropriate tissue samples and technologies are available. With microdissection and immunohistochemical analysis using small tissue specimens, cellular and molecular markers can be used to monitor the effects of dietary modifications on the altered physiological processes that may be present even prior to the diagnosis of clinical disease.

In colon cancer, several genetic alterations in the course of disease progression have been well defined and so can serve as biomarkers of carcinogenesis (70). In contrast, none of the currently available molecular biomarkers suggested for breast cancer has been accepted as a surrogate end point biomarker, although a number of cellular growth factors, markers of disordered cell signaling, markers of oncogene overexpression, and cell cycle markers are currently under study in clinical trials. Several types of biomarkers of biochemical activity or genetic alterations are currently considered promising or are in use in cancer prevention studies (74,80).

Biomarkers Involving Physiological Characteristics and Pathological Lesions

In some instances, physiological characteristics have been used as biomarkers of disease and thus may be useful in measuring the effects of nutrition interventions. Although not a biological measurement, increased breast density, which can be measured noninvasively through imaging techniques, has been used as a type of biological marker in nutrition research. Increased breast density is associated with increased breast cancer risk (81), and some studies have suggested that it may be reversible and responsive to changes in the hormonal milieu. In one clinical trial, reduced breast density was observed in association with a low-fat diet intervention (82).

Precursor lesions are known to occur in carcinogenesis, and when the lesions may be reversible, cytological and histological examination of tissues provides a useful approach to using biomarkers as a measure of efficacy of nutrition intervention. One of the best examples occurs in cervical carcinogenesis, which is characterized as a progression from cervical dysplasia to carcinoma in situ and, finally, to invasive cancer (80). In several clinical trials, the effect of nutrient supplements or dietary modification on cervical cancer risk has been monitored with serial examination of cervical tissue lesions in human subjects (83), with reversal of the lesion being the positive outcome desired. Another example of this type of approach is found in research studies on colon cancer prevention. The earliest lesion of colonic neoplasia is the polyp, and it is generally accepted that most cancers of the colon are preceded by an adenomatous polyp (71). The occurrence of polyps basically indicates an early abnormal tissue characteristic that occurs in the continuum of colon carcinogenesis. The major outcome under study in numerous colon cancer prevention trials using various nutrition interventions has been recurrence of polyps in subjects who have had them removed (84–87). A reduced rate of recurrence of these adenomatous polyps, indicating that the tissue abnormality is being corrected, would theoretically provide biological evidence suggesting a reduction in risk for colon cancer.

BIOMARKERS IN NUTRITION RESEARCH: PRACTICAL CONSIDERATIONS

Practical considerations in the use of biomarkers in nutrition research involve all the details and issues that must be addressed for the appropriate collection, handling, processing, and storage of biological samples. Before selecting the biomarkers to examine, the nutrition researcher must know what is reflected in the pool or compartment to be measured, and the various factors that might influence the interpretation of results.

Collection of Blood and Other Tissues

Although the risk involved in blood collection may be minimal, it is an invasive procedure, and subjects must be informed of all inherent risks. Trained and certified personnel must be responsible for the procedure. There are some variations in the requirements for training and certification across institutions, but a key factor to consider for subject comfort is the experience of the individual responsible for the phlebotomy and how frequently the individual performs the procedure. Experienced phlebotomists should have the knowledge and skills to cope with the challenges that can arise. For example, collecting blood from even a healthy adult can be very difficult if the subject is somewhat dehydrated. Most research studies specify a protocol (eg, how many attempts are to be made before allowing another phlebotomist to try or before a subject may be dismissed to return for another attempt at later time). When blood collections are very frequent in a very short period (say, 12 hours), an indwelling catheter enabling access without repeated venipuncture may be necessary.

The selection of the collection tube for blood collection is determined by the compartment to be measured (eg, serum, plasma, erythrocytes, or leukocytes). Tubes used for plasma collection contain various anticlotting chemicals. These chemicals may have either positive or negative effects on the constituents being measured, so the specific tube choice will be driven by the effect on the measurement. If white blood cells are needed to extract cellular constituents such as DNA, the heterogeneous "buffy coat" mixture of blood cells (the whitish layer of cells between the red blood cells and the plasma following centrifugation) is an appropriate fraction to remove and collect. If the leukocyte compartment is specifically desired, specialized cell separation tubes must be used. For many constituents of interest, especially constituents subject to oxidation by light exposure, the tube with collected blood may need to be protected from light immediately, using an amber sample bag or aluminum foil, during the processing steps when the tube is not in the centrifuge. If the erythrocyte pool is to be measured, the red blood cells remaining after the plasma has been removed typically need to be washed; this washing involves twice adding an equal volume of normal saline, centrifuging, and discarding the supernatant so that the plasma material adhering to the red blood cells is rinsed away.

The processing of the blood samples is often quite specific to the constituent to be measured. For example, extra processing steps to preserve the constituent may need to be performed immediately after the blood has been collected and before the sample is placed in cryovials for storage or analysis. Additional considerations relevant to blood sample collection involve nonfasting vs fasting samples (and how many hours postprandial are considered acceptable) and timing of the sample collection (which would be important if diurnal variations were known to occur). In planning the study design and protocol, seasonal effects on the biochemical measurement may need to be considered.

When solid tissue samples are examined or measured, the exact tissue type needs to be considered prior to collection and processing, even if normal tissue is the target. For example, a surgical biopsy sample of normal tissue from either breast or fat depots will typically include connective tissue, adipose tissue, and glandular tissue (if the sample is from the breast). Different distributions of micronutrients or other dietary constituents are usually present in these tissue types, so dissection and examination is necessary prior to static measurements of the sample. Before storage, solid tissue samples must be rinsed of blood with normal saline, and depending on the measurement to be made, a chemical preservative may need to be added before storage. If the biopsy sample is a surgical sample of a possible or known lesion, the first priority is sufficient tissue for histopathological examination for diagnosis and medical care; tissue for research purposes is considered a lower priority.

Urine Collection

Urine is an easily accessible pool for measurement of numerous biomarkers; however, urinary markers of diet generally reflect recent intake. Timing and length of collection, as well as handling and processing methods, are determined on the basis of the biomarkers being measured. Collections may vary from a "spot urine" (a convenience sample, usually less than 100 mL, collected during a clinic visit) to days of complete urine collection (24- or 72-hour urine collections). Additional collection strategies include overnight collection (approximately a 10-hour collection) or first-voided fasting morning collection (collected upon waking in the morning). A first-voided morning specimen is usually the most concentrated sample of the day and is affected least by recent dietary intake.

It is difficult to collect 24- and 72-hour urine samples in free-living individuals. The collection procedure involves significant participant burden and can impair participant recruitment, retention, and compliance. Nonetheless, these total urine collections are often necessary to provide a useful measure of dietary exposure. Participants must be provided with an adequate supply of easy-to-use, leak-proof collection containers; clear instructions for collection, labeling, and handling; and, if necessary, commode specimen systems and transport coolers. Urine collection containers may need to be pretreated with additives. For example, some biomarkers that undergo oxidation require the use of collection containers that have ascorbic acid (1 g per 1-liter bottle) added to them before collection. To monitor the completeness of a 24-hour collection, *para*-aminobenzoic acid (PABA) can be used. This compound is ingested with meals (80 mg, three times per day) and is rapidly and completely excreted in the urine (88). A urine collection containing less than 85% of the administered dose of PABA is considered incomplete.

For population studies, spot, overnight, and first-voided urine collections are more feasible than 24-hour collections. These collections are especially useful when a ratio of markers is to be determined (eg, drug metabolites to parent drug or one hormone metabolite to another). Urinary excretion of a marker also can be normalized to the creatinine content of the sample (milligrams of the marker per milligram of creatinine) to correct for diurnal variation and urine volume.

Fecal Collection

Fecal collection is less frequently used than urine and blood collection in nutrition research, in part because of the logistics of, and aversion to, collection. However, absorption studies, as well as dietary interventions with outcomes related to gut function, bile acid metabolism, and colonic microbial changes, rely on fecal samples for biomarkers. As with urine collections, minimizing participant burden is an important consideration for fecal collections. This includes devising the least offensive method of sample collection that meets the study's needs, identifying the shortest time over which samples need to be collected, and carefully arranging sample storage and transport.

Sample handling is specific to the measurements planned. Participants may need to be provided with various additives to apply directly to the specimen at the time of collection. Often, samples must be frozen immediately to prevent continued microbial degradation of dietary fiber and to preserve the bacterial community structure. Samples used for microbiological cultures may need to be collected with minimal exposure to air and processed immediately to minimize alterations in microbial populations. A careful understanding of the biology involved and testing of the collection protocol by the researchers is necessary to ensure that the samples are collected appropriately for the biomarker under investigation.

General Considerations

Unless the biological measurement is conducted immediately after sample collection, storage issues must be considered. Thawing and refreezing may promote degradation of the constituents; therefore, it is usually best to divide the sample into several aliquots for storage so that only portions of the material collected are removed for analysis at any one time. Regular laboratory refrigeration (eg, a refrigerated centrifuge) is typically at a temperature of 4° Celsius, and biological samples nearly always must be stored at −20° Celsius—or preferably at −70° Celsius to −80° Celsius—for best preservation. The ultra-low-temperature freezers necessary for better preservation have an additional compressor unit, so they are considerably more expensive. Additionally, storage in liquid nitrogen is necessary for some types of cellular samples. Stability of the biological markers to be measured should be verified in the process of planning the time span between collection and analysis. Freezers used to store biological samples for biomarker measurement should have an emergency backup power source and an alarm for notification when power is lost or the temperature rises above a preset level. Freezer space needs can be substantial in a study in which numerous aliquots are produced, and early planning can prevent later problems.

Quality Assurance

All compounds measured in biological samples have a certain amount of biological variability, reflecting the fluctuation that is inherent in the biological system because the constituents are not static but are continuously influenced by rates of metabolism and flux across body pools. For this reason, biochemical measurements may need to be replicated (if possible) or even measured in duplicate or triplicate (if the cost and effort of the measurement permit) to accurately characterize the situation. More important, knowledge of biological variability is simply a primary consideration in the interpretation of actual values obtained from the measurements; the researcher must recognize that quantified values are not absolutes but estimates, even when the best procedures and methods are in place.

Although biological variability is to be expected, other sources of variation are ideally anticipated and minimized in the measurement methodologies used (89). Biochemical methods used in the measurement of biological samples should always be tested for reliability prior to use in a research study. This aspect of quality assurance (QA) typically involves repeated measurements at several levels of set concentrations using various matrixes so that procedural sources of variation can be identified. The concentrations used to test the accuracy of the method should be in the range of the concentrations expected in the biological samples. For example, coefficients of variation obtained from QA procedures for HPLC methods produce figures for both run-to-run and day-to-day variability. External assistance with QA may be possible through the National Institute of Standards and Technology, from which samples with known concentrations of micronutrients and some other dietary constituents may be purchased for comparative testing of the validity of methods used in the researcher's laboratory. For micronutrients, the institute conducts a round-robin QA program in which samples with known concentrations are sent to participating laboratories for measurement as a type of blinded evaluation of laboratory performance (90).

Several other strategies can be used to improve the quality of biochemical measurement data produced, as well as the interpretation and conclusions based on these data. For example, conducting the analysis of samples from a given subject collected at baseline and after intervention in the same batch may help minimize the potential effect of some sources of methodological variation. However, with large numbers of samples from intervention studies that are conducted over years, it may be impossible to measure baseline and end point samples within the time span of the research project. In this case, measurements from a pooled "generic" sample (eg, aliquots of pooled plasma samples from several subjects that have been combined and stored) are obtained with each batch of samples that are measured. This allows examination of the values produced for possible shifts or errors over time so that the methods and instrumentation can be adjusted accordingly. If the nutrition researcher is considering sending samples to a service or clinical laboratory for biochemical measurements, information about these types of QA procedures should be requested for evaluation before a commitment to use the service or laboratory.

CONCLUSION

Much can be gained by the use of biomarkers in nutrition research. Advancements in both scientific knowledge and available technologies make this an area of imminent importance in nutrition research if the field is to function at a level equivalent to other areas of biomedical science. Even the biochemical measures of nutrient status, or those that provide objective evidence for an overall dietary pattern, provide powerful support for associations based on reported dietary intakes. Also, much remains to be learned about the relationship between diet and the disease process, especially at the cellular and molecular levels, and this requires the use of biological markers in nutrition intervention studies. Crucial information for establishing the biological link is obtained by the incorporation of biochemical, cellular, and molecular markers in nutrition research. Although challenges can be anticipated, a thorough knowledge of the biological markers of interest, combined with advance planning, can help to prevent or overcome problems and barriers.

REFERENCES

1. Rock CL, Flatt SW, Thomson C, Stefanick ML, Newman VA, Jones L, Natarajan L, Pierce JP, Chang RJ, Witztum JL. Plasma triacylglycerol and HDL cholesterol concentrations confirm self-reported changes in carbohydrate and fat intakes in women in a diet intervention trial. *J Nutr.* 2004;134: 342–347.

2. Polsinelli ML, Rock CL, Henderson SA, Drewnowski A. Plasma carotenoids as biomarkers of fruit and vegetable servings in women. *J Am Diet Assoc.* 1998;98:194–196.

3. Thomson CA, Giuliano AR, Shaw JW, Rock CL, Ritenbaugh CK, Hakim IA, Hollenbach KA, Childs J, Alberts DS, Pierce JP. Diet and biomarkers of oxidative damage in women previously treated for breast cancer. *Nutr Cancer.* 2005;51:146–154.

4. Meyskens FL. Principles of human chemoprevention. *Hematol Oncol Clin North Am.* 1998;12:935–941.

5. *Biosafety in Microbial and Biomedical Laboratories.* Washington, DC: US Department of Health and Human Services, Centers for Disease Control, and National Institutes of Health; 1993. HHS publication no. (CDC) 93-8395.

6. Prentice, RL. Dietary assessment and the reliability of nutritional epidemiology reports. *Lancet.* 2003; 362:182–183.

7. Clevidence BA, Bieri JG. Association of carotenoids with human plasma lipoproteins. *Methods Enzymol.* 1993;214:33–46.

8. Prentice RL, Willett WC, Greenwald P, Alberts D, Bernstein L, Boyd NF, Byers T, Clinton SK, Fraser G, Freedman L, Hunter D, Kipnis V, Kolonel LN, Kristal BS, Kristal A, Lampe JW, McTiernan A, Milner J, Patterson RE, Potter JD, Riboli E, Schatzkin A, Yates A, Yetley E. Nutrition and physical activity and chronic disease prevention: research strategies and recommendations. *J Natl Cancer Inst.* 2004;96:1276–1287.

9. Blatt DH, Leonard SW, Traber MG. Vitamin E kinetics and the function of tocopherol regulatory proteins. *Nutrition.* 2001;17:799–805.

10. Shils ME, Olson JA, Shike M, Ross AC, eds. *Modern Nutrition in Health and Disease.* 9th ed. Philadelphia, Pa: Williams and Wilkins; 1999.

11. Bowman BA, Russell R., eds. *Present Knowledge in Nutrition.* 9th ed. Washington, DC: ILSI Press; 2006.

12. Institute of Medicine. *Dietary Reference Intakes for Calcium, Phosphorus, Magnesium, Vitamin D, and Fluoride.* Washington, DC: National Academies Press; 1997.

13. Institute of Medicine. *Dietary Reference Intakes for Thiamin, Riboflavin, Niacin, Vitamin B6, Folate, Vitamin B12, Pantothenic Acid, Biotin, and Choline.* Washington, DC: National Academies Press; 1998.

14. Institute of Medicine. *Dietary Reference Intakes for Vitamin C, Vitamin E, Selenium, and Carotenoids.* Washington, DC: National Academies Press; 2000.

15. Institute of Medicine. *Dietary Reference Intakes for Energy, Carbohydrate, Fiber, Fat, Fatty Acids, Cholesterol, Protein, and Amino Acids.* Washington, DC: National Academies Press; 2002.

16. Campbell DR, Gross MD, Martini MC, Grandits GA, Slavin JL, Potter JD. Plasma carotenoids as biomarkers of vegetable and fruit intake. *Cancer Epidemiol Biomarkers Prev.* 1994;3: 493–500.

17. Rock CL, Flatt SW, Wright FA, Faerber S, Newman V, Kealey S, Pierce JP. Responsiveness of carotenoids to a high vegetable diet intervention designed to prevent breast cancer recurrence. *Cancer Epidemiol Biomarkers Prev.* 1997;6:617–623.

18. Le Marchand L, Hankin JH, Carter FS, Essling C, Luffey D, Franke AA, Wilkins LR, Cooney RV, Kolonel LN. A pilot study on the use of plasma carotenoids and ascorbic acid as markers of compliance to a high fruit and vegetable diet intervention. *Cancer Epidemiol Biomarkers Prev.* 1994;3:245–251.

19. Mazur W, Fotsis T, Wahala K, Ojala S, Salakka A, Adlercreutz H. Isotope dilution gas chromatographic–mass spectrophotometric method for the

determination of isoflavonoids, coumestrol, and lignans in food samples. *Analyt Biochem.* 1996;233:169–180.

20. Lampe JW, Campbell DR, Hutchins AM, Martini MC, Li S, Wahala K, Grandits GA, Potter JD, Slavin JL. Urinary isoflavonoid and lignan excretion on a Western diet: relation to soy, vegetable, and fruit intake. *Cancer Epidemiol Biomarkers Prev.* 1999;8: 699–707.

21. Kilkkinen A, Stumpf K, Pietinen P, Valsta LM, Tapanainen H, Adlercreutz H. Determinants of serum enterolactone concentration. *Am J Clin Nutr.* 2001;73: 1094–1100.

22. Meydani SN, Endres S, Woods MM, Golden BR, Soo C, Morrill-Labrode A, Dinarello CA, Gorbach SL. Oral (n-3) fatty acid supplementation suppresses cytokine production and lymphocyte proliferation: comparison between young and older women. *J Nutr.* 1991;121:547–555.

23. Arrab L. Biomarkers of fat and fatty acid intake. *J Nutr.* 2003; 133(suppl):925S–932S.

24. Wolk A, Vessby B, Ljung H, Barrefors P. Evaluation of a biologic marker for dairy fat intake. *Am J Clin Nutr.* 1998;68:291–295.

25. Smedman AEM, Gustafsson I-B, Berglund LGT, Vessby BOH. Pentadecanoic acid in serum as a marker for intake of milk fat: relations between intake of milk fat and metabolic risk factors. *Am J Clin Nutr.* 1999;69:22–29.

26. Gross MD, Pfeiffer M, Martini M, Campbell D, Slavin J, Potter J. The quantitation of metabolites of quercetin flavonols in human urine. *Cancer Epidemiol Biomarkers Prev.* 1996;5:711–720.

27. Coward L, Barnes NC, Setchell KDR, Barnes S. Genistein, daidzein and their β-glycoside conjugates: antitumor isoflavones in soybean foods from American and Asian diets. *J Agric Food Chem.* 1993;41:1961–1967.

28. Franke AA, Custer LJ, Cerna CM, Narala K. Quantitation of phytoestrogens in legumes by HPLC. *J Agric Food Chem.* 1994;42:1905–1913.

29. Karr SC, Lampe JW, Hutchins AM, Slavin JL. Urinary isoflavonoid excretion in humans is dose-dependent at low to moderate levels of soy protein consumption. *Am J Clin Nutr.* 1997;66:46–51.

30. Adlercreutz H, Honjo H, Higashi A, Fotsis T, Hamalainen E, Hasegawa T, Okada H. Urinary excretion of lignans and isoflavonoid phytoestrogens in Japanese men and women consuming a traditional Japanese diet. *Am J Clin Nutr.* 1991;54: 1093–1100.

31. Franke AA, Custer LJ. High-performance liquid chromatography assay of isoflavonoids and coumestrol from human urine. *J Chromatogr B Biomed Appl.* 1994;662:47–60.

32. Maskarinec G, Singh S, Meng L, Franke AA. Dietary soy intake and urinary isoflavonoid excretion among women from a multiethnic population. *Cancer Epidemiol Biomarkers Prev.* 1998:7:613–619.

33. Watanabe S, Yamaguchi M, Sobue T, Takahashi T, Miura T, Arai Y, Mazur W, Wahala K, Adlercreutz H. Pharmacokinetics of soybean isoflavones in plasma, urine, and feces of men after ingestion of 60 g baked soybean powder (kinako). *J Nutr.* 1998;128: 1710–1715.

34. Shapiro TA, Fahey JW, Wade KL, Stephenson KK, Talalay P. Human metabolism and excretion of cancer chemoprotective glucosinolates and isothiocyanates of cruciferous vegetables. *Cancer Epidemiol Biomarkers Prev.* 1998;7:1091–1100.

35. McClave SA, Snider HL. Use of indirect calorimetry in clinical nutrition. *Nutr Clin Pract.* 1992;7: 207–221.

36. Jequier E, Felber JP. Indirect calorimetry. *Baillieres Clin Endocrinol Metab.* 1987;1:911–935.

37. Owen OE. Resting metabolic requirements of men and women. *Mayo Clin Proc.* 1988;63:503–510.

38. Lusk G. Animal calorimetry: analysis of the oxidation of mixtures of carbohydrate and fat [a correction]. *J Biol Chem.* 1994;59:41–42.

39. Peronnet F, Massicotte D. Table of nonprotein respiratory quotient: an update. *Can J Sport Sci.* 1991:16: 23–29.

40. Isbell TR, Klesges RC, Meyers AW, Klesges LM. Measurement reliability and reactivity using repeated measurements of resting energy expenditure with a face mask, mouthpiece, and ventilated canopy. *JPEN J Parenter Enteral Nutr.* 1991;15:165–168.

41. Leff ML, Hill JO, Yates AA, Cotsonis GA, Heymsfield SB. Resting metabolic rate: measurement reliability. *JPEN J Parenter Enteral Nutr.* 1987;11: 354–359.

42. Seale J. Energy expenditure measurements in relation to energy requirements. *Am J Clin Nutr.* 1995;62(suppl):S1042–S1046.

43. Speakman JR. The history and theory of the doubly labeled water technique. *Am J Clin Nutr.* 1998; 68(suppl):S932–S938.

44. Sawaya AL, Tucker K, Tsay R, Willett W, Saltzman E, Dallal GE, Roberts SB. Evaluation of four methods for determining energy intake in young and

older women: comparison with doubly labeled water measurements of total energy expenditure. *Am J Clin Nutr.* 1996;63:491–499.

45. Schultz LA, Schoeller DA. A compilation of total daily energy expenditures and body weights in healthy adults. *Am J Clin Nutr.* 1994;60:676–681.

46. Halliwell B. Effect of diet on cancer development: is oxidative DNA damage a biomarker? *Free Radic Biol Med.* 2002;33:968–974.

47. Handelman GJ, Pryor WA. Evaluation of antioxidant status in humans. In: Papas AM, ed. *Antioxidant Status, Diet, Nutrition, and Health.* New York, NY: CRC Press; 1999:37–62.

48. Lemoyne M, Gossum AV, Kurian R, Ostro M, Azler J, Jeejeebhoy KN. Breath pentane analysis as an index of lipid peroxidation: a functional test of vitamin E status. *Am J Clin Nutr.* 1987;46: 267–272.

49. Kasai H, Crain PF, Kuchino Y, Nishimura S, Oostsuyama A, Tanooka H. Formation of 8-hydroxyguanine moiety in cellular DNA by agents producing oxygen radicals and evidence for its repair. *Carcinogenesis.* 1986;7:1849–1851.

50. Loft S, Vistisen K, Ewertz M, Tjonneland A, Overvad K, Poulsen HE. Oxidative DNA damage estimated by 8-hydroxydeoxyguanosine excretion in humans: influence of smoking, gender, and body mass index. *Carcinogenesis.* 1992;13:2241–2247.

51. Tagesson C, Kallberg M, Klintenberg C, Starkhammar H. Determination of urinary 8-hydroxydeoxyguanosine by automated coupled-column high performance liquid chromatography: a powerful technique for assaying *in vivo* oxidative DNA damage in cancer patients. *Eur J Cancer.* 1995;31A: 934–940.

52. Morrow JD, Harris TM, Roberts LJ. Noncyclooxygenase oxidative formation of a series of novel prostaglandins: analytical ramifications for measurement of eicosanoids. *Ann Biochem.* 1990;184:1–10.

53. Morrow JD, Roberts LJ. The isoprostanes: unique bioactive products of lipid peroxidation. *Prog Lipid Res.* 1997;36:1–21.

54. Patrono C, FitzGerald GA. Isoprostanes: potential markers of oxidant stress in atherothrombotic disease. *Arterioscler Thromb Vasc Biol.* 1997;17: 2309–2315.

55. Thompson HJ, Heimendinger J, Sedlacek S, Haegele A, Diker A, O'Neill C, Meinecke B, Wolfe P, Zhu Z, Jiang W. 8-Isoprostane $F_{2\alpha}$ excretion is reduced in women by increased vegetable and fruit intake. *Am J Clin Nutr.* 2005;82:768–776.

56. Djuric Z, Heilbrun LK, Reading BA, Boomer A, Valeriote FA, Martino S. Effects of a low-fat diet on levels of oxidative damage to DNA in human peripheral nucleated blood cells. *J Natl Cancer Inst.* 1991;83:766–769.

57. Djuric Z, Depper JB, Uhley V, Smith D, Lababidi S, Martino S, Heilbrun LK. Oxidative DNA damage levels in blood from women at high risk for breast cancer are associated with dietary intakes of meats, vegetables, and fruits. *J Am Diet Assoc.* 1998;98:524–528.

58. Mosca L, Rubenfire M, Mandel C, Rock C, Tarshis T, Tsai A, Pearson T. Antioxidant nutrient supplementation reduces the susceptibility of low density lipoprotein to oxidation in patients with coronary artery disease. *J Am Coll Cardiol.* 1997;30:392–399.

59. Habig WH, Pabst MJ, Jakoby WB. Glutathione S-transferases: the first enzymatic step in mercapturic acid formation. *J Biol Chem.* 1974;249:7130–7139.

60. Bogaards JJP, Verhagen H, Willems MI, van Poppel G, van Bladeren PJ. Consumption of brussels sprouts results in elevated alpha-class glutathione S-transferase levels in human blood plasma. *Carcinogenesis.* 1994;15:1073–1075.

61. Kashuba ADM, Bertino JS, Kearns GL, Leeder JS, James AW, Gotschall R, Nafziger AN. Quantitation of three-month intraindividual variability and influence of sex and menstrual cycle phase on CYP1A2, *N*-acetyltransferase-2, and xanthine oxidase activity determined with caffeine phenotyping. *Clin Pharmacol Ther.* 1998;63:540–551.

62. Pantuck EJ, Pantuck CB, Anderson KE, Wattenberg LW, Conney AH, Kappas A. Effect of brussels sprouts and cabbage on drug conjugation. *Clin Pharmacol Ther.* 1984;35:161–169.

63. Sinha R, Rothman N, Brown ED, Mark SD, Hoover RN, Caporaso NE, Levander OA, Knize MG, Lang NP, Kudlubar FF. Pan-fried meat containing high levels of heterocyclic aromatic amines but low levels of polycyclic aromatic hydrocarbons induces cytochrome P4501A2 activity in humans. *Cancer Res.* 1994;54:6154–6159.

64. Kall MA, Vang O, Clausen J. Effects of dietary broccoli on human drug metabolising activity. *Cancer Lett.* 1997;114:169–170.

65. Fowler BM, Giuliano AR, Piyathilake C, Nour M, Hatch K. Hypomethylation in cervical tissue: is there a correlation with folate status? *Cancer Epidemiol Biomarkers Prev.* 1998;7: 901–906.

66. Hamilton SR. Molecular genetics of colorectal carcinoma. *Cancer.* 1992;70:1216–1221.

67. Chen J, Giovannucci EL, Hunter DJ. MTHFR polymorphism, methyl-replete diets and the risk of colorectal carcinoma and adenoma among US men and women: an example of gene-environment interactions in colorectal tumorigenesis. *J Nutr.* 1999; 129(suppl):S560–S564.

68. Lauritsen K, Laursen LS, Bukhave K, Rask-Madsen J. Does vitamin E supplementation modulate in vivo arachidonate metabolism in human inflammation? *Pharmacol Toxicol.* 1987;61:246–249.

69. Ruffin MT, Krishnan K, Rock CL, Normolle D, Vaerten MA, Peters-Golden M, Crowell J, Kelloff G, Boland CR, Brenner DE. Suppression of human colorectal mucosal prostaglandins: determining the lowest effective aspirin dose. *J Natl Cancer Inst.* 1997;89:1152–1160.

70. Krishnan K, Ruffin MT, Brenner DE. Clinical models of chemoprevention for colon cancer. *Hematol Oncol Clin North Am.* 1998;12:1079–1113.

71. Boland CR. The biology of colorectal cancer. *Cancer.* 1993:71(suppl):4181–4186.

72. Einspahr JG, Alberts DS, Gapstur SM, Bostick RM, Emerson SS, Gerner EW. Surrogate end-point biomarkers as measures of colon cancer risk and their use in cancer chemoprevention trials. *Cancer Epidemiol Biomarkers Prev.* 1997;6:37–48.

73. Lipkin MH. Effect of added dietary calcium on colonic epithelial-cells proliferation in subjects at high risk for familial colonic cancer. *N Engl J Med.* 1985;313:1381–1384.

74. Bostick RM, Fosdick L, Lillemoe TJ, Overn P, Wood JR, Grambsch P, Elmer P, Potter JD. Methodological findings and considerations in measuring colorectal epithelial cell proliferation in humans. *Cancer Epidemiol Biomarkers Prev.* 1997;6:931–942.

75. Wargovich MJ, Cunningham JE. Diet, individual responsiveness and cancer prevention. *J Nutr.* 2003; 133:2400S–2403S.

76. Sinha R, Caporaso N. Diet, genetic susceptibility, and human cancer etiology. *J Nutr.* 1999;129(suppl): 556–559.

77. Kim YI, Pogribney IP, Basnakian AG, Miller JW, Selhub J, James SJ, Mason JB. Folate deficiency in rats induces DNA strand breaks and hypomethylation within the p53 tumor suppressor gene. *Am J Clin Nutr.* 1997;65:46–52.

78. Trujillo E, Davis C, Milner J. Nutrigenomics, proteomics, metabolomics, and the practice of dietetics. *J Am Diet Assoc.* 2006;106:403–413.

79. Go VL, Nguyen CT, Harris DM, Lee WN. Nutrient-gene interaction: genotype-phenotype relationship. *J Nutr.* 2005;135:3016S–3020S.

80. Ruffin MT, Ogaily MS, Johnston CM, Gregoire L, Lancaster WD, Brenner DE. Surrogate endpoint biomarkers for cervical cancer chemoprevention trials. *J Cell Biochem.* 1995;23(suppl):113–124.

81. Byrne C. Studying mammographic density: implications for understanding breast cancer. *J Natl Cancer Inst.* 1997;89:531–533.

82. Knight JA, Martin LJ, Greenberg CV, Lockwood GA, Byng JW, Yaffe MJ, Tritchler DL, Boyd NF. Macronutrient intake and change in mammographic density at menopause: results from a randomized trial. *Cancer Epidemiol Biomarkers Prev.* 1999;8:123–128.

83. Rock CL, Michael CW, Reynolds RK, Ruffin MT. Prevention of cervix cancer. *Crit Rev Oncol Hematol.* 2000;33:169–185.

84. MacLennan R, Macrae F, Bain C, Battistutta D, Chapuis P, Gratten H, Lambert J, Newland RC, Ngu M, Russell A, Ward M, Wahlqvist ML, the Australian Polyp Prevention Project. Randomized trial of intake of fat, fiber, and beta carotene to prevent colorectal adenomas. The Australian Polyp Prevention Project. *J Natl Cancer Inst.* 1995;87:1760–1766.

85. Faivre J, Bonithon-Kopp C. Effect of fibre and calcium supplementation on adenoma recurrence and growth. *IARC Sci Publ.* 2002;156:457–461.

86. Byers T. Diet, colorectal adenomas, and colorectal cancer. *N Engl J Med.* 2000;342:1206–1207.

87. Schatzkin A, Lanza E, Corle D, Lance P, Iber F, Caan B, Shike M, Weissfeld J, Burt R, Cooper MR, Kikendall JW, Cahill J, the Polyp Prevention Trial Study Group. Lack of effect of a low-fat diet on the recurrence of colorectal adenomas. *N Engl J Med.* 2000;342:1149–1155.

88. Bingham S, Cummings JH. The use of 4-aminobenzoic acid as a marker to validate the completeness of 24 hr urine collections in man. *Clin Sci.* 1983;64: 629–635.

89. Guilliano AR, Matzner MB, Canfield LM. Assessing variability in quantitation of carotenoids in human plasma: variance component model. *Methods Enzymol.* 1993;214:94–101.

90. Duewer DL, Thomas JB, Kline MC, MacCrehan WA, Schaffer R, Sharpless KE. NIST/NCI Micronutrients Quality Assurance Program: measurement repeatabilities and reproducibilities for fat-soluble vitamin-related compounds in human sera. *Ann Chem.* 1997;69:1406–1413.

18

Research Methods for Human Sensory System Analysis and Food Evaluation

Richard D. Mattes, PhD, RD, and Beverly J. Cowart, PhD

Sensory appeal is arguably the principal determinant of food selection and ingestion. In surveys, more than 90% of consumers rank taste as more influential on their food selection and ingestion choices than other factors, such as nutrition, price, or safety (1,2). Professionals in academia, industry, medicine, and government also indicate that taste takes precedence over nutrient content, price, convenience, and health concerns (3). Furthermore, concern over sacrificing the sensory pleasure of eating is a primary explanation for failure to adopt a more healthful diet. Consequently, it is vital for health care providers, and especially registered dietitians (RDs), to understand how the sensory properties of foods and the sensory abilities of humans interact to influence food choice in health and disease.

TERMINOLOGY

Taste is used colloquially to refer to the sensory properties of foods. However, to a sensory scientist, the term *taste* is restricted to those sensations arising from chemical or electrical stimulation of taste receptor cells. These cells are located on the tongue, soft palate, pharynx, epiglottis, larynx, and upper esophagus. The repertoire of taste sensations is limited. Currently five basic taste qualities are widely accepted: sweetness, sourness, saltiness, bitterness, and umami (the sensation elicited by monosodium glutamate). A detection system for dietary fat has also been proposed.

Although the evidence is still preliminary, support for a taste component to fat perception is accumulating (4).

In contrast, the array of food odors is vast, and most believe there is no limited set of primary qualities. Food odors are detected by specialized receptor cells in the olfactory neuroepithelium, located primarily at the apex of the superior turbinate. Odor molecules may reach the olfactory receptors via both the orthonasal and retronasal routes. The former pathway involves the passage of odor molecules through the nares (eg, when one is sniffing food), whereas the latter entails access of volatile compounds derived from food in the mouth to olfactory receptors through the nasopharynx. Retronasal stimulation accounts for much of the flavor of foods.

Chemically mediated irritancy (eg, the burning of pepper or the coolness of menthol) and mouth feel (eg, astringency of foods and beverages) are referred to as *chemesthesis*. This input is mediated by trigeminal innervation, which is widely dispersed throughout the nasopharyngeal region. Foods also provide an array of nonchemically mediated sensations (eg, visual, auditory, and thermal sensations).

The combination of all these inputs is referred to as *flavor*. Any alteration in a component part will result in a different flavor, much as the omission of selected pieces alters the overall appearance of a puzzle. Because we all differ in our innate and acquired sensitivities and affective responses to the plethora of chemicals in foods and beverages, the perception of flavor is idiosyncratic.

STUDY OF FLAVOR PERCEPTION

The study of flavor perception can be broadly divided into two tracks. One track concerns the sensory properties of foods and is largely the domain of food scientists. The focus is on gaining a better understanding of the physicochemical properties of foods and beverages that determine their sensory characteristics. The most widely used definition of such sensory evaluation is that it is a scientific method used to evoke, measure, analyze, and interpret responses to products perceived through the senses of sight, smell, touch, taste, and hearing (5). Generally, the approach is to identify and train a panel of judges to provide reliable and detailed information about the sensory attributes of complex stimuli (real foods). Sensory evaluation is a science based on the principles of the scientific method, including hypothesis testing through objective and reproducible measurements. The skills necessary to conduct this work are varied, but they are largely drawn from statistics, psychology, physiology, and food science. The information generated by sensory professionals in the food industry has many uses (Box 18.1). These are described more fully, along with the suitable testing methodologies, in several references (6–8).

BOX 18.1   Functions of Sensory Systems and Sensory Evaluation in Dietetics and Food Science

---

Dietary Implications of Sensory Function
  Quality of life
  Food safety
  Food selection
  Digestion and nutrient metabolism
Applications of Sensory Evaluation in the Food Industry
  New product development
  Product reformulation
  Cost reduction
  Quality control
  Quality assurance
  Monitoring the competition
  Shelf-life studies
  Assessment of raw materials
  Support of advertising claims

The second track in the study of flavor perception, referred to as *psychophysics,* is primarily concerned with the psychological perception of physical stimuli. The aim is a better understanding of the factors that influence the

TABLE 18.1   Chemosensory Disorders

Sensory System		
Taste	**Smell**	**Description**
Ageusia	Anosmia	Loss of sensation
Hypogeusia	Hyposmia	Diminished sensation
Hypergeusia	Hyperosmia	Enhanced sensation
Dysgeusia	Dysosmia (or parosmia)	Distorted sensation
Phantogeusia	Phantosmia	Sensation without known stimulation

sensory capabilities of judges (consumers). Thus, the approach is to measure individual variability in responses to standardized, typically simple stimuli (eg, a single compound in water). Such work has been dominated by psychologists, physiologists, and neuroscientists. The goal is to understand the basic mechanisms of sensory systems, as well as their contribution to, and complications from, pathological processes. Hence, psychophysical testing is useful in the clinical setting.

The array of chemosensory disorders is presented in Table 18.1. In general, olfactory disorders are much more prevalent than gustatory disorders (9,10). Anosmia and hyposmia are the most common diagnoses among patients evaluated at taste and smell centers. The majority of smell problems stem from ongoing inflammatory pathology in the nose and sinuses, prior upper respiratory infections, and head trauma. Whole-mouth diminutions in taste sensitivity, and in particular ageusia, are extremely rare, with phantogeusia being the most common form of taste dysfunction (10,11). Etiologic factors contributing to taste disorders are not well documented, but medication usage and oral health problems are the most frequently reported (10). A number of references describe the etiology, diagnosis, incidence, and management of these abnormalities (9–20).

The outcome variables for these two branches of sensory science are quite similar, but the experimental approaches often differ. Common questions in the two approaches concern (a) the minimal level of stimulus intensity that can be detected or characterized, (b) the relationship between growth of sensation and increases in physical concentration, (c) spatial-temporal influences on responsiveness, and (d) hedonic judgments. Combined, these measures characterize an individual's sensory capabilities and experiences fairly well. Individually, each measure provides information about a segment of the sensory spectrum, but because the segments are poorly correlated, knowledge of one does not provide a basis for assumptions about another. For example, as an individual recovers after radiation therapy administered to the head and neck, the ability to detect low concentrations of stimuli may return while the perceived intensities of stronger stimuli remain depressed (21). Both threshold sensitivity and responsiveness to suprathreshold stimuli hold poor predictive power for hedonic judgments, which are strongly influenced by culture and dietary experiences.

There are many methods for assessment of the different facets of chemosensory function. Several of the more common methods are described in this chapter. The interested researcher is encouraged to consult the references for a more comprehensive description of test procedures and the issues that warrant control with their use. In addition, a number of short or distance courses offer intensive training in various aspects of sensory science.

THRESHOLD MEASUREMENT

A *threshold* is a measure of the lowest limits of sensitivity of a sensory system. If the task is simply to determine whether a stimulus is present (yes/no response) or which of two or more samples contains a stimulus (forced-choice response), the threshold is called a *detection threshold.* It is not necessary to be able to characterize the stimulus; the determination of its presence alone is sufficient. If the task is to determine the lowest concentration at which the quality of the stimulus can be identified, the threshold is termed a *recognition threshold.* A *discrimination threshold* represents the increment in stimulus concentration necessary for one to detect a difference between paired samples. In actuality, a detection threshold is just one level of a discrimination threshold, where the comparison stimulus level is zero.

It is often incorrectly assumed that thresholds reflect an inherent characteristic of an individual. Rather, they are probabilistic measures that may be defined as the lowest concentration of a stimulus that can be detected (or recognized, or discriminated) at a level greater than some predetermined probability under a given set of conditions. Generally, as one is exposed to increasing concentrations of a stimulus, the likelihood of detecting its presence rises as a sigmoidal function. In yes/no tasks, a threshold is often defined as the concentration at which a subject reports a sensation on at least 50% of its presentations. In forced-choice tasks, the criterion level is customarily set somewhat above the level of chance performance for the task. For example, if two samples are presented, the probability of correctly guessing which contains a stimulus is 50%. If three samples

are presented, the probability of correct guessing is 33.3%. However, the criterion chosen is arbitrary, and if the experimenter wants to decrease the risk of a fallaciously low threshold estimate, the required correct-response level may be raised. Forced-choice formats are generally preferred because they control for individual differences in subjective criteria with regard to what constitutes a particular type of sensation. The medium in which the stimulus is to be identified is also critical. A stimulus in a simple medium, such as water, is more easily detected than the same stimulus incorporated in a complex food system. Thus, thresholds are generally lower in model solutions.

There are four common methods for measuring thresholds in sensory evaluation: the paired-comparison, duo-trio, triangle, and staircase procedures. One of these may be the method of choice when attempting to determine subtle differences in products possibly due to reformulation or processing changes, when monitoring quality control, or when performing shelf-life studies.

Paired-Comparison Test

The paired-comparison test may be directional or nondirectional. In the former, the sensory nature of the stimulus is known, and the judge is required to indicate which of the two samples presented contains the target sensory attribute (or elicits it more strongly). In this two-alternative forced-choice test, the judge must make a choice even if he or she is unsure of the correct answer. If the nature of the stimulus is not known, the judge is asked to indicate if the two samples are alike or different in the simple difference or same-different test. In both cases, pairs of samples are presented in random order. Typically, sufficient time or a means to clear the first stimulus is given prior to administration of the second (eg, rinsing with water or breathing air without a stimulus). For both tests the probability of correct guessing is 50%. Because the experimenter knows the correct response, a one-tailed test is used to establish statistical significance, which is determined by comparing the proportion of correct responses to the binomial distribution. The strengths of the paired-comparison test are that it is conceptually simple and, as a result, resistant to confusion errors, and it is quite sensitive. Because relatively few samples need to be tested, fatigue is minimized.

Duo-Trio Test

The duo-trio test involves presenting judges with three samples. One sample is labeled as a reference, and two samples are unknowns; the task is to determine which of the unknowns is most similar to the reference. The reference is sampled first, followed by the two unknowns, which are presented in counterbalanced, semi-random order over a series of trials. This test is nondirectional: the basis for making a match decision need not be specified, and it will not be known. The probability of correct guessing is 50%. Analysis is based on comparison with the binomial distribution in a one-tailed test.

The advantage of this procedure is that it can be used to assess sensitivity to changes in a product with no knowledge of what attribute of the product has changed. This characteristic is also a drawback, because the test will not provide insights on the component responsible for the difference between samples. Furthermore, it requires more sampling than the paired-comparison test, is slightly less powerful, and is more susceptible to reversal errors (ie, the judge reports which is the "odd sample" rather than the match).

Triangle Test

The triangle test entails the presentation of three samples; two are alike and one is different. The samples are presented in random order, and the task is to identify the odd sample. This test, like the duo-trio test, is nondirectional: the basis for selecting the odd sample need not be specified, and it will not be known. The probability of correct guessing is 33.3%. Analysis is based on comparison with the binomial distribution in a one-tailed test.

The advantage of the triangle test is that the probability of correct guessing is lower than for the paired-comparison or duo-trio format, so fewer subjects may be required to determine whether differences exist. This characteristic may reduce time and sample costs. The fact that it is nondirectional can be a strength (if the nature of the target sensation is not known) or a weakness (because the basis for a judgment is not known), depending on the desired outcome of testing. Because the triangle test requires exposure to more samples than does the paired-comparison test, there is a higher risk of fatigue and loss of sensitivity, especially with the use of samples that are difficult to clear from the mouth or nose.

Staircase Procedure

The staircase procedure is widely used in psychophysical studies (22), although the previously discussed methods may also be appropriate in such studies under certain conditions. In the staircase procedure, the judge is typically offered two or three samples and asked to indicate which contains a particular stimulus. If the response is incorrect, a higher concentration of the stimulus is then presented, along with one or more samples of the vehicle or medium without the stimulus. Another incorrect response is followed with a still higher concentration. This activity continues until a correct response is obtained. Because there is a 50% (or 33.3%) probability of guessing, it is common practice to present an identical concentration at least one additional time after a correct response to confirm that the stimulus was detected. Following repeated correct responses, a lower concentration is presented. If the responses to two or more matching presentations are again correct, the concentration declines again on the next trial. This procedure continues until a single incorrect response is obtained.

The concentrations at which ascending and descending trial runs originate are termed *reversal points*. The first reversal point is typically discarded as unreliable because of orienting and starting point effects. The subsequent reversal concentrations are averaged to derive an estimated threshold. Equal numbers of trials of each type, commonly two to three ascending-to-descending trials and two to three descending-to-ascending trials, are included. This rigorous method can provide a reasonable estimate of an individual's limit of sensitivity, but it can also be extremely time-consuming to administer.

General Concerns about Threshold Tests

Researchers using threshold tests should be aware of potential problems. First, all threshold procedures are in fact estimations of the ability to discriminate between a signal and a background level of stimulation (the presence of other food constituents, water, air, or whatever vehicle carries the stimulus). When there is a higher level of background stimulation, it is more difficult to detect a small increment in stimulus intensity than when there is little background noise. As an analogy, detecting the change in illumination of a room when only one light bulb is on is easier than detecting the contribution of one light bulb to a room containing 100 other lighted bulbs. Thus, the absolute value of a threshold estimate is highly dependent on the test conditions. Indeed, a reported value cannot be interpreted without knowledge of the procedural details.

Another problem with threshold tests involves learning. Familiarity with the testing procedure leads to improved performance. Thus, it is important to have a break-in period so that judge performance is confirmed to be stable before the actual testing.

General fatigue is another problem. Prolonged testing can lead to reduced attention and adaptation of sensory receptors to the stimuli under study. These effects will raise threshold levels. If feasible, it may be preferable to test individuals on two occasions so that fewer stimuli are sampled in a single session. Selecting stimulus concentration steps that are small enough to be difficult to discriminate will provide a more accurate estimate of threshold sensitivity. However, if the steps are so small that discrimination is extremely difficult, the test may take an inordinate amount of time to administer. Half- or quarter-log steps, or serial half-dilutions, often work well.

When two or more stimuli are presented, the last stimulus sampled is often rated as strongest because of memory decay. Alternatively, some judges may tend to favor one temporal or physical position (eg, they may have a bias toward selecting the stimulus on the right). Both of these problems can be avoided by counterbalancing sample presentation.

Extraneous cues may confound test results. Subtle differences in attributes not intentionally manipulated (eg, temperature, color, or viscosity), rather than in the target sensation, may be the basis of judgments. A wide array of subject attributes, including mood, alertness, hunger level, health status, and oral hygiene, may alter performance in unpredictable ways. Thus, test-retest reliability can be low. Attempts to recruit a homogeneous sample of judges or to control various relevant behaviors (eg, forbidding eating, smoking, and drinking for some period prior to testing) should reduce variability and permit identification of subtle changes that occur over time, which is often the primary dependent variable in clinical assessments.

Another concern is that sensory evaluation studies are often conducted with the objective of finding no significant difference between samples; however, failure to reject the null hypothesis in a statistical test does not demonstrate that it is true, but merely that it has not been shown to be false (which could be the result of insufficient evidence). To ensure that reasonable conclusions are drawn, it is especially critical in this case to design the test to have sufficient statistical power. This goal may be achieved by using trained judges, by lowering the critical value for significance, or by increasing the sample size.

SCALING PROCEDURES

Scaling procedures are used to evaluate the relationship between sensation and stimulus concentration at suprathreshold (above-threshold) levels. In contrast to threshold assessment, scaling procedures can provide insights into the perception of stimuli over a wide range of concentrations. Some stimuli (eg, irritants) lead to disproportionately large increments in sensation relative to gradations in physical concentration, a phenomenon termed *expansion*. The perceived intensity of many stimuli (eg, sucrose and sodium chloride) grows in approximate proportion to steps of physical concentration. Finally, for some stimuli (eg, fat and most odors), rather large changes in physical concentration are required to produce appreciable increases in perceived intensity. The latter phenomenon is referred to as *compression*. Knowledge of these relationships is vital in the food industry for product development and reformulation.

As described later, there are several response formats (eg, ranking, category and visual analog scales, magnitude estimation) for scaling stimuli, each with advantages and disadvantages. Different formats generate different levels of data. It is important to bear in mind, however, that all forms of scaling are susceptible to contextual effects. That is, humans naturally tend to judge intensity and pleasantness in a relative rather than an absolute sense; therefore, stimulus spacing, frequency, and range in the immediate experimental context can greatly influence ratings (23–28). The broader context of an individual's extra-experimental life experiences may also influence that person's ratings of experimental stimuli.

Ordinal Data

Ranking is perhaps the simplest form of scaling. It generates data at the ordinal level. The judge is asked to sample a set of stimuli and order them along a stipulated dimension (eg, odor intensity). This procedure does not require the assignment of numerical or verbal intensity ratings to the stimuli, which is an advantage in work with very young children or people unfamiliar or uncomfortable with number use. The drawback is that no information is obtained regarding the perceived magnitude of difference between successive stimuli. It is also necessary to make multiple comparisons to assign ranks, which may lead to fatigue. Thus, the number of stimuli that can be evaluated is limited. Ranked data do not meet the assumptions made in parametric statistical methods concerning the underlying distributions of response variables, so nonparametric (also known as distribution-free) tests must be used to assess test results.

Interval Data

Category scales permit the assignment of prespecified verbal or numerical responses to stimuli that reflect the

Category Scales

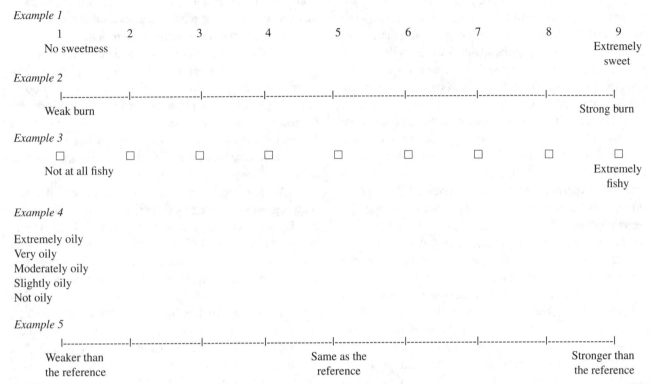

FIGURE 18.1   Examples of interval-level scales of intensity.

magnitude of differences between the stimuli. However, because these scales have no natural zero point, they yield interval-level data. Figure 18.1 shows some of the many variations of traditional category scales. Judges are presented with a set of stimuli and asked to rate each stimulus on a given scale. The samples are presented in random order, preferably in duplicate or triplicate, with allowance of adequate time or procedures to reduce carryover effects from the previous sample. Given that judges may avoid the extreme response options (end effect) (23,29), the effective scale is often reduced relative to the scale presented. Thus, three- and five-point scales provide a very limited array of response options. Scales with more than nine options (10 to 20) have a number of desirable attributes (30), but it must be confirmed that the judges are really able to make the fine discriminations that these scales imply. Given end effects, a nine-point scale can yield an adequate (seven-point) response format and is probably the most commonly used.

Using an odd number of categories makes it possible to have a bipolar scale with a neutral point in the center. This type of scale is used frequently for hedonic rating, but it can be useful for intensity judgments as well, especially if ratings are made relative to a reference sample. In this case, the center rating would indicate no difference. The choice of verbal descriptors attached to a scale is critical. They must be unambiguous to all judges, isolate a single sensory attribute (eg, intensity and hedonic terms should not be mixed), and cover the range of sensations judges will experience.

The strength of category scales is that they permit rapid acquisition of intensity judgments over a wide segment of an individual's sensory range. Furthermore, they are simple, familiar response scales that can be adapted to almost any audience. Because all judges are responding on a fixed scale, the calibration of responses is straightforward.

A drawback of category scales is that, absent a natural zero, relative intensities of stimuli cannot be determined. For example, a stimulus receiving a rating of 8 on a category scale cannot be assumed to be twice as strong as one receiving a rating of 4, just as on the Fahrenheit scale of temperature, which is an interval scale, it is not appropriate to conclude that 80° is twice as warm as 40°.

The use of verbal anchors on category scales increases the amount of information transmitted (31) and can enable within-subject comparisons of absolute perceived intensity, as well as across-group comparisons when members of the groups have been randomly assigned (ensuring no average difference in the way the groups use labels). However, it should not be assumed, as it frequently has been, that intensity labels denote the same absolute perceived intensities for groups that differ in systematic ways (eg, age, sex, clinical status) (32–34). Thus, across-group comparisons of scaled intensity (or pleasantness) are often invalid. Recent attempts to address this problem have centered on ratio scaling procedures, and are discussed next.

Finally, scales that generate interval-level data do not meet the assumptions underlying parametric statistical tests. Consequently, data derived from them are most appropriately analyzed with the use of nonparametric tests. However, the more powerful and familiar parametric tests (*t* test and *F* test) are widely applied and generally lead to comparable results if the scale used includes at least seven categorical response levels.

Ratio Scales

Ratio scales permit a judge to assign ratings to stimuli that reflect their relative intensities (ie, proportional sensation differences between stimuli). In the prototypical and most explicit ratio scaling procedure, *magnitude estimation*, judges are instructed to sample and assign a numerical intensity rating—whatever seems appropriate—to one stimulus. Subsequent samples are then rated relative to this initial assessment. If a subsequent sample is half as intense, the sample is assigned a rating half as large as the former; if it is four times stronger, it is assigned a rating four times greater.

Individual differences in number use can produce substantial variability in the data obtained. Several techniques have been proposed to reduce this noise. One approach is to determine the arithmetic mean of all sensory responses and to divide this value into 10 (an arbitrary number). The result is a factor by which each individual response is then multiplied to standardize the data. Another solution involves providing judges a reference sample with an assigned intensity score. All ratings are then made relative to the reference, so they are already standardized. The disadvantage of this approach is that judges may disagree with the number assigned by the researcher, which could bias their subsequent ratings.

Once the data are standardized, the least squares regression line for the plot of stimulus concentration vs intensity ratings is determined. The slope of the line is the metric used to evaluate the growth of sensation with physical concentration. Typically, log-log plots are used

to linearize the data (a permissible transformation only with ratio-level data), but one should use this technique only after determining the function that best describes the data. If a log transformation is used, responses of zero intensity become problematic. Suggested ways to deal with this problem include omitting any zero ratings or replacing them with a small number, although either approach can distort the data. Another method is to use the median response across judges at each concentration, but this can result in the loss of important information. In general, pilot testing should enable the experimenter to avoid stimulus levels that a substantial number of subjects consistently fail to detect on repeated presentations. Further discussions of magnitude estimation are available in a number of sources (7,29,35–37).

Magnitude estimation data show how perceived intensity grows with increasing stimulus concentration, but do not speak to absolute perceived intensity or allow comparisons in suprathreshold sensation magnitudes across individuals or groups. To address the latter issue, Stevens and Marks (38) developed the method of cross-modal magnitude matching. Briefly, stimuli from two modalities are alternated within a single experimental session. The subject is asked to assign numerical ratings to all resulting sensations using a single, common scale of perceptual magnitude. One of the modalities serves as the standard and the other as the test modality, the assumption being that individuals or groups are alike in the way they perceive stimuli from the standard modality (eg, brightness or loudness perception in patients with and without hypertension, where the test modality is salt taste perception). The responses to the standard are then used to standardize responses to the test stimuli, allowing direct comparisons between groups in the magnitude of their ratings.

Magnitude matching has been shown to reliably identify large and modest differences between groups in suprathreshold sensation; however, there is also evidence that people find it somewhat difficult to make bias-free judgments of stimuli from different sensory domains on a single scale of sensation magnitude (24). In addition, although group differences may be detected, no conclusions about exactly (or even approximately) *how* intense the sensations were perceived to be can be made. Finally, many people have difficulty assigning numbers to reflect proportional relationships.

Visual analog scales (VAS), which are widely used in pain studies, provide a continuous response format that yields ratio-level data without the need for number assignment (39). Judges are asked to place a mark along a line anchored with semantic labels that reflect their impression

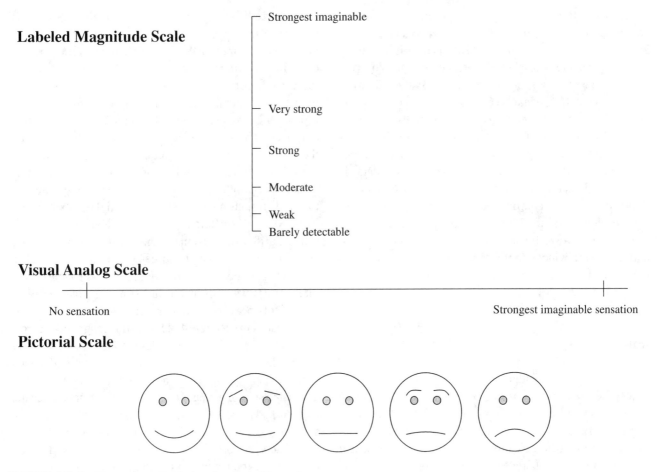

Labeled Magnitude Scale

- Strongest imaginable
- Very strong
- Strong
- Moderate
- Weak
- Barely detectable

Visual Analog Scale

No sensation   Strongest imaginable sensation

Pictorial Scale

FIGURE 18.2   Examples of ratio-level scales of intensity.

of the intensity of the attribute being rated (see Figure 18.2). Ratings are interpreted by measuring the distance from a set point (typically one anchor) to the judge's mark. Analysis is time-consuming and prone to error if done by manual measurement with a ruler. Computer-based data collection programs offer this response format and compute the distances automatically.

More recently, Green and colleagues (40,41) developed the *labeled magnitude scale* (LMS), variants of which have become the scaling instruments of choice in psychophysical studies of the chemical senses (refer to Figure 18.2). This is a continuous scale with multiple verbal anchors that was empirically derived by asking subjects to give magnitude estimates for a variety of common oral sensations together with estimates for a number of intensity descriptors, including "strongest imaginable oral sensation." It has been shown to yield ratio-level data, producing psychophysical functions equivalent to magnitude estimation. However, the addition of semantic descriptors to ratio scales does not necessarily solve the problem

of the relativity of descriptor meanings across context and experience. Although the strongest imaginable oral sensation (including pain) might be expected to be equivalent, on average, across groups of subjects, it now appears that genetically determined differences in tongue anatomy, which are associated with the ability to taste the bitter substance PROP (6-*n*-propylthiouracil), lead to systematic differences in the degree of oral pain individuals are capable of experiencing. For highly sensitive individuals, this might push down their ratings of non-painful taste stimuli on the LMS relative to those given by less pain-sensitive individuals, even if their taste sensitivity is greater. Indeed, by anchoring the top of the LMS with "strongest imaginable sensation of any kind," clearer separation of the bitterness ratings of PROP taster groups can be achieved (32–34). This generalized version of the LMS is referred to as the gLMS.

The strength of ratio scales lies in the level of data generated. Ratio-level data are amenable to potentially useful transformations and the full array of parametric statistical procedures. With some of the procedures now available, ratio scales can provide information about both the rate of growth of sensation and the perceived magnitude of sensation. The primary concern with their use lies in the level of sophistication required of judges.

For many research questions, however, the different scaling methods have comparable sensitivity and yield similar results with appropriate training of judges and control over potential biases (7). A decision about which method to use in a study should be guided by the study objectives, the nature of the study population, and the resources available for data analyses (42–46).

TIME-INTENSITY PROCEDURES

The procedures described thus far require judges to integrate the sensations derived from a stimulus over a given period of time and report the experience in the form of a single number. Consequently, all information about the time course of sensation is lost. Time-intensity procedures involve evaluation of the intensity of stimulus characteristics at specified time points (47).

Following exposure to a stimulus, there is usually a delay before it is detected. The sensation then grows in intensity to a peak and begins to decline. However, the time course of these phases differs for stimulus components because of their varying physical and chemical properties. This idea is easily illustrated for a food placed in the oral cavity. If it is a solid item, it is masticated, resulting in mechanical degradation. Volatiles are also released by this process and, in the case of cold items, by warming in the oral cavity. The speed with which the released taste and odor compounds are transported to their receptive site is determined by the degree to which they stimulate salivary flow and water-lipid-air partitioning coefficients. Chemical interactions may modify all of these steps.

To capture time-intensity information, sensory ratings may be obtained using any of the category or ratio scaling formats described earlier. Tracings of the growth and decline of sensation may also be made with the zero control of a strip-chart recorder or the joystick or sliding bar potentiometer on a computer (47). The timing of ratings will be based on the product under consideration. For example, rapid ratings are required for assessing the carbonation level of a beverage consumed under natural conditions, whereas less frequent responses are needed to trace the perceived burn of a spicy sauce or the sweetness of chewing gum over time. Because the task requires a high degree of attention to the sensory attribute under study, it is not advisable to rate more than one attribute at a time.

Analyses of time-intensity data generally focus on four dimensions: (a) time-related events, such as the delay from stimulus delivery to onset of sensation or to peak intensity; (b) rate-related parameters, such as the rate of growth or decline of sensation; (c) intensity-related attributes, including peak sensation; and (d) event-related indexes, such as breathing or swallowing. Recommendations for analyses of these parameters have been published (48–50).

Time-intensity ratings are highly susceptible to error due to fatigue, reduced motivation, and, depending on the nature of the attribute being rated (eg, odor), poor control over stimulus onset and elimination. These ratings are best obtained using trained judges. The potential biases that judges bring to the task remain largely uncharacterized (51). Thus, the data must be interpreted cautiously.

SPATIAL TESTING

Experimental exploitation of regional differences in sensation have provided new insights of clinical importance. Although the notion that there is a regional tongue map has been discredited (52), there are differences in neural innervation patterns in the oral cavity. By stimulating localized sites, it is possible to gain insights into the fundamental mechanisms of taste reception and to diagnose selective neural damage that may account for taste disorders (53,54). This stimulation is accomplished by swabbing stimuli with a cotton applicator or placing stimulus-soaked taste strips onto selected sites (55,56).

Use of spatial testing in the nasal cavity permits differentiation of the contributions of olfactory and chemesthetic components to sensations elicited by volatile compounds. This problem arises because nearly all odorants also have a pungent quality that is mediated by the trigeminal nerve. As a consequence, the diagnosis of anosmia may be complicated. Because the olfactory system does not encode spatial information, by testing a patient's ability to localize inhaled stimuli, it is possible to identify a potential contribution of the trigeminal sense to test performance (57). A blank sample is presented to one nostril, and a true stimulus is simultaneously presented to the other nostril; the patient is asked to indicate which nostril received the stimulus.

Finally, by manipulating the route of olfactory stimulation, it has been possible to better determine the nature of olfactory complaints in a range of patient populations, notably the elderly. As described earlier, odors may reach the olfactory epithelium orthonasally or retronasally. Sensory disturbances attributable to stimulant access to receptors can thus be identified by testing performance via both routes of stimulus delivery. This testing involves having individuals rate stimuli after sniffing or holding them in the oral cavity with the nose alternately pinched (which blocks retronasal flow) and open. Such studies have demonstrated that the elderly experience a greater decline in retronasal than orthonasal olfaction, and the former is the larger contributor to the flavor of food (58–60). The full potential for various forms of spatial testing to reveal insights into sensory mechanisms, flavor perception, and clinical disorders has yet to be realized.

IDENTIFICATION TESTS

As has been described, the ability of individuals to identify stimuli alone or in mixtures at threshold levels is an index of sensory sensitivity called a recognition threshold. Such a task is also used with suprathreshold stimulus concentrations in both the food industry and clinical settings. Because of common confusion among several basic taste qualities (eg, sour-bitter and salty-sour), identification tests generally are conducted with odors alone or flavors during food ingestion. Odor profiling, identification of the component parts of a complex odor, is used in the food industry for a variety of purposes, such as to evaluate a competitor's product, formulate new products, monitor quality, and check product stability. However, human beings have a limited ability to identify single odor compounds in mixtures (61,62), so odor profiling requires considerable training and may lend itself to instrumental methods.

Odor identification has gained wide acceptance as a means to diagnose olfactory disorders. Patients are presented with an array of common odors matched in intensity and are required to identify the quality. Because people are notoriously poor at retrieving the names of even highly familiar odors (63,64), a multiple-choice answer format is always used. Nonetheless, this test does place memory, language, and labeling (as well as olfactory) demands on the subject.

Descriptions of several tests have been published (65–71). The tests vary in the source (complex mixtures vs pure chemicals) and array of odors used, as well as the format of odor delivery (eg, sniffing the head space over the stimulus in a solid container or squeeze bottle or the use of scratch-and-sniff microencapsulated odors). However, similar rates of diagnosis of olfactory dysfunction in chemosensory centers using different odor identification tests suggest that variations in stimuli and procedural details may have little impact on results, at least in a clinical setting (10).

Odor identification test results generally correlate well with results of threshold tests, and they may have better reliability and require less time to administer (14,72). The primary concerns with odor identification tests are control over stimulus delivery (if stimuli differ in intensity, it may alter performance) and cognitive demands. In addition, poor odor identification ability may reflect odor quality distortions (dysosmia) rather than a simple loss of olfactory sensitivity (10).

DESCRIPTIVE ANALYSIS

Because of the diversity of products that many companies market, the increasing sophistication of food science, and the huge economic consequences of decisions based on sensory data, reliance on the expert opinions of single individuals to guide sensory evaluation in the food industry has diminished. It has been replaced by a wide array of sophisticated approaches, termed *descriptive analysis,* that involve the discrimination and description of the qualitative and quantitative attributes of products.

Broadly, descriptive analysis involves assembling a group of individuals who, through the development of a common lexicon, identify and rate the proportional contributions of salient attributes of products. Depending on the approach, the lexicon may be developed through panel consensus or more formal training with pre-established standards. The attributes rated may be determined by allowing the panel to identify the salient characteristics of the product or by using externally imposed criteria. Ratings may be made using a variety of techniques, including category or ratio scaling.

In some approaches panelists are trained to rate a limited set of products, and in others judges are trained to be generalists able to evaluate a broad range of products. In either case, considerable time and effort are typically invested to train and maintain the skills of judges. Consequently, it is essential to select panelists carefully. Criteria used include normal sensory ability judged by threshold and scaling tests, availability for training and service, and motivation. Personality is also important, because panelists must work as a team. Domineering or passive individuals may impede productivity.

Some approaches culminate in the development of a consensus report, whereas other approaches are amenable to statistical analysis. A more detailed discussion of descriptive analysis techniques may be found in the literature (73–83), and a number of professionals offer short, intensive training courses. Advertisements for these courses are published in *Food Technology* and the newsletter of the Sensory Division of the Society for Food Science and Technology.

AFFECTIVE TESTS (TESTS OF HEDONICS)

Hedonics refers to the pleasantness or appeal of stimuli (eg, foods and beverages). Some sensations seem to be inherently pleasing (eg, sweetness and saltiness) or inherently unpleasant (eg, bitterness), but in light of evidence that maternal diet during pregnancy or lactation may influence the neonate's responsiveness to flavors (84–86), delineation of the role of genetics and learning is problematic.

From a dietetics perspective, perhaps the most important point is that the affective interpretation of different forms and intensities of sensory stimulation is not immutable. It can change with physiological status, including hunger (87,88), pathological conditions (17), and dietary experience (89). Dietary experience, in particular, provides an avenue for dietary interventions. One of the most powerful but complex influences on palatability is frequency of exposure. Familiarity enhances acceptability (90). A second, related influence is culture. Foods seasoned according to the flavor principles of an individual's culture are generally well accepted, whereas other foods are not as well liked despite the lack of a clear biological basis for the superiority of any particular cuisine.

Purposeful manipulation of exposure frequency can support therapeutic diets. By restricting sensory exposure to salt, fat, or sugar, the preferred level of these flavor modifiers declines (91–93). Conversely, increased exposure will lead to a preference for higher levels of the constituents (94,95). However, exposure at too high a level can result in monotony and a decline in acceptability (96). This principle has been used therapeutically to promote reduced energy intake (eg, diets relying on free consumption of single foods). However, the success of such diets has been limited because of the overpowering desire for sensory variety and resultant diet rejection.

Another method of modifying the valence of sensory stimuli is through learned associations. If ingestion of an item is followed by malaise, its future acceptability may be diminished. Taste, odor, and texture are the attributes of food that provide the basis for this shift (97). At the same time, repeated pairing of items with positive experiences, both biological and cultural, may enhance the appeal of foods. This mechanism may be the basis for the desirability of certain items, such as the craving for chocolate when one is under stress or depressed (98).

Hedonics is a multidimensional attribute that is not adequately captured by a single test. Knowledge of the optimal level of a sensory characteristic in a food (one hedonic index) does not provide insight into the desired frequency of consumption of the item (a second index). Furthermore, knowledge of the optimal frequency of consumption of an item characterized by some sensory property does not necessarily provide insight into liking for a range of items with that particular prominent sensory attribute (a third index). Thus, attempts to capture more fully the appeal of the target product should include either carefully selected tests addressing the measure of interest or a battery of tests.

To measure the optimal concentration of an ingredient in a product, samples with graded levels of the key constituent can be presented in random order and rated for palatability. A variety of response formats may be used to capture the information. These formats include measurement of autonomic nervous system responses (eg, respiratory or heart rate) or videotaped mimetic responses to stimulus presentation in subjects unable to respond using more conventional scales (eg, infants or illiterate subjects). Pictorial scales (eg, faces) may also be used when numerical responses are not viable. Category and visual analog scales are used most commonly. Depending on the product, optimization procedures are also possible (99,100). These procedures permit the panelists to actually adjust the level of the target constituent in a food to an optimal point or to indicate how each sample of an array can be manipulated to yield a more palatable product. One potential problem is deciding which food or beverage to use as a model system, because responses to one food may not be predictive of impressions for another food. One solution is to conduct dietary surveys of the target population in order to select the products that are regularly consumed and are important components of the diet. In measuring the optimal concentration, there rarely is a single optimal level of a constituent. More commonly, there is a range of equally palatable, but sensorially distinguishable, formulations (43).

The optimal frequency of exposure to, or consumption of, a stimulus can be measured with the use of scales along with appropriate descriptors, questionnaires, food records, monitored plate waste, or garbage analysis. Such information is critical for menu planning in institutional settings.

Liking for items with a given set of sensory characteristics can be ascertained with questionnaires, analyses of diet records that include information about the predominant sensory characteristics of the foods consumed, information on intent to purchase items, or sensory testing with a broad range of products. It is important to understand that liking and preference are distinct measures. One product may be preferred over another, but both may be acceptable or unacceptable.

Frequently, researchers ask study participants to rate concurrently the intensity and palatability of stimuli. Some researchers believe that the former task confounds the latter because it creates an orientation that is more analytic than is the case under normal dietary conditions. Other researchers contend that the threat of this effect is minimal, and that it is efficient to obtain both forms of information concurrently (101). Analyses of preference testing may be based on the binomial distribution, chi-square statistic, or *z* test on proportions.

In preference testing, judges may have the option of indicating no preference. The advantages of this option are that consumers with no real preference have a logical response option, and the researcher gains insight into the proportion of judges falling into this category. However, this option complicates data analysis and interpretation. The tests previously described assume that a choice between samples is required, so "no preference" ratings must be omitted or recoded according to some arbitrary rule (eg, distributing the "no preference" scores to each product on a 50:50 basis or in proportion to the true preference choices). When judges are not required to make a decision, each judge is free to adopt subjective criteria as to how strong a feeling he or she must hold to be willing to choose one sample over the other. This characteristic introduces an uncontrolled level of variability into the data.

If preferences among a set of more than two samples are to be determined, judges may be allowed to rank the samples. The disadvantage is that the magnitude of differences is not known, and if real foods are used, the attributes upon which decisions are based are not known and may vary across samples. A strength of this approach is its simplicity, which makes it suitable for use with almost any type of sample population. Nonparametric procedures (eg, the Friedman test) are used for analysis.

The interpretation of hedonic data entails several fundamental considerations. Whereas threshold, scaling, time-intensity, and descriptive tests conducted in an industrial setting may be optimized by using trained panelists, this is not the case for hedonic testing. Here, the key outcome is to capture the impressions of potential consumers, whose responses may be based on an entirely different set of influences (eg, convenience, cost, and availability). Another consideration is the fact that hedonic data may be especially susceptible to modification by cognitive factors. For example, providing brand-name information along with test samples can markedly skew responses (102). The brand name may be important information to collect, but it is more a tool of marketing than of sensory evaluation. Health beliefs are another cognitive factor that can modify responses differentially on various scales. For example, ice cream may be regarded as more pleasant than cottage cheese, but the latter may be preferred for health reasons. Finally, hedonic judgments are strongly influenced by temporal cues. Foods customarily consumed in the morning may be less acceptable in the evening and vice versa (103).

PARTICIPANT RECRUITMENT CONSIDERATIONS

Participant selection is critical to the successful outcome of psychophysical studies and sensory evaluation. In the latter case, the expectation for all kinds of evaluation except affective testing is that judges will function as objective, sensitive, and reliable assays. Although people have a range of innate abilities, screening to identify individuals with exceptional sensitivity is not a common practice. Training and standardization of individuals with average abilities can raise performance substantially, and such individuals are more commonly encountered and may have other characteristics (eg, motivation, availability, or team spirit) that make them better suited for sensory studies.

Nevertheless, some individual characteristics may be important to consider during recruitment. These traits may include, but are by no means restricted to, the characteristics listed in Table 18.2. Other issues that vary on a daily basis should be considered, such as the judge's state of hunger, recent diet, and current health status. A judge who has eaten a large meal prior to testing may give lower hedonic ratings to foods and be less motivated to identify subtle differences between stimuli. Olfactory testing on days when an individual is experiencing nasal congestion due to allergies clearly would be inadvisable. In addition to subject characteristics, a host of

TABLE 18.2   Selected Potentially Important Individual Characteristics in Subject Recruitment for Sensory Evaluation Studies

Characteristic	Examples of Rationale
Age	There may be performance limitations at age extremes.
Gender	Sensitivity is generally slightly higher in females; expectations differ.
Smoking status	Smokers show a slight decline in sensitivity, especially olfactory sensitivity.
Genetic traits	Taste blindness and specific anosmia (insensitivity to selected taste and odor stimuli, respectively) are common and may relate to the proposed test stimuli.
Ethnic origin	Varying experience with potential stimuli or innate responsivity to them may bias reporting.
Health status	Acute and chronic health conditions may alter (generally, decrease) sensory function. Changes may be experienced in quality (eg, sweet vs bitter) or modality (taste vs smell), and may be specific or generalized.
Medication use	May alter (generally, decrease) sensory function.
Prior experience with stimuli	May influence test performance (eg, ratings for the burn of certain spices may be skewed by individuals who never use them or who regularly consume them; affective ratings for unfamiliar foods may be low because of neophobia).
Acute food constituent interactions	Recent oral exposure to spices (eg, capsaicin) may decrease the perceived intensity of other irritants.
Health beliefs	May bias judgment (eg, concern about fat, sugar, or salt may result in biased responses to stimuli containing these substances).
Dietary patterns	May influence orientation to stimuli (eg, ratings for breakfast foods may be negatively biased if this meal is not regularly consumed).

TABLE 18.3   Selected Potentially Important Testing Issues in Sensory Evaluation Studies

Testing Issue	Examples of Rationale
Time of day	Cultural norms determine appropriateness of certain stimuli (eg, alcohol or ice cream) at different times of day, and there is slight diurnal variation in sensory system sensitivity.
Nature of stimulus exposure	Stimulus consumption is more "natural" than chewing and expectorating but likely to elicit metabolic feedback that may alter responsivity over time.
Sample size	Statistical power must be balanced with allocation of resources, time, and money.
Fatigue	The number and nature of stimuli to be presented and the pace will influence sensitivity and motivation
Blinding	Unless cognitive influences are being studied, stimuli identifiers or labels that may be perceived to offer clues about their content may bias responses.
Randomization	Failure to randomize the presentation order of stimuli may lead to systematic rating biases; however, if a sample produces lingering sensations that are difficult to clear, it may be best to present it at the end of a session.
Sample presentation	To enhance the ecological validity of testing results, samples should be presented in a format that most closely resembles their intended use. All nonexperimental attributes should be uniform so that subjects rate samples on the property under study. The timing of sample presentation will be dictated by stimulus characteristics; odors and beverages may permit more rapid presentation rates than tastes of lipophilic compounds.
Data handling	Plans for data coding, storage, and analyses should be made prior to study initiation to prevent data loss or corruption.
Subject appreciation	Adequate provisions must be made for subjects to access the test center, wait comfortably and for a reasonable amount of time prior to and between testing sessions, and receive adequate compensation for their time and effort; otherwise, attrition may threaten data integrity.

issues pertaining to the testing protocol must be addressed prior to test initiation. Table 18.3 lists a few selected issues, but the relevant factors will vary according to the nature of the study.

Because psychophysical studies often seek to learn about the mechanisms of sensory function and the basis for individual differences, recruitment strategies may entail the purposeful selection of individuals with contrasting characteristics and capabilities. The same considerations of

subject and testing issues must be made before these types of studies are undertaken, although the decisions may vary from those made for sensory evaluation studies to reflect the different aims of such work. The fundamental point is that both types of study require thoughtful planning. Subtle, uncontrolled influences may invalidate entire studies.

TESTING ENVIRONMENT

A typical sensory testing facility in the food industry includes a waiting area for panelists, a food preparation area, a series of individual booths for product sampling, a group meeting area for descriptive analysis work, an office for the sensory professionals, and a sufficient amount of cold and dry storage capacity. Specifications for each of these components and other functional features have been published (7,8). The need for strict adherence to the various specifications is not clear. Indeed, facilities vary widely across industries. The most critical features are perhaps the most intuitively obvious. The environment should be free of distractions, such as noise, worker traffic, and odors.

INSTRUMENTAL ANALYSES

Interest in instrumental methods for analysis of foods and beverages, including artificial noses and tongues, is growing rapidly. Analytic methods offer a number of unique advantages. They can be used to analyze foods for nutrient composition, as well as for certain ingredients and contaminants that are not strong sensory stimuli. In addition, they can often yield data more rapidly, at lower cost, and with higher precision. They are also ideal for situations where data must be collected continuously (eg, on a processing line that runs 24 hours a day) and where information is needed on products that may contain unpleasant or dangerous constituents.

The principal disadvantage is that such data cannot reflect the affective dimension of sensory evaluation. Predictive models may be developed, but their functionality will always be tied to human sensory studies. The two approaches are complementary.

STATISTICAL ANALYSES

The outcomes of sensory studies may be the basis for multi-million-dollar decisions about product formulation or the diagnosis and management of health disorders. Consequently, conclusions drawn from sensory tests must be based on sound statistical analyses. Excellent, easily readable discussions of basic statistical treatment of commonly used sensory tests are available (7,104). Researchers who are not confident in their statistical skills should consult such references or a statistician prior to study initiation.

There is no point in conducting a poorly designed study. Chapter 28 covers statistical analysis in detail.

CONDUCTING A SENSORY TEST

The following is a general outline of the steps involved in planning and conducting a sensory test:

1. Clearly define the study objective in measurable terms.
2. Determine the appropriate testing methodology, including the types and concentrations of stimuli to be used and the number of replications. If possible, have participants rate a stimulus unrelated to the one of interest or, in the case of clinical studies, a stimulus unaffected by the patient's condition. This procedure serves as a control for test performance alone and aids in determining the specificity of responses. For example, if it is hypothesized that diabetes leads to a reduced ability to perceive sweetness, testing should include another quality, such as saltiness or sourness, to determine whether noted changes are due to a general decrement in sensory function or a decrement that is sweetness-specific.
3. Determine the risks of type I (false positive) and type II (false negative) errors, expected measurement error, within-subject variability, critical effect size, and the required sample size (see Chapters 27 and 28).
4. Estimate the costs of conducting the study.
5. Determine the availability of required resources, including space, facilities, and support staff.
6. Determine the eligibility and exclusionary criteria for subjects and the availability of individuals meeting the stipulated criteria.
7. Obtain approval to use human subjects from a local institutional review board.
8. If practical, purchase all supplies needed to complete the study. This step is especially critical if commercial products will be used, because their availability and formulation may change midway through the study. Plan for food waste.
9. Prepare all instructional materials, response forms, and consent forms, and assemble a full set of forms for each prospective participant. Set up files in a data acquisition computer, if needed. All forms should allow space for subject identification number, date, time, and testing order information.

10. Create randomization orders for subjects if different treatments will be administered, and for test stimuli presentation.
11. Create a master sheet of sample presentation orders, and label sample presentation containers with blinding codes. Use codes that cannot be perceived as conveying information about the sample.
12. Practice all test procedures, and have all response forms checked by an independent party.
13. Recruit study participants. Based on prior experience, estimate attrition rates; oversample to account for this so that the final sample will meet the projected power requirements.
14. Train participants until performance is optimal and stable. Training is not appropriate for affective testing and may not be feasible for clinical patients.
15. Prior to arrival at the test site, prepare test stimuli and portion them out to appropriately labeled containers. All stimuli should be prepared and handled similarly, because subtle differences in temperature, appearance, and other attributes not intended to vary may serve as the basis for responses.
16. Conduct the test.
17. Compile, check, and analyze data.

CONCLUSION

Sensory testing can be a powerful tool for gaining insights into how to match the sensory properties of foods with the sensory abilities of individuals to optimize food choice. Recognition of the scientific rigor required to generate reliable data and awareness of the strengths and limitations of the various methods and approaches will provide a more sound basis for interpreting and applying study findings.

REFERENCES

1. Giese J. Modern alchemy: use of flavors in food. *Food Technol.* 1994;48:106–116.
2. Glanz K, Basil M, Maibach E, Goldberg J, Snyder D. Why Americans eat what they do: taste, nutrition, cost, convenience, and weight control concerns as influences on food consumption. *J Am Diet Assoc.* 1998;98:1118–1126.
3. National Dairy Council. *Dietary Guidelines and Children's Nutrition: A Survey of Health Care Professionals.* Rosemont, Ill: National Dairy Council; 1995.
4. Mattes RD. Fat taste and lipid metabolism in humans. *Physiol Behav.* 2005;86:691–697.
5. Stone H, Sidel JL. *Sensory Evaluation Practices.* 2nd ed. San Diego, Calif: Academic Press; 1993.
6. Dethmers AE, Civille GV, Eggert JM, et al. Sensory evaluation guide for testing food and beverage products. *Inst Food Technol.* 1981;11:50–59.
7. Lawless HT, Heymann H. *Sensory Evaluation of Food: Principles and Practices.* New York, NY: Chapman and Hall; 1998.
8. Meilgaard M, Civille GV, Carr BT. *Sensory Evaluation Techniques.* 4th ed. Boca Raton, Fla: Taylor and Francis; 2006.
9. Doty RL, Bartoshuk LM, Snow JB. Cause of olfactory and gustatory disorders. In: Getchell TV, Doty RL, Bartoshuk LM, Snow JB, eds. *Smell and Taste in Health and Disease.* New York, NY: Raven Press; 1991.
10. Cowart BJ, Young IM, Feldman RS, Lowry LD. Clinical disorders of smell and taste. *Occup Med.* 1997;12:465–483.
11. Pribitkin E, Rosenthal MD, Cowart BJ. Prevalence and causes of severe taste loss in a chemosensory clinic population. *Ann Otol Rhinol Laryngol.* 2003;112:971–978.
12. Goodspeed RB, Gent JF, Catalanotto FA. Chemosensory dysfunction: clinical evaluation results from a taste and smell clinic. *Postgrad Med.* 1987;81:251–257, 260.
13. Cain WS, Gent JF, Goodspeed RB, Leonard G. Evaluation of olfactory dysfunction in the Connecticut Chemosensory Clinical Research Center. *Laryngoscope.* 1988;98:83–88.
14. Smith DV. Assessment of patients with taste and smell disorders. *Acta Otolaryngol Suppl.* 1988;458:129–133.
15. Cain WS. Testing olfaction in a clinical setting. *Ear Nose Throat J.* 1989;68:316, 322–328.
16. Snow JB, Doty RL, Bartoshuk LM. Clinical evaluation of olfactory and gustatory disorders. In: Getchell TV, Doty RL, Bartoshuk LM, Snow JB, eds. *Smell and Taste in Health and Disease.* New York, NY: Raven Press; 1991.
17. Mattes RD, Cowart BJ. Dietary assessment of patients with chemosensory disorders. *J Am Diet Assoc.* 1994;94:50–56.

18. Rankin KM, Mattes RD, Massaro EJ, eds. *Handbook of Human Toxicology.* New York, NY: CRC Press; 1997:347–368.

19. Mattes RD. Nutrition and the chemical senses. In: Shils ME, Olson JA, Shike M, Ross AC, eds. *Modern Nutrition in Health and Disease.* 10th ed. Philadelphia, Pa: Lea and Febiger; 2005:695–706.

20. Cullen MM, Leopold DA. Disorders of smell and taste. *Med Clin North Am.* 1999;83:57–74.

21. Bartoshuk LM. The psychophysics of taste. *Am J Clin Nutr.* 1978;31:1068–1077.

22. Cornsweet TN. The staircase-method in psychophysics. *Am J Psychol.* 1962;75:485–491.

23. Riskey DR. Use and abuses of category scales in sensory measurement. *J Sens Stud.* 1986;1:217.

24. Marks LE, Stevens JC, Bartoshuk LM, Gent JF, Rifkin B, Stone VK. Magnitude-matching: the measurement of taste and smell. *Chem Senses.* 1988;13:62–87.

25. Schifferstein HNJ. Contextual effects in difference judgments. *Percept Psychophys.* 1995;57: 56–70.

26. Lawless HT, Horne J, Spiers W. Contrast and range effects for category, magnitude and labeled magnitude scales in judgments of sweetness intensity. *Chem Senses.* 2000;25:85–92.

27. McBride RL. Stimulus range influences intensity and hedonic ratings of flavour. *Appetite.* 1985;6: 125–131.

28. Hulshoff Pol HE, Hijman R, Baare WFC, van Ree JM. Effects of context on judgments of odor intensities in humans. *Chem Senses.* 1998;23: 131–135.

29. Moskowitz HR. *Product Testing and Sensory Evaluation of Foods: Marketing and R&D Approaches.* Westport, Conn: Food and Nutrition Press; 1983.

30. Anderson NH. Algebraic models in perception. In: Carterette EC, Friedman MP, eds. *Handbook of Perception.* Vol 2. New York, NY: Academic Press; 1974.

31. Bendig AW, Hughes JB II. Effect of amount of verbal anchoring and number of eating-scale categories upon transmitted information. *J Exp Psychol.* 1953;46:87–90.

32. Bartoshuk LM, Duffy VB, Fast K, Green BG, Prutkin J, Snyder DJ. Labeled scales (e.g., category Likert, VAS) and invalid across-group comparisons: what we have learned from genetic variation in taste. *Food Qual Pref.* 2002;14:125–138.

33. Bartoshuk LM, Duffy VB, Green BG, Hoffman HJ, Ko CW, Lucchina LA, Marks LE, Snyder DJ, Weiffenbach JM. Valid across-group comparisons with labeled scales: the gLMS versus magnitude matching. *Physiol Behav.* 2004;82:109–114.

34. Bartoshuk LM, Fast K, Snyder DJ. Differences in our sensory worlds: invalid comparisons with labeled scales. *Curr Dir Psychol Sci.* 2005;14: 122–125.

35. Poulton EC. The new psychophysics: six models for magnitude estimation. *Psychol Bull.* 1968;69:1.

36. Moskowitz HR. Magnitude estimation: notes on what, how, when, and why to use it. *J Food Qual.* 1977;1:195–227.

37. American Society for Testing and Materials. *Manual on Sensory Testing Methods.* Philadelphia, Pa: American Society for Testing and Materials; 1968. ASTM special technical publication 434.

38. Stevens JC, Marks LE. Cross-modality matching functions generated by magnitude estimation. *Percept Psychophys.* 1980;27:379–389.

39. Price DD, McGrath PA, Rafii A, Buckingham B. The validation of visual analogue scales as ratio scale measures for chronic and experimental pain. *Pain.* 1983;17:45–56.

40. Green BG, Shaffer GS, Gilmore MM. Derivation and evaluation of a semantic scale of oral sensation magnitude with apparent ratio properties. *Chem Senses.* 1993;18:683–702.

41. Green BG, Dalton P, Cowart B, Shaffer G, Rankin K, Higgins J. Evaluating the "Labeled Magnitude Scale" for measuring sensations of taste and smell. *Chem Senses.* 1996;21:323–334.

42. Giovanni MA, Pangborn RM. Measurement of taste intensity and degree of liking of beverages by graphic scales and magnitude estimation. *J Food Sci.* 1983;48:1175.

43. Mattes RD, Lawless HT. An adjustment error in optimization of taste intensity. *Appetite.* 1985;6: 103–114.

44. Lawless HT, Malone GJ. A comparison of rating scales: sensitivity, replicates and relative measurement. *J Sens Stud.* 1986;1:155.

45. Lawless HT. Logarithmic transformation of magnitude estimation data comparison of scaling methods. *J Sens Stud.* 1989;4:75.

46. Jaeschke R, Singer J, Guyatt GH. A comparison of seven-point and visual analogue scales. Data from a randomized trial. *Control Clin Trials.* 1990;11: 43–51.

47. Lee WE, Pangborn RM. Time-intensity: the temporal aspects of sensory perception. *Food Technol.* 1986;40:71.

48. Liu YH, MacFie HJH. Methods for averaging time-intensity curves. *Chem Senses.* 1990;15:471.

49. van Buren S. Analyzing time-intensity responses in sensory evaluation. *Food Technol.* 1992;2: 101–104.

50. MacFie HJH, Liu YH. Developments in the analysis of time-intensity curves. *Food Technol.* 1992;11:92–97.

51. Lawless HT, Clark CC. Psychological biases in time-intensity scaling. *Food Technol.* 1992;11: 81–90.

52. Cowart BJ. Taste, our body's gustatory gatekeeper. *Cerebrum.* 2005;7:7–22. Available at: http://www.dana.org/pdf/cerebrum/art_v7n2cowart.pdf. Accessed February 22, 2007.

53. Lehman CD, Bartoshuk LM, Catalanotto FA, Kveton JF, Lowlicht RA. Effect of anesthesia of the chorda tympani nerve on taste perception in humans. *Physiol Behav.* 1995;57:943–951.

54. Yanagisawa K, Bartoshuk LM, Catalanotto FA, Karrer TA, Kveton JF. Anesthesia of the chorda tympani nerve and taste phantoms. *Physiol Behav.* 1998;63:329–335.

55. Bartoshuk LM, Desnoyers S, O'Brien M, Gent JF, Catalanotto FA. Taste stimulation of localized tongue areas: the Q-tip test. *Chem Senses.* 1985;10:453.

56. Mueller C, Kallert S, Renner B, Stiassny K, Temmel AFP, Hummel T, Kobal G. Quantitative assessment of gustatory function in a clinical context using impregnated "taste strips." *Rhinology.* 2003;41:2–6.

57. Wysocki CJ, Cowart BJ, Radil T. Nasal trigeminal chemosensitivity across the adult life span. *Percept Psychophys.* 2003;65:115–122.

58. Stevens JC, Cain WS. Smelling via the mouth: effect of aging. *Percept Psychophys.* 1986;40: 142–146.

59. Cain WS, Reid F, Stevens JC. Missing ingredients: aging and the discrimination of flavor. *J Nutr Elder.* 1990;9:3–15.

60. Duffy VB, Cain WS, Ferris AM. Measurement of sensitivity to olfactory flavor: application in a study of aging and dentures. *Chem Senses.* 1999;24: 671–677.

61. Laing DG, Livermore BA, Francis GW. The human sense of smell has a limited capacity for identifying odors in mixtures. *Chem Senses.* 1991;16:392.

62. Laska M, Hudson R. A comparison of the detection thresholds of odour mixtures and their components. *Chem Senses.* 1991;16:651–662.

63. Desor JA, Beauchamp GK. The human capacity to transmit olfactory information. *Percept Psychophys.* 1974;16:551–556.

64. Cain WS. To know with the nose: keys to odor identification. *Science.* 1979;203:467–470.

65. Schiffman S. Food recognition by the elderly. *J Gerontol.* 1977;32:586–692.

66. Cain WS, Krause RJ. Olfactory testing: rules for odor identification. *Neurol Res.* 1979;1:1–9.

67. Doty RL, Shaman P, Dann M. Development of the University of Pennsylvania smell identification test: a standardized microencapsulated test of olfactory function. *Physiol Behav.* 1984;32: 489–502.

68. Cowart BJ. Relationships between taste and smell across the adult life span. *Ann NY Acad Sci.* 1989;561:39–55.

69. Wright HN. Characterization of olfactory dysfunction. *Arch Otolaryngol Head Neck Surg.* 1987;113:163–168.

70. Hummel T, Sekinger B, Wolf SR, Pauli E, Kobal G. "Sniffin' sticks": olfactory performance assessed by the combined testing of odor identification, odor discrimination, and olfactory threshold. *Chem Senses.* 1997;22:39–52.

71. Doty RL, Marcus A, Lee WW. Development of the 12-item cross-cultural smell identification test (CC-SIT). *Laryngoscope.* 1996;106:353–356.

72. Cain WS, Rabin MD. Comparability of two tests of olfactory functioning. *Chem Senses.* 1989; 14:479.

73. Stone H, Sidel J, Oliver S, Woolsey A, Singleton RC. Sensory evaluation by qualitative descriptive analysis. *Food Technol.* 1974;11:24–34.

74. Schiffman SS, Reynolds ML, Young FW. *Introduction to Multidimensional Scaling: Theory, Methods, and Applications.* New York, NY: Academic Press; 1981.

75. Giovanni M. Response surface methodology and product optimization. *Food Technol.* 1983;11: 41–45.

76. Drewnowski A. New techniques: multidimensional analyses of taste responsiveness. *Int J Obes.* 1984;8: 599–607.

77. Drewnowski A, Moskowitz HR. Sensory characteristics of foods: new evaluation techniques. *Am J Clin Nutr.* 1985;42:924–931.

78. Rutledge KP. Accelerated training of sensory descriptive flavor analysis panelists. *Food Technol.* 1992;11:114–118.

79. MacFie HJH. Assessment of the sensory properties of food. *Nutr Rev.* 1990;48:87–93.

80. Stone H, Sidel JL. Quantitative descriptive analysis: developments, applications, and the future. *Food Technol.* 1998;8:48–52.

81. Szczesniak AS. Sensory texture profiling—historical and scientific perspectives. *Food Technol.* 1998;8: 54–57.

82. Schutz HT. Evolution of the sensory science discipline. *Food Technol.* 1998;8:42–46.

83. Dijksterhuis GB, Byrne DV. Does the mind reflect the mouth? Sensory profiling and the future. *Crit Rev Food Sci Nutr.* 2005;45:527–534.

84. Schaal B, Marlier L, Soussigan R. Human foetuses learn odours from their pregnant mother's diet. *Chem Senses.* 2000;25:729–737.

85. Mennella JA. Infants' suckling response to the flavor of alcohol in mother's milk. *Alcohol Clin Exp Res.* 1997;21:581–585.

86. Mennella JA, Jagnow CP, Beauchamp GK. Prenatal and postnatal flavor learning by human infants. *Pediatrics.* 2001;107:E88.

87. Pangborn RM. Influence of hunger on sweetness preferences and taste thresholds. *Am J Clin Nutr.* 1959;7:280–287.

88. Moskowitz HR, Sharma KKN, Jacobs HL, Sharma SD. Effects of hunger, satiety, and glucose load upon taste intensity and taste hedonics. *Physiol Behav.* 1976;16:471–475.

89. Mattes RD. Innate and acquired taste preferences for the macronutrients and salt. In: Guy-Grand B, Ailhaud G, eds. *Progress in Obesity Research.* London, UK: John Libbey and Co; 1999:173–185.

90. Birch LL, Marlin DW. I don't like it; I never tried it: effects of exposure on two-year-old children's food preferences. *Appetite.* 1982;3:353–360.

91. Bertino M, Beauchamp GK, Riskey DR, Engelman K. Taste perception in three individuals on a low-sodium diet. *Appetite.* 1981;2:67–73.

92. Bertino M, Beauchamp GK, Engelman K. Long-term reduction in dietary sodium alters the taste of salt. *Am J Clin Nutr.* 1982;36:1134–1144.

93. Mattes RD. Discretionary salt and compliance with reduced sodium diet. *Nutr Res.* 1990;10:1337–1352.

94. Bertino M, Beauchamp GK. Increasing dietary salt alters taste preference. *Physiol Behav.* 1986;38: 203–213.

95. Tepper BJ, Harfiel LM, Schneider SH. Sweet taste and diet type II diabetes. *Physiol Behav.* 1996;60: 13–18.

96. Schutz HG, Pilgrim FJ. A field study of food monotony. *Psychol Rep.* 1958;4:559–565.

97. Blank DM, Mattes RD. Exploration of the sensory characteristics of craved and aversive foods. *J Sens Stud.* 1990;5:193–202.

98. Weingarten HP, Elston D. The phenomenology of food changes. *Appetite.* 1990;15:231–246.

99. Moskowitz HR. Subjective ideals and sensory optimization in evaluating perceptual dimensions in food. *J Appl Psychol.* 1972;56:60–66.

100. Sidel JL, Stone H. An introduction to optimization research. *Food Technol.* 1983;11:36–38.

101. Mela DJ. A comparison of single and concurrent evaluations of sensory and hedonic attributes. *J Food Sci.* 1989;54:1098–1100.

102. Moskowitz HR. Mind, body and pleasure: an analysis of factors which influence sensory hedonics. In: Kroeze JHA, ed. *Preference Behavior and Chemoreception.* London, UK: Info Retrieval Ltd; 1979.

103. Birch LL, Billman J, Richards SS. Time of day influences food acceptability. *Appetite.* 1984;5: 109–116.

104. O'Mahony M. *Sensory Evaluation of Food: Statistical Methods and Procedures.* New York, NY: Marcel Dekker; 1985.

19

Research Methods in Appetite Assessment

Richard D. Mattes, PhD, RD, and James Hollis, PhD

Overweight and underweight are prevalent forms of malnutrition globally (1). In many regions, the latter is attributable to limited food availability. However, energy deficiency due to early satiety is also observed, especially in selected clinical populations and the elderly. Overnutrition is widely attributed to the availability of affordable, palatable, and convenient foods but also occurs in less affluent populations with relatively monotonous diets (eg, regions of Brazil, Russia, and China) (2). Recent changes of lifestyle that reduce physical activity have also been implicated in positive energy balance and weight gain. However, these observations also suggest an abnormality of appetite that, according to the body weight homeostatic model, should adjust energy intake to match expenditure. This regulatory role for appetite has yet to be verified but is widely viewed as a key component in the regulation of feeding. Thus, it is important that standardized definitions and methods of measurement be used to facilitate appetite research as well as application of the findings to preventive and therapeutic clinical and public health purposes.

This chapter begins with a discussion of the terminology used in appetite research. The methods commonly used to measure appetite are then critically reviewed. These methods include appetite questionnaires, eating behavior, biomarkers, physiological markers, and energy intake. Finally, the utility of appetite measurement and potential future developments are considered.

TERMINOLOGY

Appetite is the combination of sensations that initiate, maintain, and terminate feeding. Hunger describes the sensations that initiate the search for food and stimulate feeding. Following the initiation of an eating occasion, and as it progresses, sensations that influence the scope of the eating occasion become increasingly dominant. These sensations are termed *satiation*. Eventually, feelings of satiation will contribute to the cessation of eating and the beginning of a period of abstinence from eating. The sensations that influence the length of time between eating occasions constitute satiety. Although hunger and satiation/satiety may seem to be directly opposing sensations on a continuum, this is not the case. The sensations that promote and inhibit eating are governed by overlapping, but distinct, mechanisms. One can report a high level of satiation yet still want to eat, or indicate a strong sense of hunger but choose not to eat. Moreover, although the mechanisms that regulate hunger, satiation/satiety, and food intake have a physiological basis, these sensations are also strongly influenced by environmental and cognitive cues.

There are no widely agreed upon definitions of what constitutes a "snack" or a "meal." Both occasions serve to provide energy and nutrients to the body, but they are commonly distinguished by the timing of the act, along with the energy content and type of food consumed. However, these distinctions offer limited clarity. Some foods (eg, pizza) may be viewed as a meal by one individual and a snack by another depending on the time of day or the quantity that is ingested. Thus, in undertaking scholarly work in this area, it is preferable to refer to eating "occasions," "events," or "episodes" to avoid ambiguity.

METHODOLOGY FOR MEASURING APPETITE

Appetite is an abstract construct and is not amenable to direct measurement. Four indirect measures are widely used: questionnaires, feeding behaviors, biomarkers, and food intake.

Appetite Questionnaires

Due to the human capacity for introspection, much can be determined about subjective appetitive sensations by posing questions about them or prospective eating behaviors. Appetitive questionnaires may require participants to convey their thoughts on defined response scales or via open-ended questions. Either way, appetite is multidimensional and requires a multifaceted approach to its measurement. This fact is now widely recognized, and most appetite studies use a set of standard questions (3) encompassing sensations such as hunger, fullness, desire to eat, and prospective consumption (amount that is predicted to be consumed).

Appetite scales can be used over various intervals. Often they are completed before and after an eating episode to determine the effect of the food or beverage on satiation. Interpretation of data obtained in this manner is complicated because of the strong tendency to indicate a higher motivation to eat before an eating episode and a lower motivation afterward based solely on expectations. If appetite scales are completed repetitively over an eating episode, they can provide insights on the rate of shifts in motivation to eat over the period of ingestion. However, such a procedure is intrusive on the eating episode and may alter eating dynamics. Because appetitive sensations at one time point do not necessarily reflect sensations over a longer, more nutritionally relevant time (weeks to years), it is also possible to collect ratings at stipulated intervals (eg, hourly) over longer time periods (eg, a day or week) (4). Such studies are useful for monitoring the appetitive effects of longer-acting interventions (eg, new diets or activity protocols). This is best accomplished by providing the participant with a personal digital assistant programmed with software that presents the relevant questions and stores the responses. This poses a limited burden to participants and, because each measurement has a time and date stamp, ensures that recordings are made at the stipulated times. It also improves data accuracy by eliminating transcription errors, and it facilitates data manipulation and analyses.

Visual Analog Scales

Visual analog scales (VAS) take the form of an unbroken line, commonly 100 to 150 mm long, anchored on the ends by opposing statements. The end anchors usually represent the extremes of a single dimension (eg, hunger). The validity of the use of mixed scales (eg, from extreme hunger to extreme satiation) has not been established. Further, it should not be assumed that responses on these scales reflect linear increments by judges. As a consequence, interpretation of the magnitudes of treatment effects must be made with caution.

Category Scales

The category scale is similar to the VAS except instead of using a continuous line, participants are forced to choose a distinct category. If the number of categories is very small (eg, three to five), the scale may not allow for sufficient discrimination. However, with a large number of categories (eg, > 13), meaningful discrimination between adjacent categories is also questionable. It is unlikely that differentiation between a rating of 17 and a rating of 18 on a 100-point scale is possible. Category scales are generally constructed with end anchors representing a single dimension, but recently a mixed scale has been proposed and validated (5). It cannot be assumed that sensation grows linearly, so the use of a linear category scale to capture the information may result in anomalous responses. The difference between a rating of 2 and a rating of 3 on these scales should not be seen as the same as the difference between ratings of 8 and 9. Moreover, a rating of 8 is not twice as strong as a rating of 4.

Open-Ended Questionnaires

Open-ended questionnaires have been used to explore issues related to the location, temporal pattern, quality, time course, and intensity of appetitive sensations (6,7). The use of open-ended questionnaires is covered further in Chapter 9.

Appetite scales are frequently used as a predictor of food intake. However, the degree to which subjective ratings of appetite reflect energy intake is debatable. Laboratory studies generally show a modest relationship ($r < 0.5$) between appetite ratings and subsequent energy intake (8). Consequently, appetite scales and food intake measures should be viewed as complementary rather than as predictors of each other.

Eating Behaviors

Measurements of feeding-related behaviors have been developed in an attempt to obtain information less susceptible to the biases inherent in subjective reports captured on questionnaires. A variety of indexes have been used, including electromyographic and acoustic recordings during chewing and swallowing, videotaping, and autonomic nervous system responses. One system that has gained widespread use is the Universal Eating Monitor (UEM). This is a tool to record the amount of food a person consumes in a single eating occasion. The system consists of a set of weight scales that are hidden under a false tabletop and are connected to a computer (9). The computer can also be used to pose questions regarding motivation to eat during the test meal/snack. This system allows measurement of total food intake, rate of eating, and change in rate of eating during an eating episode. Although such measures have yielded important insights, it is difficult to interpret the results in terms of appetite because the parameters measured can be altered by removing cues that influence eating, such as vision (10). Consequently, it is not clear that the parameters measured relate to physiological sensations of appetite. It is assumed that these indexes are related to appetitive sensations, but verification is not possible because there is no gold standard for the latter.

Biomarkers of Satiation

Many physiological indexes, such as gut hormone concentrations, are being explored as biomarkers of appetite. Interest in biomarkers is based on their presumed objective relationship with appetite as opposed to the more subjective questionnaire approach to appetite assessment. For a biomarker to be useful, it must meet a number of criteria. Perhaps most important, measurement of the biomarker must be performed without incurring undue stress or requiring overly invasive procedures. It must also be sensitive to and reliably change in concert with a given appetitive sensation.

Studies of metabolic or hormonal biomarkers of appetite generally proceed in one of two ways. In one type of study, the participant is administered the relevant metabolite, hormone, or control vehicle via tube or intravenous infusion for a period of time. This dosing can be at concentrations that are physiological or supraphysiological depending on the purpose of the study (eg, understanding "normal" responses or proof of principle, respectively). Measurements of appetite are then made at stipulated times using questionnaires (11,12). The effect of the intervention on food intake can also be assessed. This type of study is useful in isolating and evaluating the independent effects of selected metabolites or hormones on appetite or energy intake. Of course, the removal of external influences means that the results from such studies cannot be directly extrapolated to more complex situations. However, these studies provide important information about the role of physiology in appetite.

Another approach is to feed participants different foods or similar foods that have been altered in their characteristics and to then measure the physiological response. In this type of study, a participant would report to the laboratory for baseline measurements. He or she would then be asked to consume a test food/beverage/meal/snack, which is followed by additional biological sample collections at stipulated times over a relevant time frame. The duration of a test will be determined by the characteristics of the dietary challenge and/or the response time of the biomarker to that challenge. Small challenges will likely exert effects for only a short time. A priori assessment of the biomarker's response characteristics is also important. The timing of measurements should reflect the time course of the expected response, with more frequent measurements made during the most dynamic period to best capture the nature of the response. A differential response between dietary challenges in their ability to change putative appetitive hormones or metabolites can then be identified. Because the observations are made under contrived conditions, interpretation of the practical implications of findings should be conducted cautiously. In addition, because many of these biomarkers interact to influence eating behavior, the measurement of an isolated biomarker is unlikely to provide useful information. A brief review of selected physiological biomarkers that reportedly influence appetite follows.

Glucose

Some researchers argue that plasma glucose concentrations are predictive of overall appetite and food intake (13,14). A role for glucose in feeding was first proposed in 1953 by Jean Mayer and was termed the *glucostatic theory of eating* (15). Since that time the concept has been modified, and limited data suggest that a transient decline in plasma glucose is associated with a spontaneous request for food (16), presumably due to hunger. Further evidence supporting a role of blood glucose dynamics in eating initiation comes from infusion studies that report a substantial postponement of eating when glucose levels are held constant (17), interpreted as a satiety effect. These studies suggest that modulation of blood glucose concentration through a dietary intervention may extend the inter-eating interval and potentially result in reduced eating frequency. However, the use of glucose as a marker for eating initiation is not tenable. First, studies demonstrating that a transient glucose decline is associated with eating initiation generally use an insulin dose infusion to artificially reduce plasma glucose. Glucose then often declines to a level not normally observed. Second, the link between the transient glucose decline and a food request is not robust, and individuals often request food in the absence of a change in blood glucose. Third, detecting a transient decline in blood glucose is technically difficult and is not a routine measure. Fourth, independent manipulation of glucose through euglycemic clamp (an experimental technique that maintains circulating levels of glucose at a predetermined, fixed level) studies does not alter either self-reported hunger or fullness (18). Blood glucose is generally correlated with appetitive sensations, but the relationship is not sufficiently reliable to support the use of blood glucose as a biomarker.

Insulin

The degree to which insulin is involved in short-term eating behavior is unclear, with studies suggesting that infused insulin increases (19), decreases (20), or has no effect on appetitive sensations (21,22). The data linking endogenous insulin to food intake is also equivocal. Several studies indicate that insulin has an appetite-suppressing effect in lean people but not in the obese (23,24). However, when glucose levels are held constant, there is no relationship between plasma insulin concentration and appetite or food intake (21,25). Thus, plasma insulin is not a useful biomarker for appetite studies.

Ghrelin

A recently proposed biomarker of appetite is the hormone ghrelin. It is released in the stomach and other parts of the gastrointestinal tract (26,27) and is the only known circulating hormone that stimulates food intake in humans (28). Ghrelin levels are depressed under conditions of positive energy balance, such as obesity (29), and are increased under conditions of prolonged negative energy balance, such as dieting (30). Under conditions of energy balance, ghrelin concentrations rise before eating initiation and then

fall after food consumption (31,32). When ghrelin is infused into humans, subsequent hunger ratings and energy intake increase (33), whereas administration of ghrelin receptor antagonists to rats reduces food intake (34). Several nutrition interventions modify the ghrelin concentration. A high-protein breakfast suppresses ghrelin concentrations more than a high-carbohydrate breakfast (35), whereas a high-carbohydrate load suppresses ghrelin more than one high in fat (36). Thus, ghrelin appears to satisfy most of the criteria for a biomarker of appetite. However, it does not act alone, and gastrectomized patients, who presumably have low ghrelin secretory capacity (30), have normal appetitive function (37). Simply monitoring this hormone is unlikely to yield reliable insights.

Cholecystokinin

Cholecystokinin (CCK) is released from the intestine due to the presence of intraluminal nutrient products. Consequently, CCK levels rise during the 10- to 30-minute period after eating and then gradually fall over the following 3 to 5 hours. CCK release is strongly stimulated by dietary fat and protein, whereas glucose causes a smaller, but still statistically significant, increase (38). A potential role for CCK in food intake was highlighted by Gibbs et al (39), who demonstrated that exogenous CCK administration in rats reduced food intake and eating duration. Since that time, CCK administration has been shown to reduce food intake across multiple species, including humans (40–42). Moreover, the appetite-suppressing effect of CCK on food intake is lost if a CCK receptor blocker is concurrently administered (43). This body of evidence suggests that CCK holds potential as an appetite biomarker. However, its association with appetitive sensations is not consistent, due in part to its relative insensitivity to carbohydrate (44), the primary source of energy in the diet. Further, the fact that there is an elaborate, redundant system of gut peptides that signal the status of substrate availability, or lack thereof, in the GI tract means that chronically increased CCK may not reduce hunger or intake. Ultimately, studies using physiological levels of CCK have found no effect on energy intake (45).

Glucagon-like-peptide-1

Glucagon-like-peptide-1 (GLP-1) is a peptide expressed in the intestinal mucosa and is thought to have a key role in the ileal break mechanism. This mechanism is activated by the presence of nutrients in the ileum and serves to inhibit gastric motility (46). It may be through this route that GLP-1 exerts its effects on appetite and energy intake, although an independent effect is also possible (47). In humans, GLP-1 levels rise after an eating episode, whereas infusion of GLP-1 reduces subjective appetite ratings and also spontaneous food intake at a subsequent eating episode (48,49). This effect is maintained when physiological levels of GLP-1 are infused (50,51). As GLP-1 is secreted in response to nutrients in the ileum, it is unlikely to be involved in eating initiation. It holds promise as a biomarker of satiation or satiety, but, like other GI peptides, it is only one in a cascade of peptides secreted in response to feeding. Thus, the redundancy inherent in the appetite system may obscure its utility for this purpose.

Peptide YY

Peptide YY (PYY) is primarily released from the distal gastrointestinal tract and acts as an agonist on the Y2 receptor in the hypothalamus. This receptor inhibits the release of neuropeptide Y, a potent hypothalamic stimulant of appetite. Intravenous infusion of exogenous $PYY_{(3-36)}$ inhibits 24-hour food intake in humans (52). This reduced food intake is mirrored by reductions in subjective ratings of appetite. To date, limited data indicate that endogenous $PYY_{(3-36)}$ is involved in appetite. Fasting and postprandial circulating concentrations of endogenous $PYY_{(3-36)}$ are lower in the obese than in lean individuals (52). This difference in plasma PYY concentrations is therefore associated with reduced sensations of satiety in the obese (53).

Although the data concerning PYY are promising, it is too early to determine if $PYY_{(3-36)}$ is a robust biomarker of appetite. The association of $PYY_{(3-36)}$ with body adiposity may dampen its sensitivity to feeding-related shifts of appetite. More research is required to elucidate the role of $PYY_{(3-36)}$ in eating behavior.

Leptin

Leptin is the product of the ob gene. Loss of function due to mutation in this gene causes severe obesity in mice and humans (54). However, such a mutation is rare and accounts for very few cases of obesity in humans (55). Leptin is largely, but not exclusively, synthesized in the adipose tissue. Its release from the stomach has also been documented and may be the better predictor of eating-related appetitive shifts. However, gastric leptin is not readily measured, and early studies noted no reliable changes in circulating leptin in the short term (ie, meal to meal). The adipose source of leptin provides information to the hypothalamus about the body's energy stores. In humans, plasma levels of leptin correlate positively with total body fat.

Studies do report a strong correlation between premeal/snack leptin concentrations and energy intake (56). Energy deficits of 24 hours result in decreased plasma leptin concentration, whereas energy surpluses over 24 hours result in increased leptin concentration (57). Consequently, leptin may prove to be a reasonable biomarker to predict the effect of a dietary intervention on body weight change.

Other Physiological Markers

Neuroimaging Techniques

The two brain imaging techniques most frequently used in appetite research are positron emission tomography (PET) and functional magnetic resonance imaging (fMRI). For PET scans, the positron-emitting radioisotope ^{15}O is administered intravenously and distributes throughout the body's tissues. This radioisotope crosses the blood-brain barrier and can be used to measure cerebral blood flow. At the site of brain activation, cerebral blood flow increases, which results in a greater uptake of the ^{15}O tracer and, consequently, an increase in the gamma rays detected in the activated area. Neuronal activity can be thereby measured. A limitation of PET is that images can be taken only every 8 to 10 minutes, which makes this method unsuitable for measuring satiation but potentially acceptable as a marker of satiety. Moreover, the spatial resolution of PET is not as high as that of fMRI. PET is also limited by the use of a radioactive tracer, which precludes multiple assessments on the same individual.

Magnetic resonance imaging works on the principle that when nerve cells are active, they consume oxygen. Therefore, active parts of the brain have a greater concentration of deoxygenated hemoglobin. Due to the magnetic resonance properties of oxygenated and deoxygenated blood, brain activity can be detected using an fMRI scanner. Typical studies involve a baseline image of the brain followed by stimulus administration and further imaging to determine the effect on brain activity. Most of the same limitations noted for PET scanning apply to the use of fMRI for identification of an appetitive biomarker. Both techniques are restricted to specialized research settings at the present time because of the limited availability of instruments and the high cost.

Gut Distention or Motility

Early studies using balloons in the stomach demonstrated a role for stomach distention in satiety (58). These studies reported that as a balloon is inflated, food intake is reduced, suggesting that stomach distention can be used as a marker of appetite. A typical experiment may involve examining the degree and length of time the stomach is distended after ingestion of a test food or meal. Several methods are available for measuring gastric distention, including ultrasound and magnetic resonance imaging.

The rate of gastric emptying is also associated with sensations of hunger or fullness (59). Slower gastric emptying prolongs stomach distention while also prolonging the time that nutrients are in the gut. Therefore, satiety signals arising from nutrients in the gut theoretically will be generated for a longer time, promoting satiety. Methods suitable for the measurement of gastric emptying include ultrasound, magnetic resonance imaging, gamma radiation cameras, radioactive isotopes, breath hydrogen, or absorption of a marker such as acetaminophen (a nonmetabolized compound that can be quantified in the blood).

Evidence indicates that these markers are highly adaptive. For example, chronic distention of the stomach leads to tolerance and loss of sensitivity. The practice of ingesting a large quantity of water just prior to or with a food load as a means to promote satiety via gastric distention has not proven effective. Thus, because measurement requires that participants be in a laboratory setting, the ecological validity of these markers is uncertain. Finally, evidence of normal appetitive responses in gastrectomized patients (33) demonstrates that the measures may, under selected conditions, be sufficient to modify appetite, but are not necessary.

Energy Intake as a Marker of Appetite

It is often assumed that appetite and energy intake are so inextricably linked that one is a measure of the other. From a nutrition perspective, energy intake is the primary outcome due to its role in the development of underweight or overweight conditions. However, energy intake is not an uncontaminated marker of appetite, and measurement requirements or environmental influences can uncouple the relationship. Nevertheless, energy intake is frequently used as a marker of appetite in both short- and long-term studies (60–63).

Time

One approach to appetite measurement is to simply record the timing of eating events. It is presumed that hunger and satiety are related to the interval between eating events in a direct and an inverse manner, respectively. However, this index is of limited value because casual observation indicates that the presumption commonly does not hold. The longest interval between eating events for most people occurs overnight, but few people indicate that they are hungrier upon rising relative to any other time of the day. Instead, appetitive sensations are closely linked to customary lifestyle. Whether this reflects an influence of behavior on physiological processes linked to energy metabolism (eg, gastrointestinal transit, hormone release), cognitive influences, or an interaction between environmental and physiological signals that influence appetite is not established. However, the orderly cycles of appetitive sensations often seen during periods of regular activity, such as patterns during the workweek, are not as prominent in less structured times, such as during the weekend (3). These limitations noted, it is common to test the effects of a particular intervention on the duration of a change in an appetitive sensation. For example, in attempting to develop a high-satiety food, it is reasonable to assess whether one food or form of food augments satiety for a longer period of time than another. However, it bears repeating that should a researcher obtain such an outcome, it cannot be assumed that the food that delays the return of hunger longer will also result in lower total energy intake. Individuals may shift the timing of eating occasions or increase the scope of the fewer eating occasions to offset the stronger satiety effect of a product.

Short-Term Studies Using Energy Intake as a Marker of Appetite

Short-term studies of energy intake are usually conducted in a laboratory environment to permit greater experimental control over relevant variables. Certain influences, such as food attitudes, are difficult to eliminate, but their effects may be reduced through the use of within-subject study designs or by screening participants using validated questionnaires to characterize potentially important traits (eg, dietary restraint, food neophobia). A further advantage of laboratory-based studies is that they permit researchers to accurately measure energy intake as opposed to relying on often-flawed self-reports of intake by free-living individuals. These advantages increase the internal validity of the study.

Typically, laboratory studies are based on the preload paradigm. This entails an initial measurement of appetitive sensations, ingestive intentions, and/or other chosen markers of appetite to establish a baseline. The conditions for this measurement are critical to the interpretation of the assessment. Participants are generally required to report to the laboratory for testing after a specified period of fasting (eg, overnight or 4 hours after the first eating episode of the day). The goal is to standardize the baseline level of hunger and to ensure that participants are willing to eat. However, such a fast does not necessarily accomplish this purpose. In the case of an overnight fast, individuals who customarily eat in the morning will likely be motivated to eat, whereas individuals who do not generally eat at this time will not. To address this issue, participants can be selected based on customary behaviors, although this will result in reduced external validity. Alternatively, the variability can be addressed during statistical analyses through the use of the baseline ratings as covariates or calculation of treatment effects as a change from baseline. The caution here is that such an approach assumes that hunger grows linearly, and this assumption has not been established. In addition, this approach may be compromised by floor or ceiling effects. For example, testing the effect of a food on hunger suppression in a person who is initially not hungry will likely yield limited information because the subject may display little change on whatever scale is used. The timing of assessments also dictates the types of foods or interventions that can be evaluated. Based on the participant's culture or lifestyle, providing him or her with food items that are not considered appropriate at the time of day that testing is conducted may lead to erroneous results. Recruiting a sample of sufficient size can minimize the impact of these sources of variability.

Following the baseline measurement, a food/beverage portion, defined by its energy content, volume, or macronutrient composition, is eaten. This is termed the preload. Depending on the aims of the study, the preload may be of a standard size for all participants (eg, providing 300 kcal or 250 g of the test food) or vary based on the energy/nutrient needs of individual study participants (eg, larger participants are provided with a larger portion of the test food). The former approach emphasizes a property of the stimulus, whereas the latter probably better reflects the nature of the physiological response system.

Too small a preload may result in a response that is not measurable, whereas one that is overly large may lead to a nonphysiological response (ie, a response that is outside normal physiological parameters and would not be encountered during normal eating behavior). A direct relationship between portion size and intake has been documented (64,65). The size and timing of preloads must be determined based on prior experience and the study goals.

In a preload paradigm, the participant is typically asked to consume the preload within an allotted time. Often the time of ingestion is fixed to standardize the challenge posed to participants and to provide a clear time point to initiate the subsequent measurement period. After preload ingestion, appetitive sensations are recorded at stipulated times. One measure of satiety is the length of time appetitive sensations are reduced (eg, hunger, desire to eat) or elevated (eg, fullness). It is also common to present a test food or meal after the preload and allow the participant to eat until comfortably full. The amount of test food/meal consumed can also be used as an index of satiety. The timing of presentation of the test food/meal can be fixed or at the request of the participant. Using a fixed presentation time is more convenient for the researcher and allows a straightforward analysis of intake of the test food/meal. However, this test food/meal is often presented at a time when participants would not spontaneously choose to eat. Consequently, its interpretation requires caution. Allowing individuals to determine the interval between preload and the next eating occasion ensures greater ecological validity. However, this interval may be elongated if the participant feels uncomfortable requesting food. The time interval between preload and first eating occasion is an index of the satiety value of the preload. The amount eaten can also be used to reflect the satiety value of the preload in this paradigm but will be complicated by the fact that different participants wait different periods of time before initiating an eating episode, and thus may do so at different levels of hunger.

There is no correct or incorrect testing paradigm; the tests convey different and complementary information. Often the test food will determine the best experimental approach. One potential intervention (intervention 1) may cause an immediate but short-lived decrease in hunger, whereas another (intervention 2) may cause a lesser but more prolonged drop in hunger. A short, fixed time span between the preload and the test food/meal would lead to the interpretation that intervention 1 has the greater effect on appetite. Conversely, a longer time period would give the impression that intervention 2 exerts a stronger effect. It is therefore appropriate to test potential interventions using several time points to fully assess their effect on appetite.

The strength of short-term laboratory-based studies is that they can control the environment in which the experiment is being conducted; this is also their main weakness. Normal eating behavior takes place in an environment that contains numerous factors that influence food intake, including the number of people present (66), the nature of the surroundings (67), and other distractions (eg, watching television or listening to the radio) (68). In natural settings, people may be exposed to foods at unexpected times and therefore eat while not hungry. Conversely, they may cognitively restrain their food intake and not eat despite being hungry. Therefore, the data obtained from laboratory studies lack external validity, which means the results must be generalized to naturalistic eating with great caution.

An additional threat to the external validity of preload studies is the nature of the test food/meal provided. By design, they are not of limiting size (ie, more food is provided than could usually be eaten). The provision of unlimited free food might encourage participants to overconsume, yielding an erroneous outcome. The use of practice trials may reduce this threat. Moreover, the food that is provided for the participant is often arbitrarily chosen by the researcher and might not be what the participant would have selected. This would likely act to reduce energy intake. Conversely, a varied selection of palatable foods has been shown to augment food intake (69).

The macronutrient content of the test food/meal may also confound interpretation. Macronutrients have differing effects on appetite, with protein being more satiating than carbohydrate or fat (70). Therefore, a participant preferentially consuming a high-protein food from a mixed meal or buffet may increase satiation and reduce food intake independent of the intervention. Providing a homogeneous dish, such as a casserole, minimizes this potentially confounding effect. At the same time, eating occurrences generally encompass a variety of foods, and because variety promotes energy intake, the use of homogeneous foods may result in an artificially reduced food intake (71).

A further concern is that under laboratory conditions, participants might eat only what they feel is a socially acceptable amount of food. To alleviate this problem, researchers have tried to disguise the amount of food that is being provided to the participant. For instance, a device has been devised that surreptitiously replaces the selected amount of soup in a bowl during ingestion (72). Other strategies have included hiding the food from participants so that they cannot use the visual cue of how much they have eaten (73), and cutting sandwiches into unusual shapes and sizes to disorient the participants. The degree to which these strategies work and the validity of responses to such artificial conditions are not known.

Taken together, short-term, laboratory-based studies can yield useful insights. However, the potential confounding factors underscore the fact that findings from such studies should not be uncritically accepted as a true reflection of appetite under free-living conditions.

Long-Term or Free-Living Studies

The use of energy intake as an index of appetite in free-living people is hampered because it is difficult to accurately measure dietary intake under these conditions. Underreporting and misreporting are rife because subjects accidentally or willfully fail to accurately convey information on foods and portions eaten (74). Undereating is also a problem when intake is being monitored. Because of the varied nature of such effects, it should not be assumed that these errors are systematic, especially in comparing the differences between lean and obese individuals (see Chapter 14). Consequently, free-living studies using diet recall methodology are more applicable to within-subject measurement.

Furthermore, the genuine effects of dietary interventions on appetite are likely to be subtle and so, methodologically, may be difficult to detect. For instance, even if the effect of the intervention is biologically significant (say, up to 300 kcal each day), this value is smaller than the errors frequently encountered with the use of diet diaries. To address this problem, it may be necessary to use larger sample sizes or to conduct longer-term studies that would allow for a measurable change in body weight. This is an end point that can be measured more precisely and so requires less statistical power. However, there are drawbacks here as well. Such an approach would require long-term, time-intensive, and expensive studies. Further, it may be difficult to ascribe noted changes to appetitive factors because changes in energy expenditure may occur and intake may be augmented or diminished by nonappetitive factors, such as the availability of foods.

Overall, longer-term studies offer the potential for greater external validity but are weakened by the difficulties of measuring actual energy intake. Ultimately, the value of feeding trials in furthering understanding of appetite is limited by the uncritical circularity of the fundamental argument that we eat because we are hungry and hungry if we eat. Hunger and eating are commonly uncoupled, so one is not a reliable proxy for the other.

CONCLUSION

Appetitive sensations are universally experienced, but there is no widely agreed upon lexicon to describe them and no assurance that they are experienced in a common way by all individuals. Hence, understanding of their etiology, management, and dietary implications is limited. To remedy this, several methods for their measurement are available. Each has its own strengths and weaknesses, and none fully captures the scope of relevant sensations and behaviors. Consequently, the results from any individual measure should be interpreted cautiously. Short-term, laboratory-based studies can demonstrate relationships between a wide array of indexes and appetite. However, the removal of the majority of the environmental factors that influence appetite hampers the extrapolation of findings to free-living behavior. Longer-term studies may be more ecologically valid but do not permit the same level of experimental control and often require large numbers of participants in order to possess adequate statistical power to detect what might be subtle effects of the intervention. Short- and long-term studies each contribute unique information and are complementary.

With their knowledge of nutrition, food science, psychology, and clinical practice, registered dietitians are well positioned to move research on appetite forward. Areas that should prove fruitful include (a) establishment of a quantitative lexicon for appetitive sensations; (b) exploration of new methodologies to better characterize and quantify appetitive sensations; (c) assessment of the environmental and cognitive signals that modulate appetite; (d) evaluation of the hormonal signal patterns that influence appetite as opposed to the effects of single hormones; (e) investigation of imaging techniques to identify the neural bases of sensations and a possible means to quantify them; and (f) ultimately, more expansive studies that integrate these approaches and processes. A more complete understanding may help in attaining the ability to modulate appetitive sensations for health promotion.

REFERENCES

1. World Health Organization. Obesity: preventing and managing the global epidemic. Report of a WHO consultation. *World Health Organ Tech Rep Ser.* 2000;894:i–xii, 1–253.
2. Doak CM, Adair LS, Monteiro C, Popkin BM. Overweight and underweight coexist within households in Brazil, China and Russia. *J Nutr.* 2000;130:2965–2971.
3. Rogers PJ, Blundell JE. Effect of anorexic drugs on food intake and the micro-structure of eating in human subjects. *Psychopharmacology* (Berl). 1979;66:159–165.
4. Mattes R. Hunger ratings are not a valid proxy measure of reported food intake in humans. *Appetite.* 1990;15:103–113.
5. Cardello AV, Schutz HG, Lesher LL, Merril E. Development and testing of a labeled magnitude scale of perceived satiety. *Appetite.* 2005;44:1–13.
6. Mattes RD, Friedman MI. Hunger. *Dig Dis.* 1993;11:65–77.
7. Friedman MI, Ulrich P, Mattes RD. A figurative measure of subjective hunger sensations. *Appetite.* 1999;32:395–404.
8. Herzog AR, Bachman JG. Effects of questionnaire length on response quality. *Public Opin Q.* 1981;45:549–559.
9. Kissileff HR, Klingsberg G, Van Itallie TB. Universal eating monitor for continuous recording of solid or liquid consumption in man. *Am J Physiol.* 1980;238:R14–R22.
10. Linne Y, Barkeling B, Rossner S, Rooth P. Eating and vision. *Obes Res.* 2002;10:92–95.
11. Naslund E, Barkeling B, King N, Gutniak M, Blundell JE, Holst JJ, Rossner S, Hellstrom PM. Energy intake and appetite are suppressed by glucagon-like peptide-1 (GLP-1) in obese men. *Int J Obes.* 1999; 23:304–311.
12. Wren AM, Seal LJ, Cohen MA, Brynes AE, Frost GS, Murphy KG, Dhillo WS, Ghatei MA, Bloom SR. Ghrelin enhances appetite and increases food intake in humans. *J Clin Endocrinol Metab.* 2001;86:5992–5995.
13. Ludwig DS. Dietary glycemic index and obesity. *J Nutr.* 2000;130(suppl 2S):280S–283S.
14. Anderson GH, Woodend D. Effect of glycemic carbohydrates on short-term satiety and food intake. *Nutr Rev.* 2003;61:S17–S26.
15. Mayer J. Glucostatic mechanism of regulation of food intake. *N Engl J Med.* 1953;249:13–16.
16. Campfield LA, Smith FJ, Rosenbaum M, Hirsch J. Human eating: evidence for a physiological basis using a modified paradigm. *Neurosci Biobehav Rev.* 1996;20:133–137.
17. Campfield LA, Brandon P, Smith FJ. On-line continuous measurement of blood glucose and meal pattern in free-feeding rats: the role of glucose in meal initiation. *Brain Res Bull.* 1985;14:605–616.
18. Chapman IM, Goble EA, Wittert GA, Morley JE, Horowitz M. Effect of intravenous glucose and euglycemic insulin infusions on short-term appetite and food intake. *Am J Physiol Regul Integr Comp Physiol.*1998;43:R596–R603.
19. Rodin J, Wack J, Ferrannini E, DeFronzo RA. Effect of insulin and glucose on feeding behavior. *Metabolism.* 1985;34:826–831.
20. Holt SHA, Miller JB. Increased insulin responses to ingested foods are associated with lessened satiety. *Appetite.* 1995;24:43–54.

21. Gielkens HA, Verkijk M, Lam WF, Lamers CB, Masclee AA. Effects of hyperglycemia and hyperinsulinemia on satiety in humans. *Metabolism.* 1998;47:321–324.

22. Woo R, Kissileff HR, Pi-Sunyer FX. Elevated postprandial insulin levels do not induce satiety in normal-weight humans. *Am J Physiol.* 1984;247: R745–R749.

23. Speechly DP, Buffenstein R. Appetite dysfunction in obese males: evidence for role of hyperinsulinaemia in passive overconsumption with a high fat diet. *Eur J Clin Nutr.* 2000;54:225–233.

24. Verdich C, Toubro S, Buemann B, Lysgard Madsen J, Juul Holst J, Astrup A. The role of postprandial releases of insulin and incretin hormones in meal-induced satiety—effect of obesity and weight reduction. *Int J Obes Relat Metabol Disord.* 2001; 25:1206–1214.

25. Lavin JH, Wittert G, Sun WM, Horowitz M, Morley JE, Read NW. Appetite regulation by carbohydrate: role of blood glucose and gastrointestinal hormones. *Am J Physiol.* 1996;271:E209–E214.

26. Asakawa A, Inui A, Kaga T, Yuzuriha H, Nagata T, Ueno N, Makino S, Fujimiya M, Niijima A, Fujino MA, Kasuga M. Ghrelin is an appetite-stimulatory signal from stomach with structural resemblance to motilin. *Gastroenterology.* 2001;120:337–345.

27. Kojima M, Hosoda H, Date Y, Nakazato M, Matsuo H, Kangawa K. Ghrelin is a growth-hormone-releasing acylated peptide from stomach. *Nature.* 1999;402:656–660.

28. Schmid DA, Held K, Ising M, Uhr M, Weikel JC, Steiger A. Ghrelin stimulates appetite, imagination of food, GH, ACTH, and cortisol, but does not affect leptin in normal controls. *Neuropsychopharmacology.* 2005;30:1187–1192.

29. Tschop M, Weyer C, Tataranni PA, Devanarayan V, Ravussin E, Heiman ML. Circulating ghrelin levels are decreased in human obesity. *Diabetes.* 2001;50: 707–709.

30. Cummings DE, Weigle DS, Frayo RS, Breen PA, Ma MK, Dellinger EP, Purnell JQ. Plasma ghrelin levels after diet-induced weight loss or gastric bypass surgery. *N Engl J Med.* 2002;346: 1623–1630.

31. Cummings DE, Purnell JQ, Frayo RS, Schmidova K, Wisse BE, Weigle DS. A preprandial rise in plasma ghrelin levels suggests a role in meal initiation in humans. *Diabetes.* 2001;50: 1714–1719.

32. Cummings DE, Frayo RS, Marmonier C, Aubert R, Chapelot D. Plasma ghrelin levels and hunger scores in humans initiating meals voluntarily without time- and food-related cues. *Am J Physiol Endocrinol Metab.* 2004;287:E297–E304.

33. Wren AM, Seal LJ, Cohen MA, Brynes AE, Frost GS, Murphy KG, Dhillo WS, Ghatei MA, Bloom SR. Ghrelin enhances appetite and increases food intake in humans. *J Clin Endocrinol Metab.* 2001;86:5992–5995.

34. Asakawa A, Inui A, Kaga T, Katsuura G, Fujimiya M, Fujino MA, Kasuga M. Antagonism of ghrelin receptor reduces food intake and body weight gain in mice. *Gut.* 2003;52:947–952.

35. Blom WAM, Lluch A, Stafleu A, Vinoy S, Holst JJ, Schaafsma G, Hendriks HFJ. Effect of a high-protein breakfast on the postprandial ghrelin response. *Am J Clin Nutr.* 2006;83:211–220.

36. Monteleone P, Bencivenga R, Longobardi N, Serritella C, Maj M. Differential responses of circulating ghrelin to high-fat or high-carbohydrate meal in healthy women. *J Clin Endocrinol Metab.* 2003;88:5510–5514.

37. Bergh C, Sjostedt S, Hellers G, Zandian M, Sodersten P. Meal size, satiety and cholecystokinin in gastrectomized humans. *Physiol Behav.* 2003;78: 143–147.

38. Liddle RA, Goldfine LD, Rosen MS, Taplitz RA, Williams JA. Cholecystokinin bioactivity in human plasma. Molecular forms, responses to feeding, and relationship to gallbladder contraction. *J Clin Invest.* 1985;75:1144–1152.

39. Gibbs J, Young RC, Smith GP. Cholecystokinin decreases food intake in rats. *J Comp Physiol Psychol.* 1973;84:488–495.

40. MacIntosh CG, Morley JE, Wishart J, Morris H, Jansen JB, Horowitz M, Chapman IM. Effect of exogenous cholecystokinin (CCK)-8 on food intake and plasma CCK, leptin, and insulin concentrations in older and young adults: evidence for increased CCK activity as a cause of the anorexia of aging. *J Clin Endocrinol Metab.* 2001;86:5830–5837.

41. Muurahainen N, Kissileff HR, Derogatis AJ, Pi-Sunyer FX. Effects of cholecystokinin-octapeptide (CCK-8) on food intake and gastric emptying in man. *Physiol Behav.* 1988;44:645–649.

42. Kissileff HR, Pi-Sunyer FX, Thornton J, Smith GP. C-terminal octapeptide of cholecystokinin decreases food intake in man. *Am J Clin Nutr.* 1981;34: 154–160.

43. Reidelberger RD, Castellanos DA, Hulce M. Effects of peripheral CCK receptor blockade on food intake in rats. *Am J Physiol Regul Integr Comp Physiol.* 2003;285:R429–R437.

44. Bowen J, Noakes M, Trenerry C, Clifton PM. Energy intake, ghrelin, and cholecystokinin after different carbohydrate and protein preloads in overweight men. *J Clin Endocrinol Metab.* 2006;91:1477–1483.

45. Lieverse RJ, Jansen JB, van de Zwan A, Samson L, Masclee AA, Lamers CB. Effects of a physiological dose of cholecystokinin on food intake and postprandial satiation in man. *Regul Pept.* 1993;43:83–89.

46. Naslund E, Gutniak M, Skogar S, Rossner S, Hellstrom PM. Glucagon-like peptide 1 increases the period of postprandial satiety and slows gastric emptying in obese men. *Am J Clin Nutr.* 1998;68: 525–530.

47. Chelikani PK, Haver AC, Reidelberger RD. Intravenous infusion of glucagon-like peptide-1 potently inhibits food intake, sham feeding, and gastric emptying in rats. *Am J Physiol Regul Integr Comp Physiol.* 2005;288:R1695–R1706.

48. Flint A, Raben A, Astrup A, Holst JJ. Glucagon-like peptide 1 promotes satiety and suppresses energy intake in humans. *J Clin Invest.* 1998;101:515–520.

49. Naslund E, Barkeling B, King N, Gutniak M, Blundell JE, Holst JJ, Rossner S, Hellstrom PM. Energy intake and appetite are suppressed by glucagon-like peptide-1 (GLP-1) in obese men. *Int J Obes Relat Metab Disord.* 1999;23:304–311.

50. Flint A, Raben A, Ersboll AK, Holst JJ, Astrup A. The effect of physiological levels of glucagon-like peptide-1 on appetite, gastric emptying, energy and substrate metabolism in obesity. *Int J Obes Relat Metab Disord.* 2001;25:781–792.

51. Gutzwiller JP, Goke B, Drewe J, Hildebrand P, Ketterer S, Handschin D, Winterhalder R, Conen D, Beglinger C. Glucagon-like peptide-1: a potent regulator of food intake in humans. *Gut.* 1999;44:81–86.

52. Batterham RL, Cohen MA, Ellis SM, Le Roux CW, Withers DJ, Frost GS, Ghatei MA, Bloom SR. Inhibition of food intake in obese subjects by peptide YY3-36. *N Engl J Med.* 2003;349:941–948.

53. Le Roux CW, Batterham RL, Aylwin SJ, Patterson M, Borg CM, Wynne KJ, Kent A, Vincent RP, Gardiner J, Ghatei MA, Bloom SR. Attenuated peptide YY release in obese subjects is associated with reduced satiety. *Endocrinology.* 2006;147:3–8.

54. Zhang YY, Proenca R, Maffei M, Barone M, Leopold L, Friedman JM. Positional cloning of the mouse obese gene and its human homologue. *Nature.* 1994;372:425–432.

55. Maffei M, Stoffel M, Barone M, Moon B, Dammerman M, Ravussin E, Bogardus C, Ludwig DS, Flier JS, Talley M. Absence of mutations in the human OB gene in obese/diabetic subjects. *Diabetes.* 1996;45: 679–682.

56. Chapelot D, Aubert R, Marmonier C, Chabert M, Louis-Sylvestre J. An endocrine and metabolic definition of the intermeal interval in humans: evidence for a role of leptin on the prandial pattern through fatty acid disposal. *Am J Clin Nutr.* 2000;72: 421–431.

57. Chin-Chance C, Polonsky KS, Schoeller DA. Twenty-four-hour leptin levels respond to cumulative short-term energy imbalance and predict subsequent intake. *J Clin Endocrinol Metab.* 2000;85:2685–2691.

58. Geliebter A. Gastric distension and gastric capacity in relation to food intake in humans. *Physiol Behav.* 1988;44:665–668.

59. Cecil JE, Francis J, Read NW. Comparison of the effects of a high-fat and high-carbohydrate soup delivered orally and intragastrically on gastric emptying, appetite, and eating behaviour. *Physiol Behav.* 1999;67:299–306.

60. Mattes RD, Hollis J, Hayes D, Stunkard AJ. Appetite: measurement and manipulation misgivings. *J Am Diet Assoc.* 2005;105(5 suppl 1): S87–S97.

61. Anderson GH, Woodend D. Effect of glycemic carbohydrates on short-term satiety and food intake. *Nutr Rev.* 2003;61(suppl):S17–S26.

62. Batterham RL, Cohen MA, Ellis SM, Le Roux CW, Withers DJ, Frost GS, Ghatei MA, Bloom SR. Inhibition of food intake in obese subjects by peptide YY3-36. *N Engl J Med.* 2003;349:941–948.

63. Alper CM, Mattes RD. Effects of chronic peanut consumption on energy balance and hedonics. *Int J Obes Relat Metab Disord.* 2002;26:1129–1137.

64. Rolls BJ, Roe LS, Meengs JS, Wall DE. Increasing the portion size of a sandwich increases energy intake. *J Am Diet Assoc.* 2004;104:367–372.

65. Rolls BJ, Morris EL, Roe LS. Portion size of food affects energy intake in normal-weight and overweight men and women. *Am J Clin Nutr.* 2002;76: 1207–1213.

66. de Castro JM, Brewer EM. The amount eaten in meals by humans is a power function of the number of people present. *Physiol Behav.* 1992;51: 121–125.

67. Meiselman HL, Johnson JL, Reeve W, Crouch JE. Demonstrations of the influence of the eating environment on food acceptance. *Appetite*. 2000;35: 231–237.

68. Poothullil JM. Role of oral sensory signals in determining meal size in lean women. *Nutrition*. 2002;18:479–483.

69. De Graaf C, De Jong LS, Lambers AC. Palatability affects satiation but not satiety. *Physiol Behav*. 1999;66:681–688.

70. Poppitt SD, McCormack D, Buffenstein R. Short-term effects of macronutrient preloads on appetite and energy intake in lean women. *Physiol Behav*. 1998;64:279–285.

71. Rolls BJ, Rowe EA, Rolls ET, Kingston B, Megson A, Gunary R. Variety in a meal enhances food intake in man. *Physiol Behav*. 1981;26: 215–221.

72. Wansink B, Painter JE, North J. Bottomless bowls: why visual cues of portion size may influence intake. *Obes Res*. 2005;13: 93–100.

73. Linne Y, Barkeling B, Rossner S, Rooth P. Vision and eating behavior. *Obes Res*. 2002;10: 92–95.

74. Hill RJ, Davies PS. The validity of self-reported energy intake as determined using the doubly labelled water technique. *Br J Nutr*. 2001;85: 415–430.

PART 7

Key Aspects of Research in Food, Nutrition, and Dietetics

20

Outcomes Research and Economic Analysis

Patricia L. Splett, PhD, RD, FADA

Across the health care system, organizations are examining the structure and processes of care, its outcomes, and its cost; they are then using these data to improve the consistency, effectiveness, and efficiency of care. These activities have taken many forms over the years, including peer review, quality assurance, total quality management, continuous quality improvement, and more recently, outcomes measurement and performance improvement. Outcomes research and economic analysis are important research approaches to apply in practice settings. Registered dietitians (RDs) along with other members of the health care team are encouraged to make outcomes research a standard part of their practice (1).

Policy makers are interested in the impact of health care, including discrete interventions as well as broader programmatic or system interventions, on the health outcomes of patients and populations (2,3). Outcomes research planned and conducted at this level is sometimes referred to as *medical effectiveness research*, and its results become part of the body of evidence used in evidence-based practice. The goal of medical effectiveness research is to shape health care policy, including reimbursement; affect clinical practice, such as through clinical practice guidelines; define programs; and, ultimately, improve health outcomes across the country. At this level, greater weight is given to the external validity and generalizability of findings so that they can be applicable across settings and population groups.

OUTCOMES RESEARCH

Outcomes and Effectiveness Research

Attention to outcomes (ie, "a change in status confidently attributable to antecedent care," according to Donabedian [4]) has greatly increased since the beginning of the outcomes movement in the late 1980s (5), and the movement continues to attract the attention of health care systems, decision makers, and practitioners (6,7). Outcomes research/medical effectiveness research (now also called *outcomes and effectiveness research*) is used to evaluate the effectiveness of preventive, diagnostic, and therapeutic procedures, treatments, and programs. It answers the following questions: Does it work? What is the magnitude of the effect? Is the effect large enough to be clinically meaningful? Outcomes research investigates the results of interventions as they are used in typical practice settings and determines their effectiveness. In contrast, randomized clinical trials conducted under tightly controlled conditions are used to establish a causal relationship and determine efficacy. Efficacy proves something "can work," whereas effectiveness verifies that it "does work" when applied in routine practice. A range of outcomes are considered in outcomes and effectiveness research. The key outcomes of interest differ depending on who (RDs, other health care providers, health care administrators, payers/buyers, policy makers, or patients) is using the information. Carefully selected evaluation and research methods are used to determine whether the procedure or care process does lead to the desired results (3). An aim of outcomes and effectiveness research is to determine what approaches work best for most patients or clients in routine settings and at what cost.

There is some debate over the types of studies used to determine effectiveness. How the conclusion is to be applied determines which study design in the hierarchy is required. When evidence of effectiveness is used to develop broadly disseminated guidelines, such as the National Institutes of Health's Obesity Guidelines, studies at the top of the hierarchy are desired (see Chapter 12 for a hierarchy of study types). This chapter takes a more liberal view of research designs for outcomes and effectiveness studies; it considers situations in which RDs conduct outcomes studies to assess the effects of nutrition interventions in a more localized environment.

Costs can also be investigated in outcomes studies. Costs include both the cost of delivering specific interventions and the costs associated with the resulting consequences, such as health care resources saved by positive health outcomes. This cost concern closely links outcomes and effectiveness research to cost-effectiveness analysis. Methods of economic analysis (discussed later in this chapter) examine effectiveness and costs to determine the cost-effectiveness of competing interventions.

The findings from outcomes research inform decisions about implementing, expanding, or changing care processes. The findings are also used, along with findings from other research approaches, to develop evidence-based protocols, clinical practice guidelines, and clinical pathway or care maps that foster the use of the most effective and cost-effective practices across the system (7–9). Outcomes research also aids planning and decision making by providing data on which to base prediction of future clinical, cost, and patient outcomes if specific interventions, procedures, or treatments are adopted.

Types of Outcomes

Three outcome categories are traditionally assessed in health care outcomes research: clinical outcomes, patient outcomes, and cost outcomes. However, to study the immediate effects of nutrition care and to elucidate the linkage of nutrition intervention to health care outcomes, additional categories organized as nutrition care outcomes (behavior and environmental outcomes, intake outcomes, and physical sign and symptom outcomes) must be included. When an outcomes study is planned, the outcomes most relevant to the study question and purpose are identified and defined as indicators for measurement. It is extremely helpful and highly recommended for researchers to draw out the hypothesized relationship between the intervention to be studied and the chain of consequences across all types of outcomes. This process is illustrated in general terms in Table 20.1 and with a specific example in Table 20.2. Although the entire chain of consequences represents potential outcomes, researchers define a few key outcomes that are operationalized as indicators and become the focus of the study. The exact outcome indicators that will be measured and the specification of clinically meaningful changes in the indicators are based on scientific studies, expert judgment, or established norms (7).

Nutrition Care Outcomes

Nutrition care outcomes are the direct consequences of nutrition intervention (eg, medical nutrition therapy [MNT], enteral or parenteral nutrition support, supplemental feeding,

TABLE 20.1   Chain of Outcomes of Nutrition Care

	Nutrition Care Outcomes			Health Care Outcomes		
	Nutrition-Related Behavior and Environmental Outcomes	**Food and Nutrient Intake Outcomes**	**Nutrition-Related Physical Sign and Symptom Outcomes**	**Clinical Outcomes**	**Cost Outcomes**	**Patient Outcomes**
	→	→	→	→	→	→
Appropriate nutrition intervention leads to:	• Changes in knowledge, attitudes, and behavior • Access to food	• Improved nutrient intake	• Changes in (normalization of) anthropometric, biochemical, and physical exam indexes	• Improvement of disease or condition • Prevention of adverse event	• Reduced diagnostic and treatment costs • Decreased hospital and outpatient visits	• Reduced disability • Increased quality of life

TABLE 20.2   Chain of Outcomes Resulting from Weight Management Program (12-Month Period)

	Direct Nutrition Care Outcomes					
	Nutrition-Related Behavior and Environmental Outcomes	**Food and Nutrient Intake Outcomes**	**Nutrition-Related Physical Sign and Symptom Outcomes**	**Clinical Outcomes**	**Cost Outcomes**	**Patient Outcomes**
	$\rightarrow$	$\rightarrow$	$\rightarrow$	$\rightarrow$	$\rightarrow$	$\rightarrow$
12-week group weight management program leads to:	• Knowledge of food choices • Awareness of eating cues and responses • Self-efficacy • Increased physical activity	• Reduced energy intake • Healthful eating pattern consistent with Dietary Guidelines	• 12-week weight loss • 12-month weight loss • Reduced waist circumference • Decreased serum cholesterol	• Improved blood pressure	• Reduced hypertension medication	• Increased quality of life • Improved self-confidence

education and counseling, or a community nutrition program). General categories of nutrition outcomes are changes in knowledge, attitude, or behavior; changes in food or nutrient intake; and changes in biochemical tests and physiological outcomes. Outcomes of interest are identified in evidence-based guides for dietetics practice, practice guidelines, nutrition care manuals, individualized patient goals, and community nutrition program goals. They are operationalized for measurement as specific indicators such as score on a knowledge test or attitude scale, servings of fruit and vegetables, glycosylated hemoglobin level, weight change, and number of hypoglycemic events.

Health Care Outcomes

Clinical outcomes.   Clinical outcomes are the health status–related outcomes such as changes in the progression or severity of signs or symptoms of disease and its sequelae, and complications resulting from the disease or condition or its treatment, including mortality. Selection of clinical outcomes for evaluation is determined by what indicators are the most relevant and important outcomes of health or disease progression in the specific life cycle stage, condition, or disease state and which ones have a logical and biologically plausible relationship with nutrition. The indicators change depending on the time horizon of the study. In some situations, clinical signs in the next few days are of interest; in other situations, the outcome of interest is disease severity or mortality several months or even years later.

Patient outcomes.   Patient outcomes emphasize the consequences of an intervention that are of concern to patients and their families. These consequences include survival, symptom relief, adverse effects of the condition or its

treatment, functional status, quality of life, and satisfaction with care (3). Nutritional status has been shown to be related to patients' functional status, including psychological and cognitive performance, psychosocial status, and performance of activities of daily living (10). Patient-related outcomes extend from the individual to community systems (11).

Assessment of patients' perceptions of nutrition care services and the effect of nutrition on quality of life are relatively new areas in nutrition research and outcomes assessment (12). An early study identified a range of health and nonhealth benefits that patients gained from nutrition counseling, including reassurance, sense of control, and relief of symptoms (13). Other studies have shown a link between nutrition-related biochemical parameters and patients' quality of life (14).

Outcomes as perceived by the patient and family are also related to the willingness of individuals and society in general to pay for health and nutrition care. If it is perceived that improved health outcomes result from nutrition intervention, then individuals and society will demand, and be willing to pay for, these interventions. Demand and willingness to pay diminish, however, if care is perceived to be of poor quality, to have little effect, and to be of high cost.

Cost outcomes.   The financial implications of a specific intervention or procedure are considered cost outcomes. Cost outcomes are derived from documented health care utilization, which can include diagnostic and treatment costs, charges for outpatient visits and hospitalization, and medical equipment costs. Some outcomes studies also include the financial impact of the disease and its treatment on patients. Technically, cost outcomes include the input cost to provide the intervention or procedure (eg, cost of course of enteral nutrition support) as well as the cost associated with the consequences of the outcomes produced—which may be positive or negative. Inclusion of the costs of inputs as well as outcomes is used in the analysis of cost-effectiveness, discussed later. Cost outcomes are of major importance to health care administrators and policy makers.

Methods Used in Outcomes Research

The challenge of outcomes research is to determine the magnitude of effect attributable to the intervention (2,3). Many designs have been used, including observational, correlational, quasi-experimental, and randomized controlled trials. All can provide information to quantify the effect, but well-designed quasi-experimental and experimental designs are needed to confirm the causal relationships linking the intervention to the outcomes.

There is debate about which methods are suitable (2,15). The essence of the debate concerns the relative merits of observational vs randomized studies. Although observational studies have the advantage of most closely approximating usual care, they cannot provide definitive answers to many questions about comparative clinical effectiveness. Trotter emphasizes that prospective studies that are naturalistic in design produce results with greater validity to actual practice than do tightly controlled trials with rigid eligibility criteria and tightly defined protocols (16). Others recommend more traditional randomized controlled designs because they overcome the potential bias inherent in observational and quasi-experimental studies (17). However, randomized clinical trials lack generalizability across the range of settings and patients encountered in usual practice. An answer to this dilemma may be prospective effectiveness trials that afford randomization of similar patients to intervention alternatives but that are conducted in routine practice settings. Other factors influencing the selection of study design are the type and amount of existing research in the practice area. Often observational studies precede randomized trials.

Observational and quasi-experimental studies have several advantages over randomized controlled trials, including lower cost, greater timeliness, and inclusion of a greater range of patients. These designs are used when there are practical or ethical barriers to conducting randomized trials. Before-and-after studies without a comparison group are weak designs whose validity are subject to many threats and generally are not recommended. If this study design is used, findings must be interpreted with great caution. Controlled before-and-after studies (in which

a population with similar characteristics serves as the comparison group, and data are collected in both populations at the same time using the same methods) can give an estimate of effect. However, this study design requires a well-matched comparison group and appropriate techniques of data collection and statistical analysis to control for intervening factors. Other quasi-experimental designs, their strengths and weaknesses, and recommended statistical analysis approaches have been described (2,15).

Two questions can be asked in considering a study design (3): How likely is it that bias could affect the findings? How certain of the results must one be in order to change policy or practice? In outcomes and effectiveness research, as in any research effort, the design and methods selected must match the research question, the planned application of the findings, and the resources available for conducting the study while minimizing threats to validity. These issues are addressed throughout this book. In spite of the controversy, a common process, outlined in Box 20.1, is used to plan and conduct outcomes and effectiveness studies.

Results of Outcomes Research

The final result of an outcomes study should be a quantitative estimate of (a) the magnitude of effect in outcome associated with, or attributed to, the studied intervention or interventions; and (b) the proportion of patients, clients, or the population who benefit from access to, and participation in, the intervention. Both the statistical and clinical significance of results should be reported. Other results that can be presented in quantitative or qualitative terms are variation in provision of the intervention, costs, client characteristics associated with positive or negative outcomes (such as risk level used in case mix analysis), other important outcomes, and intervening or confounding factors. Results can then be used to guide resource allocation to the most effective interventions.

Challenges of Outcomes Research

Outcomes research can be conducted prospectively or retrospectively. Prospective studies are carried out from the present to the future. The advantages are the ability to control for confounding factors and potential bias; as a result, a prospective study is a more powerful design for establishing cause and effect. A challenge is allocating sufficient staff and resources to implement the study and oversee its management over a period of time. Standardized measurements and consistent documentation should be used throughout the

BOX 20.1 Outcomes and Effectiveness Research: Planning and Conducting a Study

Define the research purpose and question or questions:
- Describe the intervention, procedure, or program to be evaluated.
- Identify and describe its alternatives.

Determine the key outcome or outcomes:
- Specify indicators of the key outcome and the appropriate time period for their measurement.
- Identify other important positive and negative outcomes to be tracked.

Design the study, and specify procedures for data collection:
- Define the relevant population.
- Determine the sample size and the method of sampling.
- Establish points to measure outcome and other indicators, considering the period of time necessary for the effect to occur.
- Define all data elements to be included (with the aim of "controlling" relevant elements either through design or by statistical analytic techniques), considering intervention details, patient or client characteristics, key outcomes and other outcomes, and intervening and confounding factors.
- Develop and pilot test forms and procedures for data collection.
- Determine data analysis methods.

Collect data according to procedures:
- Train data collectors.
- Monitor quality and completeness of data.

Analyze the data:
- Code and enter the data.
- Assess the clinical importance of the data.
- Assess the data's statistical significance.

Interpret and report the results.

Act on the findings.

study. A disadvantage is potential bias related to the investigator or provider when either is aware of the alternatives being studied.

Retrospective studies, which are conducted in the present and look into the past, can be divided into three general approaches: retrieval of data from source documents such as medical records; retrieval from existing databases (eg, administrative databases and payment systems); and meta-analyses, or systematic reviews of previously conducted and reported studies. The retrospective approach requires complete and consistent documentation at the time the record is created. A limitation is that important confounding variables may not have not been consistently assessed or documented in preexisting data records used and therefore cannot be controlled. It also can take considerable resources and skill to access and use archival data. Adding to the challenge of undertaking valid and reliable retrospective studies is the fact that procedures for measurement and recording can change over time, and terminology is often used inconsistently. The expansion of computerized charting and electronic databases offers promise for improving retrospective and prospective studies (18,19). Well-designed observational studies, including controlled cohort studies and case-controlled studies, can provide useful data on the effectiveness of interventions. (See Chapter 8 for information on these types of studies.)

Outcomes studies frequently involve practitioners in providing and documenting the care under study. Data collection can be done by an outside investigator, be performed by the RD, or be delegated to other nutrition staff, medical records personnel, students, or volunteers. The individuals involved must be trained in the study protocol and committed to avoiding the introduction of bias arising from their knowledge and experience and their desire for a positive study result. Study procedures must be designed and executed with the goal of preventing bias and ensuring validity (eg, unbiased selection of participants, tracking to avoid dropouts, standardized measurement methods that are used consistently across participants, and consideration of covariates and confounders).

Evaluating the effectiveness of nutrition therapy, programs, and services is challenging. There are many confounding variables (ie, factors that interfere with the hypothesized relationship between the intervention and its outcome) in nutrition care and many threats to validity in outcomes research. A study must be designed carefully and the appropriate methodologies used. The better the study design, the more valuable the results will be to the profession and to individual decision makers. However, no study is perfect; each has limitations. RDs need to tackle these challenges and go forward with outcomes research and economic analysis (1,2,7,9). Suggestions for making outcomes and economic studies a regular part of dietetics practice include planning studies to address problems encountered regularly in the patient population; selecting areas where the RD has control and will be able to implement changes shown to be effective; beginning with a small study that can be finished in a few months and building on experience to plan larger studies; collaborating with others (team members, colleagues at other facilities, and faculty at nearby colleges or universities) who have interest, experience, and expertise in research design; constructing databases; and performing statistical analysis and outcomes evaluation (20).

The Nutrition Care Process and Outcomes Research

The nutrition care process and use of standardized nutrition language support outcomes research (21,22). The nutrition care process requires the documentation of pertinent information using uniform terminology. This includes relevant assessment indicators, a specific nutrition diagnosis with etiology and signs and symptoms, an explicit intervention approach, and results of the intervention measured at specific follow-up points using standard terminology for outcomes and indicators. Consistent documentation that includes more relevant information about the nutrition care situation enables study of the effectiveness of nutrition intervention alternatives used in varying circumstances and can lead to greater understanding of the results and value of dietetics services.

ECONOMIC ANALYSIS

Economic analysis examines outcomes in relation to costs; it determines efficiency. The methods of economic analysis are used to identify the most efficient intervention, that is, the one that achieves more of the desired outcomes for the lowest or most reasonable investment of resources. Economic analysis requires a systematic process of defining, measuring, and valuing the costs and outcomes of two or more competing alternatives for accomplishing some objective (23). The six steps of economic analysis, discussed later in the chapter, are based on a synthesis of the principles and current recommendations for economic analysis (23–25).

Opportunity cost is a concept integral to economic analysis. As nutrition interventions or programs are implemented and produce outcomes, they consume resources. The consumed resources are then unavailable for other purposes. Opportunity cost is the value that would have been gained if the resource had been used for the next best alternative. Competition for scarce resources is the foundation of economic analysis.

Economic Analysis in Nutrition

Before 1979, economic evaluation was rare in the nutrition literature. At that time, the American Dietetic Association (ADA) proposed a model for estimating the economic benefits of nutrition (26).

In 1989 Disbrow (27) summarized data on costs, health status (outcomes) and economic benefits, and results of economic analysis. In 1991, following a critical analysis of existing studies in four areas of practice, the ADA published summary documents that justify nutrition care in terms of its effectiveness, intermediate-term cost savings, and economic gains (28). In that publication, research designs were proposed for assessing the effectiveness and cost-effectiveness of nutrition care defined by practice guidelines. In 1993 the Agency for Health Care Policy and Research (29) published a critique of nutrition effectiveness and cost studies, and in 1995 the ADA published a position paper summarizing the body of literature supporting the cost-effectiveness of MNT (30). In 2004 Pavlovich et al (31) reported a systematic review of the cost-effectiveness of nutrition services in ambulatory care.

During this same time, economic evaluation was increasingly used throughout health care and public health to evaluate new and old medical procedures and technology, as well as public health interventions. The methods of economic analysis as applied to health also have been evolving. In the early 1990s, the US Public Health Service convened an expert panel to review the theory and practice of cost-effectiveness analysis (CEA) and to make recommendations for standardizing CEA methodology in health and medicine (23). Staff of the Centers for Disease Control and Prevention (CDC) also reviewed methods and described methodology for CEA as it applies to public health intervention and prevention (24). Current recommended methods merge the theoretical base of economic analysis with its practical application for decision making in the health care sector. However, a recent supplement to the journal *Medical Care* explored variations in the use of CEA methodology and barriers to consistent use of CEA findings in decision making (32).

Analytic Methods Used in Economic Analysis

Several analytic methods are used in economic analysis, including cost minimization analysis, CEA, cost-benefit

TABLE 20.3   Analytic Methods Used in Economic Analysis

Method	Focus	Application Example	Outcomes	Costs	Ways to Report
Cost minimization analysis	Identifies the lowest-cost way to do something	Should an RD, DTR, or RN do nutrition assessment at hospital admission?	No data; assumes outcomes are equal	Cost analysis and comparison using cost of inputs	Costs of inputs for each alternative (dollars per activity, day, patient, or course of treatment)
Cost-effectiveness analysis	Compares the efficiency of two or more alternatives for a specified outcome	Should a special oral supplement be recommended for HIV/AIDS patients?	Biochemical, clinical, or quality-of-life measures for each alternative	Cost of each alternative or net cost (cost of inputs plus cost of consequences)	Amount of successful outcome per dollar of investment, net cost per unit of outcome, or dollars per unit of improvement
Cost-benefit analysis	Assigns dollar value to resource inputs and health outcomes; may compare alternatives with different goals	Is it cost-beneficial to initiate nutrition intervention to prevent pressure ulcers?	Dollar value assigned to outcomes	Cost of inputs over complete course of intervention	Net consumption of resources, the dollar ratio of outcomes to inputs (benefit-cost analysis), or dollar of input to dollar of outcome (cost-benefit analysis)
Cost-utility analysis	Relates cost to quality-of-life differences; other preference or satisfaction measures can also be used	Is nutrition support via enteral feeding or total parenteral nutrition worth QALY for terminally ill patients?	Weeks or months of life extended and patients' perceptions of quality of life with or without intervention	Net cost for each alternative (input cost plus cost of complications, cost of medical care for extended life, and any medical cost savings)	Net cost per QALY; dollars per QALY
Clinical decision analysis	Uses estimates from published studies or expert opinion to determine probability of events (diagnosis, treatment response, complication rate, survival)	What outcomes can be expected if elemental vs non-elemental enteral formula is used for surgical patients with hypoalbuminemia?	Intermediate and clinical outcomes	Probability estimates used to develop predictions of input costs, medical cost savings, and cost of complications for each decision alternative	Decision tree with outcome probabilities and net cost estimates

Abbreviations: DTR, dietetic technician, registered; QALY, quality-adjusted life years; RD, registered dietitian; RN, registered nurse.

analysis (CBA), cost-utility analysis, and clinical decision analysis. The objectives of the investigation determine which analytic method is appropriate. Table 20.3 compares the methods and gives examples of their application in clinical dietetics.

Cost minimization analysis and CEA are used to determine the lower-cost way to achieve a specified outcome. In cost minimization analysis, the outcomes of nutrition alternatives are assumed to be equal, and only costs are measured. In CEA, the magnitude of outcome produced by each alternative is measured, along with the cost to produce the outcome. A ratio of cost per unit of effect (outcome) is calculated for each alternative and the results are compared to determine which alternative is more cost-effective.

CBA considers the monetary (dollar) value of both inputs and outcomes. In a cost-benefit ratio, the dollar value of inputs is related to the dollar value of outcomes (positive and negative) produced. Cost-utility analysis relates costs to the patient's quality of life. Quality-adjusted

BOX 20.2   Quality-Adjusted Life Years (QALY)

Quality-adjusted life years is a universal measure of health status that is expressed as the length of healthy life. It assumes that the goal is to extend the state of good health as long as possible and to minimize periods of ill health or disability.

QALY takes two things into account:
- Length of life
- Quality or state of health (well-being) during various periods of time

---

life years (QALY) is the common unit of measure in cost-utility analysis (see Box 20.2) (23,24). Results are expressed as cost per QALY. Because of the standardized units, CBA and cost-utility analysis can be used to compare the efficiency of activities in different areas. Thus, they can be used to inform policy and resource allocation decisions across different areas of health care or different sectors of the economy (eg, health care vs education and training) or to compare many different preventive health interventions (33). Clinical decision analysis uses estimates of outcome probabilities and net cost to evaluate intervention alternatives (23–25). Economic analysis is used to inform policy decisions. It can be ex ante analysis conducted before the adoption of policy on the basis of results of pilot studies, research, or theoretical assumptions. Economic analysis can also be conducted after policy implementation using data from actual outcomes. This ex post analysis determines the true cost-benefit of the policy in real-world conditions. Before-and-after cost-effectiveness or cost-benefit estimates can be quite different.

Length of life estimates can be based on actual survival data in the study or can come from a life table of the population. Life tables specify the proportion of the population of people living and dying at each age interval.

Measures of well-being include mental, physical, and social functioning, as well as pain and suffering. Social functioning includes an individual's limitations in performing usual social roles of work, school, homemaking, and the like; physical functioning can be measured in terms of one's confinement to a bed, chair, or home because of health reasons.

Various tools have been developed to assign a quality-of-life or well-being score (a number ranging from 0.0 [death] to 1.0 [optimal health]) to an individual's functioning (12,34). Numerous disease-specific quality-of-life measures have

also been developed. QALY is calculated by multiplying years by quality of life during those years.

Steps of Economic Analysis

The process of planning, conducting, and reporting in economic analysis can be divided into six steps.

Step 1: State the Objective

Determine the objective of the economic analysis. In general terms, the objective is to arrive at an unbiased determination of how to use scarce resources most efficiently for a specific purpose. The type of intervention or program, its intended purpose (nutrition or health aims), competing alternatives, and the context for application are included in the objective. How the information will be used and the primary and other expected users of the information are also stated in the objective.

Step 2: Define the Framework for Analysis

The framework for the analysis involves decisions about perspective, alternatives, and time horizon.

Perspective.   The study perspective identifies whose resources are at stake. It is the basis for choosing the type of economic analysis to undertake, including the type of cost to include in the analysis. The perspective must be specified at the planning stage because it influences which costs and outcomes are most relevant to measure for the analysis. The perspectives of the intervention provider (the program or organization) or the payer are commonly selected in comparing medical or nutrition therapies. The perspectives of the health care sector and society are frequently used in policy analysis, health care reform, and planning (23–25).

Alternatives.   To evaluate a nutrition intervention for efficiency and effectiveness, it must be compared with one or more alternatives. All reasonable alternatives should be evaluated, but at least two are necessary. The alternatives to be included are described in detail. The selected alternatives should meet the following criteria:

- Address the same preventive or therapeutic aim.
- Represent current practice and new innovations.
- Consider available scientific evidence.
- Include alternatives that have political and professional support.

Sometimes the option of no intervention is a studied alternative.

Time horizon.   Many economic analyses track patients through a relatively short course of therapy to clinical end points. Nutrition intervention can impact longer-term outcomes, such as the patient's functional capacity at home, relapse rate, future need for health care services, or onset of disease or complications many years in the future.

When discussing the time horizon, economists use the terms *cost stream* and *benefit stream*. The cost stream is the period of time over which intervention resources must be invested. The benefit stream is the period of time over which outcomes and associated costs of consequences are accumulated. The time horizon of a study, then, refers to the defined time periods for tracking cost and benefit streams for the economic analysis. In cardiovascular disease, for example, the objective of the study could be the outcomes of care during the hospital stay for coronary artery bypass grafting, through a period of cardiac rehabilitation, or several years in the future to track cardiac events.

Step 3: Determine Costs

After the framework for analysis has been specified, the next two steps are to determine costs and to determine outcomes of the compared alternatives. These procedures are undertaken by identifying (listing and defining), measuring (quantifying the amount used or produced), and valuing (assigning units to be reported—natural units, dollars, or QALY). These steps are presented here as step 3 and step 4, but they can be conducted simultaneously.

The process of quantifying costs is called *cost analysis* or *cost identification*. It provides a systematic and defensible estimation of resources consumed, which is necessary for all types of economic analysis. Costing often focuses on the input cost of the intervention, but it is also used to determine the monetary value of outcomes for net cost-effectiveness and for CBA. The process is not complicated, but it must be approached in a systematic and careful manner (23–25).

Types of costs.   Economists traditionally categorize costs into direct, indirect, and intangible costs. The researcher decides which costs to include and how to measure them based on the objectives of the analysis and the information needs of the decision makers who will use the results.

Direct costs receive attention in most economic analyses of nutrition care and programs. Direct costs include resources consumed in the prevention, diagnosis, treatment, and rehabilitation of a disease. In nutrition, direct costs are defined as those resources used by the provider in the delivery of nutrition and related care to achieve the health goals or outcome objectives of the intervention or program. They are estimated from principal resource components incurred by the provider organization. Other perspectives for analysis would require the inclusion of other kinds of costs.

Cost analysis.   Cost analysis can be done in two ways, using either a micro costing approach, which accounts for all costs in detail, or a macro or gross costing approach, which considers only significant economic events. Cost analysis must be carried out with equal precision for all alternatives being compared. In the micro costing/cost accounting approach, principal resource components are identified, tracked, and assigned a dollar value based on prevailing market prices. Principal resource components commonly included are personnel, fringe benefits, food and nutrition products and supplies, office supplies, education materials, equipment, laboratory tests, other diagnostic and monitoring procedures, other ancillary services, continuing education and training of staff, facility/space, and administrative overhead.

Micro costing is a systematic process involving the following steps:

- List all activities.
- Identify principal resource components for activities (as previously described).
- Estimate resource consumption for each principal resource component by tracking/measuring actual utilization or using secondary data.
- Assign a monetary value to each component and activity using market prices.
- List all assumptions made for possible sensitivity analysis.
- Calculate total, average, incremental, marginal, and/or net cost.
- Perform discounting, if necessary.

Personnel costs are a large part of the costs for nutrition interventions. Time studies may be necessary to determine accurately the quantity of personnel time required for an intervention (34). Time and activity records or data from productivity studies carried out in the organization could also be used to estimate time for specific activities.

The steps of gross costing are as follows:

- Identify significant economic events relevant to the intervention (inputs) and/or outcomes. These might include outpatient care; hospitalization; nursing home placement; home health services; services of an RD, physician, or other professional; medication; and durable medical equipment.

- Measure or estimate the quantity of significant events used or produced.
- Assign values to significant events using fee schedules, actual charges, or payments.
- List all assumptions made for possible sensitivity analysis.
- Calculate total, average, incremental, marginal, and/or net cost.
- Perform discounting, if necessary.

Assigning monetary value.   The value assigned to the component or significant economic event is either the actual market price paid by the buyer or an assigned value. When the buyer is the provider or health care organization, the value can be based on the price paid for resources consumed, the amount billed (charges), or the amount received as payments or reimbursements. When the buyer is the third-party payer (eg, Medicare, an insurance carrier, or a health plan), the value assigned is usually based on records of claims paid or estimates using organization, industry, state, or national reports of health care use and cost under various circumstances. Sources of such data are described by Gold et al (23).

The value of patients' or clients' time associated with receiving the service or experiencing its consequences is an additional important cost. Time costs, including time waiting for a service to begin, travel costs, time lost from work, and child-care costs, are all potential indirect costs to patients and are important to the people receiving the service. Economists translate these indirect costs into time lost from work and lost productivity (23–25). Wages are frequently used to value indirect costs, and in spite of the potential inequities for women, minorities, and youth, wages are considered by economists to be the best measure of value. Wages must be used with caution and with the acknowledgment that indirect costs may be underestimated for some groups and overestimated for others. The perspective of the study determines whether indirect costs are included in the analysis.

The fear, grief, worry, and pain experienced by patients, clients, and family members are intangible costs that are difficult to measure. Sometimes these intangible costs are presented in narrative terms and can be influential pieces of information for decision makers.

Each alternative included in the analysis requires a cost analysis. The same types of costs and assumptions should be used in the cost analysis for each alternative; if this is not done, any differences must be described. The approaches to cost analysis and methods of valuing costs produce different results; therefore, the methods and sources used must be fully disclosed in the report. In addition, in calculating costs, assumptions are frequently used to identify relevant resource costs, estimate the amount of resources consumed, and/or assign a value to each resource component or significant economic event. All assumptions should be documented and subjected to sensitivity analysis (described in step 4).

Summarizing and reporting costs.   The findings of the cost analysis can be summarized and reported in a number of forms, including full (total) cost, average cost, marginal cost, and net cost. Full (or total) cost is the cost of the intervention over a period of time (usually 1 year or the usual course of treatment). Total costs are made up of fixed costs (stable costs not related to the volume of service) and variable costs (resource utilization that varies with the volume [number served] or intensity [frequency and type of contact] of service). Average cost is the cost per unit of output or outcome, determined by dividing total costs involved by the number of units of service (eg, cost per nutrition assessment or cost per low-birth-weight infant prevented). Incremental cost is the cost difference between one alternative and another (eg, the extra cost of managing hypercholesterolemia with pharmaceutical intervention compared with dietary intervention [35]).

When the cost of providing a little more or a little less of the intervention is calculated, it is a marginal cost calculation (eg, the added cost of a second nutrition follow-up visit for people completing a weight-loss program). Net cost (or net benefit, when positive) refers to the balance when the cost of carrying out the intervention (inputs) is added to the monetary value of positive consequences or outcomes (resources saved) and negative consequences or outcomes (additional resource consumption) (23,24,36).

Incremental or marginal costs are more relevant to economic analysis than are total or average costs because incremental or marginal costs relate to the extra resource requirements to produce each added effect (and the opportunity costs of removing those resources from other purposes). Total and unit costs are especially useful for budgeting, establishing fees, and negotiating reimbursement rates.

Special considerations in costing.   In an economic analysis covering multiple years or using cost data gathered at different times in the past, dollar values for all alternatives must be expressed in relation to a standard base year. This calculation is called *adjusting to present value*, and it uses the Consumer Price Index to adjust for inflation over time. This adjustment is made before costs are related to outcomes and before discounting is done. Sikand and colleagues (37) offer an example of this calculation in a cost-benefit study.

Discounting is a mathematical procedure used to convert future costs and future outcomes to present value. Two facts make discounting necessary in long-term analyses:

- Inflation reduces the value of money over time.
- People and institutions generally prefer to receive both dollars and benefits immediately, rather than in the future.

Discounting is discussed in greater detail after step 4 because it is applied to both costs and outcomes.

Applying cost analysis.   The following example illustrates how an RD might determine the cost of nutrition services in prenatal care from the perspective of the public health center, using data from the current program year:

1. Prepare a flowchart of all activities involved in providing nutrition services to pregnant clients, including activities such as client recruitment and outreach, nutrition assessment and diagnosis, education or counseling of clients, care coordination and referral, record keeping and scheduling, client follow-up and monitoring, and program administration and evaluation.
2. Identify the principal resource components necessary for each activity. This might include nutrition and clerical personnel, fringe benefits, nutrition education materials and equipment, laboratory tests to monitor anemia, office and clinic space, nutrition reference materials, office supplies, and administrative overhead.
3. Specify the ways costs will be measured. Use work schedules and existing reports such as service statistics or accounting records (after verifying their completeness and accuracy), conduct time studies or productivity studies, or use other methods to accurately estimate the quantity of principal resource components necessary to carry out each activity.
4. Work with the accounting staff to assign a monetary value based on the actual cost to the organization for each cost component. Keep track of all assumptions made along the way.
5. Calculate the total cost for prenatal nutrition services; then divide by the number of women served

to get an average or unit cost. If the cost analysis looked only at nutrition costs as a component of an existing prenatal care program, the cost could be considered an incremental cost (the amount added to prenatal care costs for nutrition services).

Similar steps with similar assumptions should be carried out for each alternative to be compared. For example, freestanding nutrition services delivered at a different location requiring separate staffing and facilities would likely have significantly different, and probably higher, costs.

Step 4: Determine Outcomes

Once the objectives of the service are defined and the type of analysis has been determined, the effect or benefit anticipated from the dietetics services can be identified, measured, and valued. The magnitude of the outcome (effect or benefit) associated with or attributed to the nutrition intervention is determined in step 4. The researcher must have a defensible estimate of the effect of each alternative included in the economic analysis. These estimates are made through an outcomes study, as described earlier in this chapter, or through research methods described in Chapters 8, 9, 11, and 12. In some situations, effectiveness results reported by others are used to model potential outcomes. Meta-analysis is recommended as a method for critically appraising and integrating the results of past studies into an estimate of effect (25).

Regardless of the source of outcomes data, the data must be logically and scientifically linked to the interventions being studied. Furthermore, the data must be appropriate, given the framework of the economic analysis (alternatives, perspective, and time horizon). The end point for the analysis can be short-term or longer-term results. Short- to intermediate-term outcomes might include a change in nutrition-related behaviors with an improvement in a biochemical or physiological measure, a change in the signs or symptoms of the disease, a change in the complication rate, or a change in days of hospital stay. In longer-term studies, these measures or their associated values in terms of state of health, functional ability, quality of life, and health care utilization could be used.

A series of assumptions are commonly made in dietetics practice. It is assumed that people who receive nutrition services and programs improve their nutrient intake or nutrition practices, that this change produces improved health status, and that improved health status results in reduced consumption of other medical services and therefore saves resources. These assumptions, and particularly the key outcome of interest, must be verified through scientifically sound studies—either previously reported or conducted specifically for the economic analysis. Information on the magnitude of change is required.

For CEA, a key outcome (effect) is measured and reported in natural units (eg, pounds of weight loss, percentage reduction in cholesterol, proportion of the population with diabetes who improve their blood glucose levels, or complications avoided). For CBA, important outcomes (benefits) are measured in or converted to monetary units (dollars). The magnitude of outcomes is related to cost data from step 3 for the actual economic analysis. Relating outcomes to benefits is explained in step 5.

Types of benefits.   As they do with costs, economists classify benefits as direct, indirect, and intangible. Direct benefits of nutrition care lie in the expenditures that would otherwise have been spent on health care had the intervention not been effective. Direct benefits represent all types of health resources that are not consumed as a result of the intervention; in other words, they represent resources saved or expenditures avoided because of the nutrition intervention. Direct benefits also accrue to individuals. For example, people with improved nutritional status and health outcomes may save out-of-pocket expenses when medications can be reduced.

Indirect benefits of nutrition care are improvements in functional ability and capacity to carry out the daily tasks of living and resume normal social roles (eg, worker, homemaker, or student). In some studies, improvements in work attendance and performance are used as proxies for improved health status. Estimates based on measures used in the National Health Interview Survey, the National Health and Nutrition Examination Survey, and the National Medical Expenditure Survey, among others, are useful for determining the indirect benefits of health care to consumers and to society and translating those benefits into economic consequences (23,24). The dollar savings due to indirect benefits are estimated as part of the burden of illness (38).

Improvements in the quality of life also represent important benefits that are difficult to measure. Intangible benefits express subjective judgments of well-being, improved independence and mobility, and avoidance of pain and suffering. These intangible benefits are real to the people who experience them and therefore should contribute to the decision-making process. The development of quality-of-life assessments has enabled measurement of the patients' perception of the impact of disease and disability and of the course of treatment selected on their lives and functioning (12,23,24).

All payers are interested in direct benefits because they want to reduce their expenditures. Insurance companies pay for certain services and procedures when evidence shows that savings accrue in other areas, such as hospital costs. In contrast, payers and organization administrators are less concerned about indirect benefits and intangibles because they do not produce specific dollar savings for the organization. All three categories of benefits can and do occur in the same situation; for economic analysis, however, the perspective determines which categories are measured and included in the analysis.

Study design.   After consideration of the aforementioned points, the research design and methods to measure outcomes (effects or benefits) of the compared alternatives can be determined. (See Chapter 9.) The design should include consideration of factors that could potentially confound the interpretation of the results of the effectiveness study. For example, age, race/ethnicity, socioeconomic status, smoking and other lifestyle factors, and concurrent medical care can have an effect on the measured outcome. Other factors, such as seasonal variation of illness and deaths, must also be considered. The study design should control these factors (ie, confounders) to ensure valid results.

Summarizing and reporting outcomes.   After the data are collected, they are analyzed to determine the magnitude of effect achieved by each alternative. This analysis involves aggregating the raw data into summary statistics that include a measure of variation (eg, mean with standard deviation or confidence interval), determining the statistical and clinical significance of outcomes, and making comparisons between alternatives. Appropriate statistical tests, which are determined by the design of the study and the type of variables measured, must be used. For each alternative, the following should be reported:

- Descriptive data about the sample studied and the population it represents
- Magnitude of outcome associated with, or attributed to, the intervention
- Assessment of the clinical importance of the outcome achieved
- Comparison of results between alternatives to determine if they are significantly different and/or to determine the incremental effectiveness
- Descriptive data about any intervening or confounding factors

- Statistical adjustments of the magnitude of the outcome for preexisting group differences and for intervening factors
- Quantitative or qualitative summary of other outcomes
- Relationship of the degree of outcome to the amount of exposure to the nutrition intervention

Application examples.   In CEA, two or more alternatives for achieving the same outcome objective are compared, and the units of measure are the same. Compared with CBA, CEA is easier to carry out because it uses natural units that are commonly measured and documented in health care. However, CEA can require considerable time and expense to access records and abstract data.

Economic analysis can use data that are actually measured for the study, as well as values that are estimated from other data sources. The clinical effect of MNT, for example, could be measured, but the value of the effect to an organization, third-party payers, or society might be estimated by using data from other sources. A common application of CBA is to compare the length of stay for a group of patients receiving a new or added procedure or treatment, such as MNT, with the length of stay reported for patients with the same diagnosis in a national study or existing database. The benefit then can be calculated from the cost differences if a shorter length of stay is found for the group receiving the nutrition therapy. In the CBA reported by Sheils et al, future health care utilization and resulting costs were compared between adults who had and those who did not have nutrition counseling (39).

For a societal perspective in CBA, information collected by the government through state, regional, and national studies is often used. The National Center for Health Statistics conducts the National Health Survey and publishes the results on a regular basis through the *Vital and Health Statistics* series. In CBA, the benefits are expressed in dollar terms (eg, cost per day of hospital stay), so they can be directly compared with the input costs.

Discounting costs and benefits.   Whenever the time horizon of an analysis extends beyond a year, or when data for input costs or outcome estimates for compared alternatives come from different years, the issues of present value and discounting must be addressed. The discounting procedure adjusts estimates of cost and/or outcomes that will be experienced in a future time period. This procedure should be used in a study when the time difference between investment and benefit is longer than 1 year. Computer accounting or statistical analysis software can be used for discounting. The discount rate can range between 2% and 10% per year, with 5% the most common rate (23). Economists recommend reporting a range of calculations in order to include conservative and more optimistic projections. If a low discount rate is used, the value of long-term costs and benefits is increased; in contrast, a higher discount rate increases the value of short-term costs and benefits. When necessary, cost, outcomes, or both are discounted before step 5. Present-value tables in economics and accounting reference books and in computer spreadsheet software programs simplify the process of discounting.

Step 5: Relate Costs to Outcomes

After accurate and defensible estimates of costs and outcomes have been gathered (steps 3 and 4), they are related so that judgments about the relative economic efficiency of the compared alternatives can be made. This economic analysis can be done and presented in several ways—using ratios, net benefit or net cost-effectiveness, or an array table. The method is determined based on the objectives of the study, the type of economic analysis, and the nature of the data, as well as on considerations about what form will be most understandable and helpful to potential users of the results.

Ratio.   The ratio communicates the cost for a unit of outcome and allows direct comparison between the efficiency of one alternative and the efficiency of another alternative. When a ratio is used, it is difficult to visualize the total costs of implementing the intervention. Another drawback is that the actual magnitude of change is not evident, so clinicians cannot determine whether the amount of change is clinically meaningful. Decision makers will need additional descriptive or graphic information to determine the budgetary ramifications and numbers of persons who are likely to have access to the defined nutrition intervention and to benefit from it. Additionally, various audiences may be interested in other outcomes beyond the key outcomes identified for the cost-effectiveness or cost-benefit ratio.

Array table.   Many of the drawbacks of ratio use are overcome by presenting results in an array. An array table lists the actual costs in dollars and the outcomes in their natural units of measurement. An array table is useful for reporting the findings across a chain of outcomes. It allows audiences to consider simultaneously more than one outcome measure in relation to the resource requirements to produce the outcomes. Franz et al used an array table to present the findings from a study of nutrition practice guidelines for type 2 (non-insulin-dependent) diabetes mellitus (40).

From ratio to net benefit.   A ratio is traditionally used to express the results of CBA research. It may be a cost-benefit ratio, in which the numerator is the cost of inputs and the denominator is the monetary value of benefits (outcomes), or it may be a benefit-cost ratio, in which the numerator is the benefits and the denominator is the costs:

$$\text{Cost-benefit ratio} = \frac{\text{Cost of inputs in dollars}}{\text{Benefit (outcomes) in dollars}} = 1:3$$

$$\text{Benefit-cost ratio} = \frac{\text{Benefit (outcomes) in dollars}}{\text{Cost of inputs in dollars}} = 3:1$$

Net benefit (or net cost) is equal to the dollars gained (or lost) when the monetary value of all resources consumed is subtracted from the total estimate of cost savings or averted expenditures when the alternative is implemented. It uses the same values that are used in the numerator and denominator of the cost-benefit ratio. Compared with the ratio, the net benefit calculation does a better job of communicating the magnitude of resources at stake and can be applied more directly to budgetary planning.

Presenting only the ratio conceals the magnitude of the resources at stake. For example, benefits of $3 million gained from an expenditure of $1 million results in a 1:3 cost-benefit ratio. A benefit of $3,000 from an investment of $1,000 is also a 1:3 cost-benefit ratio. However, the net benefits would be reported as $2 million and $2,000, respectively, which certainly tells a different story.

Some experts advocate presenting the results of a CEA as net cost-effectiveness. In this method, the monetary value of cost savings generated by the improved health or averted deterioration is calculated (usually using gross costing to assign value to economically significant events). From this value, the input (intervention) costs are subtracted. The resulting value is related to a key outcome presented in natural units (22,23).

Sensitivity analysis and ethical issues in economic analysis.   Before the final conclusions can be drawn, three more things must be considered: discounting (discussed earlier), sensitivity analysis, and ethical issues. Sensitivity analysis is used to check the robustness of the conclusions. It involves the reanalysis of data using different estimates for assumptions or uncertainties. It informs the researcher and

decision maker of the degree to which specific assumptions affect the results. For example, in a study of MNT in type 2 diabetes mellitus, the impact of different assumptions about RDs' salaries, variations in the use of laboratory tests, and the magnitude of glucose control outcome were assessed (40).

In sensitivity analysis, what-if scenarios are used to determine the impact of substitute assumptions (or other uncertainties) on the conclusions. Several rounds of reanalysis are done using more conservative and more liberal estimates. Reanalysis is not difficult. With the use of computer spreadsheets or statistical software programs, revised estimates can be substituted for a value used in the original analysis, and the computer quickly recalculates the results.

Reports of CEA and CBA should describe the assumptions made and how sensitivity analysis was used to explore the impact of the assumptions on the analysis and its conclusions. If a conclusion holds up under varying assumptions, it is said to be *robust*. If changing some of the assumptions used to assign value to resources significantly changes the conclusion, greater efforts should be directed toward determining the true value for the cost component or the outcome estimate. When this effort is not possible, the researcher must state explicitly that the results are "sensitive to" the value assigned to that component. In the report of a type 2 diabetes mellitus study, the authors stated, "The results indicate that cost-effectiveness conclusions were sensitive to the outcome indicator selected." They went on to report the impact of RDs' salaries, laboratory tests, and outcome variations on conclusions (40).

In reports of studies about the cost-effectiveness of nutrition services, questions can arise about assumptions used in the estimates of costs or outcomes. RDs and others conducting these studies must identify the potential areas for questioning. They must use sensitivity analysis to understand the strengths and limitations of the analysis and openly report them along with conclusions and recommendations.

The results of economic analysis indicate the preferred alternative based on the criterion of economic efficiency—that is, the alternative that produces the greater amount of outcomes for the lower cost. However, additional criteria come into play in setting policies, making administrative decisions, or recommending clinical practices. The findings of CBA or CEA could favor targeting MNT or a nutrition program to younger, more compliant patients with less severe disease. But is it ethical to withhold therapy from older or more acutely ill persons? And although delivering a nutrition program via the Internet may be efficient, is it ethical to exclude persons who cannot afford a computer or Internet access? Ethical issues like these must be considered in conducting economic analyses.

When an ethical issue, such as access to nutrition care for people without insurance, is incorporated into the objectives of the CEA or CBA, the study can be designed to measure and value the issue. Ethical issues can also come to light during the study and interpretation of results. Relevant ethical issues should be explored, identified, and discussed, even if it is not possible to measure or place a dollar value on them. Many people—especially advocates, legislators, planners, and policy analysts—who use reports about the economic implications of nutrition services and programs have no nutrition training. Ethical issues related to food and nutrition may not be evident and thus must be brought to their attention. Whenever ethical issues are identified, their implications should be explored and presented as a part of the findings. Roth-Yousey presents additional discussion of ethical issues in nutrition and their analysis (41). Chapter 3 covers ethics in greater detail.

Step 6: Interpret and Use the Results

When the analysis is complete, the last step is to interpret the findings and make recommendations for action. The results provide information about the cost, effectiveness, and efficiency of nutrition programs and services. The study and its findings must be presented to decision makers who can use the information. Clinical nutrition managers benefit from a CEA that identifies areas in which expected outcomes are not being reached or patients' health outcomes could be achieved with fewer inputs. The results can support changes in practice necessary to make dietetics services more effective and efficient. Providing results of CBA to health plans and insurance companies can support coverage of MNT (42), and CBA results are prominent factors in policy decisions at the state and federal levels (2,32).

Every study has limitations that must be acknowledged. RDs in the state of Washington, for example, collected case studies of the impact of nutrition services for children with special health care conditions and used the results to estimate health care averted and associated economic benefits. The report described limitations of the study and offered appropriate applications of the findings and identified the need for further study (43).

The report of an economic analysis must include enough information for users to be able to understand the

conclusion, judge its accuracy, and determine the context in which it can be applied. The following is a checklist of items needed in preparing reports of economic analysis or reviewing reports prepared by others.

- Statement of the purpose and objectives of the analysis
- Description of compared alternatives and why they were selected, the perspective for analysis, the time frame for inputs and outcomes, and the key outcome or outcomes
- Procedures for determining costs, cost components included, sources of data, assumptions made, costing approach, the base year for standardizing costs, the computed monetary value of inputs (and outcomes, if monetized), and discounting (if done)
- Procedures for determining effectiveness/outcome, including study design, sources of data, assumptions made, methods of statistical analysis, proportion of the target population that benefited and their characteristics, the magnitude of effect for each alternative and its variation, discounting (if done), any problems or limitations encountered, and significant intervening or confounding factors affecting the interpretation of results
- The relative efficiency of each alternative—relating costs to outcomes in a ratio, array, and/or net cost (benefit) equation—as well as sensitivity analysis to explore the robustness of conclusions under more conservative or liberal assumptions
- Ethical issues and their role in interpreting findings
- Conclusions and recommendations for action, when appropriate

APPLICATIONS IN DIETETICS PRACTICE

Economic Analysis in Clinical Nutrition

Clinical nutrition involves many options for nutrition intervention: For whom? When to provide? What type? How long? By whom? Economic analysis can provide answers to these questions. The following examples illustrate the range of opportunities for incorporating economic analysis in nutrition research and outcomes studies.

Gallagher-Allred et al (10) reviewed studies that demonstrated how appropriate nutrition support is associated with reduced morbidity and mortality and lower costs among hospital patients. Together the studies build a case for early and appropriate MNT. Specific studies, such as work by Hedberg et al (44), help quantify the resource requirements for appropriate and effective nutrition care.

Brannon et al (45) examined the cost-effectiveness of two methods of nutrition education delivered through physicians' offices for children with hypercholesterolemia. They calculated CEA ratios in two ways—one relating program costs to changes in calories consumed from fat, and another relating program costs to reduction of low-density lipoprotein cholesterol at 3 and 12 months. They noted that the findings were sensitive to the time horizon for measurement, assumptions about children's contact with primary care, and availability of someone to administer the intervention (parent or RD). They also noted that third-party payment favored one method over another.

Sikand et al (37) conducted a cost-benefit study of MNT vs lipid drug therapy for a sample of adults with hypercholesterolemia. Their comprehensive report included MNT and lipid costs; identified change in lipids, body mass index, and drug eligibility as outcomes; and reported CBA results as annualized net benefits, cost-effectiveness ratios for different intensities of nutrition care, and a cost-benefit ratio of MNT costs to drug therapy cost. The results of studies like this have been used to influence payment/reimbursement policies for MNT (42).

Shevitz et al (46) conducted a clinical and cost-effectiveness study of alternative treatments for wasting added to nutrition care in AIDS patients. In addition to clinical indicators, they assessed HIV-specific quality of life. An institutional micro cost-accounting approach was used, and the researchers also considered subjects' transportation costs as well as time (an indirect cost). The economic findings were reported as institutional costs per subject and dollars per QALY for each treatment alternative. The technically correct label for the latter analysis would be cost-utility analysis.

Braga and Gianotti (47) evaluated the cost-benefit of preoperative immunonutrition as part of a randomized clinical trial. Resources used by each patient were delineated, tracked, and assigned a value using the micro costing approach. The researchers reported postoperative complications and compared costs for patients with and without complications. Actual costs were compared with diagnosis-related group (DRG) reimbursement to determine cost-benefit.

Kruizenga et al (48) reported the incremental cost-effectiveness of nutrition screening and subsequent care for patients admitted to a medical/surgical ward. They found a higher rate of identification of malnutrition using a specific screening protocol that resulted in increased nutrition care costs but shorter length of stay. The authors reported risk adjustment by graphing individual patients' cost-effectiveness ratios to compare differences among risk levels.

Using a Continuum of Risk Evaluation (CORE) model, Caro et al (49) disaggregated health and cost outcomes for prevention of cardiovascular disease related to a patient's risk category. This approach allows decision makers to determine the incremental gains associated with intervention for successively lower risk categories. Although many analyses do not require such complexity, the authors' article serves to remind researchers about the importance of their assumptions about risk level, duration of treatment, and time horizon for outcomes in planning cost-effectiveness studies.

Sheils et al (39) used a large longitudinal database from a health maintenance organization to measure the relationship between MNT and health care spending for diabetes, cardiovascular disease, and renal disease. They used multiple regression to separate the effects of other factors that could impact health care utilization in addition to MNT. The outcome indicator was difference in health care utilization measured as change in physician visits per quarter. The cost of MNT provided by RDs was estimated using the average Medicare reimbursement rate for physicians, and Medicare claims data were used to estimate the health care utilization and its costs. The investigators found significant reductions in utilization for persons with diabetes and cardiovascular disease but not renal disease, and they projected net savings of $369.7 million beginning after 3 years of the program. This study demonstrates the use of administrative databases as the data source for economic analysis of nutrition intervention.

Following work with a CEA study, Naglak et al (50) offered advice about what to include and what to avoid in future CEA. They discussed issues of sample size, compliance with MNT and alternative therapies, the importance of following patients long enough to assess the effects of recidivism, and selection of the outcomes measure for the efficiency calculation. They also recommend consulting with a statistician early in the process. Following a systematic review of published cost-effectiveness studies of nutrition services, Pavlovich et al (31) reported additional limitations commonly found in studies, including nonrepresentativeness of patients and providers, patient self-selection, lack of patient randomization, and study periods that are too short to determine nutrition care effects on risk factors and prevention of adverse events. By recognizing these common threats to validity and building on the methods and findings of others, RDs can plan studies, and manage their implementation, to produce valuable information on the costs and outcomes of nutrition care.

Economic Analysis in Public Health

The ADA position paper on the role of dietetics professionals in health promotion and disease prevention includes potential cost savings associated with reducing the burden of chronic disease in the population through nutrition-related prevention strategies (51). Under the leadership of the CDC, extensive work has been done to link the principles and analytic techniques of economic analysis and epidemiology to improve the quality of CEA studies of prevention. *Prevention Effectiveness: A Guide to Decision Analysis and Economic Evaluation* provides extensive coverage of the topic (22). In addition, the World Health Organization has identified methods to assess the costs and health effects of interventions for improving health in developing countries (52).

CONCLUSION

Dietetics practitioners in all practice settings can contribute to knowledge about the effectiveness and efficiency of nutrition care. Using data collected for quality assurance purposes and outcomes measurement can ease the burden of conducting a CEA. RDs with management responsibilities can allocate time for staff to spend on planning, conducting, and reporting outcome studies and economic analyses.

Studies may be small and carried out in one facility, or several locations may collaborate. The ADA's Dietetics-Based Research Network is a way of involving RDs from many locations in a centrally designed study (53). This provides a means of joining resources to answer research questions about the effectiveness of nutrition care, and the results of multisite studies will have greater generalizability than outcome studies conducted at a single facility.

Outcomes research and economic analysis can be planned and implemented prospectively or conducted retrospectively using medical records and existing databases. Results from either approach will add to the information needed to refine, improve, and promote nutrition care. The results need to be shared through professional and scientific meetings and publications. It is up to RDs, along with other researchers and economists, to conduct the research and make the results available to the administrators, planners, regulators, legislators, and third-party payers who need this information to make informed decisions about the allocation of resources to nutrition care. By working with these policy makers, RDs will learn about their different information needs and thus be better able to plan, conduct, and report studies that can influence clinical administrative and policy decisions.

CEA and CBA are tools to provide more information about nutrition care and its cost and effectiveness. If used wisely, these tools will enable RDs to continue to improve their services, increase their visibility with payers and other decision makers, and provide nutrition services that will have greater impact on the health of the public.

REFERENCES

1. Pichard C, Genton L. From basic research to cost-effectiveness trials: the needed spirit to promote clinical nutrition. *Curr Opin Clin Nutr Metab Care.* 2005;8:373–376.
2. Guthrie JF, Myers EF. USDA's Economic Research Service supports nutrition and health outcomes research. *J Am Diet Assoc.* 2002;102:293–297.
3. Kane RL. *Understanding Health Care Outcomes Research.* Sudbury, Mass: Jones and Bartlett Publishers; 2006.
4. Donabedian A. Quality assessment and assurance: unity of purpose, diversity of means. *Inquiry.* 1988;25: 173–192.
5. Epstein AM. The outcomes movement—will it get us where we want to go? *N Engl J Med.* 1990;323: 266–270.
6. Byham-Gray LD. Outcomes research in nutrition and chronic kidney disease: perspectives, issues in practice, and processes for improvement. *Adv Chronic Kidney Dis.* 2005;12:96–106.
7. Splett PL. *Developing and Validating Evidence-Based Guides for Practice: A Tool Kit for Dietetics Professionals.* Chicago, Ill: American Dietetic Association; 2000.
8. Myers EF, Pritchett E, Johnson EQ. Evidence-based practice guides vs protocols: what's the difference? *J Am Diet Assoc.* 2001;101:1085–1090.
9. Jonnalagadda SS. Effectiveness of medical nutrition therapy: importance of documenting and monitoring nutrition outcomes. *J Am Diet Assoc.* 2004;104:1788–1792.
10. Gallagher-Allred CR, Voss AC, Finn SC, McCamish MA. Malnutrition and clinical outcomes: the case for medical nutrition therapy. *J Am Diet Assoc.* 1996;96:361–396.

11. Splett PL, Weddle DO. *A White Paper on Measuring Outcomes. Prepared for the Administration on Aging.* Washington, DC: Dept of Health and Human Services; 1999.

12. Barr JT, Schumacher GE. The need for a nutrition-related quality-of-life measure. *J Am Diet Assoc.* 2003;103:177–180.

13. Hauchecorne CM, Barr SI, Sork TJ. Evaluation of nutrition counseling in clinical settings: do we make a difference? *J Am Diet Assoc.* 1994;94:437–440.

14. Lemon CC, Lacey K, Lohse B, Hubacher DO, Klawitter B, Palta M. Outcomes monitoring of health, behavior, and quality of life after nutrition intervention in adults with type 2 diabetes. *J Am Diet Assoc.* 2004;104:1805–1815.

15. Cook TD, Campbell DT. *Quasi-experimentation: Design and Analysis Issues for Field Settings.* Boston, Mass: Houghton Mifflin; 1979.

16. Trotter JP. *The Quest for Cost-Effectiveness in Health Care.* Chicago, Ill: American Hospital Publishers; 1995.

17. August D. Outcomes research in nutrition support: background, methods, and practical applications. In: Ireton-Jones CS, Gottschlich MM, Bell SJ, eds. *Practice- Oriented Nutrition Research: An Outcomes Measurement Approach.* Gaithersburg, Md: Aspen; 1998.

18. Hoggle LB, Michael MA, Houston SM, Ayres EJ. Nutrition informatics. *J Am Diet Assoc.* 2006;106: 134–139.

19. Chima CS, Farmer-Dziak N, Cardwell P, Snow S. Use of technology to track program outcomes in a diabetes self-management program. *J Am Diet Assoc.* 2005;105:1933–1938.

20. Schiller MR, Moore C. Practical approaches to outcomes evaluation. *Top Clin Nutr.* 1999;14(2):1–12.

21. Lacey K, Pritchett E. Nutrition Care Process and Model: ADA adopts road map to quality care and outcomes management. *J Am Diet Assoc.* 2003;103: 1061–1072.

22. Hakel-Smith N, Lewis NM. A standardized nutrition care process and language are essential components of a conceptual model to guide and document nutrition care and patient outcomes. *J Am Diet Assoc.* 2004;104:1878–1884.

23. Gold MR, Siegel JE, Russell LB, Weinstein MC. *Cost-Effectiveness in Health and Medicine.* New York, NY: Oxford University Press; 1996.

24. Haddix AC, Teutsch SM, Corso PS, eds. *Prevention Effectiveness: A Guide to Decision Analysis and Economic Evaluation.* 2nd ed. New York, NY: Oxford University Press; 2003.

25. Petti DB. *Meta-Analysis, Decision Analysis, and Cost-Effectiveness Analysis: Methods for Quantitative Synthesis in Medicine.* 2nd ed. New York, NY: Oxford University Press; 2000.

26. Mason M, ed. *Cost and Benefits of Nutrition Care: Phase 1.* Chicago, Ill: American Dietetic Association; 1979.

27. Disbrow DD. The cost and benefits of nutrition services: a literature review. *J Am Diet Assoc.* 1989; 89(suppl 4):S3–S66.

28. Splett PL. Effectiveness and cost effectiveness of nutrition care: a critical appraisal with recommendations, Phase III: research designs for future studies. *J Am Diet Assoc.* 1991;91(suppl):S9–S35.

29. Barr JT. *Clinical Effectiveness in Allied Health Practices.* Silver Springs, Md: US Dept of Health and Human Services, Agency for Health Care Policy and Research; 1993.

30. American Dietetic Association. Cost-effectiveness of medical nutrition therapy. Position paper of the American Dietetic Association. *J Am Diet Assoc.* 1995;95:88–91.

31. Pavlovich WD, Waters H, Weller W, Bass EB. Systematic review of literature on the cost-effectiveness of nutrition services. *J Am Diet Assoc.* 2004;104: 226–232.

32. Berger ML, Teutsch S. Cost-effectiveness analysis: from science to application. *Med Care.* 2005; 43(7 suppl):49–53.

33. Tengs TO, Wallace A. One thousand health-related quality-of-life estimates. *Med Care.* 2000;38: 581–637.

34. Splett PL. *A Practitioner's Guide to Cost-Effectiveness Analysis of Nutrition Interventions.* Arlington, Va: National Center for Education in Maternal and Child Health; 1996.

35. Delahanty LM, Sonnenberg LM, Hayden D, Nathan DM. Clinical and cost outcomes of medical nutrition therapy for hypercholesterolemia: a controlled trial. *J Am Diet Assoc.* 2001;101:1012–1023.

36. Montgomery DL, Splett PL. The economic benefits of breastfeeding infants enrolled in the WIC Program. *J Am Diet Assoc.* 1997;97:379–385.

37. Sikand G, Kashyap ML, Yang I. Medical nutrition therapy lowers serum cholesterol and saves medication costs. *J Am Diet Assoc.* 1998;98:889–894.

38. Rice DP. *Estimating the Cost of Illness.* Washington, DC: US Dept of Health Education and Welfare;

1966. Health Economic Series 6, Public Health Service.

39. Sheils JF, Rubin R, Stapleton DC. The estimated costs and savings of medical nutrition therapy: the Medicare population. *J Am Diet Assoc.* 1999;99:428–435.

40. Franz MJ, Splett PL, Monk A, Barry B, McClain K, Weaver T, Upham P, Bergenstal R, Mazze RS. Cost-effectiveness of medical nutrition therapy provided by dietitians for persons with non-insulin-dependent diabetes mellitus. *J Am Diet Assoc.* 1995;95:1018–1026.

41. Roth-Yousey L. Ethics in community nutrition. In: Owen AL, Splett PL, Owen GM. *Nutrition in the Community: The Art and Science of Delivering Services.* 4th ed. Boston, Mass: WBC McGraw-Hill; 1999:568–586.

42. Smith RE, Patrick S, Michael P, Hager M. Medical nutrition therapy: the core of ADA's advocacy efforts (part 2). *J Am Diet Assoc.* 2005;105:825–834.

43. Lucas B, Nardella M. *Cost Considerations: The Benefits of Nutrition Services for a Case Series of Children with Special Health Care Needs in Washington State, Seattle.* Olympia: Washington State Department of Health; 1998.

44. Hedberg AM, Lairson DR, Aday LA, Chow J, Suki R, Houston F, Wolf JA. Economic implications of an early postoperative enteral feeding protocol. *J Am Diet Assoc.* 1999;99:802–807.

45. Brannon SD, Tershakovec AM, Shannon BM. The cost-effectiveness of alternative methods of nutrition education for hypercholesterolemic children. *Am J Public Health.* 1997;87:1967–1970.

46. Shevitz AH, Wilson IB, McDermott AY, Spiegelman D, Skinner SC, Antonsson K, Layne JE, Beaston-Blaakman A, Sheperd DS, Gorbach SL. A comparison of the clinical and cost-effectiveness of 3 intervention strategies for AIDS wasting. *J Acquir Immune Defic Syndr.* 2005;38: 399–406.

47. Braga M, Gianotti L. Preoperative immunonutrition: cost-benefit analysis. *JPEN J Parenter Enteral Nutr.* 2005;29(1 suppl):S57–S61.

48. Kruizenga HM, Van Tulder MW, Seidell JC, Thijs A, Ader HJ, Van Bokhorst-de van der Schuerer MA. Effectiveness and cost-effectiveness of early screening and treatment of malnourished patients. *Am J Clin Nutr.* 2005;82:1082–1089.

49. Caro J, Huybrechts KF, Klittich WS, Jackson JD, McGuire A; CORE Study Group. Allocating funds for cardiovascular disease prevention in light of the NCEP ATP III guidelines. *Am J Manag Care.* 2003;9:477–489.

50. Naglak M, Mitchell DC, Kris-Etherton P, Harkness W, Pearson TA. What to consider when conducting cost-effectiveness analysis in a clinical setting. *J Am Diet Assoc.* 1998;98:1149–1154.

51. Hampl JS, Anderson JV, Mullis R. Position paper: The role of dietetics professionals in health promotion and disease prevention. *J Am Diet Assoc.* 2002;102: 1680–1687.

52. World Health Organization. *Making Choices in Health: WHO Guide to Cost-Effectiveness Analysis.* Geneva, Switzerland: World Health Organization; 2003.

53. Trostler N, Myers EF. Research activities and perspectives of research members of the American Dietetic Association. *J Am Diet Assoc.* 2003;103: 626–632.

21

Research in Diet and Human Genetics

*Ruth E. Patterson, PhD, Johanna W. Lampe, PhD, RD, and
Cheryl L. Rock, PhD, RD*

Considerable research has focused on identifying exposures (eg, tobacco smoke, diet) that increase the risk of disease, but it is evident that not all individuals exposed to the same risk factors will develop the associated disease (1). For example, although it is well accepted that smoking causes lung cancer, only 10% to 15% of smokers will be diagnosed with the disease in their lifetime (2). We are beginning to understand the impact of differential genetic susceptibility in the etiology and pathogenesis of common diseases such as coronary heart disease and cancer. This new biology offers promise of an individualized approach to preventive medicine through risk profiling and the provision of information on how to modify the potential results of genetic predisposition via dietary modification or other environmental changes (3).

This chapter reviews the basic genetic mechanisms, describes the concepts underlying research in diet and human genetics, reviews important study designs for conducting research in this area, presents tools and techniques for the collection and archiving of DNA, discusses informed consent for studies involving genetic markers, and comments on the future of research in diet-gene interactions.

BASIC GENETIC MECHANISMS

To understand the new advances in human genetics, it is useful to review the fundamentals of molecular genetics.

This review is brief and therefore necessarily simplistic; we refer the interested reader to texts by Mueller and Young (4) and Alberts et al (5), from which the following overview is largely synthesized.

The genetic material within our cells contains the complete set of instructions for making an organism, called its *genome*. The human genome is organized into 46 chromosomes. Of these chromosomes, 44 are in 22 pairs (autosomes) in which 1 chromosome is inherited from the mother and 1 chromosome is inherited from the father. In addition, females inherit an X chromosome from each parent, whereas males inherit an X chromosome from the mother and a Y chromosome from the father.

Each chromosome contains many genes. A gene is a segment of a chromosome that encodes instructions allowing a cell to produce a specific protein, such as an enzyme, receptor, or carrier protein. The human genome is estimated to contain 20,000 to 25,000 genes (6). Each gene is composed of long stretches of DNA that can be divided into three separate classes (Figure 21.1) (7). The parts of a gene that actually provide the specific "instructions" (the coding region) for making a protein are called *exons*. In most genes, multiple exons are present, but they are separated by noncoding stretches of DNA called *introns*. In addition to exons and introns, each gene contains a noncoding region at its beginning (the 5′ end) that serves to regulate when, and to what extent, the gene is expressed. This is referred to as the regulatory region of the gene, and it can be envisioned as a series of on/off switches that respond to signals (eg, proteins

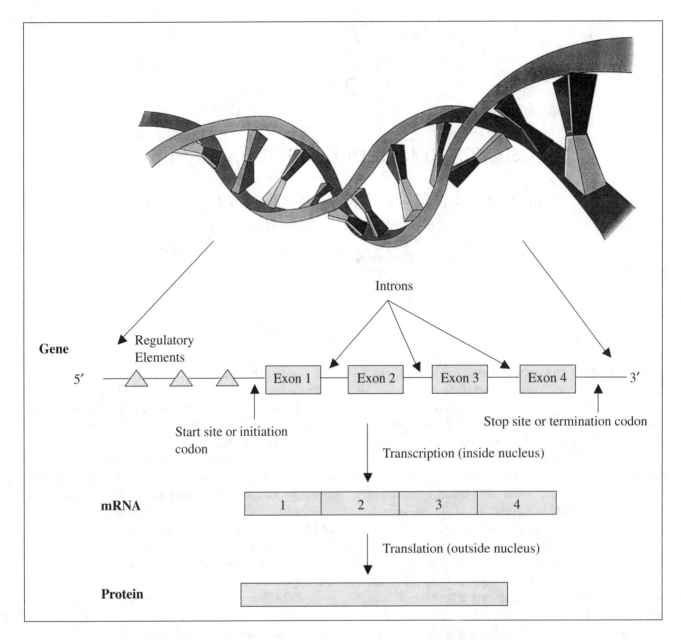

FIGURE 21.1   DNA and a diagram of a typical human structural gene. Reprinted from Patterson RE, Eaton EL, Potter JP. The genetic revolution: change and challenge for the profession of dietetics. *J Am Diet Assoc*. 1999;99:1412–1420. Reprinted with permission from the American Dietetic Association.

and hormones) from within the cell, from neighboring cells, and from more distant parts of the organism.

Genes are composed of DNA, which exists as two paired or complementary strands forming a double helix (refer to Figure 21.1). Each strand is composed of millions of chemical building blocks, called *bases*. There are four different chemical bases in DNA: adenine, thymine, cytosine, and guanine. The four bases are strung along a repetitive sugar- (deoxyribose) phosphate backbone. The two strands of DNA are held together by pairing of the

chemical bases. Adenine forms hydrogen bonds with thymine, and cytosine forms hydrogen bonds with guanine.

Every group of three bases (called a *triplet*) along a strand of DNA specifies an amino acid to be incorporated into a protein, in what is called the *genetic code*. For example, a triplet composed of the bases guanine, cytosine, and adenine, in that order, is the genetic triplet code for the amino acid alanine. Certain combinations of bases (eg, thymine adenine adenine [TAA]), called *termination* or *stop codons,* will terminate the gene product. Mathematically, four bases can form up to 64 unique triplet codes; however, there are only 20 amino acids. This redundancy in the genetic code is called *degeneracy.*

When a cell is "switched" on to make a protein, the information from a gene is copied, base by base, from DNA into a single new strand of complementary RNA. RNA differs from DNA in three ways: (a) RNA is single-stranded, whereas DNA is double-stranded; (b) the sugar-phosphate backbone of RNA is composed of ribose, whereas in DNA it is composed of deoxyribose; and (c) RNA contains the base uracil, whereas DNA contains the base thymine. This primary RNA molecule is spliced to remove intron sequences so that only the coding sequences from the exons are used to produce messenger RNA (mRNA). The mRNA travels out of the nucleus into the cytoplasm, where it directs the complex set of reactions that occur on a ribosome and result in the assembly of amino acids that fold into completed protein molecules. Two other types of RNA, transfer RNA (tRNA) and ribosomal RNA (rRNA), are used in the cell to facilitate the synthesis of proteins from the mRNA template. In addition, some RNA molecules in cells have been found to function as enzyme-like catalysts rather than serving as a template for protein synthesis.

Genes, through the proteins they encode, control all aspects of our cell function, including how efficiently we process foods, how effectively we metabolize compounds such as endogenous hormones and exogenous toxins, and how vigorously we respond to infections.

Human Genetic Variation, Mutations, and Polymorphism

Although thousands of random changes occur every day in the DNA of a cell as a result of heat energy and metabolic accidents, only a few stable changes accumulate in the DNA sequence of an average cell in a year. The rest of the changes are eliminated with remarkable efficiency by a variety of DNA repair mechanisms. Nearly all these repair mechanisms depend on the existence of two copies, or alleles, of the genetic material. If one DNA strand is accidentally changed, information is not lost irretrievably because an unaltered (complementary) copy of the altered strand remains and can act as a template to repair the damaged strand. DNA mutations that occur in germ cells (sperm or ova) are called *germ-line mutations.* These inheritable DNA mutations determine the characteristics of offspring, including their susceptibility to disease. It is important to

recognize that DNA mutations can occur in other body cells (ie, somatic cells). Somatic mutations are acquired from the environment (eg, from tobacco) and can result in the transformation of a normal cell to a malignant cell, which can then give rise to a tumor by clonal expansion. However, this overview of diet-gene interactions focuses entirely on germ-line mutations.

The effect of a change or alteration in DNA depends on a large variety of factors. If the change occurs in an intron, there may or may not be an effect on the functioning of an organism. Some intronic alterations can affect how the mRNA is processed. Furthermore, if a gene is altered, the protein encoded by that gene may or may not be modified. For example, the most common type of mutation involves a single changed base in the DNA, called a *single-nucleotide polymorphism* (SNP). However, because the triplet genetic code is degenerate, an SNP may still code for the same amino acid (called a *silent mutation*). Even if a DNA sequence alteration produces a change in an amino acid, it may not significantly affect the protein, because the amino acid may be at a site that is not crucial to the protein's function. In contrast, other DNA alterations result in protein changes that can be disabling. For example, some alterations include the loss (or gain) of a base, resulting in a frame shift mutation such that all the codons downstream are shifted out of their usual sequence of triplets. Other alterations can convert a coding triplet into a stop codon, which tells the cell to end the protein prematurely. DNA alterations can also include the multiplication or disappearance of long segments of DNA, which can severely impair (or, rarely, augment) protein function.

A genetic polymorphism is a variation in DNA that is inherited in the population at levels high enough that it could not be maintained by random DNA changes alone (conventionally defined as affecting more than 1% of the population). Studies of enzyme and protein variability have indicated that in human beings, at least 30% of gene loci are polymorphic. Polymorphisms occur with great frequency outside coding regions, where the alterations have less consequence on gene expression.

Genes and Disease Risk

The relative influences of environmental and genetic factors in disease causation are variable and result in a spectrum with diseases that are largely environmentally determined (eg, highly infectious diseases) at one end and diseases that are largely genetically determined (eg, severe inherited metabolic disorders) at the other (8). Probably the best-known genetic factors that increase risk of disease are the highly penetrant, dominant mutations associated with high disease risks. Examples of this type of mutation are breast cancer gene 1 (*BRCA1*) and breast cancer gene 2 (*BRCA2*). Although this type of genetic variation can appreciably increase the individual's risk of disease, the public health significance is less clear, because the majority of women who develop breast cancer do not have this mutation or other highly penetrant mutations that have been identified. For example, *BRCA1* and *BRCA2* mutations appear to account for 5.3% of breast cancer cases in women younger than 40 years, 2.2% of cases in women aged 40 to 49 years, and only 1.1% of cases in women aged 50 to 70 years (9). In addition, studies in low-risk populations suggest that many women with *BRCA1* or *BRCA2* do not develop breast cancer (9,10).

Compared with highly penetrant, dominant mutations, genetic variants that affect susceptibility to common diseases can have a much greater effect at the population level, even though they may pose relatively low individual risk (11). Although these genes determine susceptibility to diseases such as coronary heart disease, hypertension, diabetes, and some types of cancer, environmental factors (eg, dietary intake) determine who among the susceptible subgroup will develop the associated disease. Table 21.1

gives several examples of known or hypothesized diet-gene interactions (3,7,12,13).

One intense area of research concerns polymorphisms in genes that code for xenobiotic metabolizing enzymes (eg, cytochromes P450 and glutathione-*S*-transferases), which play an important role in activating and/or detoxifying foreign compounds, such as carcinogens (Figure 21.2) (7). Dietary constituents (including micronutrients and nonnutrient compounds) act as inducing agents through several molecular mechanisms and are well-known substrates of some of these enzymes. Interactions between these enzymes and dietary intake likely play a major role in cancer etiology (12,13). Another area of interest in susceptibility genes includes polymorphisms in apolipoproteins, which influence serum lipid responsiveness to dietary intake and thereby modify the development of cardiovascular disease (12).

Polymorphisms that alter enzyme activities often have high prevalence in the population, so even modestly increased absolute risk can lead to a rather high population-level risk when there is appropriate exposure (3). For example, McWilliams et al conducted a meta-analysis in which they concluded that deficiency of a certain enzyme (glutathione-*S*-transferase M1) results in approximately a 40% increased risk of lung cancer among smokers (14). Although the increased risk to an individual is fairly low, both cigarette

TABLE 21.1   Examples of Known and Hypothesized Diet-Gene Interactions

Polymorphism (Gene or *Gene Product*)	Gene Product Function	Environmental Exposure(s) (Risk Factor)	Associated Condition or Disease (Phenotype)
Known Diet-Gene Interactions			
Glucose-6-phosphate dehydrogenase (G6PD)	Metabolism	Fava bean consumption	Hemolytic anemia
Phenylketonuria (PKU) gene	Metabolism of phenylalanine	Dietary phenylalanine	Phenylketonuria
Hemochromatosis (HFE) gene	Iron absorption	Dietary iron	Hemochromatosis
Lactase phlorizin hydrolase (LPH)	Metabolism of lactose	Dietary lactose	Lactase nonpersistence or adult lactose intolerance
Hypothesized Diet-Gene Interactions			
Glutathione-S-transferase M1 (GSTM1)	Detoxification	Smoking combined with diet low in antioxidants	Lung cancer
Epoxide hydrolase (EH), glutathione-S-transferase M1 (GSTM1)	Detoxification	Consumption of aflatoxin (fungal contaminant, especially of peanuts)	Liver cancer
Apolipoprotein A-I and A-IV, apolipoprotein E (Apo E), apolipoprotein B	Lipoprotein metabolism	Dietary cholesterol and fat	Altered responsiveness to dietary cholesterol and fat intake
Methylenetetrahydrofolate reductase (MTHFR)	Metabolism of folate, affecting plasma homocysteine levels	Low folate status, multivitamin nonuse	Coronary heart disease, stroke, colon cancer, and neural tube defects

Source: Data are from references 3, 7, 12, and 13.

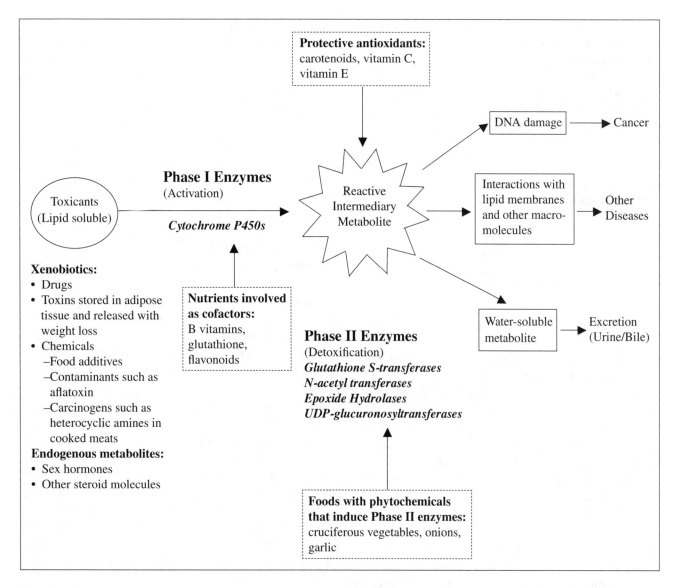

FIGURE 21.2   Interrelationships between xenobiotic biotransformation enzymes and dietary constituents in detoxification pathways. Reprinted from Patterson RE, Eaton EL, Potter JP. The genetic revolution: change and challenge for the profession of dietetics. *J Am Diet Assoc.* 1999;99:1412–1420. Reprinted with permission from the American Dietetic Association.

smoking and the enzyme deficiency are so prevalent that this polymorphism may result in approximately 29,000 new cases of lung cancer each year in the United States.

Diet-Gene Interactions

Several definitions for diet-gene interactions have been proposed. From a biological perspective, interaction between two factors (eg, genotype and dietary intake) has been defined as their coparticipation in the same causal mechanism of disease development (15,16). Alternatively, interaction is often thought of as a situation in which joint exposure to two or more factors results in a greater number of cases of disease than the sum of the separate factors, regardless of the biological mechanism (17). Interactions have also been defined as a statistical concept, relating to the statistical significance of joint-predictor variables in multivariable models of disease risk (16). This chapter uses the simplest and broadest possible definition of interaction as being two factors that act upon each other (18), in this case in the modification of disease risk.

TABLE 21.2   Hypothetical Examples Illustrating Two Different Types of Diet-Gene Interactions That Increase Disease Risk (Expressed as Relative Risks)

a. Neither dietary intake nor the genotype is an independent risk factor, but their interaction results in disease risk.

	Genotype	
Nutrient Intake	Wild Type ("Normal")	Variant
Low	1.00	1.00
High	1.00	2.00

b. Both dietary intake and the genotype are independent risk factors, and their interaction increases disease risk synergistically.

	Genotype	
Nutrient Intake	Wild Type ("Normal")	Variant
Low	1.00	2.00
High	2.00	10.00

It is also important to note that there are different biological types of gene-environment interactions. For example, in some cases, neither the genotype nor the environmental factor has any effect on disease risk in the absence of the other, but when both are present the interaction increases disease risk (Table 21.2a). An example of this kind of diet-gene interaction that is well known to RDs is phenylketonuria, in which neither the abnormal genotype nor the environmental exposure alone is sufficient to cause mental retardation (19). Alternatively, in other types of diet-gene interactions, either the genotype or the environmental factor carries some risk for disease, but their combination increases disease risk additively or even synergistically (Table 21.2b). The critical point is that the term *interaction* covers a variety of biological phenomena, and the specific form of the interaction is as important as the fact that an interaction exists.

STUDY DESIGNS FOR RESEARCH IN DIET AND HUMAN GENETICS

Research studies involving humans can be roughly divided into two types: experimental and observational. An experiment is a set of observations conducted under controlled circumstances, in which the investigator manipulates the conditions to ascertain what effect such manipulation has on the observations (16). In human studies, the main experimental study design is randomized controlled trials (RCTs), also called *clinical trials*. These controlled studies can provide definitive information on a research question, but they

are usually expensive and logistically challenging. In addition, it is not ethical to knowingly expose individuals to factors that increase their risk of disease simply to learn about disease causation. Therefore, when it is not feasible to conduct an experiment, scientists typically use observational studies to investigate what might have been learned if an experiment had been conducted (16). The primary observational study designs include cohort and case-control studies. The following discussion provides an overview of experimental and observational designs in relation to the study of diet-gene interactions.

Experimental Design: Randomized Controlled Trials

Randomized controlled trials (RCTs) prospectively examine the effect of an exposure (eg, diet) on an outcome (eg, a disease, a risk factor for a disease, or a biomarker). The two main designs are crossover and parallel arm. In a crossover study, each participant receives all test diets in a randomized order. Important considerations regarding crossover designs are the potential for carryover effects and the time between experimental conditions that is necessary to achieve baseline conditions (ie, the washout period). In a parallel-arm design, each participant is assigned at random to only one test diet, and therefore different groups of participants receive different test diets. Each design has advantages and disadvantages related to sample size, duration of the study, and design considerations (20). Both study designs lend themselves to the study of diet-gene interactions, so the design should be selected on the basis of the hypothesis being tested.

Another important consideration in the design of an experimental study is the degree of dietary control required. The stringency of dietary control (eg, a controlled diet provided by the investigators vs supplementation of a usual diet vs dietary counseling) is determined in part by the expected size of the response variable of interest and the length of the treatment period required. For instance, if the interindividual variation in the response variable is high (possibly as a result of normal dietary differences), standardizing the diet (eg, by using a controlled feeding study) may improve the capacity to detect an effect of a particular nutrient or dietary constituent. However, if the required dietary treatment period exceeds several months, a controlled feeding study is usually not logistically or financially viable.

Two different approaches to testing gene-diet interactions in RCTs are used. One approach is to select participants a priori on the basis of genotype. This requires that the investigator identify candidate genetic polymorphisms and have some knowledge or hypothesis regarding the associated phenotypic response. In studies of this type, individuals are screened for study participation, genotyped for the polymorphism of interest, and then recruited and block randomized to treatment or treatment order by genotype. This design ensures that there is adequate, balanced representation of genotypes, which is especially valuable if the frequency of the polymorphism is low.

Another approach is to select participants for a study, conduct the intervention or feeding study, genotype individuals, and test for diet-gene interactions in the statistical analysis. This approach is feasible in studies with large sample sizes and for polymorphisms that are highly prevalent. For example, if the frequency of a particular genetic variant is 50% and the variant (a) does not phenotypically influence eligibility for the study and (b) does not bias willingness to participate in the study, one would expect relatively equal representation of the wild type (ie, the "normal" genotype) and the variant. In contrast, if the variant frequency is low (eg, 10%), the distribution may be unbalanced, and it is unlikely that there will be enough individuals with the variant genotype to make it possible to test for the diet-gene interaction.

Clinical trials provide a useful platform for testing effects of genetic polymorphisms in response to particular dietary treatments, and this approach to researching diet-gene interactions is gaining popularity. A clinical trial is a rigorous study design because participants with factors that might influence the disease or other end point being studied (eg, diet quality, physical activity, or cancer screening behavior) are equally likely to be randomized into the intervention group or the control group. However, as is the case with traditional feeding studies, these projects tend to be expensive and labor-intensive and therefore may not be feasible.

Observational Design: Epidemiologic Studies

Ideally, the quality of evidence from an observational (nonexperimental) study will be as high as that from a well-designed experiment. However, in an experiment the investigator has the power to assign exposures, whereas in an observational design the investigator cannot control the exposure (16). A major limitation of all epidemiologic observational studies is the possibility of confounding, in which the exposure of interest is merely a surrogate for a different active agent. Although statistical models that control for confounding factors attempt to address this problem, an absence of confounding cannot be ensured, particularly if important confounding factors are unknown or not measured.

There are two primary types of observational study designs in epidemiology: the cohort study and the case-control study. The basics of these study designs and their application in research on diet-gene interactions are reviewed next.

Cohort Studies

The classic cohort study is a design in which one or more groups of people who are free of disease and who vary in exposure to a potential risk factor (eg, dietary intake) are followed over time and examined with respect to the development of disease. The major advantage of cohort studies is that exposure to potential risk factors is assessed before the development of disease. Therefore, risk factors, such as serum micronutrient concentrations, cannot be influenced by the disease process. In addition, these types of studies can examine many different exposures in relation to many different disease outcomes. Cohort studies are generally large enterprises because most diseases affect only a small proportion of a population, even if the population is followed for many years. These studies typically have sample sizes exceeding 50,000 and require that the cohort be followed for at least 10 years (16).

Because of the large size of these studies, the analysis of biological markers (eg, serum micronutrient concentrations or genotype) of all participants is prohibitively expensive. Therefore, these studies typically rely on specimen repositories or frozen banks of substances such as serum, white blood cells, and DNA to conduct future nested case-control studies. In a nested case-control study, a sample of cohort participants who develop a disease, such as breast cancer (cases), are matched to other individuals in the cohort who do not develop the disease (controls). Biological samples from cases and controls are then pulled from the freezer and analyzed for genetic polymorphisms. Statistical analyses are performed to determine whether there are differences in the prevalence of the polymorphism and other exposures (eg, dietary intake) between the cases and the controls. This design can be efficient and powerful, and it avoids many of the pitfalls of retrospective case-control studies (see the next section).

Case-Control Studies

In a case-control study, individuals are identified and studied according to a single disease outcome. In the classic case-control study, individuals who have recently been diagnosed with a disease (eg, colon cancer) are queried about their past exposure to diet and other risk factors, and they often provide a blood sample. A matched set of control individuals, usually drawn from the same population, are also enrolled in the study. The major advantage of this design is that an entire study can be completed in 4 years, typically with as few as 400 cases and 400 controls. However, this design can answer only questions about a single disease outcome. In addition, these studies can introduce biases that are absent in cohort or nested case-control studies. Another problem with case-control studies is that many biomarkers (eg, serum micronutrient concentrations) are affected by the disease process and therefore may not be reliable measures of predisease status (risk) in cases. However, genetic polymorphisms are not altered by disease and therefore remain valid markers of individual susceptibility to disease, even in this study design, where the cases have already developed the disease of interest.

Sample Size Considerations in Studies of Diet-Gene Interactions

A major concern in all studies of diet-gene interactions is sample size. Interaction effects can be thought of as the identification of subgroups of the population for whom the exposure of interest imparts a particularly high risk. The sample size required to study interactions is dependent on the percentage of the sample exposed to both the main effects (eg, fat intake and a particular polymorphism), the degree of increased risk conferred by each of the main effects separately, and the increased risk conferred by their interaction (21).

For example, a sample size of approximately 750 cases and 750 controls is required to detect, with reasonable statistical confidence ($\alpha = 0.05$ [one sided], $1 - \beta = 0.95$), a twofold increased risk among individuals with a variant genotype who are also exposed to a specific diet, assuming no increased risk among those exposed to diet or the genotype alone (refer to Table 21.2)—*if* 50% of the population are exposed to the genotype (21). If only 10% of the population are exposed to the genotype, the minimum study size necessary to detect the interaction effect is approximately 1,800 cases and 1,800 controls.

In general, detecting an interaction effect of the same magnitude as a postulated main effect requires an increase in the study size by approximately a factor of 4, and in some circumstances considerably more (21). Therefore, unless a study is designed to test for diet-gene interactions, it is unlikely to have enough power to detect such an interaction;

indeed, much of the published literature on diet-gene interactions has that limitation.

TOOLS AND TECHNIQUES: COLLECTING AND ARCHIVING DNA

Several factors related to the logistics and planned use of DNA specimens should be considered in choosing a method of DNA collection and storage. For example, what is the study sample size? Do you need blood for measuring other biomarkers? Where will the DNA specimens be collected? How many assays are you planning to run on the sample? Are you collecting the samples for long-term storage? How are you going to retrieve the samples from storage? Many of these considerations are generic issues that relate to the collection and storage of all types of biological specimens for biomarker measurement; however, other issues are DNA specific. Note that information on methods for analyzing polymorphisms is beyond the scope of this chapter; interested readers should refer to recent papers and texts on the topic (22).

Traditionally, DNA for genetic analyses has been extracted from white blood cells (leukocytes) collected from whole blood. This approach yields substantial amounts of DNA (approximately 100 µg DNA from 10 mL whole blood). However, to participants, venipuncture is probably the least attractive method of providing genomic DNA. It is invasive and uncomfortable, is unacceptable to some for cultural or religious reasons, and usually requires that participants come to a central location to have blood drawn. These undesirable aspects of venipuncture mean that participant refusal rates for blood collection can be high (20% to 40%) (23). In addition, for molecular epidemiologic studies, blood specimen collection is expensive and can be a logistical challenge when sample sizes are large and people are scattered geographically.

For studies where only DNA is needed (ie, blood samples are not also being collected for plasma), there are other approaches to collecting genomic DNA. Improved sensitivity in molecular biological techniques means that very small quantities of DNA are often sufficient for many assays. Thus, biological samples obtained by less invasive methods, but providing lower yields of DNA, can be sources of DNA for genotyping (Table 21.3) (23–26). DNA for genetic analysis can be extracted from urine, hair roots, finger-stick blood, saliva, and buccal cells obtained by cheek scraping, brushing, or oral rinsing. Some of these methods are moderately invasive or unpleasant (finger

TABLE 21.3 DNA Yields from Human Tissues and Body Fluids

Biological Specimen	DNA Yield (μg, Mean [Range])
Whole blood, 10 mL	~100–400
Serum, 250 μL	0.16–1.06
Plasma, 250 μL	0.16–0.37
Paraffin-embedded tissue, 5- to 20-μm sections	1–11.7
Buccal cells, mouth wash method	49.7 (0.2–134.0)
Buccal cells, 1 swab	1–2
Buccal cells, 10 swabs	32 (3.2–110.8)

Source: Data are from references 23 (buccal cells, mouthwash method), 24 (buccal cells, 10 swabs), 25 (whole blood; buccal cells, 1 swab), and 26 (serum, plasma, paraffin-embedded tissue).

stick, cheek scraping or brushing, and urine collection), or provide lower yields (urine, hair roots, and saliva) or lower-quality DNA (ie, short fragments) (23–25).

Tissues obtained at surgery that are fixed and embedded in paraffin provide another source of DNA. The ability to isolate DNA from paraffin-embedded tissues, as well as from serum and plasma, facilitates genetic analysis of archived samples from prospective cohort studies (26); however, the ethical and legal issues of analyzing archived tissues must be addressed, and appropriate institutional review board approval must be obtained. (This topic is covered in more detail later in the section "Informed Consent Issues.")

Guidelines for collecting, processing, and banking DNA have been published (26–28). Although the extraction of DNA from fresh samples is optimal, storage of whole blood for up to 3 days at room temperature does not appear to adversely affect DNA recovery (27). This fact provides researchers with some leeway when samples are collected at remote sites and shipped to a central laboratory for processing.

Currently, DNA is purified from biological samples using one of three major methods that are fast and yield good-quality DNA. These methods include salt precipitation (29), phenol/chloroform extraction (30), and solid-phase extraction (31,32); the latter can be carried out using commercially available kits. Differences in DNA extraction procedures do not appear to affect DNA yields, which are influenced more by how the blood or tissue is collected and stored (26). Carefully handled lymphocytes obtained from whole blood can be frozen in liquid nitrogen for 20 years or more without losing their viability. Thus, they can be

stored and processed at a later date, or they can be immortalized to provide a stable, indefinite source of DNA (33).

Storing or banking DNA offers researchers the option of testing new hypotheses about gene-diet interactions in relation to disease risk many years after the blood or tissue specimen has been collected. The use of DNA banks requires appropriate long-term storage conditions and meticulous record keeping (28).

INFORMED CONSENT ISSUES

Increasing knowledge regarding disease etiology and treatment is generally good for both society and the individuals whose care is improved by a more complete understanding of disease (34). Despite the desirability of increased knowledge, however, research can risk harm to the individuals who are being studied. Therefore, the prevailing legal and ethical precept is that people participate in research only after they have given their informed consent. From the perspective of individuals, consent provides information about the nature of the project and the risks and benefits that accompany participation so that they can decide whether to participate. For the investigator, obtaining informed consent reduces the risk that participants will pursue legal actions if their expectations about the study are not met (34).

Although not unique to genetic research, the issues related to potential discrimination based on genetic profiling, the retrospective use of archived tissue samples, and the adequacy of protections for privacy and confidentiality have triggered public concerns about the pace and scale of technological change (35,36). Two characteristics of genetic testing make it especially controversial. First, the implications of genetic information are both individual and familial; second, genetic testing often identifies disorders for which there are no effective treatments or preventive measures. Obtaining informed consent for genetic testing is particularly challenging in view of the complexity of the genetic information, the controversial nature of clinical options such as abortion or prophylactic surgery of unknown efficacy, and the social and psychological implications of testing (37).

Informed Consent for Genetic Testing

For conditions in which a polymorphism confers a fairly high risk of developing the associated disease, the consequences of knowledge of genotype are complex. On the basis of family history alone, individuals at risk of relatively uncommon and highly penetrant conditions (eg, Huntington's disease) have found it difficult to obtain health insurance and have faced employment discrimination. The ethical response to these concerns has been to mandate detailed informed consent with pretest, and sometimes posttest, counseling of participants (38). However, the paradigm for consent in genetic research may not be appropriate for all applications. For research on common low-risk genotypes, it is not clear that the risks to participants warrant counseling, particularly if little is known about the risk of the genotype. Hunter and Caporaso have suggested that, as in most other aspects of research, the level of consent should be proportional to the degree of risk involved, and thus less stringent consent procedures may be appropriate for low-risk genotypes than for high-risk genotypes (38).

Informed Consent for Genetic Research on Stored Tissue Samples

It is widely accepted that individuals must provide informed consent for projects that involve their direct involvement. However, the role of informed consent is much less clear for research that does not require such personal involvement but rather can be performed using stored tissue samples.

The use of banked serum samples in the study of both chronic and infectious disease has a long and distinguished history in public health and medicine (39). Many important studies in these areas came about only after stored samples provided the material to test hypotheses that could not have been formulated at the time of specimen collection. Similarly, genetic research is evolving rapidly, and most hypotheses will emerge because of future research. Suggestions have been made that specific informed consent be required for all genetic testing (34). If it were necessary to recontact participants, however, most studies could not be performed. Recontacting participants would be prohibitively expensive and time-consuming, and it would be impossible to reach many participants because of relocation or death. In addition, this process has the potential to introduce bias, threatening the validity of the research findings. One approach to this dilemma is to ask participants to approve genetic testing of their biological samples on the condition that all identifying information be removed. The results of these tests could not be matched to the individual participant in the study, at any time or by any investigator. However, even this procedure is controversial (34).

Summary: Informed Consent and Genetic Testing

The current regulations regarding genetic testing are unclear, and expert groups offer conflicting advice. A survey of informed consent forms from seven different testing facilities found that the forms demonstrated substantial variation in content and organization (40), indicating that the institutional approaches to these questions can vary substantially. It is critical that the debate on measures to prevent the misuse of genetic information in research be conducted by scientists and professional societies. Otherwise, well-intentioned, but ill-informed, efforts to protect the rights of individuals and groups could hurt everyone by blocking the progress of research.

CONCLUSION

Research on diet-gene interactions can greatly improve our understanding of the influence of nutritional factors on risks for common diseases. If only a subgroup of individuals are sensitive to dietary factors, the effect on disease risk may be diluted, or even undetectable, when the entire population is the focus of study. Continued research in this area will also clarify the underlying mechanisms of many nutritional factors by delineating their biological roles in relation to variations in enzyme activity. Eventually, increased knowledge will allow us to target disease-preventing diet interventions at those individuals most likely to benefit by diet modification, based on their genetic susceptibility.

In spite of the substantial potential benefits in this area of study, there are also notable constraints:

- There are substantial challenges involved in accurately identifying and characterizing exposures to nutritional factors in epidemiologic studies, and even the best methods for nutrition and dietary assessment used in population-based research have well-known limitations and weaknesses (41).
- Given the potential importance of recently recognized phytochemicals (eg, isothiocyanates in cruciferous vegetables) in diet-gene interactions, considerable research is needed to improve our understanding of the bioavailability and other pharmacokinetic properties of these compounds. Exacerbating the problem is the fact that in most cases, a food content database that would allow quantification of intake of these compounds is not available.

- Biomarkers and biological assays that are used to characterize the susceptibility of individuals based on genetic variation must be readily available, at low cost, with demonstrated and understood validity in the targeted populations.
- Studies must be carefully designed so that sample sizes are large enough to detect diet-gene interaction effects.

Diet-gene interactions are likely to contribute considerably to the observed individual variation in disease risk in response to nutritional factors (12,13). In the future, we will be able to define more precisely the molecular mechanisms underlying human health and disease; subdivide clinically indistinguishable diseases and conditions (eg, obesity) into more distinct entities, thereby improving our ability to choose rational preventive and treatment measures; identify genotypic markers that predict metabolic responses to dietary interventions; and stratify the population into groups at higher or lower risk of chronic diseases such as cancer, allowing dietary intervention to be appropriately targeted (42). Diet-gene interactions represent an exciting and important new interdisciplinary research area for RDs in collaboration with epidemiologists and molecular scientists.

REFERENCES

1. Khoury MJ. Genetic epidemiology. In: Rothman K, Greenland S, eds. *Modern Epidemiology.* 2nd ed. Boston, Mass: Little, Brown, and Company; 1998: 609–622.
2. American Cancer Society. *Cancer Facts and Figures 1995.* Atlanta, Ga: ACS; 1995.
3. Lampe JW, Potter JD. Genetic variation, diet, and disease susceptibility. In: Costa LG, Eaton DL, eds. *Gene-Environment Interactions: Fundamentals of Ecogenetics.* Hoboken, NJ: Wiley; 2006:321–350.
4. Mueller RF, Young ID. *Emery's Elements of Medical Genetics.* 9th ed. New York, NY: Churchill Livingstone; 1995.
5. Alberts B, Johnson A, Lewis J, Raff M, Roberts K, Walter P. *Molecular Biology of the Cell.* 4th ed. New York, NY: Garland Science Publishing Inc; 2002.
6. International Human Genome Sequencing Consortium. Finishing the euchromatic sequence of the human genome. *Nature.* 2004;431: 931–945.
7. Patterson RE, Eaton EL, Potter JP. The genetic revolution: change and challenge for the profession of dietetics. *J Am Diet Assoc.* 1999;99: 1412–1420.
8. Garte S, Zocchetti C, Taioli E. Gene-environmental interactions in the application of biomarkers of cancer susceptibility in epidemiology. In: Toniolo P, Boffetta P, Shuker DEG, Rothman N, Hulka B, Pearce N, eds. *Applications of Biomarkers in Cancer Epidemiology.* Lyon, France: IARC Scientific Publications; 1997:264. Publication 142.
9. Sellers TA. Genetic factors in the pathogenesis of breast cancer: their role and relative importance. *J Nutr.* 1997;127(suppl 5):929–932.
10. Malone KE, Daling JR, Thompson JD, O'Brien CA, Francisco LV, Ostrander EA. BRCA1 mutations and breast cancer in the general population: analyses in women before age 35 years and in women before age 45 years with first-degree family history. *JAMA.* 1998;279:922–929.
11. Perera FP. Environment and cancer: who are susceptible? *Science.* 1997;278:1068–1073.
12. Reszka E, Wasowicz W, Gromadzinska J. Genetic polymorphism of xenobiotic metabolising enzymes, diet and cancer susceptibility. *Br J Nutr.* 2006;96: 609–619.
13. Ordovas JM. Nutrigenetics, plasma lipids, and cardiovascular risk. *J Am Diet Assoc.* 2006;106: 1074–1081.
14. McWilliams JE, Sanderson BJS, Harris EL, Richert-Boe KE, Henner WD. Glutathione *S*-transferase M1 (GSTM1) deficiency and lung cancer risk. *Cancer Epidemiol Biomarkers Prev.* 1995;4:589–594.
15. Yang Q, Khoury MJ. Evolving methods in genetic epidemiology. III. Gene-environment interaction in epidemiologic research. *Epidemiol Rev.* 1997;19: 33–43.
16. Rothman KJ, Greenland S. Types of epidemiologic study. In: Rothman K, Greenland S, eds. *Modern Epidemiology.* Boston, Mass: Little, Brown, and Company; 1998:67–78.
17. Blot WJ, Day NE. Synergism and interaction: are they equivalent? *Am J Epidemiol.* 1979;110:99–100.
18. Flexner SB, Hauck LC, eds. *The Random House Dictionary of the English Language.* 2nd ed. New York, NY: Random House; 1987.
19. Elsas LJ, Acosta PB. Inherited metabolic disease: amino acids, organic acids, and galactose. In: Shils ME, Shike M, Ross AC, Caballero B, Cousins RJ, eds. *Modern Nutrition in Health and Disease.* 9th

ed. Philadelphia, Pa: Lippincott Williams & Wilkins; 2005:909–959.

20. Derr JA. Statistical aspects of controlled diet studies. In: Dennis BH, Ershow AG, Obarzanek E, Clevidence BA, eds. *Well-Controlled Diet Studies in Humans: A Practical Guide to Design and Management.* Chicago, Ill: American Dietetic Association; 1997.

21. Smith PG, Day NE. The design of case-control studies: the influence of confounding and interaction effect. *Int J Epidemiol.* 1984;13:356–365.

22. Bammler TK, Farin FM, Beyer RP. Tools for ecogenetics. In: Costa LG, Eaton DL, eds. *Gene-Environment Interactions: Fundamentals of Ecogenetics.* Hoboken, NJ:Wiley; 2006:17–49.

23. Lum A, Le Marchand L. A simple mouthwash method for obtaining genomic DNA in molecular epidemiological studies. *Cancer Epidemiol Biomarkers Prev.* 1998;7:719–724.

24. Meulenbelt I, Droog S, Trommelen GJM, Boomsma DI, Slagboom PE. High-yield noninvasive human genomic DNA isolation method for genetic studies in geographically dispersed families and populations. *Am J Hum Genet.* 1995;57:1252–1254.

25. Steinberg K, Beck J, Nickerson D, Garcia-Closas M, Gallagher M, Caggana M, Reid Y, Cosentino M, Ji J, Johnson D, Hayes RB, Earley M, Lorey F, Hannon H, Khoury MJ, Sampson E. DNA banking for epidemiologic studies: a review of current practices. *Epidemiology.* 2002;13:246–254.

26. Blomeke B, Bennett WP, Harris CC, Shields PG. Serum, plasma, and paraffin-embedded tissues as sources of DNA for studying cancer susceptibility genes. *Carcinogenesis.* 1997;18:1271–1275.

27. Austin MA, Ordovas JM, Eckfeldt JH, Tracy R, Boerwinkle E, Lalouel JM, Printz M. Guidelines of the National Heart, Lung, and Blood Institute Working Group on blood drawing, processing, and storage for genetic studies. *Am J Epidemiol.* 1996;5:437–441.

28. Yates JR, Malcolm S, Read AP. Guidelines for DNA banking. Report of the Clinical Genetics Society working party on DNA banking. *J Med Genet.* 1989;26:245–250.

29. Miller SA, Dykes DD, Polesky HF. A simple salting out procedure for extracting DNA from human nucleated cells. *Nucleic Acids Res.* 1988;16:1215.

30. Strauss WM. Preparation of genomic DNA from mammalian tissue. In: Ausubel FM, Brent R, Kingston RE, Moore DD, Seidman JG, Smith JA, Struhl K, eds. *Current Protocols in Molecular Biology, Vol. 1. Molecular Biology—Technique.* New York, NY: Wiley; 1998:10–18.

31. Hawkins TL, O'Connor-Morin T, Roy A, Santillan C. DNA purification and isolation using a solid-phase. *Nucleic Acids Res.* 1994;22:4543–4544.

32. McCormick RM. A solid-phase extraction procedure for DNA purification. *Anal Biochem.* 1989;181:66–74.

33. Louie LG, King MC. A novel approach to establishing permanent lymphoblastoid cell lines: Epstein-Barr virus transformation of cryopreserved lymphocytes. *Am J Hum Genet.* 1991;69:383–387.

34. Clayton EW, Steinberg KK, Khoury MJ, Thomson E, Andrews L, Kahn MJ, Kopelman LM, Weiss JO. Informed consent for genetic research on stored tissue samples [consensus statement]. *JAMA.* 1995;274:1786–1792.

35. Godard B, Schmidtke J, Cassiman JJ, Ayme S. Data storage and DNA banking for biomedical research: informed consent, confidentiality, quality issues, ownership, return of benefits. A professional perspective. *Eur J Hum Genet.* 2003;11(suppl): S88–S122.

36. Sterling R, Henderson GE, Corbie-Smith G. Public willingness to participate in and public opinions about genetic variation research: a review of the literature. *Am J Public Health.* 2006;96:1971–1978.

37. Burgess MM, Laberge C, Knoppers BM. Bioethics for clinicians: 14. Ethics and genetics in medicine. *Can Med Assoc J.* 1998;158:1309–1313.

38. Hunter D, Caporaso N. Informed consent in epidemiologic studies involving genetic markers. *Epidemiology.* 1997;8:596–599.

39. Kelsey KT. Informed consent for genetic research [letter]. *JAMA.* 1996;275:1085.

40. Durfy SJ, Buchanan TE, Burke W. Testing for inherited susceptibility to breast cancer: a survey of informed consent forms for BRCA1 and BRCA2 mutation testing. *Am J Med Genet.* 1998;75:82–87.

41. Willett W. *Nutritional Epidemiology.* 2nd ed. Oxford, UK: Oxford University Press; 1998.

42. Trujillo E, Davis C, Milner J. Nutrigenomics, proteomics, metabolomics, and the practice of dietetics. *J Am Diet Assoc.* 2006;106:403–413.

22

Behavioral Theory–Based Research

Geoffrey W. Greene, PhD, RD, and Colleen A. Redding, PhD

This chapter discusses the importance of behavioral theory–based research, provides guidelines on using theories in nutrition research, and describes the practical aspects of conducting research based on commonly used behavioral theories. The material is only an introduction to the behavioral theories and is not intended as a comprehensive review (1). The more established theories, such as the health belief model and social cognitive theory, are discussed only briefly because they are extensively reviewed in the literature. The newer theories, in contrast—the theory of reasoned action/planned behavior and the transtheoretical model—are discussed in greater depth to provide researchers with a better understanding of how to apply them.

IMPORTANCE OF BEHAVIORAL THEORY–BASED RESEARCH

Theory describes the mechanisms of how attitudes and beliefs related to diet and health influence behavior. Theory guides our choice of variables and intervention strategies. Theories consist of a set of variables in a specified relationship (2). Research based on a theory involves measuring variables and, depending on the study design, using interventions designed to affect those variables (3). Describing these mechanisms and relationships clearly is necessary for behavioral science to advance. Behavioral theory–based research guides an orderly investigation of these mechanisms and relationships, which results in a

better understanding of how people change from high-risk to health-promoting dietary behavior.

It is important to distinguish between theories and planning models such as PRECEDE-PROCEED (4) and social marketing (5) or intervention techniques like motivational interviewing (6). Planning models are like recipes: they provide step-by-step instructions about developing interventions. Techniques are similar to cooking skills: they are necessary to implement the recipes. However, theories provide the *why;* analogous to food science, they explain the mechanisms of behavior change.

By increasing understanding of the basic mechanisms and our ability to predict important dietary outcomes, behavioral theory–based research has the potential for increasing the efficiency and efficacy of interventions for both individuals and populations. A recent National Cancer Institute monograph stated, "Interventions based on health behavior theory are not guaranteed to succeed, but they are much more likely to produce the desired outcomes" (7 p 1). This potential also exists in qualitative research, where theory provides a starting place and a framework for qualitative designs (which may generate new or revised theories) (8), and in quantitative research, where theory provides validated instruments measuring key variables associated with behavior change (2,3). Thus, researchers can avoid "reinventing the wheel." Properly conducted theory-based research will produce meaningful results, both positive and negative, as well as study findings that are more easily interpretable. Theory-based research facilitates grant funding or approval of a thesis, as well as the publication of research results (7).

TABLE 22.1   Similarities in Key Constructs by Behavioral Theory*

	Theory			
Construct	Health Belief Model	Social Cognitive Theory	Theory of Reasoned Action/ Planned Behavior	Transtheoretical Model
Self-efficacy	†	Self-efficacy	†	Confidence/temptation
Benefits	Perceived benefits	Positive outcome expectancies	Positive attitudes toward behavior	Pros
Barriers	Perceived barriers	Negative outcome expectancies	Negative attitudes toward behavior	Cons

*The health belief model postulates (in part) that people change behavior if the perceived benefits are greater than the perceived costs. Similarly, social cognitive theory suggests that a person's belief that he or she can change a behavior (the construct of self-efficacy) is critically important in the decision to change. This table lists the names of the analogous constructs in these four theories.
†Although not part of the original theory, this construct has been added by some researchers (1).

Most theories used in nutrition have been applied to behavior change for health promotion. However, these theories may be applied to behavior change in clinical and management situations as well. The health belief model has defined *perceived severity* as a key variable predicting change. For example, if a patient does not believe that his "touch of diabetes" is likely to affect his health, he will not be motivated to change his diet. Increasing this patient's awareness of his risk for diabetic complications may increase his motivation to change.

Similarly, the transtheoretical or stages-of-change model has been applied to organizational change (9). Key variables in this model are *stage of change* and *decisional balance*. If a worksite is in the "contemplation stage" and employees perceive the disadvantages of change as outweighing the benefits, they are likely to resist change. The model suggests that management prepare for change by explaining to employees how the change will benefit them and providing mechanisms for employee input in solving or reducing problems.

GUIDELINES FOR APPLICATION OF THEORIES IN RESEARCH

Theories lay out the big picture much like a map and are defined in terms of constructs and relationships between constructs. For example, the health belief model postulates

that people change those behaviors that are threatening if the perceived benefits are greater than the perceived barriers or costs of change. Perceived benefits and barriers are key constructs in this model, as well as other models (see Table 22.1). Similarly, social cognitive theory suggests that a person's belief that he or she can change a behavior (the construct of self-efficacy) is critically important in the decision to change.

Constructs are abstract concepts that cannot be measured directly. They need to be made concrete (ie, operationalized) by variables that can be measured. In general, variables are measured by a set of questions or *items* on a questionnaire (survey instrument). Inclusion of at least three to five items that are highly correlated (ie, Cronbach $\alpha > 0.7$) will provide a relatively stable measurement of a construct, provided that expert opinion has determined that the set of items is a valid representation of the construct (10). Constructs should be measured using only reliable, validated instruments, and the instruments should be selected or developed and tested with the target population prior to the study. Although each theory includes its own distinct constructs (see Table 22.2), several closely comparable constructs are evident across different theories (refer to Table 22.1) (11).

Start by selecting the theory best suited to your goals and study it thoroughly. Then define the research question in terms of the theory (eg, the intervention will test the efficacy of a theory-based intervention, the survey will assess key constructs of a theory, or the study will develop/validate

TABLE 22.2   Distinct Key Constructs by Behavioral Theory

	Theory			
Construct	Health Belief Model	Social Cognitive Theory	Theory of Reasoned Action	Transtheoretical Model
	Perceived risk	Reciprocal determinism	Perceived norms	Stages of change
	Perceived severity			Processes of change

instruments measuring constructs). The third step is to clearly define dependent variables (eg, the percentage of energy from fat or servings of fruits and vegetables in a day). Key dependent variables are called *primary outcome variables.* In addition to primary outcome variables, the researcher can use constructs as intermediate outcome variables. Thus, even if the primary outcome goal of dietary change is not attained, you can identify change in intermediate outcomes (eg, an increase in motivational readiness to change). A fourth step is to define the independent variables (eg, the intervention group). The final step for experimental studies is to determine the expected effect size (the amount of change in the dependent variable due to the independent variable) in order to conduct statistical power calculations for the estimation of sample size (12). In general, previous studies based on the theory can provide an estimate of the effect size.

In addition to outcome analyses, you can conduct correlational analyses looking at the relationships between constructs. You also can conduct process-to-outcome analyses looking at the proportion of the variance in the dependent variable that can be explained by a construct (r^2). Cohen (12) defined a large effect in the behavioral sciences as an effect that explains at least 14% of the variance in outcome. However, any lack of precision in the assessment of dietary intake usually attenuates the effect size (13). Nevertheless, from a public health perspective, even a relatively small change in diet can have enormous economic and public health significance. Ostler and Thompson (14), for example, estimated that decreasing saturated fat intake by 1% of energy on a population basis would reduce the incidence of cardiac events by 32,000 per year for a savings of $4.1 billion.

USING MAJOR BEHAVIORAL THEORIES

Health Belief Model

The first theory in health behavior was the health belief model (15), which was developed more than four decades ago (16). The health belief model hypothesizes that individuals are more likely to change behavior if they perceive that (a) they are threatened by an adverse health condition and (b) the change will provide benefits that exceed the costs. The health belief model is defined by the constructs of perceived susceptibility, perceived severity, perceived benefits, and perceived barriers. Perceived susceptibility measures a person's belief in his or her vulnerability to the

adverse health condition (how likely it is that you will get it). Perceived severity measures a person's belief in the severity of the adverse health condition if he or she does get it. The construct of perceived benefits measures a person's belief that the behavior change will reduce threats and provide other benefits. The construct of perceived barriers measures a person's evaluation of the cost or problems associated with behavior change.

One of the difficulties in using this theory is the necessity of developing instruments that measure the constructs for the specific health problem in the target population. Other difficulties arise when there is little variance in the constructs (eg, cancer is considered by most people to have extremely severe health consequences). The strength of the model is in identifying and measuring perceived threat as an important mediating variable in predicting how people respond to perceived benefits and barriers. This model was one of the first to define benefits and barriers and how these constructs may affect change. These constructs are generally believed to be associated with behavior, as demonstrated in Table 22.1. In the past, the health belief model has not been credited with success in explaining dietary behavior change (16). However, recent data suggest that the magnitude of the correlation between its constructs and dietary variables is similar to that for other theories (17,18).

Social Cognitive Theory and Reciprocal Determinism

Bandura initiated development of social cognitive theory in 1962, defined principles of behavior modification (an application of the theory) in 1969, added the construct of self-efficacy in 1977, and broadened the scope for population-based interventions in 1978 with reciprocal determinism (19–24). Social cognitive theory postulates that behavior is not random but is a predictable result of antecedents and consequences that either increase or decrease the likelihood that the behavior will be repeated. However, the constructs of self-efficacy (the confidence one has to perform a particular behavior) and outcome expectancies (the anticipated positive and negative consequences) modulate this effect. New behaviors can be learned and old ones extinguished. The overall goal of an intervention is to increase the likelihood of performance of the health-promoting behavior and minimize the likelihood of the risky health behavior. Interventions focus on skills training designed to break down complex behaviors into small steps to maximize the chance of success and to provide practice in learning new behaviors. Practice and success will increase self-efficacy and create positive outcome expectancies, thereby enhancing the probability of successful behavior change.

Using social cognitive theory for individual change, a process referred to as *cognitive behavior modification,* involves behavioral analysis and the design of a specific, individualized intervention (20). Social cognitive theory has been successfully used in group treatment for weight control following a one-size-fits-all type of approach (25). However, this approach has been less successful with minority groups and groups with literacy challenges (25), and a greater focus on individualization and cognitive behavior therapy has been recommended (26).

Reciprocal determinism broadens the application from group to community (23,24). A strength of reciprocal determinism is that it focuses on the dynamic reciprocal relationships between person, environment, and behavior. A person both influences the environment and in turn is influenced by the environment. Environmental interventions can increase positive outcome expectancies, as well as increase "positive" antecedents (18,23,24). Social cognitive theory and reciprocal determinism have been used in a variety of community-based interventions with mixed results. Despite early promise, community-based interventions involving more than 600,000 participants found no consistent results (27), and there was no effect found for a 15-year, school-based smoking cessation intervention in 40 school districts (28). In contrast, involving parents in school-based interventions has been successful in promoting dietary change in children (29) and increasing the availability of fruits and vegetables, which is critical in increasing children's intake (24,30). Although the translation of social cognitive theory and reciprocal determinism from the individual and group to the community has been

disappointing, many of the constructs in these theories have proven to be important predictors of behavior; for example, self-efficacy has consistently been identified as a key moderating or intermediate outcome variable (18,24,31,32).

Theory of Reasoned Action/Planned Behavior

The theory of reasoned action, developed in 1967 by Fishbein and Ajzen (33,34) and modified in 1980 (35), proposes that behavior change is ultimately the result of changes in beliefs. Therefore, to influence behavior, people need to be exposed to information that will change their beliefs (36). A strength of the theory of reasoned action is that it facilitates deciphering actions by identifying, measuring, and combining beliefs that are relevant to individuals or groups in making decisions about health. Behavioral beliefs and normative beliefs are linked to behavioral intention and behavior by attitude and subjective norm (Figure 22.1) (37), resulting in the following equation (34,35):

$$Behavior = Behavioral\ intention$$
$$= Attitude + Subjective\ norm$$

The theory of reasoned action is unique in its potential for extension, with the addition of sensory factors such as taste and texture, to the link between attitude, subjective norm, and behavior, making the theory particularly attractive to food scientists (37–42).

The theory of reasoned action assumes that (a) human beings are usually quite rational and consider the implications of their actions, and (b) most actions of social relevance are under volitional control, and therefore a person's intention is the immediate determinant of the action (34,35).

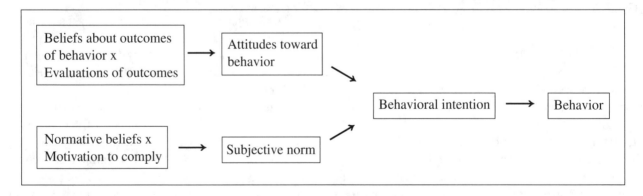

FIGURE 22.1   Model of the theory of reasoned action. Reprinted from Brewer JL, Blake AJ, Rankin SA, Douglass LW. Theory of reasoned action predicts milk consumption in females. *J Am Diet Assoc.* 1999;99:39–44. Reprinted with permission from the American Dietetic Association.

However, many researchers have added the use of measured behavior in the model to confirm intention (37–40).

A study by Brewer and coworkers (37), investigating the ability to predict consumption of four milk types (whole, reduced-fat, low-fat, and nonfat) by adult females, provides an example. The researchers added components measuring milk consumption and sensory attributes, leading to the modified equation

Behavior = Behavioral intention
= Attitude + Sensory score + Subjective norm

Constructs were represented using three to six items, which were assessed on a 7-point Likert scale.

Attitude (*A*) is the learned predisposition to respond in a consistently favorable or unfavorable manner toward an object or an act. It is the sum of the *salient beliefs* (b_i) about the outcomes multiplied by the *evaluations* (e_i) of whether these outcomes are important to the individual:

$$A = \Sigma b_i e_i$$

Health-related belief item scores for nonfat and low-fat milk were significantly higher than scores for reduced-fat and whole milk, but the opposite was found for taste-related scales. That is, milk drinkers preferred the taste of higher-fat milks. Nevertheless, evaluation scores (importance to the individual) were highest for health-related belief items. Therefore, overall attitude scores were higher for nonfat and low-fat milk than for reduced-fat or whole milk.

The *subjective norm* (*SN*) is the individual's perception of social pressure to perform a particular behavior. It is found by multiplying the *normative beliefs* (NB_j), representing what specific people or groups of people think the individual should do, by the individual's *motivation to comply* (MC_j), or how much the individual wishes to comply with his or her normative influences:

$$SN = \Sigma NB_j MC_j$$

The theory of reasoned action assumes a multiplicative relationship. That is, the likelihood and desirability of each outcome should be multiplied and their products added, reflecting the assumption that threats will be ignored if either their severity or their likelihood and desirability is zero (40). Because *SN* did not have a significant effect in this study, it was omitted in the overall predictive equation.

The hedonic testing protocol produced a *sensory score* evaluating the taste of four milks under blinded taste testing according to the attributes of overall appeal/liking using a 9-point Likert scale (1 = Like extremely to 9 = Dislike extremely). Whole milk was liked by subjects significantly more than nonfat and low-fat milk. However, sensory scores contributed minimally to the final equation (37).

Behavioral intention (*BI*) is the likelihood that a person will perform the *behavior* (*B*), which was defined as milk intake or avoidance measured by a dairy product frequency questionnaire. Intention was a strong predictor of behavior, and intention to drink nonfat milk was significantly higher than intention to drink the other milks. Therefore, in this study health concerns prevailed over beliefs about taste and sensory scores in determining milk choice by milk drinkers.

The final equation in the study was as follows:

Behavior = Behavioral intention
= Attitude + Sensory score

A regression model with behavior of "milk as a beverage" as the dependent variable explained 67% of the variability for nonfat milk use, 45% for low-fat milk use, 60% for reduced-fat milk use, and 67% for whole milk use. Correlational analyses between variables showed that attitudes for all milks correlated significantly with behavioral intention; however, the standardized regression coefficients were higher for nonfat and low-fat milk. Key findings in this study were that (a) the model was strongest in predicting whether an individual would use whole or nonfat milk, (b) intention was a strong indicator of actual milk intake behavior as reported in the dairy frequency questionnaire, and (c) attitudes and beliefs about health outweighed the sensory response in milk drinkers.

The model seems best suited to studying a specific behavior, such as drinking low-fat milk or eating low-nutrient snacks (38–40), as well as single food/nutrient consumption behavior, such as consumption of high-fat food, sugar, or milk (16,41–45). The theory of reasoned action does not specify particular beliefs about a behavior. Therefore, it is necessary to generate items for the model based on formative research (elicitation interviews) unless items have previously been validated for the target population and behavior (34,35,37).

The theory of reasoned action does not deal with behavior not under volitional control. In an effort to account for factors outside the individual's control that may affect intention and behavior, Ajzen and Madden (46) developed the theory of planned behavior as an extension of the theory of reasoned action. The theory is insightful in that it covers more diverse motivational factors (beliefs) for explaining decision making. The authors added the concept of perceived behavioral control, which is measured by the following constructs: *control belief,* defined as likelihood of occurrence of each facilitating or constraining condition, and *perceived power,* defined as the perceived effect of each condition in making behavioral performance difficult or easy. Although these additions reflect important concepts, they have not been fully validated (16,36,47,48).

Transtheoretical Model

During the last two decades, the transtheoretical model has become one of the most influential theoretical models for health-related behavior change. This model is also known as the stages-of-change model because of its key organizing construct, stages of readiness to change behavior. The model consists of four interrelated dimensions: the central organizing construct, stage of change (the temporal dimension), and the three additional dimensions of decisional balance, self-efficacy (or temptation), and process of change (49–51). Of these four dimensions, stages of change is the most widely researched dimension; during the last decade, decisional balance and self-efficacy also have received considerable attention. The least investigated dimension is process of change.

Stage of change is the temporal dimension of motivational readiness to change a health behavior. The stages are as follows: precontemplation (no intention of changing in the foreseeable future), contemplation (intending to change, but not soon), preparation (intending to change within the next few weeks), action (recent change), and maintenance (maintaining change). The stage defines when change occurs and can be used in interventions to show individuals where they are in the change process. Stages of change are both descriptive and proscriptive because different intervention strategies are important to people at different stages of change. Like all dimensions of the model, stage is a dynamic variable, and people are expected to move from one stage to another. Although stage change is sometimes conceptualized as linear, a spiral appears to best express stage movement because of the dynamic nature of change. For example, regression from preparation or action to an earlier stage may be just as likely as progression to the next stage (50,52). In the area of smoking cessation, self-changers averaged three serious quit attempts (action stage) over 7 years before succeeding (50).

Developing a good staging algorithm is critical to all applications of the model. However, to measure stage, it is necessary to define the target behavior and the criterion for effective action (53). Once the criterion is defined, the

algorithm should be constructed to allow self-assessment of whether the criterion has been met and—if it has— whether it has been met for longer than 6 months (maintenance) or less than 6 months (action). If the criterion has not been met, individuals should clearly understand the amount of change necessary to meet the criterion (behavioral distance) in order to assess whether they intend to change in the next month (preparation), they intend to change in the next 6 months (contemplation), or they have no intention of changing to meet the criterion in the next 6 months (precontemplation) (54,55).

The stages-of-change model originated from an analysis of 18 systems of psychotherapy that identify common processes of change (49). Processes are the covert and overt activities that people use to progress through the stages; they are *how* people change. Experiential processes focus on thoughts, feelings, and experiences, whereas behavioral processes focus on behaviors, social support, and reinforcement. In a study of dietary fat reduction, Greene and colleagues found that process use was lowest in precontemplation (56). Experiential process use increased sharply through preparation, peaked in action, and then decreased in maintenance. Behavioral process use remained low through contemplation, and it rose sharply and linearly through action before decreasing in maintenance.

Decisional balance measures the relative importance to the individual of the pros (advantages or benefits) and cons (disadvantages, barriers, or costs) of change. Prochaska and colleagues (57) found that for 12 health behaviors, including dietary fat reduction, pros had to outweigh cons for all behaviors before action. Progress from precontemplation to action required an increase in the pros of approximately one standard deviation (58). This progress was associated with a decrease in the cons of approximately one-half of a standard deviation. Shifting decisional balance so that pros outweigh cons appears to be important in explaining why people make a commitment to change behavior in the near future.

The self-efficacy construct represents the situation-specific confidence people have that they can engage in the desired behavior change; it is usually operationalized as confidence (59). This construct was adapted from Bandura's self-efficacy theory (20). The converse of confidence is situation-specific temptation (eg, how tempted a person feels to eat high-fat foods across different situations). Confidence and temptation have the same measurement structure, with three distinct factors: positive social occasions, negative affective situations, and challenging situations (situations in which it is difficult to obtain low-fat foods) (59,60). In a smoking cessation study, temptation predicted which self-changers would relapse and start smoking again (59). For dietary fat reduction, Greene found that temptation was low in precontemplation, rose sharply to a peak in contemplation, dipped slightly in preparation, and then declined somewhat in action and sharply in maintenance (56). The low values in precontemplation may be typical for dietary restriction; people perceive temptation as a problem only if they are trying to avoid eating something. The sharp decline in maintenance illustrates the reduced effort needed to maintain the change after 6 months.

The stage construct has been found to be an important predictor of change in several intervention studies (31,61–70). Tailoring intervention materials to stage as well as other key constructs of the model is possible using computerized expert systems to generate individualized materials (71,72). This intervention strategy has been demonstrated to be effective across a range of health behaviors, including dietary fat reduction treated both as a single risk behavior (64) and as part of a multiple risk behavior intervention (67–69). The programming and development of this computerized system and the necessity for individual assessment can make this approach expensive. However, once developed, transtheoretical model-tailored expert systems can be readily disseminated across various settings or even over the Internet, which can make them cost-effective tools to increase public health impact. As an alternative, tailoring interventions to the stage of a group (64) or an organization (9) has also been found to be effective. This strong program of transtheoretical model-based dietary research proceeded through a series of steps in the development of effective model-based interventions: studying the theory and how it applied to dietary behavior, operationalizing all key constructs and validating measures, developing tailored interventions based on those constructs, and conducting randomized efficacy trials in various populations. These steps can provide a foundation for scientific progress in dietary behaviors across theories.

In spite of the strong evidence supporting the transtheoretical model, this model has critics. Some have criticized the stages-of-change concept itself as too developmental (73) or as failing to include the most important stages (74). More specific criticism has emerged with regard to the smoking area, where some found that addiction variables accounted for more variance than transtheoretical model variables (75,76); however, limited data sets and limited sets of variables were used, tempering this criticism (77). Further analysis of transtheoretical model–tailored intervention outcomes across five studies

of smoking cessation demonstrated that both addiction variables and stages of change were strongly related to outcomes (70). Such debate can strengthen theories by challenging specific components or generating research that leads to reformulation and can result in stronger, clearer theories. This is the ideal for theoretical progress.

CONCLUSION

Although it may be difficult to operationalize all dimensions of a theory, key constructs should be measured if validated instruments exist. Constructs such as perceived benefits and barriers (which originated in the health belief model), self-efficacy (from social cognitive theory), or stage of change (from the transtheoretical model) have consistently been found to predict behavior. Theories evolve over time in part in response to new data, and new theories will be formulated. However, it is important for nutrition researchers to strive to base their studies on specific theories. Behavioral theory–based research in nutrition has the potential to explain, predict, or influence eating behavior on both an individual and a population basis. By describing the mechanisms and interrelationships between variables, behavioral theory–based research can advance the science explaining why people eat the way they do and how to help them improve their eating habits, thereby reducing their health risks and maximizing their quality of life.

REFERENCES

1. Glanz K, Rimer BK, Lewis FM, eds. *Health Behavior and Health Education: Theory, Research, Practice.* 3rd ed. San Francisco, Calif: Jossey-Bass Publishers; 2002.

2. Glanz K, Lewis FM, Rimer B. Linking theory, research, and practice. In: Glanz K, Lewis FM, Rimer B, eds. *Health Behavior and Health Education: Theory, Research, Practice.* 2nd ed. San Francisco, Calif: Jossey-Bass Publishers; 1997:19–35.

3. Redding CA, Rossi JS, Rossi SR, Prochaska JO, Velicer WF. Health behavior models. In: Hyner GC, Peterson KW, Travis JW, Dewey JE, Foerster JJ, Framer EM, eds. *SPM Handbook of Health Assessment Tools.* Pittsburgh, Pa: Society of Prospective Medicine and Institute for Health and Productivity Management; 1999:83–93.

4. Green LW, Kreuter MW. *Health Program Planning: An Educational Ecological Approach.* 4th ed. New York, NY: McGraw Hill; 2004.

5. Andereasen A. *Marketing Social Change: Changing Behavior to Promote Health, Social Development, and the Environment.* San Francisco, Calif: Jossey-Bass Publishers; 1995.

6. Miller W, Rollnick S. *Motivational Interviewing: Preparing People for Change.* 2nd ed. New York, NY: Guilford Press; 2002.

7. National Cancer Institute. *Theory at a Glance: A Guide for Health Promotion Practice.* 2nd ed. Bethesda, Md: US Department of Health and Human Services; 2005. NIH Publication 05-3896.

8. Kirby S, Baranowski T, Reynolds K, Taylor G, Binkley D. Children's fruit and vegetable intake: socioeconomic, adult child, regional, and urban-rural influences. *J Nutr Educ.* 1995;27:261–271.

9. Prochaska JM. A transtheoretical model approach to organizational change: family service agencies' movement to time-limited therapy. *Fam Soc.* 2000;81:76–84.

10. Redding CA, Maddock JE, Rossi JS. The sequential approach to measurement of health behavior constructs: issues in selecting and developing measures. *Calif J Health Promot.* 2006;4:83–101.

11. Institute of Medicine. *Speaking of Health: Assessing Health Communication Strategies for Diverse Populations.* Washington, DC: National Academies Press; 2002.

12. Cohen J. *Statistical Power Analysis for the Behavioral Sciences.* 2nd ed. Hillsdale, NJ: Lawrence Erlbaum Associates; 1988.

13. Thompson FE, Subar A. Dietary assessment methodology. In: Coulston AM, Rock CL, Monsen ER, eds. *Nutrition in the Prevention and Treatment of Disease.* San Diego, Calif: Academic Press; 2001.

14. Ostler G, Thompson D. Estimated effects of reducing dietary saturated fat on the incidence and costs of coronary heart disease in the United States. *J Am Diet Assoc.* 1996;96:127–131.

15. Becker MH, ed. *The Health Belief Model and Personal Behavior.* Thorofore, NJ: CB Flack; 1974.

16. Janz NK, Champion VL, Strecher VJ. The health belief model. In: Glanz K, Rimer BK, Lewis FM, eds. *Health Behavior and Health Education: Theory, Research, Practice.* 3rd ed. San Francisco, Calif: Jossey-Bass Publishers; 2002:45–66.

17. Kloeblen AS. Folate knowledge, intake from fortified grain products, and periconceptional supplementation patterns of a sample of low-income pregnant women according to the health belief model. *J Am Diet Assoc.* 1999;99:33–38.

18. Baranowski T, Cullen K, Baranowski J. Psychosocial correlates of dietary intake: advancing dietary intervention. *Annu Rev Nutr.* 1999;19:17–40.

19. Bandura A. Social learning through imitation. In: Jones MR, ed. *Nebraska Symposium on Motivation.* Vol 10. Lincoln: University of Nebraska Press; 1962.

20. Bandura A. *Principles of Behavior Modification.* Austin, Tex: Holt, Rinehart, and Winston; 1969.

21. Bandura A. *Social Learning Theory.* Englewood Cliffs, NJ: Prentice Hall; 1977.

22. Bandura A. Self efficacy. Toward a unifying theory of behavior change. *Psychol Rev.* 1977;84:191–215.

23. Bandura A. The self system in reciprocal determinism. *Am Psychol.* 1982;37:122–147.

24. Baranowski T, Perry CL, Parcel GS. How individuals, environments, and health behavior interact: social cognitive theory. In: Glanz K, Rimer BK, Lewis FM, eds. *Health Behavior and Health Education: Theory, Research, Practice.* 3rd ed. San Francisco, Calif: Jossey-Bass Publishers; 2002: 165–184.

25. Expert Panel on the Identification, Evaluation, and Treatment of Overweight in Adults. Clinical guidelines on the identification, evaluation, and treatment of overweight and obesity in adults: executive summary. *Am J Clin Nutr.* 1998;68:899–917.

26. Fabricatore AN. Behavior therapy and cognitive behavior therapy of obesity: is there a difference? *J Am Diet Assoc.* 2007;107:92–99.

27. Luepker RV, Murray DM, Jacobs DR. Community education for cardiovascular disease prevention: risk factor changes in the Minnesota Heart Health Program. *Am J Public Health.* 1994;84:1383–1393.

28. Peterson AV, Kealey KA, Mann SL, Marcek PM, Sarason IG. Hutchinson Smoking Prevention Project: long-term randomized trial in school-based tobacco use prevention. Results on smoking. *J Natl Cancer Inst.* 2000;92:1979–1991.

29. Luepker RV. Outcomes of a trial to improve children's dietary patterns and physical activity: the child and adolescent trial for cardiovascular health. *JAMA.* 1996;275:768–776.

30. Hearn MD, Baranowski T, Baranowski J, Doyle C, Smith M. Environmental influences on dietary

behavior among children: availability and accessibility of fruits and vegetables enables consumption. *J Health Educ.* 1998;29:26–32.

31. Campbell MK, Symons M, Demark-Wahnfried W, Polhamus B, Bernhardt JM. Stages of change and psychosocial correlates of fruit and vegetable consumption among rural African-American church members. *Am J Health Promot.* 1998;12:185–191.

32. Havas S, Treiman K, Langenberg P. Factors associated with fruit and vegetable consumption among women participating in WIC. *J Am Diet Assoc.* 1998;98:1141–1148.

33. Fishbein MH, ed. *Readings in Attitude Theory and Measurement.* New York, NY: Wiley; 1967.

34. Fishbein M, Ajzen I. *Belief, Attitude, Intention, and Behavior: An Introduction to Theory and Research.* Reading, Mass: Addison-Wesley;1975.

35. Ajzen I, Fishbein M. *Understanding Attitudes and Predicting Social Behavior.* Englewood Cliffs, NJ: Prentice Hall; 1980.

36. Montano DE, Kasprzyk D, Taplin SH. The theory of reasoned action and the theory of planned behavior. In: Glanz K, Rimer BK, Lewis FM, eds. *Health Behavior and Health Education: Theory, Research, Practice.* 3rd ed. San Francisco, Calif: Jossey-Bass Publishers; 2002:67–98.

37. Brewer JL, Blake AJ, Rankin SA, Douglass LW. Theory of reasoned action predicts milk consumption in females. *J Am Diet Assoc.* 1999;99:39–44.

38. Shepherd R, Sparks P, Belliers S, Raats M. Attitudes and choice of flavored milks: extension of Fishbein and Ajzen's theory of reasoned action. *Food Q Preference.* 1991;3:157–164.

39. Arvola A, Lahteenmaki L, Tuorila H. Predicting the intent to purchase unfamiliar and familiar cheeses, the effects of attitudes, expected liking and food neophobia. *Appetite.* 1999;32:113–126.

40. Weinstein ND. Testing four competing theories of health protective behavior. *Health Psychol.* 1993;4:324–333.

41. Freeman R, Sheiham A. Understanding decision-making processes for sugar consumption in adolescence. *Dent Oral Epidemiol.* 1997;25:228–232.

42. Mester I, Oostveen T. Why do adolescents eat low nutrient snacks between meals? An analysis of behavioral determinants with Fishbein and Ajzen models. *Nutr Health.* 1994;10:33–47.

43. Raats MM, Shephard R, Sparks P. Attitudes, obligations, and perceived control. Predicting milk selection. *Appetite.* 1993;20:239–241.

44. Stafleu A, de Graff C, van Staveren WA, de Jong MA. Attitudes toward high-fat foods and their low-fat alternatives: reliability and relationship with fat intake. *Appetite.* 1994;22:183–196.

45. Saunders RP, Rahilly SA. Influences on intention to reduce dietary intake of fat and sugar. *J Nutr Educ.* 1990;22:169–176.

46. Ajzen I, Madden TJ. Prediction of goal-directed behavior: attitudes, intentions, and perceived behavioral control. *J Exp Soc Psychol.* 1986;22:453–474.

47. Raats MM, Shephard R, Sparks P. Attitudes, obligations, and perceived control. Predicting milk selection. *Appetite.* 1993;20:239–241.

48. Park K, Ureda J. Specific motivation for milk consumption among pregnant women enrolled in or eligible for WIC. *J Nutr Educ.* 1999;31:76–85.

49. Prochaska JO, DiClemente CC. *The Transtheoretical Approach: Crossing the Traditional Boundaries of Therapy.* Homewood, Ill: Irwin; 1984.

50. Prochaska JO, DiClemente CC, Norcross JC. In search of how people change: applications to addictive behaviors. *Am Psychol.* 1992;47:1102–1114.

51. Prochaska JO, Redding CA, Evers KE. The transtheoretical model and stages of change. In: Glanz K, Rimer BK, Lewis FM, eds. *Health Behavior and Health Education: Theory, Research, and Practice.* 3rd ed. San Francisco, Calif: Jossey-Bass; 2002:99–120.

52. Greene GW, Rossi SR. Stages of change for dietary fat reduction over 18 months. *J Am Diet Assoc.* 1998;98:529–534.

53. Reed GR, Velicer WF, Prochaska JO, Rossi JS, Marcus BH. What makes a good staging algorithm: examples from regular exercise. *Am J Health Promot.* 1997;12:57–66.

54. Greene GW, Rossi SR, Reed GR, Willey C, Prochaska JO. Stages of change for reducing dietary fat to 30% of total energy or less. *J Am Diet Assoc.* 1994;94:1105–1110.

55. Hargreaves M, Schlundt D, Buchowski M, Hardy RE, Rossi S, Rossi J. Stages of change and the intake of fat in African American women: improving stage assignment using the eating styles questionnaire. *J Am Diet Assoc.* 1999;99:1392–1399.

56. Greene GW, Rossi SR, Rossi JS, Velicer WF, Fava JS, Prochaska JO. Dietary applications of the stages of change model. *J Am Diet Assoc.* 1999;99: 673–678.

57. Prochaska JO, Velicer WF, Rossi JS, Goldstein GG, Marcus BH, Rakowski W, Fiore C, Harlow LL, Redding CA, Rosenbloom D, Rossi SR Stages of

change and decisional balance for 12 problem behaviors. *Health Psychol.* 1994;13:39–46.

58. Prochaska JO. Strong and weak principles for progressing from precontemplation to action on the basis of twelve problem behaviors. *Health Psychol.* 1994;13:47–51.

59. Velicer WF, DiClemente CC, Rossi JS, Prochaska JO. Relapse situations and self-efficacy: an integrative model. *Addict Behav.* 1990;15:271–283.

60. Rossi SR, Greene GW, Rossi JS. Validation of decisional balance and temptations measures for dietary fat reduction in a large school-based population of adolescents. *Eating Behav.* 2001;2:1–18.

61. Campbell MC, DeVellis BM, Strecher VJ, Ammerman AS, DeVellis RF, Sandler RS. The impact of message tailoring on dietary behavior change for disease prevention in primary care settings. *Am J Public Health.* 1994;84:739–787.

62. Brug J, Steenhuis I, van Assema P, de Vries H. The impact of a computer-tailored nutrition intervention. *Prev Med.* 1996;25:236–242.

63. Brug J, Glanz K, van Assema P, Kok G, van Breukelen GJ. The impact of computer-tailored feedback and iterative feedback on fat, fruit, and vegetable intake. *Health Educ Behav.* 1998;25:517–531.

64. Greene GW, Rossi SR, Rossi JS, Fava JL, Prochaska JO, Velicer WF. An expert system intervention for dietary fat reduction [abstract]. *Ann Behav Med.* 1998;20(suppl):S197.

65. Marcus BH, Emmons KM, Simkin-Silverman L. Evaluation of tailored versus standard self-help physical activity interventions at the workplace. *Am J Health Promot.* 1997;12:246–253.

66. Steptoe A, Kerry S, Rink E, Hilton S. The impact of behavioral counseling on stage of change in fat intake, physical activity, and cigarette smoking in adults at increased risk of coronary heart disease. *Am J Public Health.* 2001;91:265–269.

67. Prochaska JO, Velicer WF, Rossi JS, Redding CA, Greene GW, Rossi SR, Sun X, Fava JL, Laforge R, Plummer BA. Impact of simultaneous stage-matched expert system interventions for smoking,

high fat diet and sun exposure in a population of parents. *Health Psychol.* 2004;23:503–516.

68. Prochaska JO, Velicer WF, Redding CA, Rossi JS, Goldstein M, DePue J, Greene GW, Rossi SR, Sun X, Fava JL, Laforge R, Rakowski W, Plummer BA. Stage-based expert systems to guide a population of primary care patients to quit smoking, eat healthier, prevent skin cancer and receive regular mammograms. *Prev Med.* 2005;41:406–416.

69. Velicer WF, Prochaska JO, Redding C, Rossi JS, Sun X, Rossi SR, Greene GW, Fava JL, Abrams DB, Linnan LA, Emmons KM. Efficacy of expert system interventions for employees to decrease smoking, dietary fat, and sun exposure [abstract]. *Int J Behav Med.* 2004;11(suppl 1):S277.

70. Velicer WF, Redding CA, Sun X, Prochaska JO. Demographic variables, smoking variables, and outcomes across five studies. *Health Psychol.* 2007;26:278–287.

71. Redding CA, Prochaska JO, Pallonen UE, Rossi JS, Velicer WF, Rossi SR, Greene GW, Meier KS, Evers KE, Plummer BA, Maddock JE. Transtheoretical individualized multimedia expert systems targeting adolescents' health behaviors. *Cogn Behav Pract.* 1999;6:144–153.

72. Velicer WF, Prochaska JO. An expert system intervention for smoking cessation. *Patient Educ Couns.* 1999;36:119–129.

73. Bandura A. The anatomy of stages of change. *Am J Health Promot.* 1997;12:8–10.

74. Weinstein ND, Rothman AJ, Sutton SR. Stage theories of health behavior: conceptual and methodological issues. *Health Psychol.* 1998;17:290–299.

75. Farkas AJ, Pierce JP, Zhu SH, Rosbrook B, Gilpin EA, Berry C, Kaplan RM. Addiction versus stages of change models in predicting smoking cessation. *Addiction.* 1996;91:1271–1280.

76. Abrams DB, Herzog TA, Emmons KM, Linnan L. Stages of change versus addiction: a replication and extension. *Nicotine Tobacco Res.* 2000;2:223–229.

77. Prochaska JO. Moving beyond the transtheoretical model. *Addiction.* 2006;101:768–778.

23

Research Methods for Dietary Supplementation and Complementary and Alternative Medicine

Cynthia A. Thomson, PhD, RD, and Leila G. Saldanha, PhD, RD

Awareness and use of dietary supplements and complementary and alternative medicine (CAM) have increased markedly in recent years. According to a nationwide government survey of CAM therapies commonly used in the United States released in May 2004, 36% of US adults aged 18 years and older had used some form of CAM in the past year (1). Dietary supplement usage is also high. In the 1999–2000 National Health and Nutrition Examination Survey (NHANES), more than 50% of adults reported taking a dietary supplement in the past month, and 35% took a multivitamin/multimineral (MVM), calcium, vitamin C, vitamin E, or B-complex vitamin supplement (2). Forty-seven percent of all adult dietary supplement users in NHANES took just one supplement, whereas 55% of women and 63% of adults aged 60 years or older took more than one. Most supplements were taken daily and for at least 2 years (2).

In the 1999–2000 NHANES, the prevalence of use of supplements was associated with select demographic and lifestyle characteristics (2). Users of dietary supplements were more likely to be female, be in an older age group, report higher levels of education, be of non-Hispanic white race/ethnicity, perform regular physical activity, and be normal weight or underweight. Dietary supplement users, although more likely to report frequent use of wine or distilled spirits and to be former smokers, were more likely to report their health status as excellent/very good (2–6). In a 2005 survey, 42.8% of children between the ages of 20 and 24 months received MVM supplements; 60.9% did so on a daily basis (7). Use is greater among children whose mothers have a higher level of education; however, parental age, weeks of gestation, and newborn birth weight were not different between dietary supplement users and nonusers.

Federal funding for dietary supplements and CAM reflects consumer interest and use of these modalities (8). In 2002, the National Institutes of Health (NIH) invested approximately $917 million in nutrition research and training (9) including, $181 million for dietary supplement research. From fiscal year 1999 through 2002, the number of NIH-funded dietary supplement–related research projects increased steadily from 374 to 569 projects annually; 1,749 projects were funded during the 4-year period (9).

This chapter provides information, resources, and suggestions for designing, implementing, and analyzing research in the area of dietary supplementation and, to a lesser extent, other CAM modalities. RDs interested in this area of research should make an effort to understand the regulatory environment as well as their scope of practice prior to engaging in dietary supplement research. RD involvement in collaborative research within a multidisciplinary team (ideally as the principal investigator) will build the evidence necessary to integrate dietary supplementation into clinical and public health practice.

DEFINITION OF CAM RESEARCH

CAM, as defined by the National Center for Complementary and Alternative Medicine (NCCAM) and described on the center's Web site, "is a group of diverse medical and health care systems, practices, and products that are not presently considered to be part of conventional medicine" (10). Conventional medicine is medicine as practiced by holders of MD (medical doctor) or DO (doctor of osteopathy) degrees and by their allied health professionals, such as physical therapists, psychologists, and registered nurses. Although some scientific evidence exists for some CAM therapies, well-designed scientific studies are needed specifically to address whether these therapies are safe and whether they are effective for preventing or treating the diseases or medical conditions for which they are used.

The list of what is considered to be CAM changes continually, as those therapies that are proven safe and effective become adopted into conventional health care, and as new approaches to health care emerge.

NCCAM classifies CAM therapies into five categories (10):

- **Alternative medical systems.** Alternative medical systems are built on complete systems of theory and practice. Often, these systems have evolved apart from and earlier than the conventional medical approach used in the United States. Examples of alternative medical systems that have developed in Western cultures include homeopathic medicine and naturopathic medicine. Other examples of these systems include traditional Chinese medicine (TCM) and Ayurveda.
- **Mind-body interventions.** Mind-body medicine uses a variety of techniques designed to enhance the mind's capacity to affect bodily function and symptoms. Some techniques previously considered CAM have become mainstream, such as patient support groups and cognitive-behavioral therapy. Techniques that are still considered CAM include meditation, prayer, mental healing, and therapies that use creative outlets such as art, music, or dance.
- **Biologically based therapies.** Biologically based therapies use substances found in nature, such as herbs, foods, and vitamins, often in the form of dietary supplements.
- **Manipulative and body-based methods.** Manipulative and body-based methods are based on manipulation and/or movement of one or more parts of the body. Examples include chiropractic or osteopathic manipulation, and massage.
- **Energy therapies.** Energy therapies involve the use of energy fields. They are of two types:
  - **Biofield therapies** are intended to affect energy fields that surround and penetrate the human body.

Some forms of energy therapy manipulate biofields by applying pressure and/or manipulating the body by placing the hands in, or through, these fields. Examples include qi gong, Reiki, and therapeutic touch.
  - **Bioelectromagnetic-based therapies** involve the unconventional use of electromagnetic fields, such as pulsed fields, magnetic fields, or alternating current or direct current fields.

METHODOLOGICAL ISSUES IN CAM RESEARCH

Because CAM therapies cover many modalities, challenges in performing CAM research vary. Established research techniques and statistical procedures can be used to address a majority of CAM study questions, from clinical research on therapeutic efficacy to basic science on mechanisms. Randomized controlled trials (RCTs) have an important place in the assessment of the efficacy of CAM. However, they address a limited range of questions, such as whether an intervention has an effect. RCTs do not address questions such as why the intervention works, how participants are experiencing the intervention, and/or how participants give meaning to these experiences (11). Also, concerns regarding appropriate "dose" have been expressed (12). The addition of qualitative research methods to RCTs may greatly enhance understanding of CAM interventions. Qualitative research can assist in understanding patients' beliefs about the treatment and expectations of the outcome. Finally, qualitative research may be helpful in developing appropriate outcome measures for CAM interventions.

DEFINITION OF DIETARY SUPPLEMENTS

Dietary supplements are regulated as foods under the Dietary Supplement Health and Education Act of 1994 (DSHEA) (13). Congress, through DSHEA, expanded the meaning of the term *dietary supplements* beyond vitamins and minerals to include other substances such as botanical products, fish oils, psyllium, enzymes, glands, and mixtures of these. The regulatory definition of a dietary supplement is as follows (14):

- A product (other than tobacco) that is intended to supplement the diet that bears or contains one or more of the following dietary ingredients: a vitamin, a mineral, an herb or other botanical, an amino acid, a dietary substance for use by humans to supplement the diet by increasing the total daily intake, or a concentrate, metabolite, constituent, extract, or combinations of these ingredients

- A product that is intended for ingestion in pill, capsule, tablet, or liquid form
- A product that is not represented for use as a conventional food or as the sole item of a meal or diet
- A product that is labeled as a "dietary supplement"
- Products such as an approved new drug, certified antibiotic, or licensed biologic if marketed as a dietary supplement or food before approval as a drug (eg, psyllium)

UNDERSTANDING THE CONTEXT OF DIETARY SUPPLEMENT RESEARCH IN THE PRACTICE OF DIETETICS

Given that usage of dietary supplements among patients has increased over time and that patients receiving dietary assessment and counseling should be evaluated in terms of dietary supplement use, it seems likely that RDs will become increasingly involved in dietary supplementation research. Thus, it is imperative that RDs have a working knowledge of the context for and by which they may play a role in this expanding area of nutrition science.

There are two important issues that all RDs should understand regarding dietary supplement research. The first issue pertains to the selection of subjects. Because supplements are regulated as foods, they are intended for healthy persons. When selecting subjects for a clinical trial, researchers cannot select subjects who have been diagnosed with the disease or health-related condition for which the product is being tested. Subjects can be at high risk for the disease or health-related condition, but they cannot have the disease or health-related condition. If this policy is not followed, then the intended use would make the study a drug study and not a dietary supplement study. The second issue pertains to the selection of products. Dietary supplements may be grouped into three major categories related to dietary function or origin (13):

- Substances with established nutritional function, such as vitamins, minerals, amino acids, and fatty acids
- Botanical products and their concentrates and extracts

- Other substances with a wide variety of origins and physiological roles (documentation of product quality is addressed later in this chapter)

Resources

To fully understand the complexity of dietary supplement research and the issues that surround the design of evidence-based research, one should review current government Web sites that provide extensive background information and guidance that support the development of a successful research project. Box 23.1 lists key Web-based resources for dietary supplementation research (15).

BOX 23.1   Developing Quality Research Projects on Dietary Supplementation: Key Web-Based Government Resources

---

National Center for Complementary and Alternative Medicine (NCCAM)

- Data and Safety Monitoring Guidelines for NCCAM-Supported Clinical Trials (http://nccam.nih.gov/research/policies/datasafety)
- Guidance on Designing Clinical Trials of CAM Therapies: Determining Dose Ranges (http://nccam.nih.gov/research/policies/guideonct.htm)
- Biologically Active Agents Used in CAM and Placebo Materials—Policy and Guidance (http://nccam.nih.gov/research/policies/bioactive.htm)
- Considerations for NCCAM Clinical Trial Grant Applications (http://nccam.nih.gov/research/policies/clinical-considerations.htm)

Office of Dietary Supplements
(http://ods. od.nih.gov)

Food and Drug Administration (FDA)

- FDA Guidance for Industry: Botanical Drug Products. 2004. (http://www.fda.gov/cder/guidance/4592fnl.pdf)
- Center for Food Safety and Applied Nutrition (Food and Drug Administration) (http://www.cfsan.fda.gov)

American Dietetic Association
(http://www.eatright.org)

Herb Research Foundation
(http://www.herbs.org)

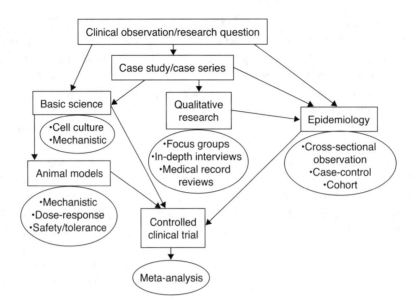

FIGURE 23.1   Key approaches to dietary supplement scientific investigation.

Dietary Supplement Research

In recent years, with the establishment of the NIH's Office of Dietary Supplements, there has been significant interest and advances in the area of dietary supplement research, in part related to the establishment of botanical research centers across the United States (16). With their knowledge of diet, food, nutrition-related biochemistry, health, and disease, RDs are uniquely positioned to participate in and contribute to this dynamic research agenda.

Figure 23.1 illustrates the key approaches to scientific investigation within the context of dietary supplement research. Research is generally initiated when a clinician observes a phenomenon that has not previously been explained or when a patient poses a question to the clinician for which no clear evidence-based explanation is available.

An arbitrary example might begin with a patient who asks an RD whether aloe vera reduces the mucositis associated with cancer chemotherapy. The patient is likely asking this question in response to having tried aloe vera or as a result of receiving information from another source (eg, a friend, relative, or the Internet) that suggests that efficacy exists. In turn, the patient may begin to use the dietary supplement despite a lack of evidence. If at a later date the patient returns to the RD's office with marked changes in clinical status, the clinician may decide to gather more information from the patient and to present the findings in the form of a case report or perhaps a case series, if data from additional patients provide the same or similar results. In addition, qualitative data may be collected in the form of in-depth, structured interviews or in the form of well-designed focus group discussions. The preliminary data generated by these approaches are insufficient to modify clinical practice. However, this type of data can serve as an impetus for basic mechanistic research to determine how biologically, physiologically, or biochemically the dietary supplement may alter the clinical outcome of interest. The data may also be used—sometimes concurrently—in efforts to identify possible associations between exposure to the particular dietary supplement and outcomes of interest in specific population groups. Once the basic mechanistic research is available and epidemiological support exists in the form of either case-control or cohort studies, then a randomized, placebo-controlled clinical trial can be conducted (see Chapters 8 and 9). Once several RCTs have been completed, investigators further substantiate the evidence for or against efficacy by conducting meta-analyses of generally homogeneous studies (see Chapter 9) or systematic reviews (see Chapter 10).

Clinical Trials

The gold standard for assessing the role of food substances in human health and disease prevention is the RCT. In medicine, the established approach for drug development and regulatory approval is to complete Phase I/II trials followed by a clinical intervention RCT; this approach is relevant to dietary supplement research as well. (See Chapters 2 and 9.)

Determination of Appropriate Dosage

The first step is determining the appropriate dosage and the safety history of the product to be tested. If animal data are available, these data are applied in estimating a starting dose as well as a dose-escalation plan for determining the maximum tolerable dose (MTD) in humans. Dosage studies include pharmacokinetic studies, which are performed to evaluate product deposition in human tissue, urinary clearance, and peak plasma/serum levels as well as time course for peak and clearance of the standardized active constituent under evaluation. All of this information is used to develop the portion of the research in which human dosage studies are paramount.

During the early stages of research regarding a specific supplement, criteria for product (in this case, dietary supplement) response evaluation and safety are used to test—in a descriptive way—and determine the safest dose, the MTD, and the most appropriate dose to achieve the expected clinical response in most patients. Criteria for establishing both a response evaluation and a safety evaluation are available for select clinical treatments, and may be adapted for research using dietary supplementation. For example, the National Cancer Institute has accepted the Response Evaluation Criteria in Solid Tumors (RECIST) approach (17) as the standard by which antitumor treatments are assessed.

Although guidelines specific to dietary supplement research have not been universally adopted, these standardized approaches are important for setting the most appropriate starting dose for the research, including future RCTs. Further, these safety-related, dose-ranging, and early-demonstration-of-effect studies allow for refinement of intervention protocols not only in terms of dose but also in terms of dose division, dose frequency, optimal administration route, patient tolerance/acceptance (including reports of adverse events), and preliminary evidence of efficacy. It is important to understand that these early studies are pilot in nature and as such are underpowered statistically to establish efficacy. The results of such preliminary research should only direct future study design and not inform clinical practice.

Determination of Product Efficacy

Once the preliminary pilot work is completed, there are numerous study design issues that clinicians should consider when developing dietary supplement intervention studies. The following is an overview of several key issues, and a summary of the clinical trial research process is illustrated in Figure 23.2.

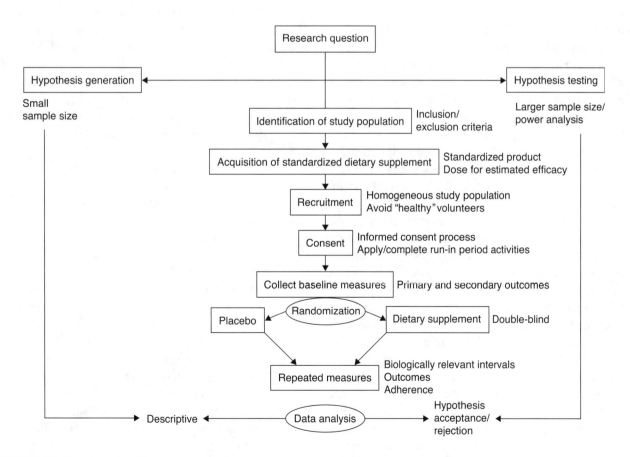

FIGURE 23.2   The scientific process: dietary supplement research model.

TRIAL DESIGN ISSUES

Trial Design in and of Itself

To have high scientific integrity, the design of a trial, from the outset, must be strong. Generally, there are three key components that researchers should strive for when designing a quality dietary supplement trial:

- Inclusion of an appropriate control or placebo group (18–21)
- Randomized assignment to the treatment group
- Double-blind approach to treatment

Inclusion of these approaches in the design of the study will support a quality outcome in terms of an unbiased assessment of efficacy. Unfortunately, these factors are often not well thought out in selecting trial designs for dietary supplement research.

Briefly, inclusion of a placebo group that is randomly assigned ensures that any placebo effect in relation to overall participation in a study is captured and evaluated separate from any specific effects attributable to the dietary supplement. A significant placebo response is not an unusual outcome in clinical trial research, particularly dietary supplement research (18). In terms of blinding, it is imperative that *both* the investigators (and staff) and the study participants be blinded as to the treatment assignment until the end of all data collection. The lack of blinding is a common limitation to dietary supplementation trials where an open-label approach is used.

In addition to the aforementioned factors, another key issue in designing dietary supplementation trials is an absolute awareness of dietary intake, particularly for the dietary supplement (in this case, nutrient or bioactive food component) of interest. This requires an assessment of dietary exposure both at baseline and throughout the intervention. It may also require a dietary restriction throughout the study to ensure that exposure is specific to the dietary supplement under study. For example, in an RCT assessing the efficacy of lycopene supplementation to reduce prostate-specific antigen levels in patients with early-stage prostate cancer, the participants may be asked to restrict dietary lycopene sources over the course of the study to reduce confounding of the results. In addition, participants interested in dietary supplementation research may be taking a number of self-prescribed supplements at the time of study enrollment. In this case, the investigator may choose to establish an exclusion criterion for study participation that states that those taking select dietary supplements cannot be considered for enrollment in the study. Another approach may be to offer a standardized MVM to all study participants to replace their self-prescribed supplements.

Supplement Product Selection

When selecting and describing a product to be used in research, investigators should adequately describe the dietary supplement so that other researchers can duplicate the study. NCCAM now requires investigators to demonstrate that the biologically active test agents and their placebos proposed for investigation are of sufficient quality. NCCAM also requires investigators to reserve test agent and placebo samples from each batch for verification at a later date of product quality, stability over time, and comparability from batch to batch. Although these are specific requirements for NIH-funded trials, they serve as excellent framework for all researchers. An abbreviated version of these requirements is described here; a complete version can be accessed from the NCCAM Web site (22).

For single-ingredient preparations (eg, nutrients, botanicals, animal-derived preparations, or probiotics), information on the raw material and final preparation is required by NCCAM. For multiple-ingredient botanical preparations, identity and quality information (eg, specifications and Certificates of Analysis for all components and for the finished product) is required by NCCAM for each individual ingredient, as well as for the mixture as a whole. Requirements include the following:

- Identification of each study agent using the scientific taxonomic nomenclature (eg, genus, species, variety [if applicable], and strain) and author citation.
- The name of the study agent supplier of the final study product. If the supplier is a middleman, the provider of the source material(s) to the supplier should be identified.
- Description of where and how an authenticated reference specimen of the source material is reserved.
- Description (macroscopic) of the parts of the plant or animal from which the product is derived.
- Description of the extraction procedure (eg, solvent[s] used, ratio of starting material to finished extract, time and temperature employed, type of extraction, whether fresh or dried material was used, whether any excipient materials were added, what percentage of the extract is native extract, and what

percentage is composed of excipients). Define the entire composition of the final extract.

- Information regarding active and/or other relevant marker compound(s) used for standardization.
- Identification of the specific pharmacopoeial monograph (eg, US Pharmacopeia) with which the material complies, or a description of suitable tests performed that are specific to the proposed study material and that can be compared to results from an authenticated reference. When no pharmacopoeial monograph exists for a study ingredient or in cases where the ingredient does not conform to the existing monograph, specifications should be provided, including all of the same tests found in the monograph.
- Information on the characterization (eg, chemical profile or fingerprint) of the agent as thoroughly as the state of the science allows.
- Any other information relevant to the standardization process of ensuring reasonably consistent material suitable for scientific study (eg, process control and chemical and/or biological standardization of ingredients).
- Information on the analysis of the product for contaminants, such as pesticide residues, heavy metals, toxic elements, mycotoxins, microorganisms, and adulterants.
- Description of bioavailability, dissolution, disintegration, and release if the information is available.
- Information on short- and long-term stability.

Population Sample

Selecting the appropriate population sample is central to maintaining the scientific integrity of the work. For example, you would not select a cohort of 20-year-old women with healthy body weights to test the role of soy supplementation in reducing serum cholesterol levels, because the likelihood that their serum cholesterol levels are high or even at risk of being above clinical recommendations in the next several years is low. Soy (or any other supplement) would be unlikely to have any significant effect on lipid levels in this circumstance. Even if the supplement did lower serum lipids slightly, the clinical relevance would be low given that the population was healthy at the time the intervention was initiated (ie, no evidence of dyslipidemia). In this case, there would be no clinical application for the research findings. Yet, it is not uncommon in dietary supplementation research to find published studies in which relatively healthy volunteers have been recruited to test the

efficacy of a dietary supplement. This "healthy volunteer effect" has been described (23). However, despite efforts to control this selection bias in dietary supplement trials (and other health intervention trials), this problem in recruitment continues. This bias commonly results in null findings even when efficacy may have otherwise been demonstrated in the setting of a clinically relevant study population sample.

Study Participant Homogeneity

Another problem in dietary supplementation research is the lack of homogeneity in selecting patients for study participation, particularly when sample size is small. For example, if sample estimates suggest that a sample size of 50 patients is sufficient to determine whether vitamin E supplementation reduces oxidative stress as measured by changes in 8-epi-prostaglandin F2α over time as compared with placebo, it is imperative that the sample population be as homogeneous as possible to reduce the likelihood that confounders are significantly modifying the response or lack of response. Although some of this error can be controlled for statistically and some will be controlled for by the randomized design, efforts should be made to keep the study population as homogeneous as possible. Characteristics that might be relevant here because they are known to vary oxidative stress include patient gender, physical activity patterns, smoking status, lean body mass, age, diet, and environmental exposures as well as concurrent use of other dietary supplements. Note that these factors, although most easily addressed in the eligibility criteria for study participation, could also be addressed in the study design.

Sample Size

Setting a statistically appropriate sample size is critical to quality research and should involve some consultation with a biostatistician working in a similar area of research (Estimating sample size is covered in detail in Chapter 27). Unfortunately, sample size is at times dictated by the research budget; however, spending any amount of funding on poorly designed science is inappropriate. One way to reduce sample size is to consider a crossover study design. This approach cuts sample size in half; however, adequate washout of the supplement/placebo between treatments is essential to deriving interpretable results.

Dietary supplement studies are frequently criticized for using small sample sizes. Many published studies are descriptive in nature because they use small samples or are pilot research. These studies do not test specific hypotheses; instead, varying doses of a dietary supplement are provided to small numbers of participants to determine tolerance, dose response, and optimal administration forms (eg, pill, capsule, powder). Although this is important preliminary work, it does not command the same level of scientific scrutiny as RCTs. As this field of research progresses and additional resources are allocated, we can expect substantial enhancement in trial design related to dietary supplementation.

Additional Key Issues for Optimal Trial Design

Other concerns regarding the body of scientific evidence for dietary supplementation stem from the lack of vigor in trial design. Among the issues that must be thoughtfully addressed are the use of run-in periods/activities to reduce participant dropout, randomization, blinding to intervention for both the subject and the investigative team, the use of a placebo group, and a crossover design that includes sufficient washout between intervention periods.

Dose

Selection of an appropriate dose for clinical trials develops from sound epidemiological, animal, or basic science evidence. In the absence of such data, researchers tend to rely on common dosages from market distribution or previously published pilot studies that are commonly of insufficient sample size to test hypotheses. If the dietary supplement is a nutrient or bioactive food constituent derived from food, evidence from studies using the whole food may provide some guidance in terms of establishing a test dose. And, in some circumstances, animal data may afford some guidance in dose setting. When the dose at which clinical efficacy is demonstrated is unclear, it is prudent for researchers to test more than one dose so that a more precise estimate is available for follow-up trials. Further explanation of the importance of multiple-dosage testing is available at the Office of Dietary Supplements Web site (24). Researchers should understand that dosage setting is critical in the clinical design decision-making process; underdosing may result in null trial findings that would not have been reached had an appropriate dose been selected, and setting dosage above levels required for clinical efficacy may result in an increase in adverse events among study participants.

Duration

Determining the length of the intervention is also of importance because premature termination of the dietary supplementation may result in a null trial. If previously published studies used the dietary supplement of interest, the duration data from trials that have shown efficacy are certainly relevant to the design of the new trial. However, null findings may indicate that a longer intervention time is needed to test efficacy. One approach to establishing duration is to understand and take into consideration the underlying biochemistry/biology that may influence the bioavailability of the nutrient or compound either systemically or at a specific tissue site of relevance to your research hypotheses. Relevant questions include the following: Is the nutrient/compound lipid- or water-soluble? What is the chemical structure of the bioactive compound of interest? Does it require substantial digestion to release the biologically active compound? Generally, it has been shown that most botanical dietary supplements (as compared with prescription medications used for a similar clinical outcome) require longer duration of use before clinical efficacy is demonstrated. Again, in the absence of strong Phase I/II data, clinical trial dose estimates involve a certain degree of guesswork in terms of establishing an appropriate duration of therapy.

Adherence

A major challenge in clinical research, regardless of whether the intervention is a dietary supplement, medication, or lifestyle intervention, is adherence or patient compliance. There are several ways to test adherence in the context of a clinical trial, and it is judicious to include more than one approach when designing your intervention trial.

Biomarkers of exposure.   Ideally, there will be a valid and reliable biomarker of exposure that can be used to test compliance. In this case, biological samples (eg, blood, urine, or toenail) are collected at baseline before the study participants take the dietary supplement and repeatedly throughout the study for measurement of the specific nutrient and/or dietary constituent present in the supplement being studied (25). Some of the commonly used biomarkers of dietary compliance are plasma carotenoids, used as biomarkers of supplementation with specific carotenoids; plasma/serum/red blood cell micronutrient levels (eg, retinol, vitamin D_3, or folate); and fatty acid composition of cell membranes as derived from fat biopsy samples. Table 23.1 lists common nutrient and phytochemical biomarkers that could have utility in dietary supplement trials as indicators of exposure/adherence.

Self-report study diaries.   In research, investigators commonly rely on self-report to evaluate whether the study

TABLE 23.1 Biomarkers of Nutrient/Phytochemical Exposure Available for Use in Dietary Supplement Intervention Trials

Nutrient Exposure	Biomarkers for Exposure Assessment
Vitamins	
Vitamin A	Plasma retinol, retinol-binding protein
Vitamin C	Plasma vitamin C, urine deoxypyrinodine
Vitamin D	Serum 25-hydroxy vitamin D_3
Vitamin E	Plasma alpha or gamma tocopherol
B vitamins	Plasma pyridoxal-5-phosphate (vitamin B-6)
	Plasma B-12 (vitamin B-12)
	Plasma folate, red blood cell folate, and plasma homocysteine (folate)
Minerals	
Calcium	Calcium retention assay, serum osteocalcin
Iron	Serum iron, serum ferritin, transferrin saturation
Selenium	Plasma or whole blood or toenail selenium
Phytochemicals	
Carotenoids	Plasma or serum carotenoids
Isothiocyanates	Urinary dithiocarbamate
Polyphenols	Urinary polyphenols (eg, EGCG, EGC, EG)

participant complied with the study medication protocol. Dietary supplementation logbooks can be used to document "pill" use as well as any adverse events observed by the participant in the course of dietary supplement use. Generally, participants maintain a pill diary throughout the clinical trial, beginning during the run-in phase as an indicator of expected compliance during the treatment phase(s) of the study. Dietary supplement logs/diaries are subsequently reviewed by study staff on a regular basis (usually weekly or bimonthly) and in conjunction with participants receiving each subsequent supply of dietary supplement. These diaries can also serve as a document of side effects, time of administration, missed doses, duplicate dosing, or other deviations from dosage protocol.

Pill counts. The use of pill counts is another way to assess adherence in dietary supplementation studies. In this approach, study participants return to the study clinic weekly with all unused dietary supplements. The investigator then documents the number of dietary supplement "pills" provided at each clinic visit, as well as the number returned, and then calculates the difference to define each study participant's pill count. Pill counts are generally estimated every 1 to 2 weeks throughout the study period. It is important to note that regardless of whether the participant is receiving

the dietary supplement or a placebo, pill counts should be kept using the same standardized approach.

Outcomes

Your original hypothesis should specify the primary outcome of your research. This outcome should not involve a medical diagnosis, but it may be clinical in nature and must have clinical relevance in terms of health. In other words, reducing neck circumference may be of interest, but if neck circumference has never been associated with risk for disease, identifying neck circumference as your primary (or even secondary) outcome would result in wasted resources. Further, if the outcome selected has clinical relevance in terms of a disease but not the disease of interest, then again resources would be wasted and inappropriate conclusions might be drawn. For example, say you are interested in testing the efficacy of fenugreek in reducing blood glucose levels, but you have no blood samples available to assess. Using urinary ketones (which are available) as a surrogate indicator of blood glucose levels would not be appropriate because these two biomarkers assess different biological processes.

When establishing outcomes, it can be helpful to consider what type of outcome specifically interests you. For example, outcomes might be exposure related or related to a specific biological or pathophysiological mechanism. Exposure outcomes would involve a measurement of the level of a given nutrient and/or bioactive food constituent in human biological samples. These exposure outcomes may be direct or indirect. For example, measurement of folate levels may involve measurement of red blood cell folate or serum folate (direct measures), or change in folate status may be assessed by measuring plasma homocysteine levels, which are known to be highly correlated with folate status.

Mechanistic outcomes can also serve as outcome measures of relevance in dietary supplement research, reflecting the functional response to dietary supplementation. These outcomes are commonly used in dietary supplement research as the premise for structure-function claims on the dietary supplement label. In this case, the outcome denotes one or more specific biological responses that are known to be of relevance in determining the absence, presence, or severity of a disease without directly measuring a disease outcome. Examples of mechanistic outcomes include reducing biomarkers of oxidative stress (8-epiprostaglandin F-2α, 8-hydroxy-deoxyguanosine), inflammation (C-reactive protein, interleukins), lowering of fasting blood glucose or serum lipid levels, increasing resting energy expenditure, bone health (density, osteocalcin) or alteration of body composition (body fat, lean mass, etc).

When designing a clinical trial to test the efficacy of a dietary supplement, it is also imperative to establish appropriate time points for baseline and repeat measurement of both your primary and secondary outcome variables. Baseline measurements must be collected before randomization and preferably before total disclosure of the intervention. Follow-up measures should be taken at intervals that are relevant to the biological processes under study and for which participant burden is not unduly increased. For most biological measurements, a minimum of 4 to 6 weeks of dietary supplementation will be required before any biological activity can be demonstrated. For outcomes such as changes in body composition, longer intervals (eg, 6 months) are generally required to show relevant changes. In addition, trial designs are generally strengthened by having several outcome biomarkers that are related in the biological effects of interest. For example, if you were interested in the role of vitamin E supplementation in modulating oxidative stress (outcome biomarker), you could consider measuring both a biomarker of DNA damage (eg, 8-hydroxy-deoxyguanosine) and one of lipid peroxidation (eg, 8-epi-prostaglandin F-2α) in order to further substantiate any effect of supplementation on oxidative stress as well as to provide more specificity in terms of the type of oxidative stress being modulated. Other examples might include multiple biomarkers of immune function, body composition, exercise tolerance, and so on.

Chapter 28 provides detailed guidance regarding statistical analysis of diet- and nutrition-related research. A few important items need to be emphasized in regard to dietary supplementation trials:

- Analysis should be driven by the a priori hypothesis.
- Depending on the hypothesis as stated at the study onset, comparisons should be made in terms of either change in outcome measure from baseline by treatment group (best) or difference between groups at the prestated time point(s).
- If subjects are removed from the analysis, sufficient description of the statistical process leading to their exclusion should be provided.
- Associations between dietary supplement use and outcome should be evaluated in the context of confounders or effect modifiers (ie, factors that may influence both the exposure and the outcome of interest).
- Subgroup analysis should be avoided or presented only as pilot data for future prospective study.

OTHER APPROACHES TO DIETARY SUPPLEMENTATION RESEARCH

Adherence to the RCT design in the development of dietary supplement trials is imperative to advancing our understanding in this area. However, the RCT is not the only scientific approach, and the quality of trials in terms of methodology employed can vary substantially. To this end, scoring systems have been developed to rate the quality of clinical research both generally (26) and in relation to dietary supplements (27). In addition, summary reports, systematic reviews, and/or meta-analytic approaches have been employed to evaluate the strength of the evidence, particularly in relation to dietary supplementation by the Agency for Healthcare Research and Quality (28). The following is a description of other research approaches that provide evidence toward our understanding of the role of dietary supplementation in health.

Epidemiological Studies

Epidemiological research is by its nature observational; such studies use statistical modeling of data collected either cross-sectionally (ie, at one given point in time) or longitudinally (ie, over an extended period of time) to evaluate associations between dietary supplement use and some health outcome. These studies do not show cause and effect as we might derive from the RCT, but they do provide indications of specific association between dietary supplement(s) and health outcomes that support more stringent experimental study. There are three common epidemiological approaches:

- Migration studies in which a population's health is assessed while they reside in their country of origin and later after they migrate to the new country/culture with differing exposures.
- Case-control studies in which dietary supplementation patterns are compared for those who demonstrate a select health outcome and those who do not.
- Cohort studies in which dietary supplement use data are collected over time within a population and the population's risk for a select health outcome is assessed in relation to the dietary supplement exposure.

Migration studies currently have limited application to dietary supplementation research because data regarding dietary supplement intake patterns in most countries are not generally collected. Case-control studies are used to assess the relationship between supplementation and health outcomes, but the risk for recall bias is high because participants are frequently asked to recall dietary supplementation patterns after a health condition has been identified. Cohort studies are the most informative of the observational epidemiological studies, but most have not collected ample data regarding dietary supplement use. Two large, prospective cohort studies that have contributed to our understanding of dietary supplementation and health are the Framingham Heart Study, which has been conducted among residents of Framingham, Massachusetts, since 1948 (29), and the Nurses' Health Study, which has been conducted by Harvard University researchers and which includes longitudinal dietary supplement data collected from approximately 120,000 US nurses (30).

Although observational epidemiological studies provide evidence of associations, they do not provide sufficient evidence to establish cause and effect. Further, a large portion of the epidemiological studies do not collect data on dietary supplement use but rather focus on only dietary intake data. The collection of reliable and accurate information regarding dietary supplementation efficacy is critical if we want to advance our understanding of the role of dietary supplementation in health.

Assessment of the use of dietary supplements among study participants is challenging, and that is likely the primary reason why these data, historically, were seldom collected in the context of health research. In recent years, the Office of Dietary Supplements at NIH has begun the labor-intensive process of centralizing data on the composition of dietary supplements available on the US market, supplements that are potentially being used by study participants and may alter study findings. This database, once available, will allow investigators to assess nutrient/phytochemical/botanical exposures in the context of ongoing research. However, researchers will also need to collect data regarding dietary supplement usage. This requires two steps:

1. Participant listing of dietary supplement inventory including what products are taken (eg, brand name and dose), amount taken per dose, dosages per day or per week, and perceived adherence frequency
2. On-site review of dietary supplements with study participant that includes photocopying of supplement labels for entry into a study database

A sample dietary supplement data collection form is provided in Figure 23.3 (31).

Animal Models

Animal models are also an important tool for testing hypotheses related to dietary supplementation. Identifying an appropriate animal model is essential. For example, if one wanted to test the role of vitamin C supplementation in reducing endothelial damage using an animal model of coronary heart disease, dogs—which endogenously synthesize vitamin C—would not be appropriate models. Thus, in selecting a model, it is important to understand how the model's nutritional biochemistry differs or resembles the human condition. In addition, much of the research uses either rat or mouse models; the reasons for this are partially related to the animals' similarities to the human condition and partially related to the reduced costs of breeding, housing, and managing these animals. Further, there have been significant advances in the development of transgenic mouse models in which specific clinical conditions and biochemical pathways of biological response have been genetically altered to mimic human disease. For a list of available animal models for potential use in dietary supplementation biological research, consult the NIH's Model Organisms for Biomedical Research Web page (32). Animal models also afford the opportunity to test hypotheses related to dose response, adverse events, and timing of exposure (eg, in life span or in relation to disease prevention vs progression).

Basic Science/Mechanistic Studies

Much of what we understand about the biological mechanisms of how dietary supplements (eg, nutrients, herbs, or food constituents) modulate human disease evolves from basic science. The tools of basic science allow us, in a somewhat controlled environment, to evaluate cell-specific response and tissue-specific response in relation to exposure to the specific dietary supplement of interest. As with human intervention trials, the strength of the evidence generated is dependent on our ability to select relevant models to test our hypotheses.

One approach to studying the efficacy or the mechanistic underpinnings of a dietary supplement is to expose a cell line, tissue culture, or tissue array to the dietary supplement at varying concentrations or under variable conditions. This approach is commonly employed in the study of carcinogenesis. Cell lines are formed from specific cancer cells collected from tumor tissue and grown in culture. Numerous cell lines exist for use in research, most derived from human cancer, but beyond cell lines, whole tissues and even tissue arrays (which combine several tissues on

Supplement	Dose	When (times/ day/week)	For How Long? (number of weeks, months, years)	For Research Use Type/Brand	Label Collected? (Y = yes, N = no)	
Multivitamin					Y	N
Multivitamin-mineral					Y	N
B complex vitamin					Y	N
Vitamin C					Y	N
Vitamin E					Y	N
Folic acid					Y	N
Calcium (including antacids)					Y	N
Magnesium					Y	N
Iron					Y	N
Selenium					Y	N
Zinc					Y	N
Coenzyme Q_{10}					Y	N
Echinacea					Y	N
Fish oil					Y	N
Garlic					Y	N
Glucosamine/chondroitin					Y	N
Mixed carotenoids					Y	N
Other:*					Y	N
Other:					Y	N
Other:					Y	N
Other:					Y	N

*Probe participant regarding the use of supplements for select conditions such as cancer, heart disease, weight control, constipation, cognitive function, energy, and so on.

FIGURE 23.3   Sample dietary supplement use data collection form. Adapted with permission from Thomson CA, Newton TR. Dietary supplements: evaluation and application in clinical practice. *Top Clin Nutr*. 2005;20:28–39.

a single "sheet") are available to test mechanisms of biological response.

Beyond selecting a cell culture, it is also important that the researcher select the appropriate scientific assay specific to the biological activity of interest. Assays exist to assess numerous biological activities, from antioxidant response to cell cycle or growth arrest to immune response to proliferation. It is imperative that the appropriate model be selected to test the hypothesis of interest.

Beyond the decision of which biological mechanism or pathway may be of interest, the researcher must also select the appropriate assay. Characteristics of a scientifically appropriate assay include reliability, specificity, sensitivity, coefficient of variation (less than 10% essential on repeat measures), and established and reported use in peer-reviewed

journals. One limitation of research in the field of dietary supplementation is the lack of scientific rigor in selecting an appropriate assay to test relevant hypotheses.

CONCLUSION

With the advent of the Office of Dietary Supplements and NCCAM, the opportunities to develop and test evidence-based research hypotheses related to dietary supplementation are unprecedented. RDs are positioned to advance this science, both in terms of leading new projects and in terms of building collaborative multidisciplinary projects. Our understanding of dietary supplement efficacy will require a translational approach, applying the best of basic science, animal science, and even epidemiological evidence to well-designed, randomized, double-blind, placebo-controlled trials. Here we provide resources, guidance, and information to assist RDs in this viable and important area of research. Thus, the following action items should be considered as dietetics professionals explore and conduct research in dietary supplementation:

- Develop a resource library of dietary supplementation research articles.
- Develop a network of advisers and colleagues who share interest and expertise in dietary supplementation research.
- Know the regulatory issues surrounding dietary supplementation use, labeling, and marketing.
- Go beyond descriptive studies to the development and testing of research hypotheses.
- Start with strong pilot data (eg, basic, animal, epidemiological, or pilot trials) that support larger, well-designed intervention trials.
- Publish to advance the science for the greater good.

REFERENCES

1. National Center for Complementary and Alternative Medicine. Statistics on CAM Use in the United States. Available at: http://nccam.nih.gov/news/camstats.htm. Accessed March 9, 2007.
2. Radimer K, Bindewald B, Hughes J, Ervin B, Swanson C, Picciano MF. Dietary supplement use by US adults: data from the National Health and Nutrition Examination Survey, 1999–2000. *Am J Epidemiol.* 2004;160:339–349.
3. Picciano MF. Who Is Using Dietary Supplements and What Are They Using? Presentation at the Food and Nutrition Conference and Exhibits, American Dietetic Association, St Louis, Mo, October 2005.
4. Foote JA, Murphy SP, Wilkens LR, Hankin JH, Henderson BE, Kolonel LN. Factors associated with dietary supplement use among healthy adults of five ethnicities: the Multiethnic Cohort study. *Am J Epidemiol.* 2003;157:888–897.
5. Gunther S, Patterson RE, Kristal AR, Stratton KL, White E. Demographic and health related correlates of herbal and specialty supplement use. *J Am Diet Assoc.* 2004;104:27–34.
6. Archer SL, Stamler L, Moag-Stahlberg A, Van Horn L, Garside D, Chan Q, Buffington JJ, Dyer AR.

7. Association of dietary supplement use with specific micronutrient intakes among middle-aged American men and women: the INTERMAP Study. *J Am Diet Assoc.* 2005;105:1105–1109.
7. Eichenberger Gilmore JM, Hong L. Longitudinal patterns of vitamin and mineral supplement use in young white children. *J Am Diet Assoc.* 2005;105:763–772.
8. Office of Dietary Supplements. ODS Celebrates Its 10th Birthday. Available at: http://ods.od.nih.gov/News/ODS_Update_-_January_2006.aspx. Accessed February 1, 2007.
9. Haggans CJ, Regan KS, Brown LM, Wang C, Krebs-Smith J, Coates PM, Swanson CA. Computer access to research on dietary supplements: a database of federally funded dietary supplement research. *J Nutr.* 2005;135:1796–1799.
10. National Center for Complementary and Alternative Medicine. CAM Basics: What Is CAM? Available at: http://nccam.nih.gov/health/whatiscam. Accessed February 1, 2007.
11. Verhoef MJ, Casebeer AL, Hilsden RJ. Assessing efficacy of complementary medicine: adding qualitative research methods to the "gold standard." *J Altern Complement Med.* 2002;8:275–281.
12. Berman J, Chesney MA. Complementary and alternative medicine in 2006: optimising the dose of the intervention. *Med J Aust.* 2005;183:574–575.
13. Hathcock J. Dietary supplements: how they are used and regulated. *J Nutr.* 2001;131(suppl):1114S–1117S.
14. US Food and Drug Administration. Center for Food Safety and Nutrition. Dietary Supplement Health and Education Act of 1994. Available at: http://www.cfsan.fda.gov/~dms/dietsupp.html. Accessed February 1, 2007.
15. Appendix D. In: Sarubin Fragakis A, Thomson CA. *The Health Professional's Guide to Popular Dietary Supplements.* 3rd ed. Chicago, Ill: American Dietetic Association; 2006:658.
16. Office of Dietary Supplements Web site. Available at: http://dietary-supplements.info.nih.gov. Accessed February 1, 2007.
17. Therasse P, Arbuck SG, Eisenhauer EA, Wanders J, Kaplan RS, Rubinstein L, Verweij J, Van Glabbeke M, van Oosterom AT, Christian MC, Gwyther SG. New guidelines to evaluate the response to treatment in solid tumors. *J Natl Cancer Inst.* 2000;92:205–216.

18. Miller FG, Rosenstein DL. The nature and power of the placebo effect. *J Clin Epidemiol.* 2006;59:331–335.

19. Kaptchuk TJ, Stason WB, Davis RB, Legedza AR, Schnyer RN, Kerr CE, Stone DA, Nam BH, Kirsch I, Goldman RH. Sham device vs inert pill: randomized controlled trial of two placebo treatments. *BMJ.* 2006;332:391–397.

20. Saunders J, Wainwright P. Risk, Helsinki 2000 and the use of placebo in medical research. *Clin Med.* 2003;3:435–439.

21. Ellenberg S. Scientific and ethical issues in the use of placebo and active controls in clinical trials. *J Bone Miner Res.* 2003;18:1121–1124.

22. National Center for Complementary and Alternative Medicine. NCCAM Interim Applicant Guidance: Product Quality: Biologically Active Agents Used in Complementary and Alternative Medicine (CAM) and Placebo Materials. Notice NOT-AT-05-004. Release date: April 29, 2005. Available at: http://grants.nih.gov/grants/guide/notice-files/NOT-AT-05-004.html. Accessed March 9, 2007.

23. Austin MA, Criqui MH, Barrett-Connor E, Holbrook MJ. The effect of response bias on the odds ratio. *Am J Epidemiol.* 1981;114:137–143.

24. Office of Dietary Supplements. Why, When, What, and How of Clinical Trials: Educational Sessions. Supplyside West International Trade Show and Conference. November 9, 2005. Las Vegas, Nev. Available at: http://ods.od.nih.gov/News/SupplySide_West_2005_Educational_Sessions.aspx. Accessed February 1, 2007.

25. Blanck HM, Bowman BA, Cooper GR, Myers GL, Miller DT. Laboratory issues: use of nutritional biomarkers. *J Nutr.* 2003;133(suppl):888S–894S.

26. Van Tulder M, Furlan A, Bombardier C, Bouter L. Updated method guidelines for systematic reviews in the Cochrane Collaboration Back Review Group. *Spine.* 2003;28:1290–1299.

27. Introduction. In: Sarubin Fragakis A, Thomson CA. *The Health Professional's Guide to Popular Dietary Supplements.* 3rd ed. Chicago, Ill: American Dietetic Association; 2006:xiv–xv.

28. Agency for Healthcare Research and Quality. EPC Evidence Reports. Available at: http://www.ahrq.gov/clinic/epcindex.htm#dietsup. Accessed July 1, 2006.

29. Framingham Heart Study Web site. Available at: http://www.nhlbi.nih.gov/about/framingham. Accessed February 1, 2007.

30. Nurses' Health Study Web site. Available at: http://www.channing.harvard.edu/nhs/index.html. Accessed February 1, 2007.

31. Thomson CA, Newton TR. Dietary supplements: evaluation and application in clinical practice. *Top Clin Nutr.* 2005;20:28–39.

32. National Institutes of Health. Model Organisms for Biomedical Research. Available at: http://www.nih.gov/science/models. Accessed March 9, 2007.

24

—ɯ—

Research in Foodservice Management

Bonnie L. Gerald, PhD, DTR, and Mary Cluskey, PhD, RD

Research is critical to the integrity of the evolving field of foodservice management. There is a rich history of research related to foodservice management, dating back to the early years of the profession. Through research, the field has continued to develop. This chapter illustrates the historical development of research in the field, presents a matrix of foodservice management research areas, and discusses current research techniques used in the field.

HISTORICAL DEVELOPMENT OF FOODSERVICE MANAGEMENT RESEARCH

The profession of dietetics formally began in 1917, and foodservice management has always been emphasized. Soon after the first publication of the *Journal of the American Dietetic Association* in 1925, an article was published by Rush (1) on job analysis in lunchrooms and cafeterias.

In the 1930s, emphasis in foodservice management was on labor (2,3), cost control (4,5), and training (6). Research also measured work effectiveness (7,8). World War II had a dramatic impact on dietetics. Research focused on the layout and design of kitchens, food cost control and rationing, and personnel management (9–12).

Work on efficiency continued through the 1960s, beginning with the publication of research in the areas of work sampling and the use of computers in foodservice (13). Computer simulations and computer use in cafeteria serving lines (14), menu planning (15), and food cost

accounting (16) were reported. Researchers evaluated food produced using different production systems (17). Employee outcomes, such as job satisfaction, also were studied (18).

Research in the 1970s continued to focus on computer applications (10–21). During this decade, research related to Hazard Analysis and Critical Control Point (HACCP) and food safety (22,23) first appeared in the *Journal of the American Dietetic Association.* Food production systems research continued (24), and behavioral science research, particularly that related to work values and job satisfaction, flourished (25–27).

In the 1980s, research themes were similar to those of the 1970s. The availability of microcomputers (ie, the personal computer [PC]) in the workplace facilitated research of computer applications for training (28,29) and information systems (30–40). Methods from business research were used to evaluate productivity (31–52). Food production systems using new technology were also compared (53–61). Research from the 1990s to the 2000s will be used as examples of research techniques discussed in this chapter.

FOODSERVICE MANAGEMENT RESEARCH AREAS

There are many ways to organize areas of foodservice management research. Olsen, Tse, and Bellas (62) developed a classification system for research and development

337

TABLE 24.1   Foodservice Management Research Area Matrix

Customer-Related Topics	Product- and Process-Related Topics	Human Resources–Related Topics
Needs and preferences • Dietary Guidelines for Americans • ADA Guidelines • Nutrition education Behavior Marketing • Product • Place • Price • Promotion Service • Style • Institutional constraints • Customer satisfaction Environmental scanning • Political • Economic • Technological • Sociological • Ecological	Menu-related issues • Nutrition • Cost: food and labor • Variety • Acceptability • Product development Procurement Production • Forecasting • Production systems • Production scheduling • Productivity • Food preparation • Food safety/HACCP • Nutrition • Equipment • Layout and design Cost Natural resources • Waste management • Water conservation • Ventilation and air quality • Energy conservation • Hazardous substances • Emergency and disaster planning Food safety • Microbiological • Chemical Environmental issues Sustainable food systems	Staffing • Competencies • Training and development • Compensation • Retention Performance • Productivity • Motivation • Satisfaction • Organizational commitment Safety and health regulations • Americans with Disabilities Act • AIDS/HIV Sociocultural factors • Multicultural diversity • Organizational culture Leadership

The authors of this chapter wish to recognize Jeannie Sneed, PhD, RD, and Mary B. Gregoire, PhD, RD, FADA, for their contributions to this table.

in the hospitality industries. Others have identified research needs relevant to specific areas, such as school foodservice (63). Sneed (64) developed a foodservice management research area matrix to provide a contemporary and comprehensive view of areas of research in the field. A revised version of this matrix (see Table 24.1) reflects current terminology and areas omitted in the earlier version. This matrix shows the breadth of research as well as research needs in foodservice management.

RESEARCH TECHNIQUES IN FOODSERVICE MANAGEMENT

Foodservice management research differs from research in other areas of dietetics. The differences are due to the complex, interrelated nature of foodservice. Researchers in this field must consider the interaction of human factors, available resources, and the physical environment when design-

ing research projects. Methods within operational units can be highly variable, limiting the ability to control variables across units. For example, Wie, Shanklin, and Lee (65) evaluated cost-effective methods of waste disposal for four types of foodservice operations. Annual costs and net present worth for disposal methods and associated labor requirements were determined for five alternative strategies. The researchers used data collected from a previous study to determine costs for labor, supplies, transportation, utilities, and fees (66). Foodservice research necessitates the use of many research techniques to answer research questions, explore research variables, and ultimately to improve practice. (See Chapters 7 and 8.)

Research Settings

Foodservice research may be conducted in the laboratory or in the field. Each setting has its advantages and disadvantages. Laboratory research has the advantage of providing for better control of research variables. However, it may not realistically reflect operational practice, and this can limit the applicability of the findings. Field studies have the advantage of being realistic, but researchers have less control over variables. Because of the inherent advantages and disadvantages of both laboratory and field settings, studies conducted in both settings are necessary to produce meaningful research outcomes.

Most laboratory research focuses on product development, product performance, or equipment testing. Daniel et al (67) compared the *trans* fatty acid content of french fries fried in hydrogenated and nonhydrogenated oils. A randomized block design was used with fryer tanks as a block and time in days as the split plot to generate cooked potatoes for fat analysis by gas chromatography. Another study evaluated the performance of various sweeteners in muffins, pound cakes, and cocoa cupcakes in a laboratory setting (68). A complete block experimental design was used to compare specific volume, surface area, tenderness, and percentage of water loss in products. Food evaluations may involve subjective and objective measures The acceptability of okra as a fat replacement in a frozen dairy dessert was evaluated in a laboratory study (69). Untrained testers used a hedonic scale to rate samples for color, flavor, odor, texture, and aftertaste. Timed observations were used to measure the dessert's melting characteristics.

Many research studies have been conducted in the field, including studies related to total waste composition in a retirement community (70), food waste in a retirement community and an elementary school (71,72), acceptance of foods in a school and an employee cafeteria (73,74), plate waste and competitive foods (75), microbiological content of foodservice contact surfaces (76), and pricing strategy in a high school (77). Researchers have conducted field observational studies to determine the time spent by schoolchildren eating either school lunches or sack lunches, using stopwatches to record data (78,79).

Data Collection

Data may be recorded either by an observation or by self-report. Researchers may use existing databases and conduct secondary analyses of data. Numerous examples of these kinds of studies are found in the foodservice management literature.

Lieux and Manning (80) observed work performance in eight senior centers and recorded 5-minute intervals of labor activities. Because the information was collected in several operations, managers scheduling labor in similar operations could learn from the data about the minutes that workers spent per meal performing various activities (such as service, processing, and cleaning). Research related to problems with salad bars (81), tray error rates (82), and decreasing plate waste (83) also used observation techniques.

Self-reporting of data is a common method whereby survey instruments solicit information that will then be analyzed. Theis and Matthews (84) asked registered dietitians (RDs) to record the amount of time spent performing management functions. In another study, Shanklin and coworkers (85) had clinical RDs document actual work time expenditures on specific client-related, administrative, professional, and nonprofessional activities, including delays and transit time. Thus, data were estimates of real time use. Results of these studies could be used by current and prospective RDs to estimate the amount of time required for various professional activities.

Examinations of existing data from secondary sources can sometimes be useful in answering research questions. Greathouse et al (61) obtained financial data (salaries, other direct costs, overhead, and total costs) from the Health Care Financing Administration to compare conventional, cook-chill, and cook-freeze foodservice systems. Cai (86) analyzed food expenditure patterns on trips and vacations, and Ham and coworkers (87) studied expenditures on food away from home using Consumer Expenditure Survey data from the Bureau of Labor Statistics. March and Gould (88) used data from the Kansas State Department of Education and the Kansas State Board of Education Division of Financial Services to compare school meal programs' financial self-sufficiency and compliance with federal nutrition guidelines. Shanklin and Wie determined nutrient contribution per 100 kcal and per penny for school lunches that used cycle menus from two elementary schools in two school districts (89). Cheung and associates (90) obtained organization charts from college and university foodservice operations and used them to evaluate the organizational levels, position titles, and lines of reporting.

Level of Analysis

For both qualitative and quantitative studies, the level of analysis is based on the research design. Qualitative analysis examine and code data in an effort to identify themes, which depict results about research questions. In quantitative studies, the level of analysis is based on how variables are measured. Data can be analyzed at the individual or the group level, depending on the research question, the type of variable, and how the data were collected. Variables at the individual level have been examined in research related to job characteristics, job satisfaction, and organizational commitment (25–27). The group level is the focus of much research in foodservice management, particularly in studies related to productivity and financial performance (61,80).

Number of Observations

Research may be a one-time observation, or it may be replicated. Most studies using survey research techniques represent one-time data collection. For example, O'Hara et al (91) asked geriatric patients to complete a survey to determine which of eight aspects of food and foodservice affected satisfaction. Wolf and Schiller (92) conducted a survey of dietetics and foodservice personnel to determine their readiness to contribute to team problem solving. Hospital administrators and hospital foodservice directors evaluated competency skill levels of RDs for hospital foodservice director positions (93). Brown (94) conducted telephone interviews of school foodservice directors to identify types of food production systems used. School foodservice directors provided information in a mail survey about factors associated with offering competitive foods and the impact of such offerings on school lunch participation (95). In all cases, data were collected at one point in time.

Researchers may combine observations with survey research. This technique compares behavior with the subjects' attitudes or beliefs. Sneed, Strohbehn, and Gilmore (96) observed food safety practices in assisted-living facilities and interviewed staff about their food safety knowledge. The staff then completed written tests of knowledge and attitudes toward food safety.

Patient satisfaction, tray accuracy, and food and labor costs were measured for a 30-day period to evaluate the implementation of a spoken menu (97). To evaluate menu performance, Connors and Rozell (98) used visual estimation of lunch and dinner plate waste for four 7-day periods over the course of 1 year. Hackes et al (71) made observations for 7 days to determine the weight and volume of service food waste in a continuing-care retirement community.

Replications of observations indicate the stability of data over time, whereas one-time observations provide snapshots of the variables studied. Replicated studies that reveal consistent results give credibility and allow for inference of results.

Research Design

The research design can be descriptive, preexperimental, quasi-experimental, or true experimental. Simulations and mathematical modeling are also used fairly extensively in foodservice management research.

Descriptive Research

Delphi technique.   The Delphi technique is a descriptive research method that brings together, in group process, individuals considered experts in their respective fields to respond to a series of questionnaires. The first questionnaire may have a few general questions; it is then followed by a second, more detailed questionnaire developed from responses gathered from input from the Delphi group. The process may include several iterations, depending on research objectives and data generated.

The Delphi technique is versatile, cost-effective, and time-efficient for participants. When using the Delphi technique, it is important to have highly motivated participants with good written communication skills as well as adequate time for collecting responses (99).

Johnson and Chambers (100) used the Delphi technique in a two-round process to identify foodservice benchmarking activities and performance measures. In round 1, 11 expert panel members responded to open-ended questions about measures for benchmarking related to four areas: operations, finance, customer satisfaction, and human resources. These results were developed into a list of benchmarking performance measures. In round 2, the panel members rated the importance of these measures.

Gregoire and Sneed (101) used a modified Delphi technique to explore the challenges and needs of school foodservice practitioners attempting to implement the US Dietary Guidelines for Americans. School foodservice practitioners attending a conference on procurement were divided into two discussion groups and asked to generate a list of barriers to implementing the guidelines along with relevant research and training needs. Their lists were used to develop a mail survey. This questionnaire asked participants to rate the importance of the items listed. This consensus-building process provided information and the motivation to develop strategies to remove barriers. Instead of using the true Delphi technique of mailing a questionnaire, these researchers took advantage of having the foodservice practitioners together to conduct the first step.

Gregoire and Sneed (102) used the Delphi technique to develop nutrition integrity standards. Forty-one participants were selected for their knowledge and expertise in child nutrition programs. In round 1, panel members provided feedback about proposed nutrition integrity standards. All responses were compiled; then a revised list of standards was generated and mailed to panel members in round 2. For this round, panelists used a five point rating scale to indicate their level of agreement with each statement. An item was retained if at least 85% of the panel members agreed or strongly agreed that it should be included.

A modified Delphi technique was used by Strohbehn, Gilmore, and Sneed (103) to identify food safety concerns and barriers to HACCP implementation in assisted-living and long-term-care facilities. In the first phase, a three-item open-ended questionnaire was sent to a national panel of 14 RDs and certified dietary managers. In the second phase, a structured questionnaire was developed based on panelists' comments from the first round and sent to the expert panel. The final version of the questionnaire was completed after the second round and mailed to a national sample of RDs and dietary managers.

Focus group.   Focus groups are used to collect qualitative information from carefully planned discussions designed to obtain perceptions and information from a small group of individuals (typically 7 to 10 people). Group members may stimulate discussion and contribute unique or divergent perspectives of which the researchers may not be aware. Open-ended questions are prepared in advance and posed to the group by a moderator. Focus groups have several advantages—this method is socially oriented, offers flexibility, has high face validity, provides quick results, and is low in cost. Like other qualitative research methods, it may be used to generate instruments to collect quantitative data.

Focus groups have been used extensively for market research and more recently for dietetics-related research. Parham and Benes (104) conducted focus groups of foodservice management educators to determine their preparation for teaching, identify which factors may contribute to teaching satisfaction and frustration, and evaluate the educators' level of research involvement. The researchers combined focus groups, survey research, input from an advisory committee, and college catalog reviews to identify development needs and strategies for facilitating roles of foodservice management faculty.

Harp et al (105) used focus groups to develop a beef appetizer for casual dining restaurants. Three consumer groups were used: university students (aged 21 to 24), young professionals (aged 25 to 30), and midcareer professionals (aged 31 to 40). In addition, an industry group was composed of managers of casual dining restaurants. The researchers developed discussion guides for the consumer and industry groups. Consumer questions addressed participants' habits and attitudes regarding beef consumption and their reactions to a beef appetizer. The industry focus group solicited input on the quality of beef available to restaurants, appetizer consumption patterns, and an appetizer preparation orientation.

Focus groups were used to determine both patient and nursing staff satisfaction with hospital foodservice (106). One postdischarge patient focus group and three nursing staff focus groups were conducted by a trained moderator. The discussion was transcribed and themes were developed using hierarchical analysis. Participants completed a validation questionnaire to evaluate whether the themes identified matched their perceptions. A questionnaire developed from the focus group themes was then used for patient interviews during meal rounds.

Survey research.   Survey research is an important technique in descriptive research. Survey research can help the researcher understand or describe a population, or test hypotheses. In studying populations, Gregoire and Sneed (107) used survey methodology to evaluate continuing education needs of various groups of school foodservice employees. Brown (108) used telephone interviews of school foodservice administrators, managers, and supervisors to characterize the prevalence of cook-chill or cook-freeze production systems.

Survey research may be used to identify best practices within a population. To assess the major predictors of satisfaction with middle and junior high school foodservice, Meyer (109) mailed questionnaires to 14 suburban high schools representing all regions of the country. School foodservice directors coordinated distribution of the survey to the students. Sheehan-Smith (110) used on-site interviews of administrative and foodservice staff to determine the best practices of hotel-style room service in four hospitals. These hospitals had similar hotel-style meal delivery systems but differed in hospital type and patient populations.

Gilbert and Sneed (111) collected data about organizational commitment, job satisfaction, productivity, turnover, and absenteeism of employees in hospitals in the United States and Canada. Chong et al (112) compared perceptions of total quality management performance among clinical and foodservice dietetics professionals. McKnight et al (113) evaluated opinions of Commission on Accreditation for Dietetics Education (CADE) program directors on the importance of financial management in all areas of dietetics practice.

Surveys used to test hypotheses are developed carefully to ensure the validity and reliability of the scales that measure the research variables. For survey scales, the Cronbach α (114) is used to check the internal consistency (or reliability) of the measure. When available, developed scales with established validity and reliability are used. Validated scales that have been used in foodservice management research include the Job Descriptive Index (115) and the National Academy for State Health Policy (116).

Researchers may want to study variables with no established scale. In these cases, the researcher must establish the scale's validity and reliability. Dienhart and coworkers (117) developed a 50-item scale to evaluate the service orientation of restaurant employees. This scale was used in later research conducted by Groves and coworkers (118). In both instances, the reliability of the scales was determined using measures of internal consistency. Kwon and Yoon (119) had an expert panel review a survey of outsourcing health care dietetics services for face validity. Based on the experts' input, a revised survey was pilot tested by a subsample of the target population. A modified survey was then mailed to all members of a dietetic practice group (DPG).

Unklesbay et al (120) developed a scale to assess attitudes toward food safety. The Cronbach α and item-total statistics were used to determine the reliability of the scale. These analyses indicated that there were two subscales. Based on the items that were related to each other, the two scales were named "personal responsibility for food safety" and "external responsibility for food safety" (which included, for example, government, food processors, and restaurants). To develop a questionnaire that would measure long-term-care residents' satisfaction with foodservice, Lengyel et al (121) reviewed previous surveys of patient and/or foodservice satisfaction. The instrument was further refined through interviews with long-term-care residents about issues in foodservice, and then the instrument was pilot tested . The survey instrument's reliability was determined by test-retest (paired sample t test) and internal consistency (Cronbach's α).

Survey research data are collected through either interview or questionnaire. Usually, survey data are collected from a subset of a population of interest; occasionally, however, data from an entire population may be sought. Sneed and coworkers (122) did a study to develop financial management competencies for entry-level and advanced-level RDs. The population of directors for CADE-approved Plan IV/V, AP4, and dietetics internship programs were included in the study. Sneed et al used a random sample of practitioners because the population for this group was very large. Canter and Nettles (123) surveyed all members of the Food and Nutrition Systems DPG to discover the prevalence of multidepartment management in health care settings and the competencies needed by multidepartment managers. Kwon and Yoon (119) mailed their dietary services outsourcing survey to all members of the Clinical Nutrition Management DPG.

Survey methods are the most frequently used research technique in the foodservice management literature. Survey methods have been used to study a variety of foodservice areas, including computer use (124,125), customer satisfaction (91,121,126–128), equipment (129,130), food safety (120,131), management decision making (132,133), personnel issues (92,134), purchasing (135), and production/delivery systems (108,109).

Survey research has many advantages as a research technique. Written surveys are relatively inexpensive and can be distributed by mail to large numbers of geographically dispersed individuals. Thus, surveys can access nationally representative samples. Individuals can respond either anonymously or confidentially, which increases the likelihood that responses will be frank. The written survey format provides each individual with the same stimulus, so the variability in data collection is minimized (114).

There are several disadvantages of survey research, most of which are primarily related to the response rate. Ideally, the survey return rate would be 100%, which would ensure that the results were representative of the sample; in reality, return rates are rarely 100%. The researcher needs to find out whether the respondents differed from nonrespondents. With a small response rate, results cannot be used to draw inferences about the population as a whole. Another concern is reading levels of the study sample. Pilot testing can show whether the individuals in the sample can read and understand the survey questions. The response format of the survey instrument may confuse respondents, making it difficult to know whether their interpretation is consistent with the researcher's. In addition, respondents may not accurately or completely respond to all survey questions; incomplete instruments may need to be eliminated, reducing the response rate (114).

Preexperimental Designs

Preexperimental designs are often used in field studies. They do not have the experimental control of quasi-experimental or true experimental designs. Preexperimental designs conducted in the field have the advantage of a naturalistic (or realistic) setting.

Examples of the one-group pretest-posttest design in foodservice management include Getlinger et al's study (72) of the impact of the timing of school recess on food waste. Sixty-six students in grades 1 through 3 made up the sample for the 5-week study. Data were collected in weeks 1 and 5. For week 1, students remained on their usual schedule of eating lunch for 15 minutes, followed by a 15-minute recess. In week 2, the schedule was reversed. A 3-week washout period was given so students could adjust to the new schedule. Plate waste data were collected for 4 days during weeks 1 and 5, using the same menu during both weeks of data collection. The researchers found that plate waste decreased when recess was given before meal time.

In a retirement community, Kim et al (70) conducted a waste composition study with a source reduction intervention and a service delivery intervention (70). After each intervention the researchers conducted follow-up analyses. They found that these interventions were effective in reducing the weight and volume of waste from the retirement community (70).

Perlmutter et al (74) conducted two interventions to study the profitability and acceptability of fat- and sodium-reduced hot entrées in one worksite cafeteria. Marketing was done to promote the modified entrées. Sales data were collected for 9 months, as was before and after acceptability data regarding the entrée modification. The researchers found that the interventions did not affect sales, but acceptability scores decreased for some modified entrées.

The efficiency and effectiveness of a new patient food system was evaluated in three phases: baseline printed menus with substitution lists; spoken-menu model with bundled meals; and spoken-menu with additional upscale items and point-of-service snack cart (136). Data were collected on labor hours, substitutions, late trays, and wasted trays.

Shatenstein and Ferland (137) measured the impact of a food delivery change in a nursing home. The centralized food delivery system was changed to a decentralized bulk food portioning system on the residents' floors. Data were collected for 3 nonconsecutive days both in the preintroduction phase and 10 weeks postintroduction. Plate waste, biochemical parameters, and anthropometric measurements were used to determine the impact of the food delivery change.

Buscher et al (138) conducted two separate studies in a university cafeteria to evaluate the effect of point-of-purchase interventions on healthy snack purchases. There was a 7-week washout period between the two interventions. Data were collected for baseline, intervention, and the follow-up periods.

French et al (77) used a variation of preexperimental design to study pricing. In another variation of preexperimental research design, Remsburg et al (139) evaluated the effect of service style on long-term-care residents' nutritional status. Individuals from a homogeneous group of residents were randomly assigned to receive either regular tray or buffet-style service for a 3-month intervention period. The data were compared with baseline nutritional status indicators.

Preexperimental designs have both advantages and disadvantages. As noted previously, one advantage is that they are conducted in actual operations, so the setting is realistic (naturalistic). This is important when the research questions are applied ones. Such questions are needed to improve operations, and they are often difficult or impossible to study with more controlled research designs.

A major disadvantage is that the researcher has little control over extraneous variables that might confound the results. This design often is viewed as a case study. To be able to generalize findings, researchers would need to replicate the study in other operations or settings.

Quasi-experimental Designs

Quasi-experimental research designs are conducted in field settings. Because it uses intact groups, this design limits the researcher's ability to assign participants to groups. It does allow the researcher to select who gets measured and decide when the measurement takes place. Costello and coworkers (140) used a quasi-experimental design to study food safety training. The research team randomly selected six stores of a quick-service restaurant chain; then they randomly assigned two of the stores as the control (no treatment), two stores as sites where employees were trained by lectures, and two stores as stores where employees were computer trained. Compared with the control group, food safety knowledge increased 29% for the lecture stores and 20% for the computer-trained stores. In another study, Endres et al (141) evaluated acceptability of soy-enhanced menus by Head Start participants at a rural site. The soy-modified items were randomly assigned over a 3-week-cycle menu period. The traditional and soy-enhanced foods were compared by nutrient content and amount consumed. Reilly et al (142) selected three closely located elementary schools to determine acceptability of soymilk as an alternative calcium-rich beverage to cow's milk. Data to measure the amounts of beverages consumed were collected for three periods: baseline, initial 2 days of soymilk introduction, and 4 days after introduction.

Quasi-experimental designs have the advantage of occurring in a naturalistic setting. This research addresses actual operational research questions, which may apply to only that operation. The lack of control (because of the limited ability to randomly select and assign treatment to groups) means that factors unrelated to the interventions may plausibly explain the study's findings. As a result, theories cannot be proved, only explored. Quasi-experimental studies often have more external validity (generalizability) than internal validity.

True Experimental Designs

True experimental designs allow the researcher to manipulate the independent variable and determine the impact on the dependent variable. There are many examples of the use of true experimental designs in foodservice management. These research studies are often conducted in laboratory settings, but there are examples of field studies as well.

Studies of energy consumption (143,144) and heat processing (145–147) have used true experimental designs. Tutt et al (143) compared the energy consumption (dependent variable) of 110,000- and 100,000-BTU convection ovens in a university and a school, respectively. The independent variables were load (full loads of 16 pans vs partial loads of 8 pans) and preheating (no preheating vs preheating). Three trials for each treatment were conducted.

There are many examples of true experimental design related to food product development and food quality. Goldmon and Brown (148) examined the effect of fat (15% and 20%) and the addition of soy fiber (0%, 4%, and 6%) on the quality of ground pork patties. The sensory attributes of the treatments were evaluated by a 10-member trained taste panel. The effects of cooking methods and other treatments of food products, particularly meat, have been studied extensively using true experimental designs (149,150). Food safety issues also have been studied using true experimental designs. Ollinger-Snyder and Matthews (151) evaluated the coliform and aerobic plate counts of turkey slices reheated in a microwave oven. Bacterial growth on wet-nested plates was compared with that on air-dried plates using cultures from swabbed plates (152). Both air-dried and wet-nested plates were inoculated with contaminated soy broth.

True experimental designs have the advantage that all the variables are controlled, and the impact of the independent variable on the dependent variable can be determined. However, many areas in which foodservice research is needed cannot be studied in a laboratory under tightly controlled conditions. Much of what we need to know occurs in operations where people work. Thus, experimental design is not often realistic for foodservice management research.

Simulations and Mathematical Modeling

Simulation. Computer simulations are used to illustrate the behavior of systems and to evaluate strategies for the operation of a system. Simulations have many applications in foodservice management and provide a model for predicting outcomes in a cost-effective manner. The use of computer simulations in foodservice dates back to the mid-1960s, when Knickrehm (153) used simulations to determine dining room seating capacity. Guley and Stinson (154) applied computer simulation techniques for production scheduling in a ready-foods system. Nettles and Gregoire (155) used computer simulations to examine the time required for tray-line flow in school foodservice.

Research on the use of computers to plan menus dates back to the early 1960s. Balintfy (156) and Eckstein (157) did much of the early work related to the use of computers for menu planning. More recently, artificial intelligence systems have been developed for computer-assisted menu planning (158).

Another type of simulation is service blueprinting, a process that looks at a service from a customer's perspective. It has been used in service marketing and in medical practice, and it has the potential to improve customer satisfaction with nutrition services. Paquet et al (159) developed a service blueprint case study of nutritional quality of food intake in institutions. The blueprint was a representation of the patient experience from nutrition assessment to meal delivery. The blueprint was developed by measurement of meal production, observations, and interviews of staff and patients. Service blueprinting may possibly ensure that all processes and resources are included in the patient's experience with healthcare services.

Mathematical modeling. Several mathematical modeling techniques, originally developed for use in business operations, have been applied successfully in foodservice management. These models use mathematical relationships to represent some aspect of reality. With mathematical models, the researcher can draw conclusions about the impact of various decisions by experimenting with the model instead of intervening in actual operations. The advantages of mathematical models are that they are a less expensive, less time-consuming, and less risky way to model the impact of a decision before implementation in an actual operation.

Mathematical models have been used to assist with foodservice decision making related to forecasting (160), food expenditures (86,87), and customer seating (161). Miller and coworkers (162) used simple mathematical models to forecast production quantity needs for a university residence hall. They developed models that provided more accurate forecasts than did the manual forecasting methods used previously. Blecher (163) applied the forecasting models to determine the most accurate method of predicting meal demand in Title IIIc congregate lunch programs.

CONCLUSION

Foodservice management research has played an integral part in dietetics practice since its early days. Research continues to be needed to provide information on ways to most efficiently and effectively run foodservice operations in a changing environment.

Many research techniques have been used to address foodservice management research questions. Much of the research conducted to date has used survey methodology to describe and compare foodservice operations. Future research should expand the use of qualitative techniques to better build theories and explore relationships. Experimental research methods in foodservice management have been limited to product development and equipment testing; expansion of the use of experimental methods in actual operational settings would be beneficial and move practice forward. The foodservice management knowledge base continues to grow through the use of a variety of techniques to explore research hypotheses. Researchers are encouraged to expand their use of a variety of data collection and analysis techniques. Environmental scanning of trends in the hospitality and marketing sectors may generate new theories with application to foodservice management in dietetics.

REFERENCES

1. Rush G. Job analysis of lunchroom and cafeteria management. *J Am Diet Assoc.* 1925;1:130–137.
2. Baker RT, Barlow M. Personnel study of dietary departments of hospitals. *J Am Diet Assoc.* 1931;6:356–359.
3. Augustine GM. Labor policies in college residence and dining halls. *J Am Diet Assoc.* 1939;15:254–272.
4. Gleiser FW, Severance GM. Budgeting the student's food dollar in a cooperative residence hall system. *J Am Diet Assoc.* 1938;14:692–696.
5. Leigh MJ. Management and food control in the college dormitory. *J Am Diet Assoc.* 1939;15:179–184.
6. Pendergast WS. Standards of postgraduate training in school lunchroom management for college graduates. *J Am Diet Assoc.* 1938;14:93–98.
7. MacDonald MF. Measuring effectiveness in the preparation and service of hospital food. *J Am Diet Assoc.* 1938;14:330–338.
8. Rogers MP. Operating lunchrooms with pupil satisfaction and financial success. *J Am Diet Assoc.* 1938;14:85–92.
9. Blaker GG, Harris KW. Labor hours and labor costs in a college cafeteria. *J Am Diet Assoc.* 1952;28:429–434.
10. Donaldson BD. Labor hours in the dietary department. *J Am Diet Assoc.* 1957;33:1239–1243.
11. McKinley MM, Augustine GM, Chadderdon H. Training employees in work simplification. *J Am Diet Assoc.* 1957;33:592–595.
12. Bloetjes MK, Gottlieb R. Determining layout efficiency in the kitchen. *J Am Diet Assoc.* 1958;34:829–835.
13. Wise BI, Donaldson B. Work sampling in the dietary department. *J Am Diet Assoc.* 1961;39:327–332.
14. Knickrehm ME, Hoffman TR, Donaldson B. Digital computer simulations of a cafeteria service line. *J Am Diet Assoc.* 1963;43:203–208.
15. Eckstein EF. Menu planning by computer: the random approach. *J Am Diet Assoc.* 1967;51:529–533.
16. Andrews JT, Moore AN, Tuthill BH. Electronic data processing in intra-departmental food cost accounting. *J Am Diet Assoc.* 1967;51:32.
17. Quam ME, Fitzsimmons C, Godfrey RL. Ready-prepared vs conventionally prepared foods. *J Am Diet Assoc.* 1967;50:196–200.
18. Tansiongkun V, Ostenso GL. Job satisfaction in hospital dietetics. *J Am Diet Assoc.* 1968;53:202–210.
19. Hoover LW, Moore AN. "Dietetic com-pak"—an educational model simulating computer-assisted dietetics. *J Am Diet Assoc.* 1974;64:500–504.
20. Orser J, Mutschler M. A computer tallied menu system. *J Am Diet Assoc.* 1975;67:570–572.
21. Wilcox MM, Moore AN, Hoover LW. Automated purchasing: forecasts to determine stock levels and print orders. *J Am Diet Assoc.* 1978;73:400–405.

22. Bobeng BJ, David BD. HACCP models for quality control of entrée production in hospital foodservice systems: I. Development of Hazard Analysis Critical Control Point models. *J Am Diet Assoc.* 1978;73:524–529.

23. Bobeng BJ, David BD. HACCP models for quality control of entrée production in hospital foodservice systems: II. Quality assessment of beef loaves utilizing HACCP models. *J Am Diet Assoc.* 1978;73:530–535.

24. Zallen EM, Hitchcock MJ, Goertz G. Chilled food systems: effects of chilled holding on quality of beef loaves. *J Am Diet Assoc.* 1975;67:552–557.

25. Swartz RS, Vaden AG. Behavioral science research in hospital foodservice. I. Work values of foodservice employees in urban and rural hospitals. *J Am Diet Assoc.* 1978;73:120–126.

26. Swartz RS, Vaden AG. Behavioral science research in hospital foodservice. II. Job satisfaction and work values of foodservice employees in large hospitals. *J Am Diet Assoc.* 1978;73:127–131.

27. Calbeck DC, Vaden AG, Vaden RD. Work-related values and satisfactions. *J Am Diet Assoc.* 1979;75:434–440.

28. Waddell KP, Rinke WJ. Effectiveness of a computer-assisted program for teaching sanitation. *J Am Diet Assoc.* 1985;85:62–67.

29. Cloninger BJ, Messersmith AM, McEwan CW. Food item inventory instructional simulation using microcomputers. *J Am Diet Assoc.* 1988;88:1090–1093.

30. Guley HM, Stinson JP. Computer simulation for production scheduling in a ready foods system. *J Am Diet Assoc.* 1980;76:482–487.

31. Fromm B, Moore AN, Hoover LW. Computer-generated fiscal reports for food cost accounting. *J Am Diet Assoc.* 1980;77:170–174.

32. Galloway ME, Kraus G. A computerized food management system for an extended care unit. *J Can Diet Assoc.* 1983;44:347–357.

33. Matthews ME, Norback JP. A new approach to the design of information systems for foodservice management in health care facilities. *J Am Diet Assoc.* 1984;84:675–678, 681.

34. Hart RA, Kolasa K, McFadden J. Computerized nutrient analysis for foodservice. *J Am Diet Assoc.* 1985;85:1337–1339.

35. McCool, AC, Garand MM. Computer technology in institutional foodservice. *J Am Diet Assoc.* 1986;86:48–56.

36. Hicks ZR, Matthews ME, Norback JP. A computer-based decision-support system aids in distribution in planning and control of foodservices. *J Am Diet Assoc.* 1986;86:1182–1188.

37. Aldrich DS, Helbig LC. A sequential procedure for implementing a computer-based information system. *J Am Diet Assoc.* 1986;86:1228–1231.

38. Hicks ZR, Matthews ME, Norback JP. Activities of and time spent by the project dietitian in implementing a custom-designed decision support system for a computer. *J Am Diet Assoc.* 1988;88:200–205.

39. Stinson JP, Guley HM. Use of the computer to determine direct costs of menu items. *J Am Diet Assoc.* 1988;88:586–590.

40. Bender JR, Matthews ME. Development of an evaluation model for computer foodservice management systems. *J Am Diet Assoc.* 1989;89:1465–1472.

41. Harper JM, Shigetomi CT, Mackin SD, Iyer PA, Jansen GR. Alternate lunch patterns in high schools. I. Labor requirements and meal costs. *J Am Diet Assoc.* 1980;77:152–159.

42. Yung LS, Matthews ME, Johnson VK, Johnson NE. Productivity in foodservice systems in fourteen nursing homes. *J Am Diet Assoc.* 1980;77:159–164.

43. Mayo CR, Olsen MD, Frary RB. Variables that affect productivity in school foodservices. *J Am Diet Assoc.* 1984;84:187–190,193.

44. Ridley SJ, Matthews ME, McProud LM. Labor time code for assembling and microwave heating menu items in a hospital galley. *J Am Diet Assoc.* 1984;84:648–654.

45. Block AA, Roach FR, Konz SA. Occurrence sampling in a residence hall foodservice: cleaning times for selected vegetables. *J Am Diet Assoc.* 1985;85:206–209.

46. Campbell CA. The enhanced productivity program. *J Am Diet Assoc.* 1985;85:1479–1482.

47. Maloney S, Zolber K, Burke K, Connell B, Shavlik G. Work function analysis of vegetarian entrée production. *J Am Diet Assoc.* 1986;86:237–241.

48. Matthews ME, Zardain MV, Mahaffey MJ. Labor time spent in foodservice activities in one hospital: a 12-year profile. *J Am Diet Assoc.* 1986;86:636–643.

49. Choi VL, Roach FR, Konz SA. Occurrence sampling in a residence hall foodservice: entrée production times. *J Am Diet Assoc.* 1986;86:1698–1701.

50. Eden SH, Wood SM, Ptak KM. Development and implementation of a human accuracy program in

patient foodservice. *J Am Diet Assoc.* 1987;87: 492–495.

51. Murray IP, Upton EM. Labour productivity in hospital foodservice. *J Can Diet Assoc.* 1988;49:178–181.

52. Lieux EM, Winkler LL. Assessing productivity of foodservice systems in nutrition programs for the elderly. *J Am Diet Assoc.* 1989;89:826–829.

53. Dahl CA, Matthews ME, Marth EH. Cook/chill foodservice system with a microwave oven: aerobic plate counts from beef loaf, potatoes and frozen green beans. *J Microw Power.* 1980;15: 95–105.

54. Dahl CA, Matthews ME. Effect of microwave heating in cook/chill foodservice systems. Some data on temperature, yield, moisture, and fat content of typical foods. *J Am Diet Assoc.* 1980;77:289–295.

55. Upton EM, Glencross PD. Convenience food use in eight hospitals in Ontario. *J Can Diet Assoc.* 1981;42: 39–46.

56. Sawyer CA, Pestka JJ. Foodservice systems: presence of injured bacteria in foods during product flow. *Annu Rev Microbiol.* 1985;39:51–67.

57. Hoffman CJ, Zabik ME. Current and future applications of microwave cooking/reheating. *J Am Diet Assoc.* 1985;85:929–933.

58. Puckett RP, Boe DG, Medved CK. Management of engineering principles applied to foodservice operation. *J Am Diet Assoc.* 1987;87:770–774.

59. Garey JG, Simko MD. Adherence to time and temperature standards and food acceptability. *J Am Diet Assoc.* 1987;87: 1513–1518.

60. Greathouse KR, Gregoire MB. Variables related to selection of conventional, cook-chill, and cook-freeze systems. *J Am Diet Assoc.* 1988;88:476–478.

61. Greathouse KR, Gregoire MB, Spears MC, Richards V, Nassar RF. Comparison of conventional, cook-chill, and cook-freeze foodservice systems. *J Am Diet Assoc.* 1989;89:1606–1611.

62. Olsen MD, Tse E, Bellas C. A proposed classification system for research and development activities within the hospitality industries. *Hospitality Educ Res J.* 1984;9:55–62.

63. Matthews ME, Bedford MR, Hiemstra S. Report on school food service research needs—1985. *School Food Serv Res Rev.* 1986;10:35–39.

64. Sneed J. Research needs in foodservice management. In: Sneed J, Holdt C, eds. *Issues for the 1990s: Americans with Disabilities Act, Cultural Diversity, and Research. Proceedings of the 17th Biennial Conference of the Foodservice Systems Management Education Council.* Hattiesburg: University of Southern Mississippi; 1993:73–79.

65. Wie S, Shanklin CW, Lee KE. A decision tree for selecting the most cost-effective waste disposal strategy in foodservice operations. *J Am Diet Assoc.* 2003;103:475–482.

66. Wie S, Shanklin CW. Cost-effective disposal methods and assessment of waste generated in foodservice operations. *Food Serv Res Int.* 2001; 13:17–39.

67. Daniel D, Thompson LD, Shriver BJ, Wu CK, Hoover LC. Nonhydrogenated cottonseed oil can be used as a deep fat frying medium to reduce trans-fatty acid content in french fries. *J Am Diet Assoc.* 2005;105:1927–1932.

68. Soliah L, Walter JM, Parks T. Laboratory performance of sweeteners: implications for recipe and menu development. *J Nutr Recipe Menu Develop.* 1998; 3:53–66.

69. Romanchik-Cerpovicz JE, Costantino AC, Gunn LH. Sensory evaluation ratings and melting characteristics show that okra gum is an acceptable milk-fat ingredient substitute in chocolate frozen dairy dessert. *J Am Diet Assoc.* 2006;106:594–597.

70. Kim T, Shanklin CW, Su AY, Hackes BL, Ferris D. Comparison of waste composition in a continuing-care retirement community. *J Am Diet Assoc.* 1997;97:396–400.

71. Hackes BL, Shanklin CW, Kim T, Su AY. Tray service generates more food waste in dining areas of a continuing-care retirement community. *J Am Diet Assoc.* 1997;97:879–882.

72. Getlinger MJ, Laughlin CVT, Bell E, Akre C, Arjmandi BH. Food waste is reduced when elementary-school children have recess before lunch. *J Am Diet Assoc.* 1996;96:906–908.

73. Borja ME, Bordi PL, Lambert CU. New lower-fat dessert recipes for the school lunch program are well accepted by children. *J Am Diet Assoc.* 1996;96:908–910.

74. Perlmutter CA, Canter DD, Gregoire MB. Profitability and acceptability of fat- and sodium-modified hot entrees in a worksite cafeteria. *J Am Diet Assoc.* 1997;97:391–395.

75. Templeton SB, Marlette MA, Pamemangalore M. Competitive foods increase the intake of energy and decrease the intake of certain nutrients by adolescents consuming school lunch. *J Am Diet Assoc.* 2005;105:215–220.

76. Sneed J, Strohbehn C, Gilmore SA, Mendonca A. Microbiological evaluation of foodservice contact surfaces in Iowa assisted-living facilities. *J Am Diet Assoc.* 2004;104:1722–1724.

77. French SA, Story M, Jeffery RW, Snyder P, Eisenberg M, Sidebottom A, Murray D. Pricing strategy to promote fruit and vegetable purchase in high school cafeterias. *J Am Diet Assoc.* 1997;97:1008–1010.

78. Bergman EA, Buergel NS, Joseph E, Sanchez A. Time spent by schoolchildren to eat lunch. *J Am Diet Assoc.* 2000;100:696–698.

79. Buergel NS, Bergman EA, Knutson AC, Lindaas MA. Students consuming sack lunches devote more time to eating than those consuming school lunches. *J Am Diet Assoc.* 2002;102:1283–1286.

80. Lieux EM, Manning CK. Productivity in nutrition programs for the elderly that utilize an assembly-serve production system. *J Am Diet Assoc.* 1991;91:184–188.

81. Diaz-Knauf K, Favila E, Vargas D, Sommer R. Behavioral problems at a student-managed salad bar. *J Coll University Foodserv.* 1993;1:55–62.

82. Dowling RA, Cotner CG. Monitor of tray error rates for quality control. *J Am Diet Assoc.* 1988;88:450–453.

83. Donnelly JE, Jacobsen DJ, Legowski P, Johnson S, McCoy P. Family-style foodservice can meet US Dietary Guidelines for elementary school children. *J Am Diet Assoc.* 2000;100:103–105.

84. Theis M, Matthews ME. Time spent in state-recommended functions by consulting dietitians in Wisconsin skilled nursing facilities. *J Am Diet Assoc.* 1991;91:52–56.

85. Shanklin CW, Hernandez HN, Gould RM, Gorman MA. Documentation of time expenditures of clinical dietitians: results of a statewide time study in Texas. *J Am Diet Assoc.* 1988;88:38–43.

86. Cai LA. Analyzing household food expenditure patterns on trips and vacations: a Tobit model. *J Hospitality Tourism Res.* 1998;22:338–358.

87. Ham S, Hiemstra SJ, Yang IS. Modeling US household expenditure on food away from home (FAFH): logit regression analysis. *J Hospitality Tourism Res.* 1998;22:15–24.

88. March L, Gould R. Compliance with the School Meals Initiative: effect on meal programs' financial success. *J Am Diet Assoc.* 2001;101:1199–1201.

89. Shanklin CW, Wie S. Nutrient contribution per 100 kcal and per penny for the 5 meal components in school lunch: entrée, milk, vegetable/fruit, bread/grain, and miscellaneous. *J Am Diet Assoc.* 2001;101:1358–1361.

90. Cheung M, Gregoire MB, Downey RG. College and university foodservice organization charts. *NACUFS J.* 1990–91;15:5–11.

91. O'Hara PA, Harper DW, Kangas M, Dubeau J, Borsutzky C, Lemire N. Taste, temperature, and presentation predict satisfaction with foodservices in a Canadian continuing-care hospital. *J Am Diet Assoc.* 1997;97:401–405.

92. Wolf K, Schiller MR. Dietetics and foodservice personnel are ready for team problem solving. *J Am Diet Assoc.* 1997;97:997–1002.

93. Gregoire MB, Sames K, Dowling RA, Lafferty LJ. Are registered dietitians adequately prepared to be hospital foodservice directors? *J Am Diet Assoc.* 2005;105:1215–1221.

94. Brown DM. Prevalence of food production systems in school foodservice. *J Am Diet Assoc.* 2005;105:1261–1265.

95. Probart C, McDonnell E, Hartman T, Weirich E, Bailey-Davis L. Factors associated with the offering and sale of competitive foods and school lunch participation. *J Am Diet Assoc.* 2006;106:242–247.

96. Sneed J, Strohbehn C, Gilmore SA. Food safety practices and readiness to implement HACCP programs in assisted-living facilities in Iowa. *J Am Diet Assoc.* 2004;104:1678–1683.

97. Folio D, O'Sullivan-Maillet J, Touger-Decker R. The spoken menu concept of patient foodservice delivery systems increases overall satisfaction, therapeutic and tray accuracy, and is cost neutral for food and labor. *J Am Diet Assoc.* 2002;102:546–548.

98. Connors P, Rozell SB. Using a visual plate waste study to monitor menu performance. *J Am Diet Assoc.* 2004;104:94–96.

99. Delbecq AL, Van de Ven AH, Gustafson DH. *Group Techniques for Program Planning.* Glenview, Ill: Scott Foresman and Company; 1975.

100. Johnson BC, Chambers MJ. Expert panel identifies activities and performance measures for foodservice benchmarking. *J Am Diet Assoc.* 2000;100:692–695.

101. Gregoire MB, Sneed J. Barriers and needs related to procurement and implementation of the Dietary Guidelines. *School Food Serv Res Rev.* 1993;17:46–49.

102. Gregoire MB, Sneed J. Standards for nutrition integrity. *School Food Serv Res Rev.* 1994;18: 106–111.

103. Strohbehn CH, Gilmore SA, Sneed J. Food safety practices and HACCP implementation: perceptions of registered dietitians and dietary managers. *J Am Diet Assoc.* 2004;104: 1692–1699.

104. Parham ES, Benes BA. Development needs of faculty in foodservice management. *J Am Diet Assoc.* 1997;97:262–265.

105. Harp SS, Hoover LC, Crockett KL, Wu CK. Development of a beef appetizer concept for casual dining restaurants: application of focus group interviews and consumer sensory evaluation. *J Hospitality Tourism Res.* 1998;21:43–60.

106. Watters CA, Sorensen J, Fiala A, Wismer W. Exploring patient satisfaction with foodservice through focus groups and meal rounds. *J Am Diet Assoc.* 2003;103:1347–1349.

107. Gregoire MB, Sneed J. Continuing education needs of district school nutrition directors/ supervisors. *School Food Serv Res Rev.* 1994; 18:16–22.

108. Brown DM. Prevalence of food production systems in school foodservice. *J Am Diet Assoc.* 2005;105: 1261–1265.

109. Meyer MK. Top predictors of middle/junior high school students' satisfaction with school foodservice and nutrition programs. *J Am Diet Assoc.* 2000;100: 100–103.

110. Sheehan-Smith L. Key facilitators and best practices of hotel-style room service in hospitals. *J Am Diet Assoc.* 2006;106:581–586.

111. Gilbert N, Sneed J. Organizational culture: does it affect employee and organizational outcomes? *J Can Diet Assoc.* 1992;53:155–158.

112. Chong Y, Unklesbay N, Dowdy R. Clinical nutrition and foodservice personnel in teaching hospitals had different perceptions of total quality management performance. *J Am Diet Assoc.* 2000;100:1044–1049.

113. McKnight LE, Dundas ML, Girvan JT. Dietetics program directors affirm the importance of teaching financial management concepts in all areas of practice. *J Am Diet Assoc.* 2002;102: 82–84.

114. Cronbach L. Coefficient alpha and the internal structure of tests. *Psychometrika.* 1951;16: 297–334.

115. Smith P, Kendall L, Hulin C. *The Measurement of Satisfaction in Work and Retirement.* Chicago, Ill: Rand McNally; 1969.

116. Chao S, Hagisavas V, Mollica R, Dwyer J. Time for assessment of nutrition services in assisted living facilities. *J Nutr Elderly.* 2003;23:41–55.

117. Dienhart JR, Gregoire MB, Downey R. Service orientation of restaurant employees. *Hosp Res J.* 1990;14:421–430.

118. Groves J, Gregoire MB, Downey R. Relationship between the service orientation of employees and operational indicators in a multiunit restaurant corporation. *Hospitality Res J.* 1995;19: 33–43.

119. Kwon J, Yoon BH. Prevalence of outsourcing and perception of clinical nutrition managers on performance of health care dietetics services. *J Am Diet Assoc.* 2003;103:1039–1042.

120. Unklesbay N, Sneed J, Toma R. College students' attitudes, practices, and knowledge of food safety. *J Food Protect.* 1998;61:1175–1180.

121. Lengyel CO, Smith JT, Whiting SJ, Zello GA. A questionnaire to examine food service satisfaction of elderly residents in long-term care facilities. *J Nutr Elderly.* 2004;24:5–18.

122. Sneed J, Burwell EC, Anderson M. Development of financial management competencies for entry-level and advanced-level dietitians. *J Am Diet Assoc.* 1992;92:1223–1229.

123. Canter DD, Nettles MF. Dietitians as multidepartment managers in healthcare settings. *J Am Diet Assoc.* 2003;103:237–240.

124. Chien C, Hsu CHC, Huss JJ. Computer use in independent restaurants. *J Hospitality Tourism Res.* 1998;22: 158–173.

125. Yoon BJH, Huss JJ, Brown NE. Computer use and training preferences of school foodservice managers in Iowa. *J Child Nutr Manage.* 1998;22: 6–12.

126. Lau C, Gregoire MB. Quality ratings of a hospital foodservice department by inpatients and postdischarge patients. *J Am Diet Assoc.* 1998;98: 1303–1307.

127. Meyer MK, Conklin MT. Variables affecting high school students' perceptions of school foodservice. *J Am Diet Assoc.* 1998;98: 1424–1428,1431.

128. Gregoire MB. Quality of patient meal service in hospitals: delivery of meals by dietary employees vs delivery by nursing employees. *J Am Diet Assoc.* 1994;94:1129–1134.

129. Meyer MK, Conklin M, Nettles MF, Carr D. School foodservice kitchens: are they equipped to meet the challenges of the new millennium? Part one: equipment availability. *J Child Nutr Manage.* 1998;22:68–72.

130. Meyer MK, Conklin M, Nettles MF. School foodservice kitchens: are they equipped to meet the challenges of the new millennium? Part two: age, condition, and frequency of equipment use. *J Child Nutr Manage.* 1998;22:73–78.

131. Giamalva JN, Redfern M, Bailey WC. Dietitians employed by health care facilities preferred a HACCP system over irradiation or chemical rinses for reducing risk of foodborne disease. *J Am Diet Assoc.* 1998;98:885–888.

132. Nettles MF, Gregoire MB, Canter DD. Analysis of the decision to select a conventional or cook-chill system for hospital foodservice. *J Am Diet Assoc.* 1997;97:626–631.

133. Myers EF, Gregoire MB, Spears MC. Quality delegation grid: a decision tool for evaluating delegation of management tasks in hospital departments. *J Am Diet Assoc.* 1994;94:420–424.

134. Barrios J, Boudreaux J. Foodservice managers' perceptions of issues related to the employment of individuals with disabilities. *J Child Nutr Manage.* 1998;22:3–5.

135. Wittenbach SA, Shanklin CW. Health care foodservice directors' perception of the importance of value-added services offered by foodservice distributors. *J Am Diet Assoc.* 1997;97:1152–1154.

136. Oyarzun VE, Lafferty L, Gregoire MB, Sowa DC, Dowling RA, Shott S. Evaluation of efficiency and effectiveness measurements of a foodservice system that included a spoken menu. *J Am Diet Assoc.* 2000;100:460–465.

137. Shatenstein B, Ferland G. Absence of nutritional or clinical consequences of decentralized bulk food portioning in elderly nursing home residents with dementia in Montreal. *J Am Diet Assoc.* 2000;100:1354–1360.

138. Buscher LA, Martin KA, Crocker S. Point-of-purchase messages framed in terms of cost, convenience, taste, and energy improve healthful snack selection in a college foodservice setting. *J Am Diet Assoc.* 2001;101:909–913.

139. Remsburg RE, Luking A, Baran P, Radu C, Pineda D, Bennett RG, Tayback M. Impact of a buffet-style dining program on weight and biochemical indicators of nutritional status in nursing home residents:

a pilot study. *J Am Diet Assoc.* 2001;101:1460–1463.

140. Costello C, Gaddis T, Tamplin M, Morris W. Evaluating the effectiveness of two instructional techniques for teaching food safety principles to quick service employees. *J Foodserv Syst.* 1997;10:41–50.

141. Endres J, Barter S, Theodora P, Welch P. Soy-enhanced lunch acceptance by preschoolers. *J Am Diet Assoc.* 2003;103:346–351.

142. Reilly JK, Lanou AJ, Barnard ND, Seidl K, Green AA. Acceptability of soymilk as a calcium-rich beverage in elementary school children. *J Am Diet Assoc.* 2006;106:590–593.

143. Tutt M, McProud L, Belo P, Ferlin B, Neil C. Comparison of energy consumption of fully and partially loaded institutional forced-air convection ovens: preheated and nonpreheated. *School Food Serv Res Rev.* 1989;13:146–149.

144. Cremer ML, Pizzimenti KV. Effects of packaging, equipment, and storage time on energy used for reheating beef stew. *J Am Diet Assoc.* 1992;92:954–958.

145. Sandik K, Unklesbay N, Unklesbay K, Clarke A. Simulating convective heating with bentonite models. *J Foodserv Syst.* 1997;9:229–244.

146. Tsai S, Unklesbay N, Unklesbay K, Clarke AD. Effect of convective heating profiles on water absorption properties of restructured beef products. *J Foodserv Syst.* 1997;10:51–71.

147. Mahadeo M, Unklesbay N, Unklesbay K, Sandik K. Effects of alternate foodservice heat processing methods on thermophysical properties of restructured beef products. *J Foodserv Syst.* 1992;7:15–28.

148. Goldmon DC, Brown NE. Effects of fat level and addition of soy fiber on sensory and other properties of ground pork patties. *J Foodserv Syst.* 1992;7:1–14.

149. Berry BW. Effects of formulation and cooking method on properties of low-fat beef patties. *J Foodserv Syst.* 1997;9: 211–228.

150. Pringle TD, Williams SE, Johnson LP. Quality grade, portion size, needle tenderization and cookery method effects on cooking characteristics and palatability traits of portioned strip loin and top sirloin steaks. *J Foodserv Syst.* 1998;10:73–88.

151. Ollinger-Snyder PA, Matthews ME. Cook/chill foodservice system with a microwave oven: coliforms

and aerobic counts from turkey rolls and slices. *J Food Protect.* 1988;51:84–86.

152. Hautenne-Dekay D, Mullins E, Sewell D, Hagan DW. Wet-nesting of foodservice dishware: investigation and analysis of potential bacterial contamination. *J Am Diet Assoc.* 2001;101: 933–934.

153. Knickrehm ME. Digital computer simulation in determining dining room seating capacity. *J Am Diet Assoc.* 1966;48:199–203.

154. Guley HM, Stinson JP. Computer simulation for production scheduling in a ready foods system. *J Am Diet Assoc.* 1980;76:482–487.

155. Nettles MF, Gregoire MB. Use of computer simulation in school foodservice. *J Foodserv Syst.* 1996;9:143–156.

156. Balintfy JL. Menu planning by computer. *Commun ACM.* 1964;7:255–259.

157. Eckstein EF. Menu planning by computer: the random approach. *J Am Diet Assoc.* 1967;51: 529–533.

158. Petot GJ, Marling C, Sterling L. An artificial intelligence system for computer-assisted menu planning. *J Am Diet Assoc.* 1998;98: 1009–1014.

159. Paquet C, St-Arnaud-McKenzie D, Ferland G, Dube L. A blueprint-based case study analysis of nutrition services provided in a midterm care facility for the elderly. *J Am Diet Assoc.* 2003;103: 363–368.

160. Messersmith AM, Moore AN, Hoover LW. A multi-echelon menu item forecasting system for hospitals. *J Am Diet Assoc.* 1978;72:509–515.

161. Luckhardt WE. A waiting line model: determining the number of seats needed in dining areas. *J Coll University Foodserv.* 1993;1:25–37.

162. Miller JL, McCahon CS, Bloss BK. Food production forecasting with simple time series models. *Hospitality Res J.* 1991;14:9–21.

163. Blecher L. Using forecasting techniques to predict meal demand in Title IIIc congregate lunch programs. *J Am Diet Assoc.* 2004;104:1281–1283.

25

The Art and Science of Consumer Communications: Using Consumer Research to Create Nutrition and Health Messages that Work

Susan T. Borra, RD, Shelley Goldberg, MPH, RD, and Michele M. Tuttle, MPH, RD

Most consumers say they are trying to eat healthfully, yet current health statistics tell a different story. In 2005, more than half of consumers (57%) queried in an on-line survey said that they had made a change to improve the healthfulness of their diet in the past 6 months (1). In fact, most consumers admit that they should weigh less, eat more fruits and vegetables, eat less fat and more fiber, and increase their physical activity (1–3). The question asked by many nutrition educators is, "If they know *what* to do, why aren't they taking action?"

This chapter provides an overview of how consumer research methods can be used appropriately to answer this question as well as other "why" and "how" questions that can improve the effectiveness of health communication messages, materials, and programs.

CONSUMER RESEARCH: A TOOL FOR BETTER UNDERSTANDING A TARGET AUDIENCE

It is not surprising that most health professionals see little connection between what they do and what marketers and advertisers do. Yet, in reality, health professionals are often in the role of "selling" or "marketing" disease prevention or health to their patients in the same way that commercial marketers strive to sell products and services. Health professionals focusing on one-on-one interventions might use a brochure or handout, whereas an advertising director may be attempting to reach people through a colorful print ad in a magazine. In both cases, the goal is to deliver a message that motivates their "customer" to change a behavior. By understanding the research methods utilized by marketing professionals, nutrition educators can learn to hone their own messages and programs so that they can reach their "customers" as well.

Consumer research, used mostly by marketers, is the study of how consumers think and behave in terms of buying products or services (4). The information gathered helps marketers to better understand their target audience's values, perceptions, and attitudes. This understanding is then used to help design and refine key messages of an advertising or communications campaign to ensure that they are understood by the target audience. Finally, additional consumer research can help advertisers evaluate whether the campaign messages and materials were effective in changing customer behaviors or sales.

Recently, consumer research has been used by health educators and communicators to promote health and wellness through social marketing. In its book *Making Health Communication Programs Work,* the National Cancer Institute defines social marketing as "the application and adaptation of commercial marketing concepts to the planning, development, implementation, and evaluation of programs that are designed to bring about behavior change to improve the welfare of individuals or their society" (5 p.251).

Examples of "products" that might be "sold" by social marketing include encouraging people to eat more fruits and vegetables, increase physical activity, or stop smoking. Social marketing campaigns that have received

BOX 25.1   Social Marketing Programs

- **VERB:** This national, multicultural social marketing campaign was launched in 2002 and is coordinated by the Centers for Disease Control and Prevention (CDC). VERB encourages young people ages 9 to 13 years ("tweens") to be physically active every day. The campaign combines paid advertising, marketing strategies, and partnership efforts to reach the distinct audiences of tweens and adults/influencers (6).

- **5 A Day for Better Health:** First launched in 1991, this program used research from interviews and surveys to study the preferences and habits of audience segments and developed messages to encourage fruit and vegetable consumption. It is currently managed as a public-private partnership between the CDC, the National Cancer Institute, and the Produce for Better Health Foundation (7).

- **Kidnetic.com:** This healthful eating and activity Web site, created in 2002, was designed for youths ages 9 to 12 years and their families. It was developed by the IFIC Foundation and the partners of ACTIVATE, based on findings from focus groups, one-on-one interviews, and ethnographic studies with children, parents, and teachers (8).

- **It's All About You:** Created in 1996 by the Dietary Guidelines Alliance, this program conducted extensive qualitative research with consumers to create messages that tie "core values" to physical activity and nutrition. Core values are the underlying beliefs that drive consumers to make the choices they do. The campaign consists of five main messages with corresponding action-oriented tips that encourage adults to make healthier food and activity choices consistent with the Dietary Guidelines for Americans (9).

national attention include the Centers for Disease Control and Prevention (CDC) VERB program, 5 A Day for Better Health, and the International Food Information Council (IFIC) Foundation's Kidnetic.com program (6–9). See Box 25.1 for descriptions of these programs. Each of these programs was developed using extensive consumer marketing research that explored the perceived needs and wants

of the target audience. In addition, materials were pretested with consumers and adjustments were made based on consumer feedback. Finally, the materials and messages were communicated and promoted through channels that were consistent with the target audience's lifestyle.

Reaching consumers with health and nutrition information that they will find relevant requires planning, material and message development, program delivery, and evaluation. Each of these processes can benefit tremendously from an understanding of the target audiences' culture, lifestyle, behaviors and motivations, interests, and needs. Consumer research can help nutrition communicators move beyond a general impression of their target audiences to an in-depth characterization of the consumers they are trying to reach.

There are generally two types of research that are helpful in creating nutrition materials and programs: qualitative and quantitative (see Table 25.1) (5). Both types of research can be applied during different stages of program development. Typically, qualitative research, including focus groups and in-depth interviews, is used at the beginning of program development to gain insights into the approaches, messages, and delivery channels that will work best. Qualitative research is also used when developing and refining messages. Quantitative research, which includes various types of surveys, is used toward the end of program development or during program evaluation to assess how the messages and program elements are working with the target audience.

Focus groups and in-depth interviews allow participants to explain their thoughts and opinions about topics, often contributing ideas that the researchers have not

TABLE 25.1   Qualitative vs Quantitative Research Methods

Qualitative Research	Quantitative Research
Provides in-depth understanding; probes individual reactions and insights into behavior	Measures levels of actions and behaviors
Is exploratory: asks "Why?" and "How?"	Asks "How many?" and "How often?"
Is subjective; studies underlying motivations and behavioral drivers	Is objective
Results cannot be quantified; findings may not reflect findings of larger audiences	Results can be quantified to provide "proof"; results are reflective of larger audiences
Is more directional than definitive	Is definitive

Source: Adapted from reference 5.

considered. Quantitative research allows study participants to respond to the researcher's specific questions with only numeric answers, so they cannot contribute new ideas. Also, even with the use of pretesting, quantitative researchers can never be completely sure that respondents have interpreted their questions correctly. In qualitative research, a skilled moderator can immediately recognize when respondents do not understand a question, and can reframe the question, if necessary. In addition, qualitative research offers the opportunity for the moderator to spontaneously follow up and probe into relevant issues that arise during the discussion.

QUALITATIVE RESEARCH

Although there are several types of qualitative research, focus groups, in-depth interviews, and ethnographic studies are the ones most frequently used in nutrition communications. Qualitative research is the use of carefully facilitated discussions or interviews to gather insights and information from an intended target audience (10). The data gathered are words, phrases, and themes of conversation rather than numbers, statistics, or other measurable types of data. Qualitative research methods are described in detail in the following sections.

Focus Groups: Description and Uses

Typically, a focus group is a 1- to 2-hour discussion led by a trained moderator with 6 to 10 participants (10). The participants are carefully recruited using a detailed questionnaire, or screener, so that the focus group will reflect the intended target audience of the messages or program that is being created (eg, primary grocery shoppers or mothers with toddlers). Research participants are usually paid or offered some kind of an incentive to make sure that they attend the group.

The moderator works from a written discussion guide that lists the questions to be asked and any activities the group will do to generate discussion on the topics. A good moderator keeps the discussion on track yet allows participants to talk spontaneously so that attitudes, thoughts, and opinions can flow freely. As participants discuss their ideas, the moderator asks follow-up questions to gain clarity and to explore relevant issues that can affect program or message development. In addition, effective moderators are skilled at eliciting involvement and discussion from all participants in a focus group. Typically, participants are not

told what organization has sponsored the research; this helps eliminate respondent bias about the topic.

Focus groups can be held in a variety of settings, including focus group facilities, conference rooms, or wherever 6 to 10 people can comfortably gather and talk. Focus group facilities offer several advantages over other locations. Because they usually provide two rooms separated by a one-way mirror, it is possible for clients or observers to unobtrusively watch the discussions. In addition, facilities are equipped to provide state-of-the-art recording so that written transcripts can be easily generated after the groups meet. Because most of the "data" from a focus group consists of the quotes, phrasing, and words used by participants, recording the group sessions is essential. In addition, videotaping the groups allows the moderator to review all or parts of the discussion when analyzing focus group findings. A visual recording means that the researcher can note the tone, nuances, or body language of participants in addition to hearing what was said.

The number of focus groups to conduct depends on the magnitude of the program and the number of distinct target audience segments. Typically, at least two groups are conducted with each audience segment in each market segment location. An example might be the development of a brochure intended for mothers with children between the ages of 4 years and 6 years that will be distributed statewide at community health fairs. Depending on how the different audience segments (ie, lower income vs higher income, urban vs rural) are expected to respond to the information, one might conduct two groups with mothers of all backgrounds or decide to conduct four groups, two with lower-income mothers and two with higher-income mothers. Alternatively, if the defining issue is community setting rather than income, two groups might be conducted with rural mothers and two with urban mothers.

Recently, some qualitative researchers have begun offering Web-based focus groups. Like traditional focus groups, respondents are carefully screened and recruited. Rather than gathering at a facility, participants and the moderator log on to a private chat room in which the moderator posts questions for respondents to answer. This method has several advantages over conventional focus groups, as well as some limitations:

- Web-based groups are more convenient for respondents because they can participate from home; this also allows for more people to participate.
- Transcripts are immediately available because responses are typed.

- Web-based groups are less expensive to conduct, and they facilitate research in multiple markets.
- Web-based groups can effectively reach geographically diverse populations, as well as individuals who value saving time.
- Web-based groups/respondents have the ability to be completely anonymous.
- Finally, because participants must answer each question prior to viewing other participants' responses, Web-based groups encourage unbiased responses.

The primary challenges of online focus groups are similar to those of telephone interviews: the moderator cannot observe nonverbal reactions, and the group dynamics that occur in traditional focus groups is lost (10). In addition, respondents must have a computer and Internet access to participate.

In-Depth Interviews: Description and Uses

Like focus groups, in-depth or one-on-one interviews are conversations conducted by trained moderators or interviewers. The researcher uses a discussion guide outlining the topics to be discussed, probing for detail and following up on unexpected yet relevant themes. Questions asked are typically open-ended, allowing respondents to provide more than "yes" or "no" answers. In-depth interviews can last from 30 minutes to an hour or longer depending on the number of topics to be covered.

In-depth interviews can be done in a variety of settings but are best done where they can be recorded. Face-to-face interviewing is best, but requires that interviews be scheduled and conducted in a manner convenient for the respondents, typically in the evening or on weekends. Telephone interviewing is convenient for both researchers and respondents, but has the drawback that nonverbal behavior cannot be observed.

Typically, 10 in-depth interviews are conducted per audience segment to be tested. For example, if messages about grocery shopping for healthier foods are to be tested with the primary grocery shoppers in households, 10 interviews might be conducted with male primary shoppers and 10 with female primary shoppers.

In-depth interviews are particularly useful for sensitive topics that people might be hesitant to discuss in groups. For example, if the topic is eating disorders or aberrant food habits such as pica, talking with respondents individually rather than in groups might work well. Although an in-depth interview does not allow for interaction among group members that can lead to richer detail and insights, it does allow the researcher an opportunity to better understand issues that cannot easily be explored in other ways. For example, topics such as physical or mental abuse or sexual practices may be too sensitive for most people to discuss either in groups or face-to-face. However, in-depth telephone interviews might work well for either of these topics.

Ethnographic Observational Studies

Ethnographic research is the observation of people behaving in their "natural environments" (4). It is a research method adapted from the fields of sociology and anthropology in which the target audience is observed doing and saying the things that they normally do in a given environment. By observing how people interact with products, services, or each other, it is possible to gain insights into the subtleties of how consumers really feel and behave. For example, to understand why people prepare certain foods for dinner, it might be helpful to observe people grocery shop and prepare meals on several nights throughout a given month. In focus groups, people answer questions based on their memories of their behaviors. Ethnographic research gives the researcher the ability to watch people behave a certain way and ask questions about what led to the behavior (11).

Analyzing and Applying the Results of Qualitative Research

Focus groups and in-depth interviews are analyzed in similar ways. First, the recorded groups or interviews are transcribed. Next, the moderator or research assistant reviews the transcripts, looking for general opinion trends in the discussion themes. Themes and opinions about topics may come up at any point during the interview or focus group, so it is important for the researcher to review and connect ideas that are related. The researcher looks for general discussion themes and agreement about topics and notes the range of opinions that participants expressed. Typically, representative quotations and phrases are gathered from each transcript and used to support the researcher's findings and conclusions in a final report.

If large numbers of focus groups have been conducted with many different participant subgroups, it may be more feasible to analyze the group using computer software. This type of analysis does not take the place of "human" analysis but can streamline the process of "coding" different conversation themes.

Qualitative reports will include summarizations and findings of all the key discussion themes. Based on these findings, researchers may make recommendations on steps to take or changes to make in materials or messages. For example, if half the respondents in three out of four focus groups do not care for the graphics or the font size used, the researcher would suggest that the graphics be changed. On the other hand, if only two people in four groups react negatively to the brochure's layout while others react favorably, the researcher will note the divergent opinion but would probably not recommend that the brochure be changed.

Qualitative research is subjective by nature. The experience of the researcher and the program developer will frequently determine how and whether the findings of the research are applied. For example, despite careful planning and message creation, there are times when focus groups and in-depth interviews are not able to generate clear directions for action. In such a case, the client or program planner must either proceed based on his or her own judgment or review the steps taken in the early stages of program planning to make sure the correct target audience and program goals were selected.

QUANTITATIVE RESEARCH

Quantitative research also has some important uses in developing effective consumer messages. Surveys, the most common quantitative research method used in message development, can be used at several points in the process of program or message development. At the start of the process, quantitative research can help to assess the target audiences' attitudes, knowledge, or behaviors. Prior to launching a messaging campaign, quantitative research can be useful for measuring audience reactions to messages that have been created based on focus group research. Once a program is in place or messages have been disseminated, quantitative research can be used to measure usage or awareness of materials or messages with the intended audience.

Types of surveys vary in their methods, advantages, disadvantages, and cost (see Table 25.2) (5). Typically, a research firm is hired to conduct the survey. Most research firms will have expertise in questionnaire design, will advise on the best survey methods to use in order to capture the desired data, and will have the software required to analyze the results. Although some research firms may have in-house capabilities to conduct the survey, others will

TABLE 25.2   Types of Quantitative Research

Survey Format	Pros	Cons
Mailed questionnaire	• Can reach hard-to-access populations (rural, homebound) • Convenient for respondents	• Not appropriate for respondents with low literacy skills • Low response rate may require follow-up by mail or telephone • Requires data entry for analysis
Telephone questionnaire	• Can be used with all literacy levels because conducted with an interviewer • Interviewer can enter answers directly into the computer • May be easier for respondents to talk truthfully about sensitive issues by phone rather than face-to-face	• Cannot sample respondents without telephones • Many respondents refuse to participate
In-person questionnaire	• Can be used with all literacy levels • Can be used with difficult-to-reach populations (eg, homeless, difficult-to-sample populations) • Interviewer can clarify questions for respondents when necessary	• More expensive than self-administered or telephone questionnaires • Not appropriate for topics that are sensitive, threatening, or controversial because respondents may not answer truthfully
Internet questionnaire	• Eliminates data entry • Very convenient for respondents with Internet access	• Not appropriate for audiences with low literacy skills or those who are uncomfortable with computers • Respondents must have access to the Internet

Source: Adapted from reference 5, pp 158–159.

contract out for services such as computer-assisted telephone interviewing or omnibus studies. An omnibus survey is one in which questions are tacked onto an ongoing national survey or poll that may be conducted on a regular basis with a preselected group of respondents. Typically, national surveys are conducted with a sample representative of the

US population based on Census data. However, when necessary, special populations can be oversampled to obtain statistically valid data.

Once the results have been collected and analyzed, program planners and message developers can use the information to fine-tune messages or make program adjustments. However, because quantitative data may not reveal the nuances of why certain messages did not appeal to people or the specific barriers that prevented participation in a program, additional focus group research may be necessary to further improve message or program outcomes.

CONSUMER RESEARCH: REACHING OUT TO OVERWHELMED CONSUMERS

There are many reasons why consumers do not respond to health and nutrition information—after all, eating patterns are comprised of many complex behaviors. According to one study, the typical consumer makes more than 200 food-related decisions every day (12). However, consumer research results from both focus groups and surveys mention two barriers more often than any others: confusion about making more healthful choices and lack of time.

It is not surprising that consumers are confused about making more healthful choices. Consumers today are continually bombarded with communication from an incredible array of sources and devices that compete for their attention. Over the course of a typical day, Americans encounter messages and information from neighbors, friends, spouses, coworkers, children, and health professionals. The information is delivered in any or all of the following formats: television programs and newscasts, books, magazines, newspapers, in-person conversations, e-mail, voice mail, regular mail, deliveries from private shipping companies, telephone calls at home and work, Web sites, billboards, posters, and radio programs. At any given moment, consumers may be juggling information ranging from a coworker's advice regarding the benefits of a weight-loss program to the latest findings of a scientific study on why certain foods or ways of eating may be harmful or beneficial to health. It is no wonder that 42% of people surveyed say the food and health information they get from different sources is contradictory (1). Sorting through all of these information sources and channels is a major feat; deciding to act on the information presented is another hurdle altogether.

Although some people think that there is too much confusing nutrition information on the news (2), others say they simply do not have enough time for healthful eating or exercising. According to a 2005 nationwide study of primary grocery shoppers ($n = 1,003$), 63% said "being too busy to take the time" was either a major or minor reason that they did not eat more healthfully (2).

Another reason why consumers fail to take action on nutrition knowledge may have to do with their perception that information about what constitutes a healthful diet is likely to change. According to a nationwide survey conducted in 2005 by the Food Marketing Institute and *Prevention Magazine,* 30% of respondents who felt that their diet could be more healthful thought that conflicting information was a major barrier to taking action (2). The same study found that 45% of shoppers think that in the next 5 years it is very likely that the experts will have completely different ideas about which foods are healthful and which are not.

To a certain degree, these consumers have a point. Nutrition science, as with all research disciplines, is an ever-changing, evolving body of information. Messages about some foods and some aspects of diet have changed (eg, advice about eggs, butter, or margarine). However, the true source of consumer confusion may be that many consumers have time for a headlines-only approach to nutrition information. Unfortunately, the explanation of how the new findings fit into established scientific consensus about healthful eating typically appears in the middle or at the end of an article or news piece—long after most consumers have already tuned in to something else. Although health professionals understand that the findings of one research study do not warrant a change in dietary advice, consumers may not (13,14).

The Importance of Health Professionals as Health Communicators

Health professionals such as registered dietitians (RDs) and doctors are uniquely suited to communicate with consumers. One national survey indicated that although consumers most frequently consult magazines (46%), the Internet (46%), and television (38%) for nutrition information, doctors are the most trusted source of this type of information (3). Consumers give high ratings to doctors and RDs in terms of providing health and nutrition information in an understandable way, according to consumer research conducted in 2005 (2). In addition, 19% of people said that they made diet-related changes based to a great extent on information received from a health professional (1). It is clear that health professionals are an incredibly important link in the "communications chain" that exists between scientists and consumers.

Because health professionals are so trusted, they can get messages through to consumers with face-to-face visits, use of educational materials, or public health programs. Such information gets through only when consumers feel that it is relevant and actionable within the current context of their lives. One way to ensure that consumers "hear" health information is to consider their needs, values, and preferences before creating and promoting messages, materials, or programs. As described earlier, social marketing uses the research methods and tools developed by people who are in the business of getting paid to get messages across to consumers: marketers and advertisers. Health professionals can use these methods as well.

Applying Consumer Research to Message and Program Development

Successful nutrition messages and programs are consumer-oriented and understandable by their target audience (see Table 25.3) (15,16). By using a combination of qualitative

TABLE 25.3 Essential Characteristics of Successful Messages

Core Message Attribute	Examples of Consumer-Tested Message
Be positive	Share the experience—split dessert with a friend or take half home to enjoy the next day.
Keep it short and simple	Stash packets of instant oatmeal and some juice boxes in your desk.
Make it specific and manageable	Prepare one new recipe each month from a favorite magazine or newspaper article.
Provide a "payoff"	Take a brisk 10-minute walk on your lunch break—you will feel good and have more energy, too.
Create it just for me	Love the taste of whole milk? Balance it with lower-fat foods such as reduced-fat cheese, low-fat sour cream, or fat-free salad dressing.
Talk food *and* fun	Try fun snacks such as fruit kabobs dipped in your favorite fruity yogurt, or baked tortilla chips with zesty black bean dip.

Source: Adapted with permission from International Food Information Council Foundation. Tools for Effective Communication: Beginning a New Conversation with Consumers. Available at: http://www.ific.org/tools/intro.cfm. Accessed November 2, 2006.

and quantitative research, program planners and nutrition communicators can gain an understanding of what consumers know, believe, and value, as well as how they behave in regard to food, diet and nutrition, and other health issues.

Using this information about the target audience, it is possible to first create and then test message or program concepts. One such process, used by IFIC for many of its consumer messaging programs, is the Consumer Message Development Model presented in Box 25.2 (16). This model was originally adapted from one used by Wirthlin Worldwide, a market research firm that is now part of Harris Interactive. As Box 25.2 shows, qualitative and quantitative research are essential elements used during key stages of the process.

Using Consumer Research in Different Settings

It may seem that consumer research is something that can be conducted by only government agencies or for-profit companies, but in fact, consumer research can be done on a more limited scale in community or clinical settings such as health departments, health clinics, doctor's offices, hospitals, schools, and community program centers. In community settings, program implementers typically have good access to their target populations. It is possible to conduct on-site surveys, interviews, focus groups, or even ethnographic studies depending on what information is sought. Program planners can either hire consultants to help conduct the research or conduct it themselves. There are many books and guides that offer further advice about conducting both quantitative and qualitative research. See the Additional Resources section at the end of this chapter.

CONCLUSION

Consumer research is a powerful communications tool that can be used to better target, craft, and evaluate nutrition education messages and programs. Qualitative research such as focus groups, in-depth interviews, and ethnographic research can answer how and why questions that quantitative surveys and other types of research may not be able to address. Ultimately, judicious use of qualitative research methods can provide insights that will help nutrition communicators create messages that help consumers think in new ways, take action, and permanently adopt more healthful behaviors.

BOX 25.2   Consumer Message Development Model

Step 1: Define the Issues

Prior to developing broad message concepts, it is imperative to understand the underlying issues that surround the health or nutrition problem that will be addressed. For example, if the nutrition topic to be addressed is obesity, it is important to understand how the target audience views the problem, their beliefs about what they can do about it, their perceived barriers to addressing the problem, and what might motivate them to take action.

Step 2: Develop Initial Message Concepts

Based on what is learned in step 1, message concepts can be drafted to address and encourage specific actions and behaviors. For example, if the initial research shows that consumers, especially female consumers, value taking care of their families above all other concerns, initial message concepts can include ideas that tie health to improving the ability to take care of one's family.

Step 3: Assess the Message Concepts

Once the message concepts or program materials have been drafted and refined to a certain degree, they can be tested with consumers in the target audience to make sure that the information is being "heard" or interpreted correctly. If more than one message or program concept has been developed, testing provides an opportunity for consumers to select the one they prefer and to discuss the reasons for their choices. Questions that might be asked at this stage of the message or program development include the following:

- What does this message or program encourage you to do?
- How likely are you to take action toward changing your behavior based on the information presented by this message or program?
- How does this message or program fit with other priorities in your life?

Step 4: Fine-Tune Messages

The message or program assessment may indicate that few, if any, changes are necessary. Often, program elements need only minor word changes or small adjustments. However, some messages and program ideas are not well received by consumers. In that case, it is necessary to go back to step 2 and revise the initial message or program concepts based on the consumer feedback from step 3.

Step 5: Validate Messages

This is typically the last step taken before the message or program is launched. Validation means confirming that the message or program is meaningful to large numbers of people in the target audience. Because the focus group research from steps 1 and 3 cannot be generalized to larger audiences, conducting a quantitative survey with a larger sample size will indicate whether the message or program will be successful in delivering the health information to be shared. If this validation step is successful, the program or message is ready to be disseminated. Otherwise, it may be necessary to review information gathered in steps 1 and 3 and make sure that the messages and program concepts are aligned with the values and priorities of consumers. Further fine-tuning can then be done followed by retesting, or the program may need to be revamped entirely.

Although this research can be expensive, it can be much more costly to spend the money to print and disseminate ineffective materials and messages. Because most organizations have limited resources, it may be tempting to skip testing materials, messages, or programs with their intended audiences. Taking the time to plan and test messages, materials, and programs thoroughly does not completely guarantee success, but it does make it much more likely.

Source: Adapted with permission from International Food Information Council Foundation. Tools for Effective Communication: Beginning a New Conversation with Consumers. Available at: http://www.ific.org/tools/intro.cfm. Accessed November 2, 2006.

REFERENCES

1. *Food & Health Survey: Consumer Attitudes toward Food, Nutrition & Health.* Washington, DC: International Food Information Council Foundation; 2006.

2. *Making Sense of Nutrition News and Health Claims.* Washington, DC: Food Marketing Institute and Prevention Magazine; 2005.

3. *U.S. Grocery Shopper Trends: 2005.* Washington, DC: Food Marketing Institute; 2005.

4. Armstrong G, Kotler P. *Marketing: An Introduction* (custom edition for AIU Online). Boston, Mass: Pearson Custom Publishing; 2003.

5. National Cancer Institute. *Making Health Communication Programs Work.* Bethesda, Md: National Institutes of Health; 2001.

6. Centers for Disease Control and Prevention. Youth Media Campaign. Available at: http://www.cdc.gov/youthcampaign/research/index.htm. Accessed November 1, 2006.

7. For Health Professionals: About the 5 A Day Program. Available at: http://5aday.gov/health_professionals/about.html. Accessed November 2, 2006.

8. What Is Kidnetic.com? Available at: http://www.kidnetic.com/Whatis.aspx. Accessed November 1, 2006.

9. Dietary Guidelines Alliance. *Reaching Consumers with Meaningful Health Messages: A Handbook for Nutrition and Food Communicators.* Chicago, Ill: Dietary Guidelines Alliance; 1996.

10. Greenbaum T. *The Handbook for Focus Group Research.* 2nd ed. Thousand Oaks, Calif: Sage Publications; 1998.

11. Burke J, Kirk A. Ethnographic Methods. Available at: http://www.otal.umd.edu/hcirm/ethno.html. Accessed November 2, 2006.

12. Wasink B. *Mindless Eating: Why We Eat More Than We Think.* New York, NY: Bantam Books; 2006.

13. Improving public understanding: guidelines for communicating emerging science on nutrition, food safety, and health. *J Natl Cancer Inst.* 1998;90: 194–199.

14. Miller G, Cohen N, Fulgoini V, Heymsfield S, Wellman N. From nutrition scientist to nutrition communicator: why you should take the leap. *Am J Clin Nutr.* 2006,83:1272–1275.

15. International Food Information Council Foundation. Tools for Effective Communication: Beginning a New Conversation with Consumers. Available at: http://www.ific.org/tools/intro.cfm. Accessed November 2, 2006.

16. Borra S, Kelly L, Tuttle M, Neville K. Developing actionable dietary guidance messages: dietary fat as a case study. *J Am Diet Assoc.* 2001;101: 678–684.

ADDITIONAL RESOURCES

Morgan D, Krueger R. *The Focus Group Kit.* Thousand Oaks, Calif: Sage Publications; 1998.

Prevention Communication Research Database. Available at: http://www.health.gov/communication. (A searchable collection of audience research conducted or sponsored by Health and Human Services agencies. Covers key prevention issues, such as physical activity, healthy eating, tobacco use, and substance abuse.)

Social Marketing National Excellence Collaborative. The Basics of Social Marketing: How to Use Marketing to Change Behavior. Available at: http://www.turningpointprogram.org/Pages/pdfs/social_market/smc_basics.pdf.

26

Dietetics Education Research

Mary B. Gregoire, PhD, RD, FADA

Dietetics education involves the preparation of entry-level practitioners with the knowledge and skills needed to compete effectively in evolving job markets (1). The formal education of dietitians began in the 1920s (2). At nearly the same time, research on dietetics education began as a way to find reliable answers to education questions, discover the best ways of educating future dietitians, and establish principles for dietetics education. The first issue of the *Journal of the American Dietetic Association,* published in 1925, contained a questionnaire from the education section of the American Dietetic Association (ADA) designed to solicit information on the courses given to student dietitians in hospitals (3).

This chapter categorizes research in dietetics education, discusses techniques used when conducting dietetics education research, and suggests future directions for dietetics education research. This chapter is not intended to be an exhaustive review of the research that has been conducted on dietetics education but rather cites selected studies as examples within each section.

CATEGORIZATION OF DIETETICS EDUCATION RESEARCH

In Chapter 2 of this text, the authors categorize research as descriptive or analytic. Descriptive research describes what exists at a given point in time; analytic research involves

testing hypotheses. Nearly all the research done in dietetics education would be categorized as descriptive, with only a small percentage of published research categorized as analytic.

Descriptive Research

Descriptive research studies include qualitative research, case reports, and survey research. The survey has been the predominant descriptive research design used in dietetics education research since its beginning in the 1920s. Surveys have been used to describe attitudes, beliefs, or practices related to dietetics education. These descriptive studies have focused on issues of concern to dietetics educators at particular points in time.

For example, Plan IV was adopted as the model for minimum competencies for dietetics education programs in 1974. Following its release, several survey projects were published addressing issues related to the determination of essential entry-level competencies (4–9). The introduction of the coordinated undergraduate program (CUP) prompted a series of descriptive studies to examine the quality of graduates from both the newer CUP and the traditional internship programs. Studies included evaluations of internship program (10,11) and CUP (12–16) graduates and comparisons of the graduates of both programs (17,18). More recent examples of descriptive studies include a focus on program content (19–28) and perceptions of cost-effectiveness (29).

Case studies also have been used to report results of descriptive studies related to dietetics education. These case studies (30–34) usually describe teaching techniques and innovative course content implemented at an individual dietetics education program.

Qualitative research, such as that described in Chapter 7, has only begun to be used as a methodology for dietetics education research. Kruzich et al (35) used qualitative techniques with practicum preceptors to evaluate a dietetics internship.

Analytic Research

Very little of the dietetics education research could be categorized as analytic. The studies that have been structured as more experimental, with the goal of hypothesis testing, have focused primarily on the testing of methods for teaching information to students.

Only two analytic dietetics education research articles were published in the *Journal of the American Dietetic Association* between 1995 and 2005 (36,37). Both focused on evaluation of the effectiveness of computer-based simulations or instruction.

DATA COLLECTION TECHNIQUES

A variety of data collection techniques have been used in dietetics education research. Questionnaires have been the most commonly used data collection technique, but the use of tests, interviews, and observations is also reported in the literature. This section gives examples of dietetics education research studies using each technique and discusses potential concerns.

Questionnaires

Questionnaires are the most common data collection technique reported in dietetics education research. Recent research studies have used questionnaires to collect data from students (19,26,28,38,39), preceptors (19,29,38), program directors (19–22,25), and practitioners (19,31) to address issues related to dietetics education.

The accuracy of data collected using a questionnaire can be jeopardized when a question's meaning is misinterpreted. Guides for effective questionnaire development in Chapter 13 and the text by Dillman (40) provide valuable information for individuals using this technique for data collection. Pretesting the questionnaire can help reduce the chances of misinterpretation of questions (40).

Tests

According to Ary et al (41), a test is a set of stimuli or questions to be answered by the study sample members and to which a numerical score can be assigned. Tests can be developed by researchers for particular studies, or standardized tests can be obtained or purchased from other researchers. Tests are categorized as being either norm-referenced or criterion-referenced. A *norm-referenced* test allows for comparison of a particular respondent's performance against a reference group, a normative group. A *criterion-referenced* test will describe what the individual respondent can or cannot do compared with the criterion, but these results cannot be compared against others.

Standardized tests have consistent and uniform procedures for administration and for scoring and interpreting behavior and have been demonstrated to have strong validity and reliability (42). Moore (43) suggests that tests that are not standardized usually do not have an established procedure for administration and have not been constructed using procedures to minimize error.

Numerous standardized tests have been developed for measuring such things as personality, reading, intelligence, behavior, and achievement. The most common references that list standardized, commercially available measuring instruments are the *Mental Measurement* yearbooks (44) and their companion volume, *Tests in Print* (45).

Purchased standardized tests are not commonly used in dietetics education research. However, Mitchell and Nyland (26) used the Learning Styles Inventory to compare learning styles of dietetics students and faculty, and Arendt and Gregoire (28) used the Student Leadership Practices Inventory to identify leadership behaviors in dietetics students.

The use of researcher-developed standardized tests is commonly reported in dietetics education research. Researchers who have developed their own tests have documented the steps taken to ensure the reliability and validity of the tests. A common use of researcher-developed tests is to measure knowledge or behavior before and after an educational program is initiated. Miller and Shanklin (46), for example, developed a test to measure behavioral objectives related to forecasting. The test was given before and after completion of a self-instructional module on food-service forecasting, and data analysis focused on the change in test scores.

Dietetics education researchers collecting data using tests must be concerned about the effect of retesting, test anxiety, and floor and ceiling skewness (41,47). The retesting effect is of primary concern in designs that use a pretest and a posttest as part of the methodology. The retesting effect is the improvement in test scores that occurs on subsequent tests because a previous test had been taken on the same material. The amount of this effect varies depending on the type of test, the sophistication of the test taker, and the amount of time between the two testings. Anderson et al (47) suggest that although reduction of the retesting effect may be difficult, having a control group that takes both the pretest and the posttest provides researchers with a way to statistically control for the effect of retesting.

Test anxiety is a concern because it may affect the meaning of test scores, and thus influence inferences based on those scores. Test anxiety is believed to have both cognitive and emotional components. The cognitive (worry) component has been shown to impact performance on tests: the greater the level of worry, the poorer the test performance (48). Dietetics education researchers can try to reduce the likelihood of test anxiety before data are collected by having students use techniques such as relaxation or positive self-talk. Alternatively, researchers can try to assess the level of test anxiety and then take its influence into account in analysis and interpretation.

Floor effect error occurs when a test is written at a difficulty level that is too hard for most of the participants, so most score poorly on the test; hence, a subject's poor performance on a test is a result of the test's difficulty rather than of his or her actual ability. Ceiling effect error can occur when a test is so easy that everyone does well; as a result, the test does not measure as high as a subject could have performed. The likelihood of either error can be reduced by thorough pilot testing of the test prior to its use with the study sample.

Interviews

Gay and Airasian (49) define an *interview* as "the oral, in-person administration of a questionnaire." Interviews vary in the amount of structure imposed and thus are categorized as structured or unstructured. Friebel and coworkers (50) used interviews of clients to obtain information on the effectiveness of students as nutrition counselors.

Dietetics educators must consider the possible increased cost involved in using interviews and the bias the interviewer can create. Training and using skilled interviewers is expensive, and the time involved is often long.

Interviewer training is critical, however, to help reduce bias. When several people serve as interviewers, interrater reliability must be assessed to reduce potential rater bias in the results (43).

Observation

As a data collection technique, observation allows researchers to document visual perceptions of behavior as it occurs rather than rely on self-reports of behavior in tests, questionnaires, and interviews. Observation can be of situations as they exist or of contrived, simulated conditions (41). Research by Vickery and associates (51) is an example of the use of observation in dietetics education research. The authors videotaped students conducting diet counseling interviews. Trained observers documented 61 skills using a scale ranging from 0 (absent) to 3 (excellent).

Ary et al (41) and Anderson et al (52) indicate that observation data can be collected using ratings, systematic observation, coding scales, or sequential narratives. *Ratings* are subjective assessments made on an established scale (52). *Systematic observation* instruments include two types of recording systems: sign and category. *Sign systems* list a large number of variables, and each variable that occurs during a given period of observation is marked. For example, a list of classroom behaviors might include the following: "student asks question," "teacher gives directions," and so forth. An observer using a sign system type of observation instrument would check each of the behaviors observed. Behaviors that occur more than once during the observation period are checked only once. *Category systems* generally include a more restricted number of variables. These variables are recorded continuously as often as they occur to produce an ongoing record of behaviors. In the classroom example just cited, the observer would record continuous behavior, documenting each time the student asks a question, each time the teacher provides direction, and so on. Data collected using the category system of observation would include a sequence of events in the classroom and the frequency of occurrence of particular behaviors. *Coding scales* are used to help describe classroom behaviors observed. Classic work by Flander (53), for example, provided the following options for coding teacher talk:

- Accepts feelings
- Praises/encourages
- Accepts ideas of students
- Asks questions

- Lectures
- Gives direction
- Criticizes or justifies authority

Sequential narratives are written descriptions of all behaviors that occur during an observation session (43).

Dietetics education researchers who choose to use observation techniques for data collection must consider the potential for several sources of error, including the Hawthorne effect, halo effect, generosity error, and error of severity (39,49). The *Hawthorne effect* refers to changes in behavior that occur when participants in an experiment or evaluation are aware of their special status. Students may work more eagerly or teachers teach more enthusiastically, perhaps because they feel they have been specially chosen. To help reduce the Hawthorne effect, researchers often need to minimize the newness of the program to students or find ways to make both the treatment and the control groups feel they are receiving something special. The *halo effect* occurs when raters allow their general impressions to influence their judgment when documenting observations. *Generosity error* occurs when raters give the subject the benefit of the doubt and tend to give a more positive rating on behavior being observed. The other extreme, the *error of severity,* occurs when a rater has a tendency to give less positive ratings on all characteristics. Thorough training of observers usually is needed to help reduce the impact of the halo effect and generosity or severity errors.

FUTURE RESEARCH NEEDS

Dietetics education researchers may choose to explore and replicate research strategies used in the field of education. Anderson (52) proposes four levels of education research: descriptive, explanatory, generalization, and basic. Moving dietetics education research from its reliance on descriptive-level research toward the generalization and basic levels would improve its quality. According to Anderson (52), descriptive research is used to describe either what has happened in the past or what is happening currently. Research methods such as case studies, needs assessments, program evaluations, and survey research are often used to describe past or current practice. Statistics are often used to quantify and simplify description by grouping observations.

The major questions addressed in explanatory research are the following: What is causing this to happen? Why did it happen? Research methods used to address

these questions often include case studies, comparative or correlational studies, observation, or time-series analysis. Explanation focuses on what is happening in a specific setting rather than on the implications for the world at large (52).

Determining whether the same thing will happen in different circumstances is the goal of generalization research. Experimental, quasi-experimental, meta-analysis, and predictive approaches are often used in this level of research (52). Very few dietetics education research studies reach the level of generalization research.

Basic or theoretical research attempts to determine whether there is an underlying principle to explain an observed phenomenon. Such research often involves experiments, meta-analysis, or time-series analysis (52).

Research in dietetics education is important to the growth and development of the profession of dietetics, and it is essential if the education of future registered dietitians (RDs) is to be effective. The 1994 Future Search Conference (54) set forth the challenge for the dietetics profession, including dietetics education researchers, to create excellence. The 1998 ADA environmental scan (55,56) encouraged dietetics education researchers to look to the future and develop projects that would help provide the information needed to better guide dietetics education. In 2004, the ADA research committee included dietetics education as one of nine research priorities (57). The committee specifically encouraged research to determine knowledge and skills that differentiate levels of practice in dietetics, effective teaching methods and strategies, career paths and employment trends in dietetics, and strategies for retention of dietetics professionals.

Nearly all the dietetics education research conducted to date has been very quantitative. Future research of a more qualitative nature might provide new insights into understanding the underlying intentions and feelings of students that affect the dietetics education process. Interdisciplinary research projects conducted with education researchers could produce information on why students learn and factors that help motivate students in the learning process.

Dietetics education research has provided valuable information for dietetics educators. Most of the dietetics education research conducted to date would be categorized as descriptive rather than analytic. Research has focused on strategies and program outcomes. Many studies have focused on a single program, which limits generalization beyond that program. A variety of errors can impact the generalizability of dietetics education research results.

CONCLUSION

Researchers in dietetics education to date have focused primarily on descriptive methods for collecting and analyzing data. Dietetics education research in the future must expand from this descriptive level to more analytic approaches. Continuing to explore the most effective ways to provide dietetics education and determining the underlying principles of how students best learn will be important.

Researchers exploring dietetics education must always be aware of the potential for error in their research projects. Developing studies that minimize the chance for error will strengthen the research results.

REFERENCES

1. Commission on Accreditation for Dietetics Education. *Accreditation Handbook.* Chicago, Ill: American Dietetic Association; 2002.
2. Chambers MJ. Professional dietetic education in the US. *J Am Diet Assoc.* 1978;72:569–599.
3. Questionnaire for the education section. *J Am Diet Assoc.* 1925;1:31.
4. Loyd MS, Vaden AG. Practitioners identify competencies for entry-level generalist dietitians. *J Am Diet Assoc.* 1977;71:510–516.
5. Meeks DK, Zallen EM. Dietitians' perceptions of administrative competencies gained during professional education. In: Zallen EM, ed. *Structuring Education Experiences in Foodservice Systems Management: Proceedings of the Tenth Biennial Conference of the Foodservice Systems Management Education Council.* Norman: Oklahoma University; 1979.
6. Morales R, Spears MC, Vaden AG. Menu planning competencies in administrative dietetic practice: I. The methodology, II. Menu planning competencies. *J Am Diet Assoc.* 1979;74:642–650.
7. Parks SC, Kris-Etherton PM. Practitioners view dietetic roles for the 1980s. *J Am Diet Assoc.* 1982;80:574–577.
8. Holmes RW. Essential competencies for baccalaureate dietetic programs. *J Am Diet Assoc.* 1982;81:573–576.
9. Bedford MR. The affective domain: behaviors important in entry-level practice. *J Am Diet Assoc.* 1984;84:670–675.
10. Stanford JR, McKinley MM, Scruggs M. Graduates of hospital dietetic internships: I. Employment and administrative experiences in internships, II. Perceptions of administrative experiences in internships. *J Am Diet Assoc.* 1973;63:254–263.
11. Wenberg BG, Ingersoll RW, Donner CW. Evaluation of dietetic interns. *J Am Diet Assoc.* 1969;54:297–300.
12. Roach F, Hoyt D, Reed JG. Evaluation of a coordinated undergraduate program in dietetics. *J Am Diet Assoc.* 1976;68:154–158.
13. Johnson CA, Hurley RS. Design and use of an instrument to evaluate students' performance. *J Am Diet Assoc.* 1976;68:450–453.
14. Ingalsbe N, Spears MC. Development of an instrument to evaluate critical incident performance. *J Am Diet Assoc.* 1979;74:134–138.
15. Shanklin CW, Beach BL. Implementation and evaluation of a competency-based dietetic program. *J Am Diet Assoc.* 1980;77:450–454.
16. Fiedler KM, Beach BL, Hayman J. Dietetic performance evaluation: establishment of validity and reliability. *J Am Diet Assoc.* 1981;78:149–151.
17. Rinke WJ, David BD, Bjoraker WT. The entry-level generalist dietitian: I. Employers' general opinions of the adequacy of educational preparation in administration, II. Employers' perceptions of the adequacy of preparation for specific administrative competencies. *J Am Diet Assoc.* 1982;80:132–144.
18. Gregoire MB, Vaden AG, Hoyt DP. Comparative evaluation of graduates of internship and coordinated undergraduate programs. *J Am Diet Assoc.* 1986;86:1082–1089.
19. Marsico C, Borja M, Harrison L, Loftus M. Ratings of food courses and culinary training components in dietetics education. *J Am Diet Assoc.* 1998;98:692–693.
20. Gates G, Sandoval W. Teaching multiskilling in dietetics education. *J Am Diet Assoc.* 1998;98:278–284.
21. Hergenroeder A, Morrow S. Interdisciplinary adolescent health training in supervised dietetic practice programs across the southern United States. *J Am Diet Assoc.* 1999;99:1450–1452.
22. Scheule B. Food-safety educational goals for dietetic and hospitality students. *J Am Diet Assoc.* 2000;100:919–927.
23. Lorenz RA, Gregory RP, Davis DL, Schlundt DG, Wermager J. Diabetes training for dietitians: needs assessment, program description, and effects on

knowledge and problem solving. *J Am Diet Assoc.* 2000;100:225–228.

24. Rhee LQ, Wellman NS, Castellanos VH, Himburg SP. Continued need for increased emphasis on aging in dietetics education. *J Am Diet Assoc.* 2004;104: 645–649.

25. Short JE, Chittooran MM. Nutrition education: a survey of practices and perceptions in undergraduate dietetics education. *J Am Diet Assoc.* 2004;104: 1601–1604.

26. Mitchell AW, Nyland NK. Learning styles differ between senior dietetics students and dietetics faculty members. *J Am Diet Assoc.* 2005;105:1605–1608.

27. Vickery CE, Cotugna N. Incorporating human genetics into dietetics curricula remains a challenge. *J Am Diet Assoc.* 2005;105:583–588.

28. Arendt SW, Gregoire MB. Dietetics students perceive themselves as leaders and report they demonstrate leadership in a variety of contexts. *J Am Diet Assoc.* 2005;105:1289–1294.

29. Gilbride JA, Conklin MT. Benefits of training dietetics students in preprofessional practice programs: a comparison with dietetic internships. *J Am Diet Assoc.* 1996;96:758–763.

30. Brehn BJ, Rourke KM, Cassell C. Enhancing didactic education through participation in a clinical research project. *J Am Diet Assoc.* 1999;99: 1090–1093.

31. Hampl JS, Herbold NH, Schneider MA, Sheeley AE. Using standardized patients to train and evaluate dietetics students. *J Am Diet Assoc.* 1999;99: 1094–1097.

32. Litchfield RE, Oakland MH, Anderson JA. Improving dietetics education with interactive communication technology. *J Am Diet Assoc.* 2000;100: 1191–1194.

33. Wolf KN, Dunlevy CL. Impact of preceptors on student attitudes toward supervised practice. *J Am Diet Assoc.* 1996;96: 800–802.

34. Smith AR, Christie C. Facilitating transdisciplinary teamwork in dietetics education: a case study approach. *J Am Diet Assoc.* 2004;104:959–962.

35. Kruzich LA, Anderson J, Litchfield RE, Wohlsdorf-Arendt S, Oakland MJ. A preceptor focus group approach to evaluation of a dietetic internship. *J Am Diet Assoc.* 2003;103:884–886.

36. Raidl MA, Wood OB, Lehman JD, Evers WD. Computer-assisted instruction improves clinical reasoning skills of dietetic interns. *J Am Diet Assoc.* 1995;95:868–873.

37. Turner RE, Evers WD, Wood OB, Lehman JD, Peck LW. Computer-based simulations enhance clinical experience of dietetic interns. *J Am Diet Assoc.* 2000;100:183–190.

38. Barrow EP, Jeong M, Parks SC. Computer experiences and attitudes of students and preceptors in distance education. *J Am Diet Assoc.* 1996;96: 1280–1281.

39. Kobel KA. Influences on the selection of dietetics as a career. *J Am Diet Assoc.* 1997;97:254–257.

40. Dillman DA. *Mail and Internet Surveys.* 2nd ed. New York, NY: Wiley; 2000.

41. Ary D, Jacobs LC, Razavieh A. *Introduction to Research in Education.* 6th ed. Belmont, Calif: Wadsworth/Thomson Learning; 2002.

42. McMillan JH. *Educational Research.* 2nd ed. New York, NY: HarperCollins; 1996.

43. Moore GW. *Developing and Evaluating Educational Research.* Boston, Mass: Little, Brown and Co; 1983.

44. Spies RA, Plake BS, eds. *The Sixteenth Mental Measurements Yearbook.* Lincoln: University of Nebraska Press; 2005.

45. Murphy LL, Spies RA, Plake BS, eds. *Tests in Print VII.* Lincoln: University of Nebraska Press; 2006.

46. Miller JL, Shanklin CW. Status of menu item forecasting in dietetics education. *J Am Diet Assoc.* 1988;88:1246–1249.

47. Anderson SB, Ball S, Murphy RT. *Encyclopedia of Educational Evaluation.* San Francisco, Calif: Jossey-Bass Publishers; 1975.

48. Cassady J. The stability of undergraduate students' cognitive test anxiety levels. *Practical Assessment, Research & Evaluation* (online journal). 2001;7(20). Available at: http://pareonline.net. Accessed February 22, 2007.

49. Gay LR, Airasian P. *Educational Research.* 7th ed. Upper Saddle River, NJ: Prentice Education; 2003.

50. Friebel DM, Sucher K, Lu NC. University wellness program: the effectiveness of students as nutrition counselors. *J Am Diet Assoc.* 1988;88: 596–598.

51. Vickery CE, Cotugna N, Hodges PA. Comparing counseling skills of dietetics students: a model for skill enhancement. *J Am Diet Assoc.* 1995;95: 912–914.

52. Anderson G. *Fundamentals of Educational Research.* 2nd ed. Bristol, Pa: Falmer Press, Taylor and Francis; 1998.

53. Flander NA. *Analyzing Teacher Behavior.* Boston, Mass: Addison-Wesley; 1970.

54. Parks SC, Fitz PA, Maillet JO, Babjak P, Mitchell B. Challenging the future of dietetics education and credentialing—dialogue, discovery, and direction: a summary of the 1994 Future Search Conference. *J Am Diet Assoc.* 1995;95:598–606.

55. Maillet JO, Rops MS, Small J. Facing the future: ADA's 1998 environmental scan. *J Am Diet Assoc.* 1999;99:347–350.

56. Bezold C, Kang J. Looking to the future—the role of the ADA environmental scan. *J Am Diet Assoc.* 1999;99:989–993.

57. Castellanos VH, Myers EF, Shanklin CW. The ADA's research priorities contribute to a bright future for dietetics professionals. *J Am Diet Assoc.* 2004;104:678–681.

PART 8

~m~

Application of Statistical Analysis in Nutrition and Dietetics Research

27

—m—

Estimating Sample Size

Carol J. Boushey, PhD, MPH, RD

Sample selection, discussed in Chapters 6 and 8, and sample size are two determinants of whether an investigation is worthwhile. An otherwise excellent study can fail to detect an important effect just because the sample size is too small. The results of such studies confuse the issue under investigation and can lead to misleading or patently wrong conclusions.

THE LOGIC OF SAMPLE SIZE CALCULATIONS

The process of estimating the required sample size involves several steps and can be technically complex; it is always wise to seek the help of a knowledgeable statistician. An understanding of the basic elements of estimating the sample size will facilitate interaction with a statistician. This chapter highlights the issues underlying the logic of sample size calculations, outlines the general procedure that is common to all situations, describes the procedures specific to common research situations, and provides references for further information (1).

The use of statistics allows the investigator to estimate the unknown. By using statistics, the investigator can estimate characteristics of a population based on observations of a sample drawn from it. The size of the sample largely determines the accuracy or precision of the estimates from the sample. The larger the sample, the more information provided about the population and the more precise the estimate. Uncertainty always exists. The investigator, however, can specify

in advance the amount of uncertainty that is acceptable for the study and perform appropriate sample size calculations.

Two hypotheses, the null hypothesis and the alternative hypothesis, provide the framework for the logic of sample size calculations. Before an investigation is undertaken, an alternative hypothesis that serves as the basis of the investigation is formulated (2). The null hypothesis—that there is no difference or effect—serves as a standard of comparison. Statistical analysis is conducted to determine whether the results of the study are consistent with the underlying null hypothesis. If the results do not demonstrate the presence of a difference or an effect, it is concluded that the data fail to refute the null hypothesis.

When drawing conclusions from statistical results, there are four possible outcomes, two correct and two incorrect (Table 27.1). First, one can correctly conclude that there is no difference or effect when there is none (probability = $1 - \alpha$). (For convenience, in sample size calculations, it is assumed that failure to reject the null hypothesis is the same as concluding that the null hypothesis is true; however, this assumption is not appropriate when interpreting results.) Second, one can conclude that there is a difference or effect when there is none (probability = α, false-positive, type I error). Third, one can conclude that there is no difference or effect when there is one (probability = β, false-negative, type II error). Finally, one can conclude that there is a difference or effect, which is truly present (probability = $1 - \beta$, power). All four possible outcomes are expressed statistically as probabilities of reaching the appropriate conclusions.

TABLE 27.1   Possible Outcomes when Drawing Conclusions from Statistical Results

		Truth about Study Hypothesis	
		True (alternative, H_1)	False (null, H_0)
Statistical test results about	**True** (reject H_0)	Correct $(1-\beta$, power)	False positive (type I error, α error)
hypothesis	**False** (do not reject H_0)	False negative (type II error, β error)	Correct $(1-\alpha)$

The type I error, or α error, is also known as the significance level of the study; its complement, $1-\alpha$, is the correct conclusion if the null hypothesis is true. By convention, α is usually set at 5%, or $P = .05$. This means that the maximum acceptable risk of drawing a false-positive conclusion is 5%. Obviously, the smaller the α, the lower the risk of drawing a false-positive conclusion. The investigator specifies the α level during the planning of the study and compares the resulting P value with α at the end of the study. If the observed P value is less than α, the result is considered to be statistically significant.

The type II error, or β error, expresses the probability of missing a difference; its complement is power, or $1-\beta$. If the null hypothesis is not true and a difference or effect exists, the β probability quantifies the risk of missing that difference, and power quantifies the chance of finding it. As β decreases, power increases. The investigator specifies β during the planning of the study, and the value of β then determines power. For example, if the risk of missing a difference were set at 20%, the chance that the study would find a real difference would be 80%.

The probability that if a true effect exists, a study will detect it (ie, power) largely depends on the sample size. Increasing the sample size increases the power. At the same time, increasing the sample size decreases the risk of a false-negative conclusion (ie, β or type II error) because the ability to detect a true difference is increased.

The power of a study also depends to some degree on the true magnitude of difference or effect under study. For any given power, a large difference can be detected with a smaller sample size more easily than can a small difference. Accordingly, for any given sample size, the study will be more likely to detect a large difference than a small difference. The investigator determines in advance the magnitude of difference or effect that is important, and this becomes the research hypothesis for the purposes of power and sample size calculations.

There is a general relationship among sample size, power, and the magnitude of the difference or effect sought. The required sample size is inversely related to the magnitude of the difference and the type I error rate, and it is positively related to the standard deviation and desired power. This relationship may be expressed as follows (3):

$$\text{Sample size } (n) > 2 \, [(\alpha \text{ error} + \beta \text{ error} \times SD)/\text{Difference}]^2$$

where the α and β errors are mathematically converted to the standardized normal deviates (Z values) for the probabilities, SD is the estimated standard deviation, and Difference is the absolute value of the magnitude of the measured change. For example, a change in low-density lipoprotein cholesterol levels from 5.19 mmol/L to 4.87 mmol/L would be a difference of −0.32 mmol/L, or an absolute difference of 0.32 mmol/L.

If the sample size is not restricted, the investigator will want to determine the sample size required to ensure a high probability of detecting a meaningful difference or effect. If, in contrast, the sample size is limited (ie, predetermined), the investigator can use sample size calculations to determine the probability (power $= 1-\beta$) that the study will be able to detect a meaningful difference. In practice, the final determination of the size of the research project will be a judicious balance of power and economics.

GENERAL PROCEDURE FOR SAMPLE SIZE CALCULATIONS

Sample size estimates are based on a number of assumptions about the conditions of the study. It is not possible for an investigator to know in advance what the conditions of the study will be; thus, the calculations provide only an estimate. The general procedure for calculating the required sample size involves seven steps.

Step 1

Choose the main end point of interest and the method by which it is to be measured. A series of sample size calculations may be performed if there is more than a single important end point for the study. In such cases, the largest estimated sample size is generally used. Note that α may need to be adjusted for the increased number of simultaneous significance tests (see step 5 later in this section).

Step 2

Choose the statistical test that is appropriate for the data and the research question. It is best to consult with a statistician at this point (see Chapter 28).

Step 3

Specify the magnitude of the difference or effect that is meaningful to detect. The magnitude of the difference or effect selected should be practical—that is, an important difference in practice. Additionally, it should be sufficiently small that a negative study outcome (ie, no significant difference) would be assurance that if a true difference existed, it would be too small to be of practical importance.

Step 4

Estimate the expected variability—that is, the estimated SD. Preferably, this value comes from a pilot study conducted earlier. However, it can also come from published research results. Lacking either of these, a "best guess" must be made.

Step 5

Specify the maximum acceptable risk of a false-positive conclusion (α, or type I, error). Alterations in α concomitantly alter both power and β. As α is lowered, power decreases and β increases; as α is increased, power increases and β decreases. By convention, the α probability is set at .05, although the situation may warrant setting a lower or higher risk. The seriousness of a false-positive conclusion determines whether the maximum acceptable risk should be set lower. Only under rare circumstances is α set greater than .05, because doing so can compromise the ability of the results to be convincing. An increased α would be warranted, however, in circumstances in which there were serious consequences of a false-negative conclusion (β error) and it was desired to decrease β without increasing the sample size beyond what was feasible.

Another consideration in choosing α is whether the statistical test is to be one-tailed or two-tailed (see Chapter 28). A one-tailed α is more liberal than a two-tailed α, as it tests for a difference in only one direction. The more conservative approach of applying a two-tailed significance test enables the investigator to test for a difference in either direction from the null and is generally preferred.

When there is more than a single primary end point for the study, it is important to test each with the same level of rigor, that is, $\alpha = .05$ or lower. Some (but not all) statisticians believe that the appropriate way to ensure that the α level remains $\leq .05$ (or desired level) for all significance tests is to account for more than one test. Accounting for more than a single primary outcome is usually achieved by dividing the desired α by the number of significance tests being conducted. For example, if we planned to test the difference between treated and control groups on three primary outcomes, and we chose $\alpha = .05$ as acceptable, we would compute the sample size based on $.05/3 = .017$ to preserve the type I error probability of .05.

Step 6

Specify the probability of successfully detecting the difference or effect, if it exists (power $= 1 - \beta$). Alternatively, the probability of a false-negative conclusion can be specified (β, or type II, error). By convention, power is usually set at .80 to .90, and β is set at .20 to .10, respectively. Again, the seriousness of a false-negative conclusion guides the decision.

Step 7

Apply the appropriate calculations (see the following examples and calculations). The estimated sample size may be larger than what is feasible under the actual circumstances and with available resources. If this is the case, the power of the study should be calculated according to the number of subjects feasible with available resources. The procedure for calculating the power of a study with a fixed sample size prior to undertaking it is similar to that just given. Steps 1 through 7 should be performed, substituting the fixed sample size for power in step 6 and solving for power instead of sample size in step 7.

SAMPLE SIZE DETERMINATION FOR SPECIFIC RESEARCH SITUATIONS

Continuous Data

All results from the following methods are based on the assumption that either the outcomes arise from a normal distribution or the sample size is sufficiently large that the normal approximation is valid. These formulas can give improper results if the assumption of normality is not valid.

Paired Observations

A paired t test is usually used in an investigation in which a continuous response measure is observed before and after the subject receives a treatment or an investigation in which observations in two groups are linked by pairing. In this instance, the sample size formula accounts for the correlation between the measurements within the pairs (4,5).

An example might be a study to assess whether a particular intervention will decrease dietary cholesterol intake as measured by 3-day food records (step 1). For the before and after study design, an experimental effect can be tested with a paired t test (step 2). Using the data of Cohen and associates (6), it can be determined that a change of -75 mg would be meaningful and practical (step 3). Furthermore, the SD of the difference (SD_{diff}) can be estimated (step 4) as 158.9 mg, according to the study of Van Horn and coworkers (7), which used 3-day food records.

In this example, α is specified in advance with a two-tailed test (step 5) as .05. The decision is made to set power, or $1 - \beta$, at .80, making $\beta = .20$ (step 6). The appropriate calculations (step 7) can now be applied. The calculation of the sample size needed to conduct a test with a significance level of α and a power of $1 - \beta$ follows:

Formula 27.1

$$n = \{[(Z_{1-\beta} + Z_{1-\alpha}) \times SD_{diff}]/(Mean_1 - Mean_2)\}^2$$

The quantities $Z_{1-\alpha}$ and $Z_{1-\beta}$ are values from the standard normal distribution that correspond to the desired probabilities of type I (α) and type II (β) errors. Table 27.2 gives selected values of $Z_{1-\alpha}$ and $Z_{1-\beta}$ corresponding to commonly used values of α and β. Therefore, using Formula 27.1, and using the values previously given, $SD_{diff} = 158.9$ mg, and $Mean_1 - Mean_2 = 75$ mg; the sample size for a two-sided test can be estimated as follows:

$$\begin{aligned} n &= \{[(Z_{1-\beta} + Z_{1-\alpha}) \times SD_{diff}]/(Mean_1 - Mean_2)\}^2 \\ &= \{[(0.84 + 1.96) \times 158.9]/75\}^2 \\ &= (444.92/75)^2 \\ &= 35.2, \text{ or } 36 \text{ subjects} \end{aligned}$$

If the investigators also planned to measure the difference in other nutrients (eg, saturated fat intake), these calculations would be repeated for each nutrient of interest,

TABLE 27.2 Unit Normal Deviates Z_α and Z_β for Selected Values of α and β

α or β	Two-Sided Test*	
	$Z_{(1-\alpha/2)}$	$Z_{(1-\beta)}$
.01	2.58	2.33
.025	2.24	1.96
.05	1.96	1.64
.10	1.64	1.28
.20	1.28	.84
.30	1.04	.52

*If using a one-sided test, the $Z_{1-\alpha}$ values would be the same as in the $Z_{1-\beta}$ column.

using $\alpha = .05/k$, where $k =$ number of nutrients of interest. The final sample size would correspond to the calculation with the highest n. Finally, the investigators would enroll extra participants to allow for attrition during the intervention without compromising the study's power (see the later discussion of dropout rates and noncompliance).

Tables are available by which sample size and power can be estimated for a variety of differences and levels of α and β errors (4,8). An increasingly wide variety of choices of computer programs for performing sample size calculations are also available. A downloadable program, *PS: Power and Sample Size Calculation,* is offered by Dupont and Plummer (8). There are other sample size calculators available on-line. One example was created with support from the National Institutes of Health, General Clinical Research Center Program (9). Other programs can be found by using an on-line search engine to find "sample size calculators."

The examples in this section use continuous variables; for discrete variables, the formulas would be slightly different (10) and are discussed later. Chapter 28 clarifies the issue of continuous or quantitative variables vs discrete or categorical variables.

Independent Groups

Study designs addressing nutrition questions usually involve a comparison of two samples. Investigations often are planned to observe the response measures on subjects who receive either of two treatments, typically an experimental treatment and a control treatment. The response variable (eg, high-density lipoprotein cholesterol) is measured on a continuous scale. A specified magnitude of difference is set at a level thought to be important with a particular power. The comparison is usually made by the two-sample t test for independent samples.

An example might involve members of the dietetics department of a health maintenance organization (HMO) who are concerned that the agency's current screening criteria for anemia using the hemoglobin value may need to be revised. The article by Nordenberg and colleagues (11) suggests that hemoglobin cutoff values should be adjusted upward for smokers. The HMO collects detailed smoking information on each new enrollee and determines hemoglobin value as well, so an investigation is planned to determine whether women smokers and nonsmokers between the ages of 18 and 44 years have significantly different hemoglobin values. One of the study components involves comparing the mean hemoglobin values of a random sample of smokers with those of a random sample of nonsmokers.

In this case, the main end point of interest is hemoglobin, a continuous variable (step 1). To compare the means of the two randomly selected groups, an independent *t* test can be used (step 2). The results reported by Nordenberg and colleagues (11) indicate that the mean hemoglobin value among female smokers is 137 g/L and is 133 g/L among female nonsmokers. The calculated difference of interest is 4 g/L (step 3). A standard error of 0.4 g/L for smokers and 0.5 g/L for nonsmokers was reported (11). By converting these values (step 4) to their corresponding SDs (standard error = SD/square root of *n*), setting α at the conventional .05 (step 5) and power at 90% (step 6), and applying the appropriate formula, the sample size for the two groups can be determined. The formula for a two-sided test (assuming unequal variances) is as follows (10):

Formula 27.2

$$n = (SD_1{}^2 + SD_2{}^2)(Z_{1-\beta} + Z_{1-\alpha/2})^2/(Mean_2 - Mean_1)^2$$

The values for $Z_{1-\beta}$ and $Z_{1-\alpha/2}$ can be found in Table 27.2. The SDs for smokers and nonsmokers are 12.37 and 17.37, respectively. The difference of interest, $Mean_2 - Mean_1$, is 4 g/L. According to Formula 27.2, the sample size is as follows:

$$n = (17.37^2 + 12.37^2)(1.28 + 1.96)^2/(-4)^2$$
$$= (454.7338)(10.4976)/16$$
$$= 298 \text{ in each group (596 total)}$$

However, the funding is limited to 175 subjects in each group (350 total). Lack of sufficient funds is common. As a consequence of various constraints, a sample size analysis often begins with a fixed value for *n*. In this case,

the resulting power $(1 - \beta)$ can be determined by rearranging Formula 27.2 and solving for $Z_{1-\beta}$:

Formula 27.3

$$Z_{1-\beta} = \sqrt{\frac{(Mean_2 - Mean_1)^2 \times n}{(SD_1^2 + SD_2^2)}} - Z_{1-\alpha/2}$$

Using all the values determined previously, but substituting 175 for *n*, the study power is calculated as follows:

$$Z_{1-\beta} = \sqrt{\frac{(4^2 \times 175)}{(17.37^2 + 12.37^2)}} - 1.96$$
$$= \sqrt{6.157} - 1.96$$
$$= 2.48 - 1.96$$
$$= 0.52$$

Table 27.2 indicates that $Z_{1-\beta} = .52$ corresponds to $\beta = .30$, so $1 - \beta = .70$, or 70% power. The investigators conclude that the 175-subject sample size will provide adequate power, and they continue with plans for the study.

The actual formula for calculating sample size based on the *t* test can be solved using computational iterative methods; therefore tables have been constructed for use (4,8). These tables provide sample sizes necessary to detect a range of differences with varying degrees of power. Additional tables indicate the power provided by various sample sizes and magnitudes of differences, and the text that accompanies them describes their use in detail (4). As has been mentioned, various statistical software manufacturers offer computer software for determining sample size and power analyses. Investigators should review products carefully and consult with a statistician before using unfamiliar statistical software.

Three or More Independent Groups

Studies that compare a continuous response measure in more than two groups usually use an analysis of variance model for data analysis rather than several *t* tests. Based on analysis of variance, Day and Graham (12) provide a nomogram to estimate the required sample size when comparing three or more treatment groups.

More Complex Designs

Nutrition studies commonly employ designs, such as prospective cohort or retrospective case-control, which evaluate the association of a risk factor with some outcome of interest. The measure of association estimated from these studies is the relative risk or odds ratio. Procedures appropriate for the prospective cohort study are given by Phillips and Pocock (13), and procedures appropriate for the case-control study, by Lubin and coworkers (14).

In some nutrition studies, especially certain clinical trials, the time when an end point occurs is important. It is especially important if it is believed that an intervention may result in a shorter duration of illness or that the desired outcome may occur sooner. Such studies are called *time-to-event investigations*. Usually the analysis uses survival analysis methods instead of more simple statistical approaches. Sample size procedures for such studies using a specialized computer program are described by Shih (15).

Reliability Studies

An examination of the reliability of methods of assessing dietary intake is common in nutrition and dietetics. In these studies, reliability is often estimated by the coefficient of intraclass correlation from an analysis of variance. Sample size requirements for reliability studies are discussed by Donner and Eliasziw (16) and by Walter et al (17). Both references provide either power contours or tables to guide in the planning. Donner (18) provides sample size formulas and tables for the design of studies that compare two or more coefficients of interobserver agreement. For inferences regarding agreement for dichotomous variables, the κ statistic is used; Donner and Eliasziw (19) present a discussion of sample size procedures for studies using the κ statistic.

Proportions

Independent Groups

In an investigation in which a dichotomous or categorical response measure is observed in two independent groups, the frequencies of response are compared between groups, usually by the chi-square test in a two-way contingency table. As with the procedure for the *t* tests, the investigator must guess about an unknown quantity—in this case, one of the proportions. The investigator then is asked, as usual, to specify the smallest difference from this amount that is important to detect, as well as the α and β errors that are acceptable. With these quantities, the investigator can estimate the required sample size. A major distinction between power calculations for the *t* test and comparing two proportions is that for discrete outcomes, the variance (or SD) is a function of the proportions being compared. In other words, with discrete outcomes, the variance is a function of the mean.

For the example of anemia (hemoglobin < 120 g/L) among smokers and nonsmokers, a two-way contingency table based on the data reported by Nordenberg and colleagues (11) can be constructed (Table 27.3). The proportions can be quantified; for example, 46/956 = 4.8%

TABLE 27.3   Two-Way Contingency Table: Anemia among Women Smokers and Nonsmokers

		Anemia (Hemoglobin Value < 120 g/L)		
		+	−	
Smoker	+	46	910	956
	−	101	1106	1207
		147	2016	2163

Source: Data are from reference 11.

prevalence of anemia among smokers. The prevalence of anemia among nonsmokers is 8.4%; therefore, the difference of interest could be 3.6 or any value specified as meaningful in the population.

Although formulas are available to calculate sample size (5,20,21), a simpler and perhaps more informative method is to use graphs (22,23) or tables (24,25). Tables and graphs have the advantage of providing, at a glance, the required sample sizes for several combinations of proportions and differences. Several computer programs, such as the one by Dupont and Plummer (8), also perform the required calculations. A public domain program available through the Centers for Disease Control and Prevention, Epi Info, is available on-line (http://www.cdc.gov/epiinfo); investigators can download the software at no charge. A function within Epi Info includes calculations designed for studies in which the results are proportions. Additional formulas and tables are compiled and carefully reviewed by Sahai and Khurshid (26).

Paired Observations

An investigation that employs a matched design, pairing observation from a case with observation from a control (eg, a matched case-control study), is analyzed in a manner that accounts for pairing, such as McNemar's test for paired studies (27). Procedures for sample size determination are provided by several authors (24,27–29) and reviewed by Lachenbruch (30).

More Complex Designs

The analysis and sample size determination are more complicated when the investigation involves more than two groups and more than one response measure. The analysis generally uses some form of the chi-square test in a multiway contingency table. Lachin (31) provides the statistical rationale and methods for determining the required sample size for such studies for the statistically inclined investigator; investigators who are less mathematically inclined should consult a statistician.

Related classes of studies common in nutrition epidemiology are studies of more than two risk factors that are dichotomous measures, such as cohort or case-control studies of the association of several risk factors with a chronic disease. Clinical trials can also evaluate more than two treatments simultaneously. Studies of this type generally employ discrete multivariate analysis methods (eg, multivariate contingency tables and unconditional logistic models). A general method for sample size determination in this class of study is described by Greenland (32). A modified method is applied to prospective studies by Phillips and Pocock (13) and to cohort and case-control studies by Lemeshow and associates (33). Again, investigators who are unfamiliar with these techniques should consult a statistician.

Performance Characteristics of Laboratory Tests

Registered dietitians often employ tests to classify persons or to screen them for certain characteristics or risk factors. The use of anthropometry to assess nutritional status and screen for patients at risk of malnutrition at hospital admission is one example. Tests are often compared with one another to determine their performance characteristics and relative usefulness in classifying persons, especially when one test is more expensive or labor-intensive. The important performance characteristics are the positive and negative predictive values (described in Chapter 6), two proportions that determine the practical usefulness of tests (34,35). Power and sample size requirements of studies of this nature are presented by Arkin and Wachtel (35).

Additional Considerations

Loss of Subjects from Dropouts and Noncompliance

It is rare that investigators can manage a study in which all participants are able to complete the study with total compliance to the study protocol. Knowing this, it is wise to anticipate some rate of noncompliance when determining sample size. Investigators can look to past experience with similar studies—their own or the studies of others—to estimate dropout rate and noncompliance (R). Sample size can be adjusted by the simple method of Lachin (5), $N_d = N/(1 - R)^2$, where N_d is the sample size needed to account for dropouts, and N is the sample size calculated without accounting for dropouts.

Repeated Measures or Longitudinal Designs

When the outcome is measured at a single point in time, the equations given previously can be relied upon to give useful estimates of sample size. They are not useful, though, when the outcome is measured more than once (ie, repeated measures) or for longitudinal study designs. Repeated measures designs are efficient in determining treatment effect in many applications (36); that is, they can require smaller sample sizes than comparable studies that do not employ repeated observations. Repeated observations on the same individual are usually positively correlated; thus, sample size estimates and data analysis must account for this correlation. Procedures related to sample size estimation are provided for both continuous (37) and discrete or binary outcome variables (37,38).

Recalculating the Sample Size during the Study

Sometimes investigators have no pilot data and results from published studies are not available. In this case, there is no information upon which to base an estimate of the variance of the outcome or response. Researchers then simply guess about the variance for sample size calculations, and thus the experiment is based on a guess. The result may be an underpowered study. In an effort to correct for this situation, statisticians developed sequential study designs—that is, designs in which data are analyzed when preset numbers of responses have occurred. Underlying this class of designs is the practical effect that after gathering an initial sample, the investigators recalculate the final sample size based on the current observed variance in the response (39). Investigators interested in this type of design should consult a statistician.

Determining Power Retrospectively

The ability of a study to detect a difference that truly exists is power. Determining the power of the study after a study is completed is crucial for interpreting the findings when the results are negative (eg, concluding that the intervention had no effect or that there was no association between variables). As readers, we want to know the likelihood that this finding was the result of a type II error. An author's claim that there was no difference in response between groups or that groups were equivalent in some characteristic may be based on a study that was underpowered to detect a meaningful difference. Readers (and investigators) can apply the previously described procedures to either (a) compute the sample size that would have been required to show a difference and compare this number with the study sample size or (b) calculate the power of the study with the reported sample size (40). With either procedure, the reader can then determine whether the negative findings reflect the lack of a meaningful difference or simply insufficient study power.

Clinical and Statistical Significance

Sample size and power calculations incorporate the concepts of both clinical and statistical significance. Of these two concepts, clinical significance is more important. The finding that the effect of two treatments is statistically significantly different is of little value if the size of the difference is of no practical importance. When planning a study, clinical or practical significance should be the driving force (1,41).

There are several methods to determine the degree of difference or strength of association needed to obtain clinical significance. Commonly, investigators use information from published reports or references, or data from pilot studies recently conducted. Lacking either of these, investigators can look to their own experience or that of colleagues as a basis for a meaningful outcome. Lindgren et al (42) describe a procedure for choosing a size of treatment effect that is based on the underlying distribution of the measurement of interest in the target population. This procedure has the benefit of minimizing any subjectivity in selecting clinical significance and is useful in generating a range of values to use for the size of the effect.

CONCLUSION

Researchers want to avoid performing a study that may fail to find a statistically significant difference when a true difference does exist. This is an example of a type II error, and such a result can be avoided through the use of sample size calculations during the design of the study. The calculation provides the researcher with the number of individuals needed in each group of study participants to produce statistically significant results. The specific calculation needed will be dependent upon the type of study and the outcome measure. There are many resources available to aid the researcher, including sample size calculators and consulting a statistician. Before using any resource, the researcher needs to estimate the level of outcome that would be meaningful and the variation surrounding the outcome measure. This can be achieved through a review of the literature or performing pilot studies.

REFERENCES

1. Browner WS, Newman TB, Cummings SR, Hulley SB. Estimating sample size and power: the nitty-gritty. In: Hulley SB, Cummings SR, Browner R, Browner WS, Grady D, Newman TB, eds. *Designing Clinical Research: An Epidemiological Approach.* 2nd ed. Philadelphia, Pa: Lippincott Williams & Wilkins; 2001:65–91.

2. Moore DS, McCabe GP. Introduction to inference. In: *Introduction to the Practice of Statistics.* 5th ed. New York, NY: WH Freeman; 2006:381–447.

3. Armitage P, Berry G, Matthews JNS. Analysing means and proportions. In: *Statistical Methods in Medical Research.* 4th ed. Malden, Mass: Blackwell; 2002:83–137.

4. Dixon WJ, Massey FJ Jr. *Introduction to Statistical Analysis.* 4th ed. New York, NY: McGraw-Hill; 1983.

5. Lachin JM. Introduction to sample size determination and power analysis for clinical trials. *Control Clin Trials.* 1981;2:93–113.

6. Cohen NL, Laus MJ, Stutzman NC, Swicker RC. Dietary change in participants of the Better Eating for Better Health course. *J Am Diet Assoc.* 1991;91:345–346.

7. Van Horn L, Moag-Stahlberg A, Liu K, Ballew C, Ruth K, Hughes R, Stamler J. Effects on serum lipids of adding instant oats to usual American diets. *Am J Public Health.* 1991;81:183–188.

8. Dupont WD, Plummer WD Jr. Power and sample size calculations: a review and computer program. *Control Clin Trials.* 1990;11:116–128. Available at: http://biostat.mc.vanderbilt.edu/ twiki/bin/view/ Main/PowerSampleSize. Accessed May 29, 2007.

9. Statistical considerations for clinical trials and scientific experiments. Massachusetts General Hospital Biostatistics Center. Available at: http://hedwig.mgh. harvard.edu/sample_size/size.html. Accessed May 29, 2007.

10. Rosner B. *Fundamentals of Biostatistics.* 6th ed. Belmont, Calif: Duxbury/Thomson Brooks/Cole; 2006.

11. Nordenberg D, Yip R, Binkin NJ. The effect of cigarette smoking on hemoglobin levels and anemia screening. *JAMA.* 1990;264:1556–1559.

12. Day SJ, Graham DF. Sample size and power for comparing two or more treatment groups in clinical trials. *BMJ.* 1989;299:663–665.

13. Phillips AN, Pocock SJ. Sample size requirements for prospective studies, with examples for coronary heart disease. *J Clin Epidemiol.* 1989;42:639–648.

14. Lubin JH, Gail MH, Ershow AG. Sample size and power for case-control studies when exposures are continuous. *Stat Med.* 1988;7:363–376.

15. Shih JH. Sample size calculation for complex clinical trials with survival endpoints. *Control Clin Trials.* 1995;16:395–407.

16. Donner A, Eliasziw M. Sample size requirements for reliability studies. *Stat Med.* 1987;6:441–448.

17. Walter SD, Eliasziw M, Donner A. Sample size and optimal designs for reliability studies. *Stat Med.* 1998;17:101–110.

18. Donner A. Sample size requirements for the comparison of two or more coefficients of inter-observer agreement. *Stat Med.* 1998;17:1157–1168.

19. Donner A, Eliasziw M. A goodness of fit approach to inference procedures for the kappa statistic: confidence interval construction, significance-testing and sample size estimation. *Stat Med.* 1992;11: 1511–1519.

20. Casagrande T, Pike MC. An improved approximate formula for calculation of sample sizes for comparing two binomial distributions. *Biometrics.* 1978;34: 483–486.

21. Fleiss JL, Tytun A. A simple approximation for calculating sample sizes for comparing independent proportions. *Biometrics.* 1980;36:343.

22. Feigl P. A graphical aid for determining sample size when comparing two independent proportions. *Biometrics.* 1978;34:111–122.

23. Aleong J, Bartlett DE. Improved graphs for calculating sample sizes when comparing two independent binomial distributions. *Biometrics.* 1979;35:875.

24. Fleiss JL, Levin B, Paik MC. *Statistical Methods for Rates and Proportions.* 3rd ed. New York, NY: Wiley; 2003.

25. Cohen J. *Statistical Power Analysis for the Behavioral Sciences.* 2nd ed. Hillsdale, NJ: Lawrence Erlbaum Associates; 1988.

26. Sahai H, Khurshid A. Formulae and tables for the determination of sample sizes and power in clinical trials for testing differences in proportions for the two-sample design: a review. *Stat Med.* 1996;15:1–21.

27. Rosner B. Hypothesis testing: categorical data. In: *Fundamentals of Biostatistics.* 6th ed. Belmont, Calif: Duxbury/Thomson Brooks/Cole; 2006: 385–447.

28. Schlesselman JJ. *Case-Control Studies: Design, Conduct, Analysis.* New York, NY: Oxford University Press; 1982.

29. Fleiss JL, Levin B. Sample size determination in studies with matched pairs. *J Clin Epidemiol.* 1988; 41:727–730.

30. Lachenbruch PA. On the sample size for studies based upon McNemar's test. *Stat Med.* 1992;11: 1521–1525.

31. Lachin JM. Sample size determinations for r X c comparative trials. *Biometrics.* 1977;33:315.

32. Greenland S. Power, sample size and smallest detectable effect determination for multivariate studies. *Stat Med.* 1985;4: 117–127.

33. Lemeshow S, Hosmer DW Jr, Kiar J. Sample size requirements for studies estimating odds ratios or relative risks. *Stat Med.* 1988;7:759–764.

34. Weiss NS. *Clinical Epidemiology: The Study of the Outcome of Illness.* 3rd ed. New York, NY: Oxford University Press; 2006.

35. Arkin CE, Wachtel MS. How many patients are necessary to assess test performance? *JAMA.* 1990; 263:275–278.

36. Jensen DR. Efficiency and robustness in the use of repeated measures. *Biometrics.* 1982;38:813–825.

37. Rochon J. Application of GEE procedures for sample size calculations in repeated measures experiments. *Stat Med.* 1998;17:1643–1658.

38. Lipsitz SR, Fitzmaurice GM. Sample size for repeated measures studies with binary responses. *Stat Med.* 1994;13:1233–1239.

39. Betensky RA, Tierney C. An examination of methods for sample size recalculation during an experiment. *Stat Med.* 1997;16:2587–2598.

40. Streiner DL. Sample size and power in psychiatric research. *Can J Psychiatry.* 1990;35:616–620.

41. Browner WS, Newman TB, Hearst N, Hulley SB. Getting ready to estimate sample size: hypotheses and underlying principles. In: Hulley SB, Cummings SR, Browner R, Browner WS, Grady D, Newman TB, eds. *Designing Clinical Research: An Epidemiological Approach.* 2nd ed. Philadelphia, Pa: Lippincott Williams & Wilkins; 2001:51–63.

42. Lindgren BR, Wielinski CL, Finkelstein SM, Warwick WJ. Contrasting clinical and statistical significance within the research setting. *Pediatr Pulmonol.* 1993;16:336–340.

28

—ᴍ—

Fundamentals of Statistical Applications

*Carol J. Boushey, PhD, MPH, RD, Jeffrey Harris, DrPH, MPH, RD,
Barbara Bruemmer, PhD, RD, and Sujata L. Archer, PhD, RD*

electing the statistical method to apply to research data can be a challenge for the nonstatistician. Guidance from a statistician during the planning of the research project and as necessary throughout the research effort is useful. To facilitate communication with a statistician, the investigator should be familiar with the fundamentals of statistics and their applications. This chapter reviews the fundamentals of statistical analysis, outlines the general procedure involved, provides suggestions for analysis of several common research situations, and illustrates the procedure with a detailed example of applying statistical methods to a typical study design.

FUNDAMENTALS OF STATISTICAL ANALYSIS

Elements that guide the selection of a statistical method include the research question, the scale of measurement in which the data are collected, the relationship among samples, and the number of samples to be evaluated. Additional considerations relate to characteristics of the statistical test and include the test's assumptions about the normal distribution (also referred to as the *Gaussian distribution*) and whether the test should be applied as a one-sided or two-sided test of significance.

Most, if not all, research questions in dietetics can be categorized into one of two main categories: comparative or relational. The statistical methods for these two types of research questions are not the same because the purposes of the analyses differ. The comparative question asks the

statistical analysis to determine whether differences exist; the relational question asks the statistical analysis to determine whether associations exist. Statistical analysis methods for comparative questions detect differences in means or medians, for example, and may use tests such as the paired *t* test or the Wilcoxon rank sum test. Methods for relational questions assess correlations or associations, for example, and may use tests such as the Pearson correlation or the chi-square test.

Comparative Research Question

One example of a comparative research question is, "Does vitamin C supplementation elevate serum oxalate levels in patients with renal disease?" In a hypothetical study designed to answer such a question, patients could be randomly assigned to receive either the standard vitamin preparation that includes vitamin C or a similar vitamin preparation that excludes vitamin C. The analysis evaluates the difference, particularly the amount of increase, in serum oxalate levels between patients who receive vitamin C supplementation and patients who do not receive vitamin C supplementation.

Relational Research Question

A relational research question might be, "Is vitamin C supplementation associated with an increased risk of hyperoxalemia among patients with renal disease?" In a study designed to answer this type of question, all patients in a given clinic could be examined to determine serum oxalate levels and interviewed about use of vitamin C supplements. The analysis evaluates whether vitamin C supplement use is associated with the presence of hyperoxalemia.

Scale of Measurement (Type of Data Collected)

The measurements collected in research are referred to as *variables.* Variables can be classified in a number of ways to help determine the method of data analysis to use. Variables that are not inherently numerical—that is, for which only a few possible values exist—are considered *discrete* random variables (1) as would be the case for gender. Variables that have numerical meaning, as would be the case for blood pressure, are referred to as *continuous* or *quantitative* random variables (1). The statistical methods used for discrete variables differ from the methods used for continuous variables.

Discrete Variables

Although the symbol used to represent discrete information may be a number, these data are categorical—that is, they represent or name categories. A discrete datum may be further classified by whether it is nonordered, termed *nominal,* or ordered, termed *ordinal.* Nominal data correspond to a limited number of categories that have no ordered meaning. Nominal variables that fit into two categories, such as "present" and "absent," are termed *binary.* Ordinal data are ordered by categories, but the space between the categories is undefined. Treatment groups may be considered ordinal if the different treatments differ by dosage of a particular supplement. For example, binary measurements might include gender (female, male) and disease status (present, absent). Race (several categories, no order) is a nominal measure. Clinical stage of cancer (1 through 4) is an ordinal measure.

Continuous Variables

Continuous variables have a numerical value and the space between the values is defined and can be measured. Common examples of continuous data are height, weight, and energy intake.

The Relationship among Samples

Independent Samples

The assumption underlying many statistical tests is that the sample measurements are independent. Samples are independent when the data points in one sample are unrelated to the data points in the second sample. For example, an investigator may be interested in the relationship between smoking and hemoglobin levels in women between the ages of 18 and 44 years. If the investigator identifies a group of smokers and a group of nonsmokers from a prepaid health plan and measures their hemoglobin levels, the two samples would be completely independent because the data were obtained from unrelated groups of women.

Dependent Samples

Measurements in samples that are related are dependent; that is, they are inherently correlated. A number of situations in research produce related measurements and thus do not meet the assumption of independence. For example, an investigator may be interested in the change in hemoglobin levels in women between the ages of 18 and 44 years before and 6 months after a smoking cessation program. If the investigator measures their hemoglobin levels before the program and again 6 months later, the two measures would be completely dependent because the data were obtained from the same group of women.

Pairing and matching.   Pairing or matching in the study design can relate samples. An example of a common study design that uses pairing is the crossover trial, a study that uses subjects as their own controls. In a crossover trial, an initial observation is compared with a second observation measured on the same subject after the completion of some intervention by the investigator.

Related observations are also obtained when the subjects are matched. In the usual matched study, each subject in one group is matched with a subject in another group by one or more factors, such as age and gender. Specially designed statistical tests that account for the pairing and its resulting dependence among measurements must be used. Examples of such tests are the paired *t* test and the sign test, which are described by standard statistics textbooks (2,3).

Serial measurements.   Besides matching and pairing, another situation giving rise to dependent measurements is the practice of obtaining repeated or serial measurements on individual subjects. It is common to repeat measurements of a variable at several points in time and to evaluate the change from baseline or how the measurement varies over time. In the study of more than one group, the variation over time must also be compared between groups.

The dependence inherent in serial measurements is not widely appreciated in the nutrition literature. Such studies are frequently analyzed by applying paired *t* tests at each time period. Because the measurements are related, this procedure is not appropriate. This approach also may present the problem of multiplicity (see the following section, Number of Samples). A simple approach to the analysis described by Matthews and associates (4) is a two-stage method that summarizes the observations of the individual responses over time and then analyzes the summary measure by standard techniques. Another method would be to use repeated measures analysis of variance to determine whether groups differ in their responses over time. Investigators who are not familiar with this procedure should consult a statistician.

Replicate measurements.   Replicate measurements, or several measurements taken without regard to time, are also related observations. Analysis of variance can be used for replicate measurements of a continuous variable, provided the number of observations is the same for each subject. If this is not the case, the analysis is more complex, and statistical advice should be obtained (5). The distribution-free Friedman test is useful to analyze several related discrete observations or continuous data that are not normally distributed (see the later discussion of the assumption of normality).

Number of Samples

Statistical tests are designed to compare one sample, two samples, or more than two samples. Tests are so designed because as the number of groups increases, the number of possible pairwise comparisons increases. For two groups, only one comparison is possible; for three groups, three comparisons are possible; for four groups, six comparisons are possible; and for five groups, 10 comparisons may be made. The chances of finding a spurious significant result increases as the number of tests applied to a single set of data increases, giving rise to the statistical problem of *multiple comparisons,* or *multiplicity.*

More Than Two Groups

In the multiplicity situation, the level of statistical significance, or α level, increases dramatically with the number of groups compared. Instead of the chances of a false-positive result at the conventional 5% level (α = .05), the chance of a false-positive or an apparently significant result is greater—almost 15% in the case of three groups (three comparisons) and up to 40% in the case of five groups (10 comparisons) (6). Clearly, the possibility is great that conclusions will be incorrect.

For this reason, the common procedure of using the paired *t* test to examine each pair in such studies is not appropriate because the *t* test does not account for multiplicity present in the study design. Multiple-comparison techniques are described by Godfrey (6) and detailed in standard statistics texts. In general, when more than two samples are being compared, the appropriate statistical procedure is to first determine whether an overall difference is present using a test designed to do so, such as analysis of variance. After finding that a statistically significant difference does exist, researchers should apply the appropriate multiple-comparison technique to determine which individual pairs of samples differ. Examples of multiple-comparisons methods are the Bonferroni, Scheffe, Tukey, Newman-Keuls, and Duncan tests.

Unrestrained Significance Testing

Multiplicity is also present in a situation in which group comparisons are done on a large number of variables, as is common in nutrition research. Inappropriate methods for multiple comparisons, particularly the unrestrained repeated use of *t* tests, are frequently seen in nutrition literature and are no doubt responsible for a number of the claims of statistically significant results (7,8). If many variables are compared (eg, all the dozens of nutrients assessed by a nutrient analysis program of dietary intake), the problem of multiplicity will be present. The multiplicity problem exists because there is a 1-in-20 chance of finding a significant difference at a .05 significance level, even if no true difference exists. Furthermore, the chances of spurious significant findings (ie, false-positive results) increase as the number of tests increases.

To avoid this problem, the conventional α level should be applied only to tests that address the research questions. Results of significance tests applied to the hypotheses that serve as the basis of the study should carry the greatest weight (5,8). If other tests are performed, they should be regarded as exploratory, and a more conservative α level should be used. Adjusting the criterion of statistical significance downward will reduce the chances of spurious false-positive results. This downward adjustment can be made using a technique such as the Bonferroni, in which the α level is made more conservative by dividing it by the number of comparisons (9,10). For example, if 20 comparisons were made, the significance level would be .05/20 = .0025 instead of the conventional .05.

Other Considerations

Assumption of Normality

The validity of many statistical tests depends on the assumptions that the data are from a normal distribution and that the variability within groups is similar. Tests that depend on these assumptions are termed *parametric* and are, to some degree, sensitive to violations of those assumptions. Violating the assumptions does not necessarily rule out the use of parametric statistical methods because many parametric methods are robust (8,11); however, the nonstatistician usually does not know the consequences of doing so. In general, parametric statistical procedures applied to data that form a skewed distribution can yield misleading results (12). When parametric assumptions are clearly not met, it is better to be cautious and choose a method that accounts for the violations. There are two common options for doing so: transformations and nonparametric methods.

Transformations.   One option in accounting for violations in parametric assumptions is to transform the data to induce normality in the distribution and then apply the statistical test to the transformed data (8,12). A data set that has extreme observations may be transformed to an approximately normal distribution by scale transformation, such as a logarithmic conversion (eg, natural log or log base 10). After transformation, the investigator can plot the transformed data using a histogram to determine whether the transformation resulted in an approximately normal distribution. The drawback of this option is that interpretation of the results may not be straightforward.

Nonparametric methods.   The second option in accounting for violations in parametric assumptions is to use a nonparametric or distribution-free statistical method. Nonparametric statistical tests do not depend on the normal distribution and thus are valid with skewed data or with data that are collected in categorical form. These tests are easy to apply, and most require minimal calculation. The major disadvantage is that nonparametric tests are usually somewhat less powerful than their parametric counterparts, especially if the assumptions for the parametric tests are met and the parametric method can be applied (8). Nonparametric tests generally are less sensitive in finding effects and produce wider confidence intervals (CIs). However, nonparametric statistical methods are useful and should be considered when the sample size is small, when the distribution is skewed, or when categorical data are used. Several resources provide details on the use of nonparametric methods (13,14).

One-Sided and Two-Sided Significance Tests

Departures from the mean (or other parameter of interest) can occur in two possible directions: either above or below it, or in the observed direction and its opposite. A one-sided significance test evaluates departures in only one direction, whereas a two-sided significance test evaluates departures in both directions.

In the majority of situations, the two-sided test should be used. A one-sided test is justified only when the difference is expected to be in a specified direction (stated in advance), and a difference in the opposite direction is either not possible or of no interest. Because one-sided tests are less stringent, the validity of their results should be questioned if the results are marginally significant and the conclusions would change if a two-sided test were applied (15).

GENERAL PROCEDURE FOR STATISTICAL ANALYSIS

Whether the research question is comparative or relational, the investigator first describes the data and then makes inferences about the population from which the sample was drawn. This procedure is performed statistically by use of descriptive statistics, followed by the application of inferential statistical tests. The procedure involves three steps: summarize, estimate, and assess statistical significance.

First, the observations are summarized using a summary statistic or set of statistics (eg, the mean, frequency, or range of the observations in the sample or samples). Summary statistics show the distribution of experiences or characteristics and provide information about the characteristics of the underlying population from which the sample was drawn.

Second, the investigator uses the observations to estimate the magnitude of the difference in the comparison or the strength of the relationship (eg, how large the difference is or how strong the association is). The estimate provides information about the clinical or practical importance of the difference or association. A small difference may be of no consequence, whereas a large difference may make a major impact.

Third, the answer is assessed by determining its statistical significance—in other words, how likely it is that the observed difference or association would be obtained if no difference or association existed. The assessment provides information about the probability that the answer is due to chance alone rather than a true condition.

Step 1: Creating Statistical Summaries

Plotting the Data

Regardless of the type of data collected, plotting the data first and then summarizing it numerically is the best approach to summarizing observations. For comparative questions, construct a frequency distribution of the data, and examine its shape. For relational questions, construct a scatter plot of the two variables of interest (see the hypothetical clinical example later in this chapter).

Summarizing the Plot

The shape of the distribution or plot may clarify the correct summary statistic to use. The idea of summarizing is to convey concisely and accurately the characteristics of the shape of the distribution curve or scatter plot.

Summarizing discrete observations.   For discrete variables , summarize the frequency distribution by simply providing a single number: the frequency. The frequency describes the distribution of the group completely. Often the frequency is presented as a proportion of the total observations. If the sample size is sufficient (at least 100), a percentage can be presented, along with the numerator and denominator from which the percentage was derived. Differences among groups can be expressed simply as the difference between the group frequencies or group proportions.

Summarizing continuous observations.   Statistical summaries of continuous variables are more complex than statistical summaries of discrete variables. The frequency distribution or histogram forms a shape, usually approximating a curve. It is clear from examining the shape of the distribution that a single number does not describe any curve adequately. In this case, it is better to describe the distribution of observations by using at least two numbers— one describing the curve's height or central location (eg, mean or median) and another describing its width or variation (eg, standard deviation [SD] or range).

Determining the standard deviation.   The shape of the distribution determines the appropriate summary statistic. If the distribution is generally normal, with a shape approximating a normal bell-shaped curve, summarize it by using the mean and SD. A normal distribution has the convenient property that 95% of the sample observations lie within the mean ±2 SD. If the distribution is asymmetrical or skewed, as is common in nutrition research, the mean and SD are less accurate summary statistics. For skewed distributions, more than two summary statistics may be necessary. The median and the range are helpful additional summaries, as are the values of the 5th and 95th percentiles.

Step 2: Estimating in Statistics

Statistical procedures are concerned with estimates and uncertainties. Because it is rarely feasible for an entire population to be measured, it is generally agreed that characteristics about populations cannot be determined directly but must be estimated from samples drawn from the population. The summary statistics—such as mean, median, correlation coefficient, and relative risk—are single-value or point estimates derived from samples.

Because a point estimate varies to some extent even among samples drawn from the same population, it is useful to quantify the "precision" of the estimate in some manner. Precision is measured statistically by calculating the standard error (SE) and the CI.

Determining the Standard Error

If a number of random samples of sufficient size (usually $n > 30$) were taken from a population, the sample means would determine a normal distribution. The height or center of the distribution of sample means—that is, the mean of the means—would be near the true population mean. The width of the distribution—that is, the SD of the means—expresses the variation among the sample means. As with any normal distribution, 95% of all the sample means are within 2 SDs of the population mean.

The SD of the means is estimated from the sample by the standard error of the mean (SEM) or the SE. The SE is calculated by dividing the sample SD by the square root of the sample size. Consequently, the SE is inversely related to the sample size, a convenient property of a measure of precision. As the sample size increases, the SE decreases; that is, as the amount of information about the population increases, the variation in the estimate of the mean, although not the mean itself, decreases.

The SD is used to describe the variation among individual subjects in a sample, whereas the SE is used to describe the uncertainty in a sample estimate about a population parameter, such as a mean (16,17). The terms are not used interchangeably. When you are describing a sample distribution, the SD is a more useful statistic than the SE. However, when you are comparing differences among samples, the SE is helpful. The SE allows probability statements about the population mean (or other estimated parameter) to be made—that is, "Given the sample data, how likely is it that the population parameter is the value estimated by the sample?" This question is best answered using the SE to calculate a range of probable values or the CI.

Determining the Confidence Interval

The CI is the estimated range within which it is likely (eg, with 95% probability) that the point estimate (eg, the true mean, difference, or correlation coefficient) exists. Because the CI is calculated using the SE derived from the study sample, it is dependent in part both on the variation in the factor of interest and on the sample size. The CI is also dependent on the degree of confidence assigned to the results, conventionally placed at the 95% level ($\alpha = .05$). Mathematically, the CI is generally expressed as shown in Formula 28.1:

Formula 28.1

$$CI = \text{Point estimate} \pm \text{"Confidence } (1 - \alpha) \text{ level"} \times SE$$

The CI shows the range from the smallest to the largest values of the parameter that is consistent with the sample data. It is presented alone with the point estimate. A wide CI indicates that the sample's point estimate (eg, mean or correlation coefficient) lacks precision, and the true value could actually be any one of a large range of values. A narrow CI indicates that the sample's point estimate is relatively precise, and the true value is likely to be one of a few possible values. The width of the CI is inversely related to the sample size, indicating that as the amount of information about the population increases, the precision in the estimate increases.

The CI provides additional information about magnitude that is useful for interpreting results. For example, it answers the questions, "By how much did the diet alter the hemoglobin levels?" and "What was the increase in risk associated with cholesterol intake?" Instead of offering a single value by which to interpret the magnitude of a difference or association, the CI offers a range of values that are plausible, given the data in hand. This information is especially helpful when evaluating the practical importance of results. The use of the CI is illustrated in the hypothetical clinical example, later in this chapter. Gardner and Altman (16) provide an excellent review of the importance of the CI in reporting and interpreting study results and show methods for calculating the CI for a number of situations. Guyatt and colleagues point out the importance of the CI in interpreting the results of clinical studies (17).

Step 3: Assessing Statistical Significance

Statistical procedures are concerned with uncertainties, so an investigator makes assumptions about the underlying populations prior to initiating the study. The investigator then tests the hypotheses using the research observations. Formally, the hypotheses are known as the *statistical hypothesis* and the *working hypothesis*.

The research question generates the statistical hypothesis. This hypothesis defines the distributions in the populations under study. An example would be the hypothesis that a parenteral amino acid solution rich in branched-chain amino acids enhances nitrogen retention, as compared with a standard parenteral solution.

The null hypothesis is the working hypothesis. The null hypothesis states that there is no difference or no relationship among the factors under investigation or that there is no difference in the distributions in the study populations. In an investigation of a parenteral amino acid solution rich in branched-chain amino acids and its effect on nitrogen retention, the null hypothesis (H_0) would be that the branched-chain solution has the same effect on nitrogen retention as a standard amino acid solution. The study or alternative hypothesis (H_1) would be that the branched-chain solution enhances nitrogen retention as compared with a standard amino acid solution.

Testing Hypotheses

Because the two hypotheses assume different characteristics about the underlying population distributions, the hypothesis-testing procedure employs statistical tests to compare the expected distribution, defined by the null hypothesis, with the observed distribution, estimated by the study results. The statistical test assesses statistical significance that the results are consistent with the null hypothesis. The statistical significance test asks the question, "How likely is it that the values for the distribution characteristics given by the sample will be observed if the null hypothesis is true?"

Results yielding a P value that is less than α indicate that the study data provide evidence to reject the null hypothesis and to support an alternative hypothesis. Results yielding a P value that is greater than α indicate that the study was unable to detect evidence that is contrary to the null hypothesis.

Interpreting Statistical Probability Values

Caution and common sense must guide the use and interpretation of statistical probability values. Although statistical significance is important to assess, it is not the primary result of a data analysis. Statistical hypothesis testing is used to determine whether results are consistent or not consistent with the null hypothesis and, as noted by Rothman and others, artificially classifies results into a dichotomous outcome of significant or not significant (17,18). This answer is not adequate as a guide for decisions in many practical situations (17). It completely ignores the size of any effect that was observed and whether the study was able (ie, had sufficient power) to detect statistically significant results. A finding of statistically nonsignificant results does not mean the findings are necessarily insignificant. Likewise, a finding of statistically significant results does not mean the findings are necessarily meaningful.

Significance values must be interpreted in relation to other aspects of the study, including design characteristics, sample size, missing values, biases in sampling and measurement, and compliance to study requirements and treatment, if given. In addition, the size of the differences or effects must be considered when interpreting results. The CI provides the information about size, and the CI, along with P values and point estimates, should be presented to allow a meaningful conclusion to be made.

ANSWERING THE RESEARCH QUESTION

This section describes in general terms how the three-step process just described would be applied to several of the most common research situations. Because readers are most familiar with studies of differences, these applications are briefly outlined in a format that will serve as a ready reference for future use. Methods used for evaluating associations are provided in a more detailed, narrative form. The reader is urged to use these descriptions and suggested applications as a foundation for further study of the topic; to refer to the references to determine whether a suggested statistical method is appropriate for the application at hand; and, when possible, to consult with a statistician. A hypothetical clinical example illustrating both comparative and relational applications follows later in this chapter.

Comparisons and Differences

When comparing differences between samples or groups, select the statistical method based on the type of variable considered (eg, binary, ordinal, or continuous). Suggested statistical methods for evaluating differences for these types of variables are outlined in Table 28.1 (2,3,14,16,19–21).

Relationships and Associations

Relationships are summarized by a variety of procedures. If the data are discrete, frequency plots that are classified by categories can be used. Such plots are summarized simply by constructing contingency tables (2 × 2 tables or

R × C tables [tables with more than two rows and more than two columns]) of the cross-category frequencies. The section "Comparison of Proportions," presented later in this chapter, describes the 2 × 2 table and shows an example. The association between variables in a 2 × 2 table can be assessed statistically by the chi-square statistic described in standard statistics texts (2,3).

As previously noted, the statistical assessment of the association is not adequate by itself. It conveys no information about the degree of association or its practical importance, and because the P value is dependent in part on the sample size, an association of little strength may be statistically significant if the sample is large enough. For this reason, it is also important to estimate a measure of the strength of the association.

Discrete Data

The strength of the association among binary variables can be measured by various methods, depending on the type of study design. For behavioral and educational studies, the φ coefficient is popular despite its deficiencies. Calculated from a 2 × 2 table, the φ coefficient is interpretable as a correlation coefficient ranging from −1 to +1, with values near zero indicating little or no association between the two variables. However, Fleiss (19) cautions that the φ coefficient has serious deficiencies and should be avoided in areas of research requiring a comparison of findings among investigations.

Fortunately, better measures of association exist. Two of the most useful measures are the relative risk and the odds ratio. The relative risk is used when the investigation is a cohort or prospective design, and the odds ratio is appropriate for investigations that are of case-control or cross-sectional design. Both measures describe the degree of association between an antecedent factor and an outcome event, such as morbidity (22), so both are important in observational analytic studies that evaluate potentially causal relationships. Methods for calculating and interpreting the relative risk and the odds ratio are discussed in Chapter 8. Readers are also referred to Fleiss et al (19) for details on deriving the CIs for both measures and for assessing statistical significance.

Continuous Data

The relationships among continuous variables are commonly explored by scatter plot and summarized with linear regression or correlation coefficients. Although they are related, regression and correlation analysis are used for different purposes and thus are interpreted differently. Linear regression expresses the relationship between two

TABLE 28.1   Suggested Statistical Methods for Evaluating Differences between Samples or Groups

Sampling Situation	Variable Type	Hypothesize	Summarize	Estimate	Assess	References
Two independent samples	Binary	Proportions are equal	Frequency table (2×2 table)	Difference in proportions with its CI	x^2	2,3,16,19
	Ordinal	Medians are equal	Median, interquartile range	Difference in medians with its CI	Mann-Whitney test, Wilcoxon rank sum test	14,20,21
	Continuous	Means are equal	Mean, SD	Difference in means with its CI	Independent t test	2,3,16,20
Several independent samples	Binary	All proportions are equal	Group frequencies (contingency table)	Difference in proportions; pairwise CI from multiple comparisons	Global x^2 followed by multiple-comparison analysis	19
	Binary, but groups are ordered	Proportions are equal	Group frequencies (contingency table)	Difference in proportions	Bartholomew's test	19
	Ordinal	All medians are equal	Medians, interquartile range	Difference in medians	Kruskal-Wallis (Jonckheere), nonparametric test	21
	Continuous	All means are equal	Group means, SDs	Difference in means; pairwise CI after multiple-comparison analysis	One-way analysis of variance followed by multiple-comparison methods	6,20
Crossover, measures taken at two times in a single group	Nominal or ordinal	Medians of time periods do not differ	Medians, interquartile range	CI for median change	Wilcoxon sign rank test	14,20,21
	Continuous	Means of time periods do not differ	Means, SD	Difference in means with its CI	Paired t test	2,3,20
Two independent groups, change in measures taken at two times (eg, before and after treatment)	Binary	Proportion improved is equal	Group frequencies (2×2 table)	Difference in proportions with its CI	Normal approximation to binomial or x^2 test; matched study— McNemar's test	16,19
	Continuous	Change in measures is equal	Mean, SD of changes	Difference in mean change with its CI	t test of mean changes, or analysis of covariance (see hypothetical clinical example)	29,30,31
Two independent groups, serial measures, difference in the response over time	Continuous	Response over time is equal	Plot response over time to determine how response changes over time (peaked or growth curves); then select appropriate summary	If appropriate, difference with its CI	t test of mean difference (from summary), or repeated measures analysis of variance, or multivariate analysis of variance	2,3,4,25

Abbreviations: CI, confidence interval; SD, standard deviation.

variables by a mathematical model describing a straight line. The correlation coefficient measures the degree of linear association between the two variables. Regression analysis is used most commonly to quantify the association between two variables and to make predictions based on the linear relationship. The correlation coefficient is used to measure the strength of the linear association and provides little other descriptive information. Guyatt et al provide helpful illustrations of the use of regression and correlation in the medical literature (23).

The first step in regression or correlation analysis is to plot the data. In regression analysis, a scatter plot is constructed with the dependent variable on the vertical axis (ie, *y*-axis) and the independent variable on the horizontal axis (ie, *x*-axis). The plot will help determine whether a straight-line model is appropriate for the data. In both regression and correlation analysis, any outlying observations can seriously affect the analysis, and a scatter plot assists in detecting those observations. If the scatter plot appears to be nonlinear, methods other than linear regression should be used.

Regression analysis. In regression analysis, after plotting the data, the investigator calculates the regression equation to summarize the plot. This method is particularly useful when an investigator wishes to predict the value of one variable from that of another. The regression equation summarizes the straight-line relationship between two variables by the equation $y = a + bx$. The equation is expressed conceptually as follows:

Predicted variable = Intercept + (Slope × Predictor variable)

The equation provides coefficients for the intercept (*a*), slope (*b*), and the correlation. The intercept is the estimated value of *y* when $x = 0$. The slope describes the average value of *y* at each value of *x* and is thus dependent on the units in which *x* and *y* are measured. Therefore, the slope can be used to predict the change in *y* that is associated with each unit change in *x*. Both the intercept and the slope have error terms (ie, variances) that are used to calculate additional significance tests and CIs for the coefficients.

The correlation coefficient has a special interpretation in regression analysis. When squared (R^2), it expresses the proportion or percentage of the variation in *y* that is explained by the linear regression with *x*. This interpretation is different from that of the correlation coefficient (*r*), which is covered later.

In addition to the coefficients, the degree to which the data points cluster around the regression line is also

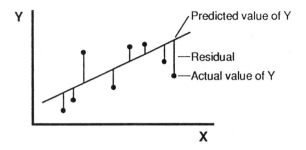

FIGURE 28.1   The difference between the observed values of *y* and the fitted regression line (predicted values of *y*).

important to quantify. The difference between the actual observed value of *y* and the value predicted by the regression equation is known as the *residual* (Figure 28.1); thus, the quantity of interest is the *residual variance*. The residual variance measures the amount by which the actual values of *y* differ from the predicted values. A good regression equation minimizes the residual variance.

It is important to verify, at least roughly, that the regression equation accurately summarizes the data (24). Briefly, the procedure involves examining the residuals by plotting them on the *x*-axis with the predicted values on the *y*-axis and determining whether a pattern exists. A relatively accurate regression equation exhibits no distinctive pattern, whereas a less accurate equation shows a systematic trend, such as a V-shaped spread. The regression equation requires further refinement if a trend is detected. Details on residual analysis are provided by Kleinbaum et al (25) and Godfrey (24); the procedure usually is done by computer analysis. The important summary statistics of regression analysis are the regression equation, the coefficients and variances of the slope and intercept, the variance of the residuals, and the proportion of the variation in the dependent variable explained by the regression equation (R^2).

Correlation. The product moment, or linear correlation coefficient (*r*), is a measure of the strength of the linear association between two variables. It is dependent on the slope and the sample size and does not depend on the units of measurement of the original observations. The correlation coefficient ranges from -1 to $+1$. When the correlation coefficient is zero, the slope of the regression line is also zero. A value of either -1 or $+1$ indicates that the data approximate a straight line and that the slope of the line is not zero. A positive coefficient indicates a positive relationship: that *y* increases as *x* increases. A negative coefficient indicates the opposite: a negative or inverse relationship in which *x* increases as *y* decreases.

The correlation coefficient can be useful in indicating whether y is related to x, but it provides no other quantitative information to describe the linear relationship. It does not describe the amount of change in y that occurs for each unit change in x, as did the previously described coefficients in the regression equation. Furthermore, because of its dependence on the slope and variance, the correlation coefficient can be influenced by both the steepness of the line and the degree to which the data points cluster about the regression line. Because it does not distinguish between these two components, it is difficult to interpret the correlation coefficient correctly when it is presented alone (26). A large value can be misleading. For example, it is possible for a correlation coefficient to be large simply because the axes are scaled in such a way that the slope is steep. For this reason, it is better to interpret the correlation coefficient when it is paired with a plot of the data or with the regression equation, including the slope and variances. The purpose of the analysis determines which statistical analysis method to include. If the purpose of the analysis is predicting y, regression analysis is used; if the purpose is determining whether a linear relationship is present, correlation analysis is used.

Correlation analysis assumes that the observations are independent. Observations of x and y are taken on each subject, but each subject contributes only one x-y pair. A common error in correlation analysis is to compute correlation coefficients on data that are related. A frequently seen example of this error is the correlation analysis of serial measurements. For example, if serum magnesium and magnesium intake are measured on each subject at several points in time, it is not valid to pool all the data to calculate the correlation coefficient for the relationship between magnesium intake and serum magnesium because measurements taken on the same person are related.

Correlation for discrete variables. A scatter plot also can be used for ordinal, or ordered, categorical data. Unlike continuous data, however, ordinal data should not be analyzed by the product moment correlation normally used. Data of these types are better summarized with a distribution-free correlation procedure, such as the Spearman or Kendall correlation coefficients.

A HYPOTHETICAL CLINICAL EXAMPLE

The application of the statistical methods described in this chapter can be demonstrated using a study undertaken to determine whether the use of a glucose polymer could enhance magnesium absorption as determined by serum magnesium levels. (Charuhas and coworkers [27] reported such a study, and their results are modified here for the purposes of illustration.) The subjects were 40 patients with hypomagnesemia who required daily magnesium supplementation until their serum magnesium levels were normal. The patients were randomized into two groups ($n_1 = 20$, $n_2 = 20$) to receive their magnesium supplementation with either a solution containing a glucose polymer or a placebo solution that was identical in appearance and taste. Measuring the patients' serum magnesium levels after 7 days of treatment and comparing the increase in serum magnesium of the patients receiving the glucose polymer with that of the patients receiving the placebo determined the effectiveness of the glucose polymer. The hypothetical raw data are presented in Table 28.2.

Comparison of Proportions

A number of approaches to the analysis of this study are possible. The calculations, figures, and tables that follow are useful in assessing the data but for the most part would not be submitted for publication. A simple method would be to describe the proportion of patients in the two groups whose serum magnesium levels improved to at least 0.65 mmol/L (Table 28.3).

The simple difference in the proportions is calculated as follows:

$$\text{Difference} = \frac{9}{20} - \frac{1}{20}$$

$$= \frac{8}{20} \text{ or } 0.40, \text{ or } 40\%$$

CIs for differences between two proportions can be constructed similarly to those for continuous variables (see Formula 28.1) using the SE:

Formula 28.2

$$SE_{diff} = 2 \overline{\left(P_1 Q_1 / n_1 \right) + \left(P_2 Q_2 / n_2 \right)}$$

where: P_1 = proportion improved in group 1, $Q_1 = 1 - P_1$, P_2 = proportion improved in group 2, and $Q_2 = 1 - P_2$.

This procedure is useful for samples of sufficient size (eg, 50 per group) and with proportions within the range 0.1 to 0.9 (15). Smaller sample sizes require more accurate, but complex, procedures that may necessitate consultation with a statistician. Readers are referred to

TABLE 28.2   Example of Study Data on Serum Magnesium Levels

Subject	Baseline (mmol/L)	Final (mmol/L)	Change* (mmol/L)	% Change
Placebo Group				
1	0.51	0.56	0.05	10.6
2	0.55	0.58	0.03	4.5
3	0.59	0.62	0.03	4.9
4	0.54	0.60	0.06	11.5
5	0.59	0.64	0.05	8.3
6	0.55	0.61	0.06	11.2
7	0.55	0.59	0.04	8.3
8	0.56	0.59	0.03	5.9
9	0.50	0.58	0.08	14.8
10	0.57	0.60	0.03	5.8
11	0.59	0.64	0.05	8.3
12	0.50	0.59	0.09	17.2
13	0.52	0.57	0.05	10.2
14	0.58	0.62	0.04	7.8
15	0.55	0.61	0.06	10.4
16	0.54	0.58	0.04	8.4
17	0.53	0.60	0.07	12.4
18	0.56	0.61	0.05	9.6
19	0.58	0.62	0.04	6.4
20	0.60	0.69	0.09	14.4
mean =	0.55	0.60	0.05	9.5
SD =	0.031	0.029	0.017	3.40
Glucose Polymer Group				
1	0.59	0.62	0.03	4.2
2	0.52	0.58	0.06	11.1
3	0.51	0.59	0.08	15.2
4	0.58	0.67	0.09	15.7
5	0.60	0.65	0.05	8.2
6	0.52	0.61	0.09	17.5
7	0.51	0.62	0.11	22.0
8	0.54	0.64	0.10	19.2
9	0.58	0.66	0.08	13.4
10	0.56	0.65	0.09	15.3
11	0.52	0.64	0.12	22.0
12	0.56	0.67	0.11	19.1
13	0.58	0.68	0.10	17.0
14	0.58	0.69	0.11	19.3
15	0.51	0.63	0.12	22.4
16	0.55	0.64	0.09	17.3
17	0.59	0.69	0.10	17.6
18	0.53	0.62	0.09	17.8
19	0.57	0.64	0.07	12.9
20	0.57	0.67	0.10	17.4
mean =	0.55	0.64	0.09	16.2
SD =	0.031	0.030	0.023	4.57

*Change = Final value − Baseline value.

Source: Data are adapted from reference 27.

TABLE 28.3 Number of Patients Showing Improvement by Treatment Group

Treatment	No. Improved (%)	Total (n)
Glucose polymer	9 (45)	20
Placebo	1 (5)	20
Overall	10 (25)	40

Gardner and Altman (16) and Fleiss et al (19) for details and examples of the usual procedure. Because the example data do not meet the size requirement, a CI is not constructed for this point estimate.

To assess statistical significance, the usual approach when the sample size is large would be to apply the z-test or the chi-square test, described in standard statistics texts. However, if an expected frequency is small (eg, approximately 5), the chi-square test may not be accurate (12).

To compute the expected frequencies for the glucose polymer response trial, see Table 28.4, which gives the observed values for these data. The row totals are 20 and 20; the column totals are 10 and 30; and the grand total is 40. Thus:

$$
\begin{aligned}
E_{11} &= \text{Expected number of units in the (1,1) cell} \\
       &= 20(10)/40 = 5 \\
E_{12} &= \text{Expected number of units in the (1,2) cell} \\
       &= 20(30)/40 = 15 \\
E_{21} &= \text{Expected number of units in the (2,1) cell} \\
       &= 20(10)/40 = 5 \\
E_{22} &= \text{Expected number of units in the (2,2) cell} \\
       &= 20(30)/40 = 15
\end{aligned}
$$

Because the expected frequency of two cells is small (no greater than 5), a more accurate significance test is given by use of the Fisher exact test. Although the assumption of this test—that all marginal frequencies are fixed—is rarely

TABLE 28.4 Data for Patients Receiving Magnesium Supplementation with and without Glucose Polymer

	Response Improved (Serum Magnesium Level $\geq$ 0.65 mmol/L)		
Treatment	+	−	Total
Glucose polymer	9	11	20
Placebo	1	19	20
Total	**10**	**30**	**40**

met in nutrition research, the test is commonly used for studies in which two of the marginal frequencies are fixed, as in this study ($n_1 = n_2 = 20$). Details of the Fisher exact test for 2×2 tables are given by Matthews and Farewell (28) and others (12,19), and computer programs are available to complete this test. When applied to this table as a two-tailed test, the P value is .008.

The statistically significant result indicates that it is unlikely that a difference of this magnitude (40%) would be observed if there were no true difference in the underlying populations. The magnitude, 40%, implies that of every 100 patients given a placebo (in whom an improvement of 5% is expected), an additional 40% would be expected to achieve serum magnesium levels of at least 0.65 mmol/L within 1 week given the glucose polymer. This degree of improvement was considered important by the clinic staff, which concluded that glucose polymer is superior to the standard therapy as an adjunct to magnesium supplementation in the treatment of patients with hypomagnesemia.

Analysis of Continuous Variables

Another approach to the analysis would be to evaluate the response as a continuous variable. First, summarize the baseline magnesium levels by graphing them using a histogram, and examine the shape of the curve (Figure 28.2). The histogram helps assess whether the two groups are similar in the distribution of baseline measurements. Figure 28.2 shows that the distributions of the two groups are also similar, indicating that randomization was successful in making the two groups comparable in this baseline measure. The distributions appear to be approximately bell-shaped, indicating that parametric statistical methods are appropriate for these data.

A simple analysis of the difference in group means of the final serum magnesium measurement by an independent t test may be misleading (eg, 0.60 vs 0.64, as shown in Table 28.2) because the final measurement may be related to the initial measurement. For example, the final value for patients with low baseline levels may be lower than the final value for patients with higher baseline levels. It is best to plot the final measure with the baseline measure to determine whether they are related (29). As is evident in the scatter plot of these data (Figure 28.3), this is the case.

The final measurement of serum magnesium is linearly related to the baseline measurement. The correlation coefficients (r) are also indicative of the relationship;

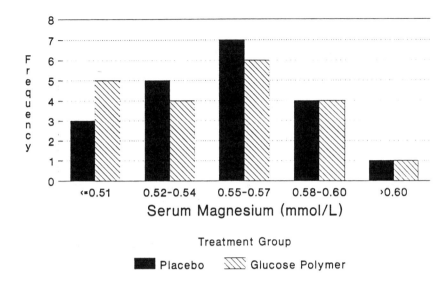

FIGURE 28.2   Histogram of baseline magnesium measurements ($n = 20$ subjects per group).

$r = 0.70$ ($P = .0006$) and $r = 0.83$ ($P = .0001$) for the glucose polymer and placebo groups, respectively. The correlation coefficient and scatter plot confirm a linear relationship.

When the two measurements are related, some adjustment for the baseline measurement is necessary. A common approach is to compute the change value—that is, the difference between the final and first measurements—and then apply statistical methods to this value. The difference computed for each subject is shown in the Change column in Table 28.2.

In some situations, investigators may be tempted to use percentage change instead of the value of the change between the two measurements. The choice between change and percentage change is not arbitrary. Kaiser (29) provides guidance on choosing between the two values. Briefly, plot change and percentage change vs the baseline for each treatment group, and then choose the one that shows little dependence on the baseline value (29). Scatter plots for the study data are shown in Figures 28.4 and 28.5.

The scatter plots and r values shown in Figures 28.4 and 28.5 indicate that the value of change is less dependent on the baseline values than percentage change, so it is this value that should be compared between groups. Compute the CI for the difference in the mean change, and assess its

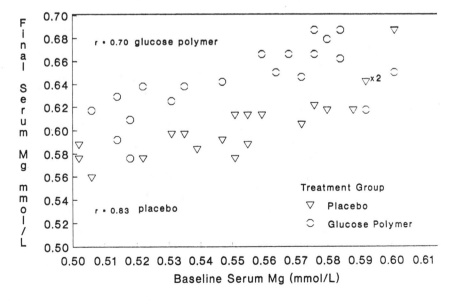

FIGURE 28.3   Scatter plot of the final measurement with the baseline measurement.

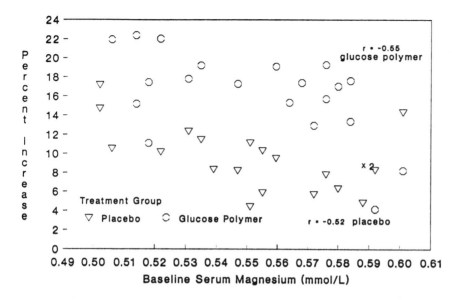

FIGURE 28.4   Scatter plot of percentage change in serum magnesium and baseline measurement.

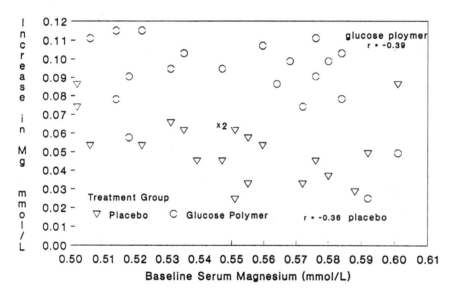

FIGURE 28.5   Scatter plot of the change and baseline measurements.

statistical significance by the independent *t* test. Results are shown in Table 28.5.

From the standard tables of the *t* distribution, the value of the Student *t* at $\alpha = 0.05$ and 38 degrees of freedom (*df*) is 2.021. The 95% CI of the difference between the means can be calculated using Formula 28.1.

$$95\% \text{ CI} = \text{Difference} \pm t \times \text{SE difference}$$
$$= 0.04 \pm 2.021 \times 0.0065$$
$$= 0.027, 0.053 \text{ (or } 0.03, 0.05)$$

The pooled variance is used because the sample variances are similar. As a general rule, variances may be considered to be similar if the ratio of the sample variances is less than 2 (12). The statistical significance test for the hypothesis that the mean change is the same for both groups is given by the standard two-tailed independent samples *t* test, which results in $t = 5.652$ and $P < .0001$.

These results provide evidence to reject the null hypothesis and to conclude that the mean change in serum magnesium levels differs between the groups. The size of the difference is estimated from the study to be 0.04 mmol/L, although the data are consistent with a difference of as little as 0.03 mmol/L and a difference as large as 0.05 mmol/L. It is a matter of judgment by the investigators and the readers whether this is a clinically meaningful difference.

TABLE 28.5   Mean Change in Serum Magnesium Measurements by Intervention Group

Group	Mean Change in Serum Magnesium, mmol/L		
	Mean	**SD**	**SE**
Placebo	0.05	0.017	0.004
Glucose polymer	0.09	0.023	0.005
Difference	0.04	0.0206*	0.0065*

Abbreviations: SD, standard deviation; SE, standard error.
*Pooled SD or SE.

Analysis of Covariance

Although the independent *t* test of the difference between initial and follow-up measurements among groups is the most common approach to analyzing data from a study of this type, another method of analysis should be considered here as well. Analysis of covariance is generally a more efficient statistical test than the independent *t* test when the response measurement is related to the initial measurement, as is the case with these data (29,30). Briefly, analysis of covariance involves computing the linear regression of the final measurement data (dependent variable) vs the initial measurement data (independent variable) and testing the difference between groups by comparing the distance between the regression lines (25). The procedure, described for medical investigators by Egger and associates (31), produces a parallel-lines analysis of covariance model by first testing whether the slopes of the regression lines for the two groups are equal and then, if the slopes are not significantly different, testing whether the intercepts of the two lines differ (Figure 28.6). This procedure warrants consideration and at times may be preferred to the more common analysis previously described. Readers are referred to Egger and associates (31) for details regarding the procedure's use and misuse, although readers who are unfamiliar with analysis of covariance also should consult a statistician.

Analysis of covariance is applied to these data to illustrate this powerful technique. Kleinbaum et al (25) present the topic with an emphasis on application rather than theory, and their text is particularly helpful for the non-statistician investigator.

The results of analysis of covariance for the example study data are shown in Table 28.6. Three questions are relevant to the analysis, and three regression models are constructed from these data to provide the components for answering the questions. The independent variables of baseline serum magnesium (x), treatment group indicator (z), and an interaction variable (xz) that is a product of the other two variables are associated with the regression coefficients: β_1, β_2, and β_3, respectively. This relationship can be shown by the following equation:

$$y = \beta_0 + \beta_1 x + \beta_2 z + \beta_3 xz + \text{Error term}$$

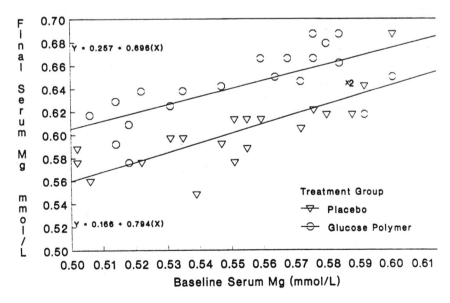

FIGURE 28.6   Plot of serum magnesium values for completing analysis of covariance.

TABLE 28.6   Analysis of Covariance Results for Example Data

Source	df^a	Sum of Squares	Mean Square^b	F Value^c
Regression $(x)^d$	1	0.019762	0.019762	27.38
Residual	38	0.027418	0.000722	
Regression $(x, z)^e$	2	0.0333357	0.016679	44.60
Residual	37	0.013823	0.000374	
Regression $(x, z, xz)^f$	3	0.033443	0.011148	29.18
Residual	36	0.013737	0.000382	

$^a df$ = degrees of freedom.
^{b}Mean square = (Sum of squares/df).
$^c F$ value = (Regression mean square/Residual mean square).
^{d}Where x = initial serum magnesium value (mmol/L).
^{e}Where z = 0 if placebo group, 1 if glucose polymer group.
^{f}Where xz = interaction term $x \times z$ (ie, 0 for placebo, which is initial serum magnesium for glucose polymer group).

The first question is this: "Is the relationship between the initial value and the final value the same for both groups?" This question is answered by determining whether the lines are parallel or nearly parallel, because if they were not, another method of analysis would be necessary (seek statistical advice). A test of the hypothesis that the regression coefficient β_3 is equal to zero assesses whether the regression lines are parallel. The testing procedure is detailed by Kleinbaum et al (25). The results, as shown in Table 28.7a ($F = 0.22$; 2,36 df; $P > .10$), indicate that there is no evidence to show that the two lines are not parallel. Figure 28.6 also shows that the lines appear parallel.

The second question is, "Are both the slopes and the intercepts the same in the groups?" It is important at this step to determine whether the two lines are actually the same line. The test of the hypothesis that both regression coefficients β_2 and β_3 equal zero assesses whether the lines are coincident. The results in Table 28.7b ($F = 17.91$; 1,36 df; $P < .001$) provide strong evidence that the two lines are not coincident.

The third question is, "Is there a difference in the mean scores?" The first and second questions indicate that the lines are parallel but not coincident, so the logical next step is to determine whether the distance between the lines is great enough to provide evidence of a difference between them. The test of the hypothesis that the regression coefficient β_2 equals zero is a measure of the distance and determines whether there is a difference in means between the

TABLE 28.7   ANOVA Tables for Analysis of Covariance Models (Using Results from Table 28.6)

Source	df^*	Sum of Squares	Mean Square	F Value
a. With the Interaction Variable				
Regression (x, z)	2	0.033357	0.016679	43.66
$(xz / x, z)$	1	0.000086	0.000086	0.22
Residual	36	0.013737	0.000382	
Total	**39**	**0.047180**		
b. For Coincident Lines				
Regression (x, z)	1	0.019762	0.019762	51.73
$(xz / x, z)$	2	0.013681	0.006841	17.91
Residual	36	0.013737	0.000382	
Total	**39**	**0.047180**		
c. For Difference of Means Between Groups				
Regression (x, z)	1	0.019762	0.019762	52.84
$(xz / x, z)$	1	0.013595	0.013595	36.35
Residual	37	0.013823	0.000374	
Total	**39**	**0.047180**		

*df indicates degrees of freedom.

TABLE 28.8   Parameters from the Analysis of Covariance

Variable	Coefficient	Estimate	SE Estimate*
Intercept	β_0	0.193257	0.056963
Initial magnesium level	β_1	0.744974	0.102725
Group	β_2	0.036873	0.006112

*SE indicates standard error.

groups. The results in Table 28.7c ($F = 36.35$; 1,37 df; $P < .001$) indicate that the means of the placebo and glucose polymer groups are significantly different. These results confirm the results of the independent t test and reject the null hypothesis at the level of less than 1%.

As with all methods of analysis, assessing statistical significance is only one part of data analysis in the analysis of covariance; estimating the size of the difference is also important. Analysis of covariance is a linear regression procedure, so it produces coefficients that express the linear relationship of the variables of interest. The parameters resulting from analysis of covariance (omitting xz and its related regression coefficient, β_3) are shown in Table 28.8.

In the example study, the coefficient of interest is β_2, or the coefficient associated with the group (ie, treatment) variable. The β_2 coefficient estimates the difference between the two mean scores after removing (in part) the influence of the initial magnesium value. Analysis of covariance estimates the difference to be 0.037 mmol/L, close to the estimate (0.04 mmol/L) from the simple analysis using the mean change values. The CI can also be computed in the usual way from the SE of the coefficient:

$$95\% \ CI \ for \ \beta_2 = 0.036873 \pm 1.96(0.06112)$$
$$= 0.0249, 0.0488 \ (or \ 0.03, 0.05)$$

These results are nearly identical to those derived by the previous method and would be interpreted in the same way. The benefit of using analysis of covariance, however, is that it can be a more efficient analysis than the independent t test (as indicated by the narrower CI) when the initial and final measurements are linearly related and the sample size is sufficient (ie, approximately greater than 20) (30,31).

It is useful to consider the conclusions possible if the significance test resulted in a statistically nonsignificant P value. As pointed out by Rothman (18), and more recently by Guyatt and colleagues (17), the CI becomes key to the interpretation in such a case. The CI shows the readers the range of values that are plausible, given the data in hand. If the CI were to range from −0.02 to +0.10, the interval

would include zero, which corresponds to a nonsignificant P value. However, most of the values extend into the range of increased mean values. The CI shows that although the data are consistent with no real difference, the data are also consistent with an increase in serum magnesium levels that generally suggests a favorable result of the treatment. A more meaningful interpretation of the data is possible when the CI is reported along with the P value. Readers then have the information to consider whether the position of the interval warrants a conclusion other than "not significant." In reporting the results, it is sufficient to present a simple table of descriptive statistics and a statement of the analysis of covariance statistics (F value, df, and P value).

CONCLUSION

This chapter focused on the area of statistics that deals with analyzing and drawing conclusions from data. The field of nutrition and dietetics offers many opportunities to carry out research. This introduction to statistical methods is intended to enhance the investigator's skills in this area, as well as facilitate communication with statisticians in planning and completing research projects. Numerous references were cited to encourage further reading on this topic and provide guidance for developing a resource library. The basic steps discussed in this chapter will help with the many decisions that need to be made in approaching and executing successful research.

REFERENCES

1. Rosner B. Discrete probability distributions. In: Rosner B, ed. *Fundamentals of Biostatistics.* Belmont, Calif: Duxbury, Thomson Brooks/Cole; 2006:82–83.
2. Moore DS, McCabe GP. *Introduction to the Practice of Statistics.* New York, NY: WH Freeman; 2006.
3. Rosner B. *Fundamentals of Biostatistics.* Belmont, Calif: Duxbury/ Thomson Brooks/Cole; 2006.
4. Matthews INS, Altman DG, Campbell MJ, Royston P. Analysis of serial measurements in medical research. *BMJ.* 1990;300:230–235.
5. Altman DG, Gore SM, Gardner MI, Pocock SI. Statistical guidelines for contributors to medical journals. *BMJ.* 1983;286:1489–1493.
6. Godfrey K. Comparing the means of several groups. *N Engl J Med* 1985;313:1450–1456.

7. Ried M, Hall IC. Multiple statistical comparisons in nutritional research. *Am J Clin Nutr.* 1984;40: 183–184.

8. Horgan GW. Statistical analysis of nutritional studies. *Br J Nutr.* 2001;86:141–144.

9. Tukey W. Some thoughts on clinical trials, especially problems of multiplicity. *Science.* 1977;198: 679–684.

10. Guyatt G, Jaeschke R, Heddle N, Cook D, Shannon H, Walter S. Basic statistics for clinicians: 1. Hypothesis testing. *Can Med Assoc J.* 1995;152:27.

11. Moore DS, McCabe GP. Inference for distributions. In: Moore DS, McCabe GP, eds. *Introduction to the Practice of Statistics.* New York, NY: WH Freeman; 2006:462–463.

12. Armitage P, Berry G, Matthews JNS. *Statistical Methods in Medical Research.* Oxford, UK: Blackwell Publishing; 2002.

13. Siegel S, Castellan NJ. *Nonparametric Statistics for the Behavioral Sciences.* New York, NY: McGraw-Hill; 1988.

14. Higgins JJ. *Introduction to Modern Nonparametric Statistics.* Belmont, Calif: Duxbury Press; 2003.

15. McKinney WP, Young MJ, Hartz A, Lee MB. The inexact use of Fisher's exact test in six major medical journals. *JAMA.* 1989;261:3430–3433.

16. Gardner MI, Altman DG. Confidence intervals rather than P values: estimation rather than hypothesis testing. *BMJ.* 1986;292: 746–750.

17. Guyatt G, Jaeschke R, Heddle N, Cook D, Shannon H, Walter S. Basic statistics for clinicians: 2. Interpreting study results: confidence intervals. *Can Med Assoc J.* 1995;152:169–173.

18. Rothman KJ. A show of confidence. *N Engl J Med.* 1978;299: 1362–1363.

19. Fleiss JL, Levin B, Paik MC. *Statistical Methods for Rates and Proportions.* New York, NY: Wiley; 2003.

20. Rimm AA, Hartz AJ, Kalbfleisch JH. *Basic Biostatistics in Medicine and Epidemiology.* New York, NY: Appleton-Century-Crofts; 1980.

21. Forrest M, Anderson B. Ordinal scale and statistics in medical research. *BMJ.* 1986;292:537–538.

22. Jaeschke R, Guyatt G, Shannon H, Walter S, Cook D, Heddle N. Basic statistics for clinicians: 3. Assessing the effects of treatment: measures of association. *Can Med Assoc J.* 1995;152: 351–357.

23. Guyatt G, Walter S, Shannon H, Cook D, Jaeschke R, Heddle N. Basic statistics for clinicians: 4. Correlation and regression. *Can Med Assoc J.* 1995;152: 497–504.

24. Godfrey K. Simple linear regression in medical research. *N Engl J Med.* 1985;313:1629.

25. Kleinbaum DG, Kupper LL, Muller KE, Nizam A. *Applied Regression Analysis and Other Multivariable Methods.* Boston, Mass: Duxbury Press; 1997.

26. Moore DS, McCabe GP. Looking at data relationships. In: Moore DS, McCabe GP, eds. *Introduction to the Practice of Statistics.* New York, NY: WH Freeman; 2006:123–127.

27. Charuhas PM, Cheney CL, Aker SN, Stern JM, Barale KM. Effect of glucose polymer on serum magnesium in adult allogeneic marrow transplant recipients. *FASEB J.* 1989;3:A1071.

28. Matthews DE, Farewell VT. *Using and Understanding Medical Statistics.* Basel, Switzerland: S. Karger Publishers; 1996.

29. Kaiser L. Adjusting for baseline: change or percentage change? *Stat Med.* 1989;8:1183–1190.

30. Samuels ML. Use of analysis of covariance in clinical trials: a clarification. *Controlled Clin Trials.* 1986;7:325–329.

31. Egger MJ, Coleman ML, Ward JR, Reading JL, Williams HJ. Uses and abuses of analysis of covariance in clinical trials. *Controlled Clin Trials.* 1985;6:12–24.

In memoriam: This chapter was originally written by Carrie L. Cheney, PhD, RD, a talented researcher, writer, and educator. Carrie played an important role in five of the chapters of the first and second editions of *Research: Successful Approaches.* Her premature death made poignant the production of this edition, and especially this chapter that covered her passion—statistical analyses. The current authors updated terminology and references and reworked some of the transitions. However, they purposely maintained nearly all of Carrie's wise advice and excellent examples as a salute to her years of dedication to teaching research methods.

PART 9

—ɯ—

Presentation of Research Data

29

—ᗰ—

Techniques and Approaches for Presenting Research Findings

Judy A. Driskell, PhD, RD, and Elaine R. Monsen, PhD, RD

Before research is initiated, the researcher(s) should give some thought as to where and in what format the research findings should be presented and/or published. The results of the research should add to current knowledge in an area of importance. The time spent in conceiving, designing, conducting, analyzing, and evaluating the research will be beneficial when researchers prepare their findings for oral and written presentations. Methods needed to conceive, design, conduct, analyze, and evaluate research were discussed in previous chapters. Ethical issues are of importance in the research process and are discussed in Chapter 3.

Research findings are presented orally and in written form using various techniques and approaches. The intended audience who will listen to or read the research findings presentation must be taken into consideration when planning effective presentations. It may be that the same research findings will be presented to dietetics and related health professionals or lay audiences, and in this case, the presentations should be different so as to be of interest and informative to the specific audience, sometimes referred to as the target audience. The research findings should be presented to audiences at audience-appropriate technical levels, using audience-appropriate visuals and/or writing formats and styles. When researchers can select the professional conference/meeting or the professional journal to which they submit their research findings, usually as an abstract or a manuscript, the interests of the audience that typically goes to the conference/meeting or that typically reads the journal should be considered in making this

selection. What you present on paper and how you present it reveals your knowledge, the quality of your thinking, and your standards of excellence (1). The same is also true of what is presented orally.

Good visuals and graphics are excellent tools for researchers attempting to express ideas, show patterns, and give results. Good written and oral communication gives depth, substance, and understanding to the visuals (2). Much planning goes into giving effective oral and written presentations of research findings. The following is a discussion of major types of presentations and suggestions for organization and professional communication.

TECHNICAL REPORTS

There are many times and many reasons that dietetics professionals need to prepare technical reports such as proposals for equipment and/or program support, interim reports, summary reports, and evaluations. Each type of report requires a specific emphasis. It is important, in the preparation of a report, to become familiar with the guidelines and requirements of the agency or group to which the report will be submitted.

In writing the report, consider carefully your aim. Draft the report clearly in light of your goals. It is wise to outline the report. In fact, a highly effective step is to develop several different outlines that you then evaluate, selecting the one that best suits your purpose. Once you accept an outline, use it and write with an eye toward your audience.

In the technical report, state the issues or problems, provide useful data, and give constructive resolutions. Devising effective headings is helpful in presenting the material you have selected. Using keywords in your headings will add to the impact of your report. Provide useful figures, graphs, tables, and, if appropriate, a bibliography. Review and revise your report. Remember, you can revise the report for a different audience if needed at a future date.

One technique report writers find useful is to start with a well-stated question. The ending of the report can summarize the tentative answers to the proposed question, including the how, why, and what. A concise abstract may be useful, if appropriate and if allowed. Such an abstract can be set apart, thereby alerting the reader of its importance. Appendixes and glossaries can also be developed as needed, but be sure that they add substantially to the report. And, of course, people and institutions aiding the research should be graciously acknowledged. The last sentence or section should give a strong summation and indicate the value of the report.

An excellent reference for report writing is Reinking and von der Osten's *Strategies for Successful Writing: A Rhetoric, Research Guide, Reader and Handbook* (3). Key features of several types of reports are described in the pages that follow.

Proposals

Clarity and focus are prime objectives of a good proposal. Focus on what you are proposing and requesting. If appropriate, indicate connections with other research. Potential benefits of the research can be stated. Proposals may require justification of proposed costs, the need for new programs and personnel, cost benefits, expected outcomes, and projected timelines. Assess carefully the guidelines of the group to which the proposal will be submitted. A useful Web site for government-related grants is Grants.gov (4). Chapter 4 discusses how to write proposals to successfully obtain funding.

Interim Reports

Interim or progress reports are usually required by granting agencies, and those agencies provide guidelines as to the structure and content of the reports. The purpose of these reports is to show how the goals and objectives of the original proposal have been met during a specified time frame. Explain the methods used and provide key results to date. Review prior work that you mentioned in earlier interim reports to place the current report in context. Discuss your results in light of the goals of the project. You may wish to complete your interim report with a statement of the next steps in your research and the potential benefits.

Summary Reports

A summary report is usually required at the end of a grant or project. This report follows the same structure as the interim report, but it may also contain a discussion of problems encountered and how they were solved or recommendations for solving those problems in future studies or projects. Present the sequential steps in your research, based on a clear explanation of the methods. Where possible, use strong visual presentations in graphs and tables for key results. Complete the summary report with a conclusion based on your findings, indicating future directions and the potential value of your research. Be sure to interpret your results in meaningful ways, emphasizing key points.

Evaluation Reports

One of the more exciting reports to prepare is an evaluation. Usually, an evaluation report is done at the end of the project, but one also may be needed during the project, and definitely before further requests and proposals are made. Evaluations often serve as a basis for proposals. Evaluation reports summarize the data and put the data and their implications into context. Issues to consider in developing your evaluation include why you did the research, what your research was, what is unique about your work and your results, how your results relate to the work of others, and what next steps you propose. It usually is appropriate to indicate, clearly, the value of your findings. Adding comments about future research needs is usually appropriate and will be valuable later on when you prepare related proposals.

PRESENTATION ABSTRACTS

Frequently, researchers and others submit abstracts to professional organizations for review and possible presentation at a professional conference/meeting, such as the Food and Nutrition Conference and Exposition (FNCE) sponsored by the American Dietetic Association (ADA). Generally, professional organizations require that abstracts be original research or material and that the findings have not been previously presented at national or international meetings and have not been published elsewhere. Researchers who have completed research projects and wish to submit abstracts for presentation at a professional conference/meeting should first decide to which professional organization they wish to submit the abstract. These individuals are encouraged to investigate which professional organizations have members who would be interested in their research findings. Also, the locations and dates that the professional conferences/meetings are to be held should be taken into consideration. Obviously, you should not submit an abstract or presentation for a conference/meeting that you cannot attend.

Today, most health-related professional societies have information on their Web sites about when and where their conferences/meetings will be held. Their Web sites most often also contain information about what their expectations are of abstracts submitted for presentation and submission deadlines. Most professional organizations publish the abstracts presented at their meetings. Researchers can also look at an organization's published abstracts from the previous year in deciding whether the organization is appropriate for presentation of their research findings.

Research is the foundation of the dietetics profession (5). In 2007, the ADA indicated that "an abstract is a brief written summary of the specific ideas or concepts to be presented, and a statement of their relevance to practice or research" (6). Also in 2007, the ADA called for submission of the following two types of presentation abstracts (6):

- Research abstracts [that] include a brief description of the author's original research methodology, including design, subject characteristics and procedures, major findings, and conclusions or implications for dietetics practice
- Project or program reports abstracts [that] contain information about the need or purpose for such a program, project, or tool development; the theory or previous research upon which it is based, or setting for its use, if appropriate; the unique characteristics of the project, program, or tool; the characteristics of subjects or target audience involved; and the type of evaluation or proposed use for the tool or instrument development

Organization of Abstracts

Most professional organizations, including the ADA, have written instructions as to what information should be included in an abstract submission, as well as the required or suggested format for the abstract. These instructions are generally given on the organizations' Web sites, although some professional organizations mail instructions to their members.

Most professional organizations reject a submitted abstract in which the authors did not follow the written instructions. Most professional organizations will also reject submitted abstracts in which the research is still in progress and the submitted abstract does not contain research results and/or conclusions.

Professional organizations frequently request that abstracts be submitted in certain topic categories. If this is the case, be sure the topic of the abstract you wish to submit is in one of these topic categories; otherwise it may be rejected. Most professional organizations allow those submitting abstracts to indicate whether they prefer a poster, oral, or either type of presentation; usually oral and/or poster presentations must be in specific topic categories. It may be that the topic of the abstract you wish to submit should be submitted to another professional organization. In many instances, manuscripts submitted to professional organizations must be prepared using specific fonts and font sizes, such as Times New Roman, 12-point font. If tables are permitted in the abstract, these tables may have to be prepared in a certain manner, such as using Word's Table feature, and be within the abstract's allotted space.

Writing a good abstract for submission takes time and effort. Several drafts of the abstract are usually prepared before the abstract has the allocated number of words or is the correct length for the space yet contains the essential research objectives, methods, findings, conclusion, and, sometimes, applications.

Submitting Abstracts

Some professional organizations require that one of the submitting authors be a member of their organization or that a member of their organization sponsor the abstract submission; this information is generally given in the call for abstracts. Individuals who made substantial intellectual contributions to the research should be listed as coauthors on the abstract, and all coauthors should participate in the writing of the abstract. Multiple authors are typically listed in an order indicating which individuals have made the most substantial contributions; however, in university settings, frequently the name(s) of the major professor or senior investigator(s) is listed last and the names of the graduate and/or postdoctoral students most involved with the research project are listed first. Researchers should identify prospective coauthors during the process of initiating their research projects.

Abstracts must be submitted by established published deadlines. If an abstract is to be mailed, contributors should note whether the deadline is a postmarked or a received deadline. Many professional organizations require that abstracts be submitted electronically at given Web sites by certain deadlines. Before putting abstracts on these Web sites, you should read and understand the rules that these professional organizations have for electronic submissions, particularly noting whether authors can make changes to posted abstracts before submitting the abstracts for consideration of presentation. Currently, some professional organization Web sites allow authors to save before submitting, whereas others do not. These Web sites are generally busy the last few days before the submission deadlines. You should allow sufficient time to resolve any technical problems that may occur during the electronic submission process.

Professional organizations sometimes publish the dates when abstracts that are submitted for presentation will be accepted. Professional organizations usually inform the submitting author whose name is listed first in the author listing or the author who is sponsoring the abstract submission whether the abstract has been accepted or rejected for presentation. Some professional organizations give the first or sponsoring author the reasons for rejection. It may be that the abstract was not properly prepared and submitted or that the subject of the research was not appropriate for presentation at the meeting of that specific professional organization. You should make every effort to submit an abstract that will be accepted for presentation at the selected professional conference/meeting.

PRESENTATIONS

Research findings may be presented at meetings/conferences as poster or oral presentations. First authors or coauthors of accepted presentation abstracts must attend the meeting where the presentation will be given. If an emergency arises, other coauthors can give the presentation. If none of the authors attend the meeting, the first or senior author must contact the individual in charge of presentations and let him or her know that their presentation will be canceled or request permission to have a nonauthor present or post the poster presentation or give the oral presentation. Failure to show up for a presentation jeopardizes

one's future acceptance of submitted abstracts for up to 3 years by some professional organizations, including the ADA (7). One's professional integrity is of utmost importance in this regard.

Presentation materials should be prepared with the expected audience in mind. If the presenter has not previously attended a meeting of the group or organization, he or she should seek guidance from individuals who have attended the meetings, particularly recent meetings. Presenters should consider the expertise of their audience with regard to their presentation topic when planning the visuals as well as the oral portion of the presentations.

If an abstract was submitted and accepted for a presentation, the presenter should base the oral or poster presentation on the information given in the abstract. Complete details of the research study generally are provided later in a manuscript submission.

Good layout of visual materials, including posters, requires consideration of page and poster dimensions, horizontal or vertical orientation of the visual, use of design templates, consistency (eg, type font and size, colors, background design, and layout), size and number of components, and use of white space (8). Additional information on the preparation of visuals is found in the next chapter. Keep visuals simple (9). The use of primary colors generally provides good color contrasts for presentation visuals (10). Color can also be used effectively in figures to demonstrate the effects of treatments on various measurements. Figures, diagrams, and photos add visual interest and may save space (11). Check to see if your university or company has an instructional design center that can help in the preparation of posters and other visual materials.

Once the visual materials are prepared, presenters should prepare themselves to answer the questions of presentation attendees. Presenters should refresh their memories as to the details of the methods as well as the results. Presenters should practice giving their presentations to individuals as similar as possible to the expected audience and answering questions that audience members might have. The individuals listening to and/or viewing the presentation might give the presenters some tips regarding their presentation materials and ask questions that the audience may be expected to ask the presenter. Practice makes for a better presentation.

Presenters should never put their posters and/or other visual materials in checked luggage when going to a meeting. Visual materials should be transported in carry-on briefcases, tubes, or other types of luggage when you travel to a meeting by plane, train, or bus. You may also want to take copies of the abstract and some business cards.

Presenters should wear appropriate clothing at the meeting/conference, especially when giving their presentations. You should treat the members of the audience with respect. Presentations provide an opportunity for professional networking.

After the presentation, you should evaluate how the presentation went and what questions people had (8). Doing so will enable you to do a better job the next time that they give a presentation, especially one to the same audience.

Presenters sometimes have printed handout materials that are made available to audience members attending oral and poster presentations. Generally, presentation abstracts of meetings/conferences are published in a program book or as a supplement to a professional organization's journal. Handout materials include reproductions of visual materials, pathways, questionnaires, detailed methods, and reference lists. You should decide whether handout materials are appropriate for their presentation and what types of information the audience might like to have available to them as a handout. You might also investigate whether handout materials are generally expected to be available at a specific meeting/conference. If handout materials are to be available, these materials should be typed and be visually attractive. Not every member of the audience will want handout materials, so if you have handouts, these handouts should be available for interested individuals to pick up if they desire.

POSTER PRESENTATIONS

Research findings are frequently presented at professional meetings/conferences, including those of the ADA, as a poster. Poster presenters should be by their poster for the entire time that the poster is scheduled for presentation. Posters on the same or similar subject areas are generally presented during the same session or time frame.

Poster sessions provide a forum for presenting research findings or other informational materials to professional or lay audiences. These sessions provide a setting for interaction with colleagues and others. Posters can be used in many settings and are easily updated as well as being portable. They should inform the audience of the whole research story—abstract, introduction, objectives, methods, results, conclusions, and, sometimes, applications or implications.

Professional organizations usually provide guidelines for preparation and presentation of posters. Posters may be mounted on bulletin-type boards of a certain size or on tabletops. Sometimes poster presenters have to supply their own display boards; if so, panels made with corkboard or such materials are usually used and the poster or poster components are mounted using pushpins or Velcro circles or squares. Posters are generally constructed using lightweight cardboard, poster board, or such materials that can be easily transported. Protective coatings can be put on poster construction materials that will later be posted for several months.

Posters are visual presentations of the research or other type of project. The layout of the poster should visually direct the viewer's eye through the research project. The Federation of American Societies for Experimental Biology, which includes the American Society for Nutrition, provides tips for poster presentations for their 2007 Experimental Biology meetings on the Federation Web site (12). A sample layout for a poster presentation is given in Figure 29.1

When taking a poster to a meeting/conference for presentation, be sure to take such materials as pushpins, pens, pencils, permanent markers, tape, glue, and written copies of poster materials. It may be possible to correct or update information on the poster if compact discs containing the poster materials are available. You may also wish to take wrapping paper or cloth to cover a discolored mounting board or to enhance the visible appearance of your poster.

At the meeting/conference, you should talk with others in attendance, especially those presenting in the same topic area. Meetings provide an excellent opportunity to network.

ORAL PRESENTATIONS

Research findings are frequently presented at professional meetings/conferences, as well as at meetings of lay groups, as oral presentations. Oral presentations should be prepared with the expected audience in mind. Some professional organizations have guidelines for oral presentations given at their meetings/conferences. Practically all organizations have an established length of time allocated for the presentation and for questions regarding the presentation. Some universities and companies provide training for employees and students who are to give presentations.

Organization of Oral Presentations

As with poster presentations, oral presentations should inform the audience of the whole research story, briefly giving the introduction, objectives, methods, results, and

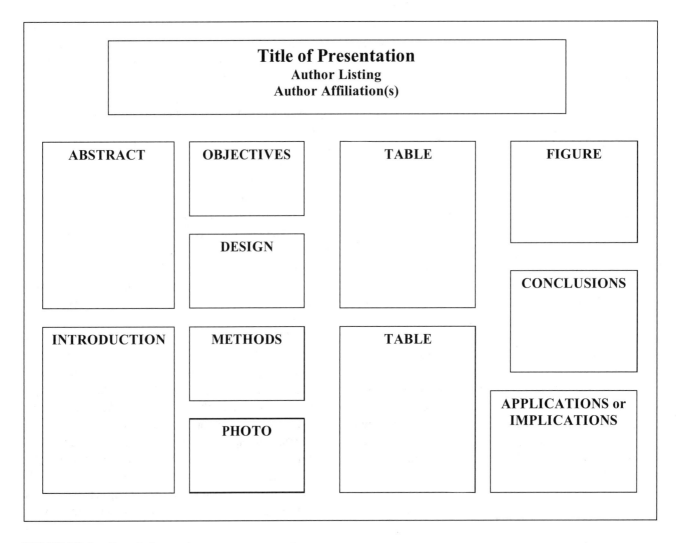

FIGURE 29.1   Sample layout for a poster presentation.

conclusions; sometimes applications or implications are also described. All of these should be covered briefly. You should focus on the important results in your oral presentations.

Developing Visual Materials

As a speaker, you should develop visual materials that support the oral portion of your presentation. First, draft the visuals you plan to use in your presentation. After the drafting is completed, reconsider the informational content of the proposed visual. Is each visual necessary? Are the visual materials written in such a manner that they can be understood by the expected audience? Once you have decided on the information to be presented on the visuals, start designing the visuals. Find out what types of equip-

ment are available for use in the room where the presentations are to be given. Equipment typically used for effective visual presentations of information includes overhead projectors, slide projectors, and computer projectors. Videotape and film may also be used in oral presentations. After developing the visual materials, verify that these visuals project well using the equipment. You also need to practice using the selected visual equipment so that you know how to manipulate the controls for the equipment and to project your visual materials on the screen; you should also evaluate your materials for readability.

Overhead Projection

Transparencies displayed on an overhead projector are easy and fast to prepare and transport to meetings. All the words on transparencies should be typed, and the print size should be large enough to allow audience members at the back of the room to read the words. The print should not be smudged and should have good contrast with the background, which is usually projected as white. Color may be used for emphasis. Photos, tables, and figures should be easy to read.

A disadvantage of using an overhead projector is that transparencies have to be placed and replaced manually by the speaker or another person. In larger rooms, the speaker is usually at a podium, which may be some distance from the overhead projector. Presenting research findings using an overhead projector is more appropriate for use in small than large rooms; overhead projection also works well in interactive lectures and workshops. You can write on transparencies while speaking using wet-erase pens. The marks made with these pens can be removed later, restoring the transparency to its original appearance.

Slide Projection

Slides, generally $2'' \times 2''$, are sometimes used for oral presentations in both small and large rooms. Today, slide projectors are occasionally used in presentations involving visual projections of photographs.

Computer Projection

Computer software such as PowerPoint or Word is frequently used in preparing visuals for presentation. These visuals are projected in the meeting room via a projector that is connected to a computer. Remote-control slide advance devices are generally available in meeting rooms so that you can control the order and speed at which visual materials are projected. Computer projection is currently the method of choice for the presentation of visual materials in oral presentations in most, if not all, professional meetings/conferences.

Before you begin using computer software to prepare your visual materials, you need to be aware of computer operating systems and software that will be available during the presentation. At meetings of smaller groups, speakers generally provide their own laptop computers and projectors, but this generally is not true when presentations are given in larger rooms. Professional organizations usually have oral presentation guidelines that indicate what types of computers, operating systems, and software are available in the meeting rooms so that speakers do not need to bring their own laptop computers. You should check the professional organization's oral presentation guidelines with regard to whether the use of personal laptop computers is permitted during these presentations.

Individuals at universities and companies who are scheduled to give oral presentations frequently can get help preparing their visuals from design or communication centers once they have a rough draft of their visual materials. Tips for creating a better PowerPoint slide show are given in Box 29.1 (13).

Oral presentations that incorporate visual materials developed through the use of computer software can be either effective or distracting. Be careful not to give the visual materials the center stage. Fancy slide transitions and fly-ins (eg, moving inserts) can be distracting. Sounds and movies can add some excitement to presentations but may not work. You should always consider your audience. Remember the following four things when preparing visual materials for technical presentations: simplicity is not simple, visual communication means thinking visually, visual materials support your presentation and information, and project your visuals in a test run before the formal presentation (2).

Most large meetings/conferences provide practice rooms where speakers can practice their oral presentations. These rooms have the equipment that is available in the meeting rooms. Speakers should use these practice rooms and verify that their visual materials project as expected and are readable.

Videotape and Film

Oral presentations may consist of or include videotapes and film. These multimedia components are used more often when presentations on the same topic are given many times or to demonstrate procedures or behaviors. A renowned expert's presentation may be recorded using videotape or film so that many audiences could view the videotape or film and thus obtain information from the expert. Videotape and film can enhance some types of oral and poster presentations, although they are expensive to produce and require that certain equipment be available for the presentation. Sometimes, but not often, videotape and film are used to present research findings at professional dietetics meetings. Videotape and film can also be used in poster presentations. However, videotapes, in particular, are most often used in various types of instructional programs.

Oration Techniques

After preparing the visual materials, most speakers, particularly less experienced speakers, draft the oral portion of their presentations. Writing down the oral portion helps speakers organize their presentations and allows speakers

BOX 29.1   Tips for Creating a Better PowerPoint Slide Show

1. **Think visually.** Keep text to a minimum and add a visual component to enhance communication.
2. **Use readable fonts.** Use sans-serif fonts (such as Arial or Helvetica) as these are easier to read on the screen than serif fonts (such as Times New Roman or Garamond). Avoid using italics and underlining; use color, bonding, or a different font to make a word stand out.
3. **Choose your background color based on a room's lighting and always make sure there is high contrast between the background color and the text color.** If you are not sure of the lighting level of the room where your presentation will be given, you may want to take along two versions of your slide show—one with a dark background and one with a lighter background.
4. **Type your slides' text content in the Outline View.**
5. **Insert images into PowerPoint.** All images must be inserted directly into PowerPoint through the Insert > Picture command. If you use copy-and-paste to add an image, you may corrupt your file.
6. **Duplicate a slide.** Duplicate a slide if used more than once or if much of the slide is used a second time.
7. **Prevent the audience from "reading ahead" in your slide show.** Do this by bringing in the bulleted text (or other object) one at a time. Use the Custom Animation feature to create this effect.
8. **Use the Reapply option to "delete" a layout or format change.** Use the Reapply option to "delete" a layout or format change on an individual slide and return to the template or Master slide default setting.
9. **Create presentation notes for yourself.** With your slide show open, select View > Notes Page. Enter desired text. Use the Page Down key to move to the next slide. Select File > Send to > Microsoft Word. Then select the "Notes next to slide" option and click OK.
10. **Make a copy of linked Web pages.** If you use the Hyperlink option to create a link to a Web page(s), you may want to create a local copy of the Web page. Having a local copy will help in case there is an Internet connection problem or in case the Web server is unavailable.
11. **Start your slide show from the desktop.** With your slide show open, go to File > Save As. In the Save As dialog box, change the Save As type option to "PowerPoint show (*.pps)." Change the "Save in" location to Desktop.
12. **Create your slide show using the same equipment as you use in your presentation.** All mediums do not show color the same; plus if you use a different computer, it may not have the same fonts (and bullets) you used to create the slide show. If the fonts are not on the computer used for the slide show, PowerPoint will make an automatic (and unannounced) font substitution. If there is a question if the fonts will be available, you can use the "Pack and Go" feature to include font files with your slide show file. Be sure to preview your slide show on the equipment you will use during the presentation.

Source: Reprinted with permission from Johnson L, Peters P. Tips for Creating a Better PowerPoint Slide Show. Available at: http://cit.information.unl.edu/tips/ppt-creating.htm. Accessed April 28, 2006.

to ensure that all important points are covered (10). Key points may be typed, usually in bold, in the PowerPoint notes page area or on index cards or paper. These notes should be typed in a sufficiently large font to allow you to easily read them. Never read a presentation or memorize it.

The most helpful thing you can do to ensure a successful oral presentation is to practice. Practice enables you to spot problems in the presentation and to get rid of them. Practice also enables you to transition from section to section instead of having awkward starts and stops (2). If possible, rehearse your presentation in front of colleagues. Videotaping practice sessions may also be beneficial so that you can

identify difficult words or phrases as well as any distracting mannerisms you may have. Avoid using slang as well as stalling, hesitant speech ("ums," and "uhs"). You should time your presentations. Videotaping or audiotaping, if videotaping equipment is not available, will help you build confidence.

You should display enthusiasm for your presentation topic, project your voice, exhibit voice inflections, pace the presentation so that it is not too slow or too fast, use effective visual materials, maintain eye contact with the audience, and appear relaxed (10). Pay attention to the amount of time allocated to your presentation. Some organizations will stop the speaker after the time limit has expired. Speakers should be considerate of the time allocated to their presentations.

Speakers presenting their own research findings should be highly confident (10). They have reviewed the relevant literature, designed and conducted the research, and assessed and evaluated the results, and their presentation abstract has been prepared, usually peer-reviewed, and accepted for presentation. Thus, they know more about their own research than anyone else does.

The visual materials used during the presentation will help keep you from deviating too much from the planned presentation. However, you should not have your back to the audience for prolonged periods as they view information on the visuals (2). Generally, you should not have to point out items on well-developed visual materials.

If possible, visit the room where you will give your presentation in advance. Also, if possible, stand at the podium and test the audiovisual equipment that you will use later during your presentation. It is also helpful, if possible, to watch other speakers giving earlier presentations at the same meeting.

After you are introduced, you should walk to the podium, locate the controls to the visual equipment, arrange your notes, thank the individual who introduced you, and look at the audience briefly before starting your presentation. While at the podium, relax and slightly spread your feet so as not to appear stiff. Attempt to exhibit good posture. Many experienced speakers find it helpful to place their hands on the sides of the rostrum.

Most members of an audience choose to attend a presentation. Early on in the presentation, you have the opportunity to convince them that they made a good choice (2). However, if people leave during the presentation, you should not let their leaving disturb you. Frequently many presentations are going on at the same time, or some individuals in the audience may need to do other things.

Be prepared to answer questions following your presentation. Acknowledge the question, paraphrase it for the audience if needed, and answer it concisely. As noted earlier, having colleagues pose practice questions can help prepare you to answer audience questions. Frequently no or little time is available for questions following presentations, and in this case, you should stay after the meeting and be available for discussion with individuals.

PUBLISHING RESEARCH FINDINGS

Researchers should publish their research findings if they believe that their study was well done and that their research findings would add to knowledge in the subject area and would be of interest to others in the profession. Research findings may be published in various types of research or extension bulletins, book chapters, books, and journal articles. All of these publications are generally peer-reviewed, or viewed for quality by one's peers, and hence would be referred to as refereed publications.

Individuals who made valuable intellectual contributions to the research should be coauthors of the publication. All coauthors should participate in the writing of the publication.

Other individuals who did not contribute intellectually to the project, such as those who assisted with data collection, coding, computer programming, and writing, are listed by name in the Acknowledgments section of the publication. In addition, the subjects are frequently thanked for their participation in a research project in the Acknowledgments section. A discussion of which individuals should be included as authors and which should be acknowledged is included in Chapter 4. The International Committee of Medical Journal Editors created uniform requirements that discuss the ethical principles relating to publishing and evaluating manuscripts in the biomedical area (14); the *Journal of the American Dietetic Association* follows these principles.

Writing for publication is time-consuming and demands attention to detail and commitment. However, the publication of one's research findings adds to the body of knowledge in the subject area. After the research findings have been published, the vast majority of researchers are pleased that they have shared their research findings in writing with interested colleagues as well as with others who may in the future be interested in the area.

Research and extension bulletins, book chapters, books, and journal articles usually must be written according to certain guidelines. These guidelines may be obtained from the proposed publisher or from the publisher's or sponsoring organization's Web site. This chapter covers the process of publishing a research article in a refereed journal, such as the *Journal of the American Dietetic Association*. However, the process of publishing is rather similar for research and extension bulletins, book chapters, and books. Generally an article is referred to as a manuscript until it has been published.

Writing a research publication takes considerable time and effort. Researchers should develop a reasonable writing schedule for themselves and stick to it. Suggestions for writing a research publication follow:

- Identify small goals within the overall project that can be easily accomplished.
- Set target dates that are reasonable for achieving each goal.

- Reward yourself in some way each time you reach one of your goals.
- Seek regular feedback from individuals with expertise.
- Allow time in your schedule for at least two to three revisions.

Publications represent a permanent way to disseminate research findings. The time taken to prepare publications is well worth the effort from professional satisfaction and advancement viewpoints.

Selecting the Journal

Potential authors need to spend some time deciding which journal might publish their findings. Which journals have published research findings that are in the same subject matter area as the proposed article? Journals have specific readerships, or audiences that subscribe to that journal. If the authors have given a presentation at a meeting/conference sponsored by a professional organization, the authors may be required to submit the manuscript for that project to that organization. Read several recent issues of the journal to make sure that it is the right place to submit the manuscript.

Once you have decided which journal to submit your manuscript to, acquire the most recent guidelines for authors for that journal and obtain a copy of an article or two on a topic similar to the one you wish to write that has been published in that specific journal. Reading and following these guidelines is important and will save time in manuscript preparation. It is easier and better to prepare a manuscript according to directions given in the guidelines than to reformat the manuscript after it has been written (15). For example, the *Journal of the American Dietetic Association* accepts three types of peer-reviewed research articles: research, research and professional briefs, and research editorial. Current guidelines are available on the ADA Web site under the Publications header (16).

Planning a Research Manuscript Submission

Obviously, researchers must first have research data that they wish to publish. Research studies may generate data for more than one publication. The manuscript that one wishes to have published generally addresses one major theme.

As with other writings, outlining the manuscript is helpful. If the research findings have already been submitted or published in abstract form, this abstract will be useful in helping one outline the manuscript. Most journals have preferred or required formats and related information that should be presented in each section of the manuscript. Manuscripts usually contain the following sections: Introduction, Methods (sometimes called Materials and Methods or Subjects and Methods), Results, Discussion, and References (sometimes called Literature Cited). Sometimes the Discussion contains the Conclusions and Applications/Implications, and sometimes these are separate sections. In some journals, Results and Discussion are combined as one section. The *Journal of the American Dietetic Association* publishes a detailed overview of the components of a research manuscript on its Web site (15).

Most manuscripts also have abstracts. An abstract provides a brief overview of the research study's design and findings. Abstracts should be understandable without reference to the text. The *Journal of the American Dietetic Association* requires structural abstracts for manuscripts submitted in the Research category and conventional (ie, unstructured) abstracts for those submitted as Research and Professional Briefs (16).

Researchers should draft a tentative title for their manuscript. The title should be specific and informative yet brief. Some journals limit the number of characters that can be in the title. Some journals also require a running title, or shortened title, with less than a certain number of characters, which will be printed on some of the pages of the printed article.

Writing the Manuscript

Preparing the first draft of a manuscript is a challenge; notes may be useful. It may be easier to write the manuscript text if the tables and figures that are to be included in the manuscript are drafted first. This helps researchers to focus on their research findings. Many researchers find it easier to then draft the Methods section, followed by the rest of the sections of the manuscript. References should be included in the first draft in a shorthand that the authors understand, not be numbered. Frequently authors use software, such as EndNote, for keeping track of references.

After the manuscript text has been drafted, it is beneficial to put the manuscript away for a week or so. During this time, you can reflect on what you have written and perhaps get new ideas. Carefully review the journal's guidelines for authors before reading the first draft with a fresh objective view. You should then revise the manuscript, being sure to evaluate whether the manuscript contains all the information about the study so that the reader can understand why the research was conducted. You should state the objectives, describe all methods in detail and reference them as needed, reveal the findings and compare them with the findings of others, explain what the findings mean, and describe the applications and implications derived from the findings. The manuscript text should flow logically. To accomplish this, you may need to move a portion of the manuscript forward or backward in the manuscript.

After the second draft, the manuscript should be read by a knowledgeable colleague or two, particularly those who have published recently in that specific journal or in similar journals. Colleagues' suggestions should be used in strengthening the manuscript. Their suggestions should be viewed as constructive. Coauthors are also responsible for the quality of the paper. Coauthors may provide portions of the first and second drafts of the paper.

The manuscript should be revised as many times as deemed necessary. Pay close attention to details such as commas, colons, semicolons, and table and figure formatting; you may need to make some corrections. The reference formatting in the text needs to be appropriate for the journal to which the manuscript is being submitted (eg, 1, 2, 3; Adams *et al.,* 2003; or Adams et al 2003). The reference style should be that of the journal. After polishing the manuscript, authors should once again put it away for a week or so, and then evaluate it for correctness.

Writing manuscripts is not easy. Even experienced authors often struggle with the writing process. However, experienced writers generally are better able to accept suggestions and take criticism than the less experienced.

Submitting the Manuscript

Today manuscripts are generally submitted online. Most journals publish checklists for authors to use to prepare their manuscripts for submission. Usually page and sometimes line numbers must be added on the manuscript text. Journals also require that manuscripts be submitted in conjunction with copyright forms. Currently the *Journal of the American Dietetic Association* indicates that manuscript submissions should contain the following (as appropriate): cover letter, abstract, author page, manuscript, tables and/or figures (attached as separate files), acknowledgment page (if any), copyright/authorship/conflict of interest form, and funding disclosure (16).

Peer Review of Manuscripts

Having colleagues review the manuscript before submission is beneficial. Journal editors or associate editors select peer reviewers who agree to review specific manuscripts with regard to their content, originality, scientific accuracy, clarity, completeness, and contribution to new knowledge. Many journals have anonymous reviewers. Some journals permit authors submitting manuscripts to suggest reviewers, and one or more of these suggested reviewers may be selected, usually along with reviewers selected by the editor or associate editor, to review the manuscript. Peer reviewers are most often recognized experts in the same specific research area of the submitted manuscript. Frequently one of the reviewers of a submitted manuscript is a member of that journal's editorial board, such as the *Journal of the American Dietetic Association*'s Board of Editors. Reviewers make suggestions and ask questions that are meant to be helpful to the authors.

After peer review, usually 1 to 3 months following submission, the corresponding author will be notified whether the manuscript has been accepted, will be reconsidered for acceptance following revision, or is rejected. If the manuscript is to be reconsidered for acceptance following revision, you should revise the manuscript in accordance with suggestions made by the reviewers and editor in a timely fashion and resubmit the revised manuscript to that journal. If the manuscript is rejected, you should carefully consider the comments of the reviewers. In most cases, the manuscript can be revised and submitted to another appropriate journal for publication; you will probably need to reformat the manuscript according to the new journal's author guidelines. Many inexperienced authors feel like failures when their manuscripts are rejected. Perhaps the manuscript should have been submitted to another journal anyway. All authors who have published extensively have likely had a manuscript rejected.

Between Acceptance of Manuscripts and Publication of Articles

A lag of 6 months to 12 months is typical between the acceptance of a manuscript and its publication. Copy editors of the journal will edit the accepted manuscript for style, grammar, and other items specific to that journal. The corresponding author will receive page proofs, also known as galleys, of the edited manuscript to proof carefully before publication of the article. Generally, authors are given only a few days to indicate corrections that need to be made on the page proofs because publishing deadlines must be met. These requested corrections are generally sent to publishers electronically. Most publishers also require that authors pay page costs (unless page costs were waived by the journal) and order reprints at or near the time that the page proof corrections are requested. Most publishers or journals hold the copyright on materials that are published by them.

CONCLUSION

Research findings may be presented orally or in written form. Researchers should consider their intended audience when preparing research presentations. Visuals and graphics are components of most presentations.

Technical reports—including proposals, interim reports, summary reports, and evaluative reports—should be clearly written, with an emphasis on objectives. The importance of the findings should also be addressed.

Frequently research findings are presented at professional conferences/meetings, generally prior to publication. Writing a good abstract takes time and effort; abstracts are usually drafted several times and must be submitted, often on-line, by published deadlines. Once accepted, these abstracts are generally published.

Research and program findings may be presented at meetings as poster or oral presentations. Presenters should consider the layout of visual materials for both poster and oral presentations. Visual materials should be easily readable and understood. Presenters should also prepare themselves to answer questions from the audience. Practice makes for better presentations. The complete research story—abstract, introduction, objectives, methods, results, conclusions, and, sometimes, applications or implications—should be covered in poster and oral presentations. Often professional organizations provide guidelines for poster and oral presentations.

Research findings should be published if the research was well done and adds knowledge in the subject area. These findings are typically published in professional journals, research or extension bulletins, and book chapters. Peer-reviewed journals publish research of good quality. Authors need to consider which journal to submit their manuscripts to. After that decision is made, the guidelines for authors for that journal should be obtained. An outline of the manuscript is prepared, and then the various sections of the manuscript are drafted; these sections usually include the abstract, introduction, methods, results, discussion (or results and discussion), and often conclusions or implications. After the manuscript has been drafted, it should be reviewed again after 1 week or 2 weeks and revised. If possible, have knowledgeable colleagues read the manu-

script and give their suggestions for revisions. Once you are satisfied that the best manuscript possible has been prepared and that it meets the journal's guidelines, the manuscript should be submitted to the journal, where it usually is peer-reviewed. Frequently authors are requested by the journal editor to revise manuscripts and resubmit them. Sometimes the manuscripts are rejected; when that occurs, authors should revise their manuscripts and resubmit them to another appropriate journal. More often than not, revised manuscripts are accepted and published in the journal.

REFERENCES

1. Leady PD, Ormrod JE. *Practical Research: Planning and Design.* 8th ed. Upper Saddle River, NJ: Pearson Prentice Hall; 2005.

2. Rupnow JH, King JW, Johnson LK. Thinking verbally: communication tips for technical presentations. *Food Technol.* 2001;55:46–48.

3. Reinking JA, von der Osten R. *Strategies for Successful Writing: A Rhetoric, Research Guide, Reader and Handbook.* 7th ed. Upper Saddle River, NJ: Pearson Prentice Hall; 2004.

4. Department of Health and Human Services. Grants.gov: Find. Apply. Succeed. Available at: http://grants.gov. Accessed May 23, 2007.

5. American Dietetic Association. Research: Foundation of the Dietetic Profession. Available at: http://www.eatright.org/cps/rde/xchg/ada/hs.xsl/career_914_ENU_HTML.htm. Accessed May 23, 2007.

6. American Dietetic Association. The 2006 Call for Abstracts. Available at: http://www.eatright.org/fnce. Accessed May 23, 2007.

7. American Dietetic Association. *FNCE Poster Presentation Guide.* Chicago, Ill: American Dietetic Association; 2007.

8. King JW, Johnson LK, Rupnow JH. Thinking visually: graphic tips for technical presentations. *Food Technol.* 2001;55:49–56.

9. Institute of Food Technologists. *Call for Abstracts.* Chicago, Ill: Institute of Food Technologists; 2006.

10. Chernoff R. Techniques and approaches for presenting research data. In: Monsen ER, ed. *Research: Successful Approaches.* 2nd ed. Chicago, Ill: American Dietetic Association; 2003:419–431.

11. Maltby HJ, Serrell M. The art of poster presentation. *Collegian.* 1998;5:36–37.

12. Federation of American Societies for Experimental Biology. Poster Presentation Guidelines. Available at: http://www.faseb.org/meetings. Accessed May 23, 2007.

13. Johnson L, Peters P. Tips for Creating a Better PowerPoint Slide Show. Available at: http://cit.information.unl.edu/tips/ppt-creating.htm. Accessed May 23, 2007.

14. International Committee of Medical Journal Editors. Uniform Requirements for Manuscripts Submitted to Biomedical Journals: Writing and Editing for Biomedical Publication. Available at: http://www.icmje.org. Accessed May 23, 2007.

15. Lawrence DJ, Mootz RD. Research agenda conference 3: editor's presentation: streamlining manuscript submission to scientific journals. *J Neuromusc Syst.* 1998;6:161–167.

16. American Dietetic Association. Information for Authors. Available at: http://www.adajournal.org/authorinfo. Accessed May 23, 2007.

30

Illustrating the Results of Research

Shortie McKinney, PhD, RD, FADA

Just as research becomes valuable when shared through scientific dissemination channels, research gains power and influence when conveyed in ways that are easy to understand. The combination of an understandable text and a clear presentation of the data helps the author make a stronger connection with the consumers of research.

Transforming data into meaningful formats is an important skill for researchers to develop. Careful review of scientific journals can help point to more or less effective approaches to presenting data. In addition, researchers can learn from their colleagues at scientific meetings through oral and poster presentations of research.

Effective presentation of research results can make the most complex research study understandable. Achieving this goal poses a challenge to even the most experienced investigator. This chapter addresses the use of illustrations—tables, graphs, distribution maps, photographs, algorithms, and flowcharts—to enhance communication of research results. The basic methods of conveying research outcomes involve tables and graphs. Researchers need to use the basics well but should also be knowledgeable about other graphic methods that may more effectively communicate the findings.

This chapter emphasizes the most widely used types of illustrations—tables and graphs—as they are used in published works. In addition, lesser used methods will be discussed as well as concepts to consider when developing illustrations.

The usefulness of illustrations in enhancing text (especially for textbooks) has been the subject of considerable study (1–4); however, an extensive search of the literature reveals that relatively little research has been directed toward the types of illustrations used in reporting research results. In addition to the published references listed in this chapter, you are encouraged to use the Internet to find online sources that show examples of various types of illustrations and resources to develop professional-looking illustrations.

PURPOSES OF ILLUSTRATIONS

Illustrations are used to make information more understandable; depict relationships; add needed emphasis; or allow the presentation of important, exact data in a clear and compact form. Types of illustrations and their functions are listed here:

- **Table:** Representation of exact data in compact form
- **Graph:** Display of trends or relationships in quickly interpretable form
- **Distribution map:** Display of the location of data
- **Photograph:** Accurate representation of the appearance of the subject (eg, a clinically observable disorder, microorganisms, or newly developed equipment)
- **Algorithm, flowchart:** Display of the steps in a procedure that lead to one or more outcomes
- **Other diagrams:** Simplified representation of the subject

In a set of guidelines for statistical reporting in medical journals, Bailar and Mosteller (5) state, "Restrict tables and figures to those needed to explain the argument of the paper and to assess its support. Use graphs as an alternative to tables with many entries; do not duplicate data in graphs and tables." These noted statisticians argue for economy in presentation as a method of increasing the chances that an article will be read. At the same time, authors need to consider the role of graphics in enticing the casual reader to look more closely at the text. The type of illustration selected should contain enough information to stand alone without referring to the text.

Illustrations will vary depending on the intended purpose. Published works, posters, slides, or transparencies should be prepared differently to support the method of viewing. Although all types of illustrations are generally suitable for inclusion in research articles, some are unsuitable for display in a poster or on a screen where the goal is to share the message quickly. For these purposes, research results must be greatly simplified. Guidelines for preparing materials for posters (6–8) and slides (9–11) focus on simplicity and clarity.

MESSAGES TO BE CONVEYED BY ILLUSTRATIONS

In deciding on illustrations for research articles, investigators should focus on the messages they wish to convey concerning the data, both in general and illustration by illustration. Different kinds of illustrations send different messages and serve different functions. Varying methods for illustrating similar data sets just to introduce variety in an article is inappropriate. Extreme complexity in illustrations should be avoided. Authors should strive to simplify as much as possible. Consider the audience and design the illustrations to match with the knowledge base of the audience. Too many speakers in professional meetings apologize for the complexity of their data slides; generally this is because they have used a published table or figure without consideration of the intended audience. You would be wiser to spend time revising illustrations to match the mode of presentation than use inappropriate graphs and charts that were designed for a different purpose.

ILLUSTRATIONS AS A SET

The number of illustrations included in a research article should be kept to a minimum so that the reader can easily comprehend the article's overall message and the data that support it. In fact, most journals advise authors to keep illustrations to a minimum, and reviewers frequently recommend that some illustrations be deleted or condensed. More extensive illustration may be appropriate for monographs, technical reports, and some types of scientific books.

Consistency adds clarity. Scientific journals therefore specify a style for tables and require its use. However, many journals do not have rigid specifications for graphs and other figures. Because these journals reproduce the figures submitted with the manuscript, authors are advised to give special attention to consistency, accuracy, and scale when preparing a set of figures. A consistent use of symbols is recommended, along with similar proportions and style. For example, a series of graphs comparing food use by different ethnic groups should represent these groups using consistent symbols in line graphs or types of fill in bar graphs.

When deciding the order in which comparison groups are to be presented, as in tables or bar graphs, consistency is often undesirable. Instead, the order of presentation ordinarily should be determined by the message to be conveyed, as illustrated in Figure 30.1 (12,13). The preferred order appears in Figures 30.1C and 30.1E; this approach places the groups in rank order for ease of comparison. (The category "Other" remains at the end because it includes many different groups with low individual rankings.)

GUIDELINES FOR PREPARING USEFUL TABLES

Many style manuals, such as the *Chicago Manual of Style* (14), give extensive guidelines for preparing tables. However, these manuals tend to deal only superficially with substantive issues in handling data. Day (15) provides a number of examples of both poorly designed and well-executed tables. Colton (16) and Ehrenberg (17), both statisticians, and Clark (18), a noted editor, present complementary suggestions for making the data in tables more understandable. Many of these suggestions are listed in Box 30.1 (16–19).

Essential Categories of Information

Clark specifies the categories of information that should be included in a table to provide a complete picture of the data (18). She recommends organizing information before actually preparing a table by producing a descriptor set that uses the categories in the far left-hand column of Table 30.1. This table also includes examples of Clark's approach using a

A. Original Graph

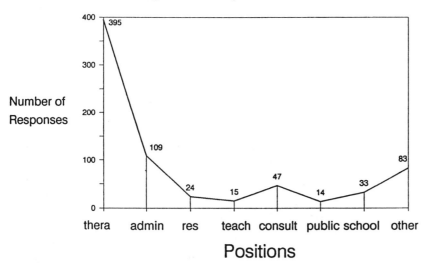

B. Direct Conversion of Data in Figure 23.1A to Bar Graph

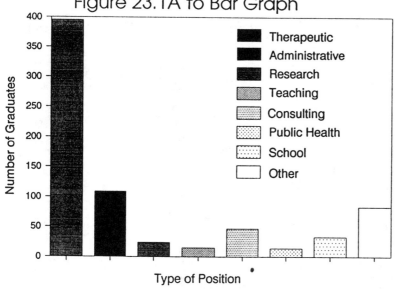

FIGURE 30.1   Examples of original and improved methods of depicting the same data. Example A is not a recommended method for several reasons: the implication of being a frequency polygon is misleading, abbreviations are used that are not standard and may not be clear to all readers, arrangement of the data is not in a logical order, and the actual frequencies are given on the graph. Example B is an improved version of the same graph. However, this version would be even better if the order were changed so that the positions (ie, type of employment) appeared in descending order of frequency, if the shading reflected the relative frequency, and if the vertical axis displayed the percentage of graduates in each type of position, rather than absolute numbers.

hypothetical data set. An additional item to include is identification of the sample size, which is necessary for interpretation of the generalizability of the data.

Stages of Table Reading

Table reading is an important skill to aid the reader in quickly interpreting data. Clark (18) identifies three stages of table reading: scanning, reading and primary comparisons, followed by second-level comparisons. In the

scanning stage, the reader looks across the column heads and down the stub (ie, descriptive labels in first column on left side of table). More experienced readers will scan more intently. Clark asserts that, in the reading stage, readers glance across the rows of data, and they assume that the column heads are the categories being presented for comparison, even if that was not the intent of the author. Ehrenberg advises authors to present the numbers to be compared in columns rather than in rows (17). No scientific basis was found for choosing one approach over the other, but if authors are formatting data in columns and readers are

C. Improved Bar Graph

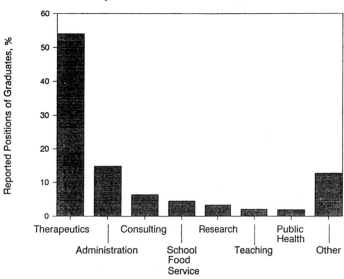

Type of Position

FIGURE 30.1   *(Continued)* Example C depicts some of these changes and uses an alternative approach for labeling. The names of the positions have been changed slightly to be more consistent in style and more informative. Example D shows how a vertical bar graph can aid in labeling. This graph was made with default settings, which used vertical grid marks and data labels. Example E shows the same graph customized to delete grid marks and labels, which cluttered the graph. Example A is reprinted from Fiedler KM, Raguso A, Morgan G, Renker L. A retrospective study of graduates of a coordinated internship/master's degree program. *J Am Diet Assoc.* 1990;90:591–596. Reprinted with permission from the American Dietetic Association.

D. Revised Bar Graph (Preliminary)

Type of Position

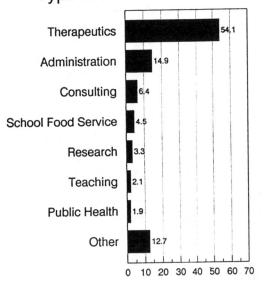

Reported Positions of Graduates, %

E. Revised Bar Graph (Preferred)

Type of Position

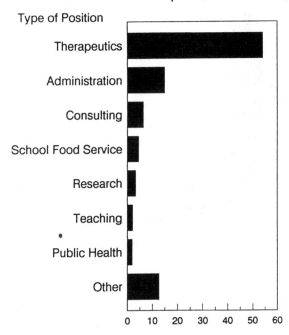

Reported Positions of Graduates, %

expecting to compare rows, likely misinterpretations will result. Authors should carefully consider the best approach to organizing rows and columns for their particular data. Depending on the type and complexity of data, transposing columns and rows may be more or less difficult.

A major advantage of placing the data to be compared in columns is to facilitate labeling. And the use of consistent units of measure for all items in a column is preferable. Nutrient comparisons generally do not follow this guideline; nutrients are listed down the stub, which keeps nutrient

BOX 30.1   Tips for Creating Clear Tables

Provide complete information in the table:
- Label clearly, making sure to include a label for the stub list (ie, the far left-hand column of the table) and the column heads. Difficulty in identifying a suitable label is likely to indicate a problem in organization of the data.
- Clearly indicate units of measurement.
- Indicate totals, where applicable, to summarize the data in the table and to help reconcile the data with those in other tables and material in the text.
- Show in which direction the percentages add to 100% in order to inform the reader how the percentages in the table were derived.
- Use tables when they promote a clearer summary of results than would prose.
- Avoid complex tables.

Carefully consider table layout and organization:
- Provide a visual focus by giving means for the rows and columns. (Often this procedure is not possible for the types of data displayed in dietetics journals.)
- Arrange the columns and rows in a logical order; facilitate comparisons when relevant.
- Round appropriately to reflect the precision of the data collection instrument (ie, round the mean to no more than one decimal place beyond the data summarized, and the standard deviation to no more than two decimal places).
- Use the text to lead the reader to important patterns and exceptions.

Source: Data are from references 16–19.

TABLE 30.1   Categories of Information Necessary for a Complete Representation of Data in Tables

Category	Definition	Example (Comment)
Current source of the table	Author, publication date	From Smith et al, 1990 (necessary only for data taken from sources apart from an original research effort; especially necessary in review articles)
Source of the data	Data collector and period of data collection	Statewide Preschool Nutrition Survey, 1981–1982
Observer	Respondents: Who reported the values?	Food intakes by preschoolers as reported by their mothers and day-care providers
Matter	Entities involved in the event covered in the table	Preschoolers ages 3–5 yr; milk consumption
Function	Nature of the event covered and factors that may influence it	Milk intake; race; income
Space	Location of the event	Large state, such as Alaska; the United States
Time	Period when the event occurred	1981–1982 (in studies examining past events—or exposures, as in case-control studies—this time may be much earlier than the time given by the period of data collection)
Aspect	What was measured and to what topic does this point?	Mean intake in grams in a single 24-hour period; points to weight of all forms of fluid milk
Domain	Range of values	0, . . . , 790 g
Sample size	Number of subjects (total and in subgroups)	$n = 100$; males = 60, females = 40

Source: Data are from reference 18.

data tables from becoming excessively wide and favors comparisons across the rows.

Sometimes a table can be laid out to convey a strong visual message; the use of graphic symbols within the table visually strengthens the message. A more visual approach is shown with a more standard approach in Table 30.2 (20). In this example, incompatibility of vitamin/mineral preparations with enteral feeding mixtures was originally shown

TABLE 30.2   Alternative Approaches to Presenting the Same Information in Tabular Form

30.2A.   Slightly Modified Excerpt from a Table by Burns PE, McCall L, Wirsching R (21)

Physical Compatibility of Vitamin/Mineral Preparations with Products X, Y, and Z

Medication	Degree of Compatibility*		
	Product X	Product Y	Product Z
Vitamin/mineral preparations			
Feosol	4	4	C
Gevrabon liquid	4	4	C
KCl elixir	C	C	C
Fleet Phospho-soda	1	4	C
Neucalglucon syrup	3	4	C
Theragran liquid	C	C	C
Zinc sulfate capsules	4	4	C

*C indicates *compatible*. Incompatibility is measured on a scale of 1 to 4, with 4 being the most incompatible or hardest to unclog.

30.2B.   Example of a More Visual Presentation of the Same Data

Physical Compatibility of Vitamin/Mineral Preparations with Products X, Y, and Z

Medication	Degree of Compatibility†		
	Product X	Product Y	Product Z
Vitamin/mineral preparations			
Feosol	• • • •	• • • •	C
Gevrabon liquid	• • • •	• • • •	C
KCl elixir	C	C	C
Fleet Phospho-soda	•	• • • •	C
Neucalglucon syrup	• • •	• • • •	C
Theragran liquid	C	C	C
Zinc sulfate capsules	• • • •	• • • •	C

†C indicates *compatible*. Incompatibility is measured on a scale of 1 to 4, with 4 dots (• • • •) being the most incompatible or hardest to unclog.

Source: Both tables are adapted from Burns PE, McCall L, Wirsching R. Physical compatibility of enteral formulas with various common medications. *J Am Diet Assoc.* 1988;88:1094–1096. Adapted with permission from the American Dietetic Association.

using letters related to the level of incompatibility. In the revision, solid black dots represent the level of incompatibility and more effectively highlight the problem visually.

USE OF COMPUTER GRAPHICS SOFTWARE

Computer graphics programs have been beneficial to researchers because they have made it easier for authors to enter data into a spreadsheet program and then graph it in a variety of ways. This ease of graphing data has likely reduced the need for highly skilled (and often expensive) illustrators to manually plot data and has increased the volume of illustrations starting from elementary school upward (21). With graphics software, researchers can quickly flip through a series of illustration methods with the click of the mouse. Unfortunately, the visually attractive results of these programs do not always convey an appropriate message.

Researchers may need to experiment with a variety of software programs to find one that will have the desired graphics outcomes. The best of these software packages are relatively expensive, so care should be taken in evaluating the one to purchase. Although most spreadsheet programs have a graphing capability, they typically have more limitations than a program designed specifically for developing illustrations. Try software before purchasing it to determine whether the program will offer the variety of illustrations required and sufficient flexibility to customize images. Graphing programs have changed a great deal in the past several years so check the capabilities of current versions. Be sure the software matches the type of data and illustrations you seek. No one program will work for all researchers.

Increased computer capabilities have resulted in rapid developments in the graphic display of results from multidimensional modeling. Suggestions for avoiding unintentional misrepresentation of data or other common problems that may be associated with the routine use of graphics software are incorporated in this section.

Guidelines for Preparing Useful Graphs

When adding text to graphs, use initial capital letters only, rather than all uppercase letters. Words written in lowercase letters are easier to read (13,22,23). Avoid using bold, italic, and underline in graphs unless the emphasis helps to guide the reader in understanding the graph. Unless data are three-dimensional, do not use multidimensional computer graphs that imply a z-axis, when the data are plotted along only the x- and y-axes.

Choice of Graph Type

Standard graph types include line graphs, scatter graphs, histograms, frequency polygons, bar graphs, stacker bar graphs, and pie charts. Texts such as *Illustrating Science: Standards for Publication* (13) are good sources of information on the appropriate use of each type of graph. Determine the message you want to convey and select graphs that will support that goal.

Graphs serve two general purposes: to examine data and to communicate data to others. Stem and leaf diagrams and scatter plots are types of graphs that are useful for finding out whether a few data points are strongly influencing measures of effect. Such graphs are useful for data interpretation, but they are seldom used in communicating the results of studies. Box plots depict important aspects of the distribution of data (24). (See articles by Hebert and Waternaux [25] and by Worthington-Roberts and associates [26] for examples of the use of a box plot graph for reporting the results of nutrition research.)

Important Characteristics of Graphs

According to Tufte (23), "graphical excellence is the well-designed presentation of interesting data—a matter of substance, of *statistics,* and of *design.*" He demonstrates ways to achieve clear, precise, and efficient communication of complex ideas and emphasizes displaying truthful messages with the data. He objects to graphs that have a small ratio of data to ink—as is the case with many bar graphs, for example. (See Figure 30.2 [27] for a superior alternative to such bar graphs.) Tufte compiled a useful list of suggestions for enhancing the visual display of statistical information:

- Choose proper format and design.
- Use words, numbers, and drawing together (eg, short messages that help explain the data).
- Produce a balanced, well-proportioned graph with a relevant scale.
- Display complex detail (ie, the data) in a simple manner (ie, avoiding abbreviations and elaborate codes).
- Tell a story with the data, if appropriate.
- Draw the graph in a professional manner.
- Avoid decorations and moiré effects (eg, hatched lines).

Colton (16), in turn, emphasizes three important characteristics of graphs:

- Graphs should aid the reader's comprehension of the material. A large number of variables are generally confusing, even with ingenious graph design.
- The axes of graphs should be clearly labeled and include the units of measure. A glance should suffice for alerting the reader to what is being illustrated and the units of measurement. More complete labeling (eg, "Percentage of Iron Absorbed") helps convey the message, whereas cryptic labeling of the vertical axis of graphs (eg, only the word "Percentage") should be avoided.
- Graphs should be scaled to represent the data and their importance accurately. Often only a small portion of the scale is used, which may overemphasize the difference between groups.

Improper or misleading scaling often occurs unintentionally, especially when graphics programs are used. Computer default settings are designed to be user-friendly by providing the user with standard preset elements. For graphics programs, default settings for the range, the scales of the *x*-axis and *y*-axis, the typeface, and so forth, are intended to make it easy to produce standard graphs that look good (at least to the casual observer). Default settings for the range of the vertical axis are based on the range of the data being displayed. Therefore, these settings minimize unused space, which is generally a desirable outcome. However, the net result is that the default settings often use an inappropriately high scale that makes minor differences appear major. The researcher should make sure that the reader can easily tell if a scale does not start at zero and whether the scales represent arithmetic or mathematical (eg, logarithmic) change. The investigator also should make sure that scales correspond exactly if graphs are to be compared. In all cases, you must inspect all graphs visually for completeness, clarity, and accuracy before using them.

Achieving Consistency in Graphs

To achieve visual consistency, the same computer software should be used to prepare all the graphs for a given report. If two or more programs must be used, special steps may be required to achieve consistency in the use of symbols, fill, and lettering. Use of the same software to prepare all the graphs in a set does not ensure consistency of scale for graphs that are likely to be compared. For example, the linear distance in millimeters between tick marks on graph A should be identical to that on graph B. To achieve this consistency, the preparer of the graphs must avoid the use of default settings for the vertical axis and be sure to specify

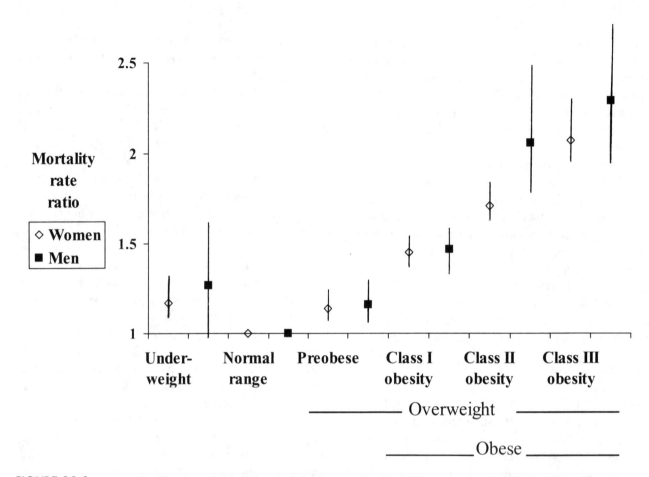

FIGURE 30.2   Rate ratios for death from all causes in white men ($n = 57,073$) and women ($n = 240,158$) by World Health Organization body mass index categories (underweight ≤ 18.4; normal range = 18.5 to 24.9; preobese = 25.0 to 29.9; class I obese = 30.0 to 34.9; class II obese = 35.0 to 39.9; class III obese ≥ 40). Values were adjusted for age, education, and physical activity. All values were significantly different from normal range at $P < .001$.

This graph illustrates the display of comparisons of means along with standard error (SE) among different categories of a factor. This graph is superior to bar graphs in displaying parameters of continuous variables, such as means, medians, and the accompanying standard error, standard deviation, or percentiles. Note that the parameters of interest are clearly shown, as is the range of values within the error bars, and that the graph does not distort the size of the differences between categories; a maximum ratio of data to ink is used, as recommended by Tufte (23). A bar graph, in contrast, uses a small ratio of data to ink; the bars do not represent data points or any specific parameter from the data, and the relative size of the bars is not proportional to the difference among the categories compared. A bar graph is useful for frequency data (ie, number or proportion of a discrete scale variable). A point graph, as shown, more clearly shows the parameters of interest (here, the rate ratios along with SE). Reprinted with permission from Stevens J, Cai J, Juhaeri, Thun MJ, Wood JL. Evaluation of WHO and NHANES II standards for overweight using mortality rates. *J Am Diet Assoc.* 2000;100:825–827. Reprinted with permission from the American Dietetic Association.

the same range for all graphs to be compared (eg, "0% to 100%" or "2.0 mmol to 6.0 mmol"). Some graphics software allows the user to change the size of the graph. If this feature is used, identical changes in size should be made in all graphs that are to be compared. Furthermore, the authors must specify that identical reductions be made in preparing the art for printing.

Illustrating Science: Standards for Publication (13) contains an outstanding set of guidelines for the preparation of graphs, including detailed methods for improving visual clarity. The book advises individuals preparing graphs to choose symbols for data points that reproduce clearly and are easily discernable. See Chapter 29 for detailed information about presenting research findings.

Graphical Perception

Graphical perception involves the way graphical information is interpreted and visually decoded by the reader; differences in line lengths, size of pie chart segments, and color saturation can be used to quickly convey information to the reader (28). According to Cleveland and McGill (28), the elementary tasks in graphical perception can be ranked from most to least accurate, as shown in Table 30.3. Because a graph is successful only if it is accurately and efficiently decoded, researchers should keep abreast of new developments in this rapidly changing field of study. The Internet has accelerated the expansion of visual media. As society moves to more graphical information sharing, researchers will need to incorporate graphical techniques that resonate with the more visual nature of readers.

Marcus (29) describes principles of visual organization and the limits of perception that can be useful to know in developing clear displays of complex relationships. Among his recommendations are the use of sans serif typefaces such as Arial or Helvetica; simplified imagery to delete unnecessary details; open spaces to guide the eye; and consistency of design, including reliance on a grid of implied lines. Marcus recommends that similar things be arranged in similar ways and that items be positioned to make the visual hierarchy clear. He further recommends that lines and symbols in charts have a relationship to the information to which the chart refers. For example, represent relatively imprecise data by relatively thin, rather than thick, lines. Visual emphasis can be achieved through the use of heavier lines, larger type, and gray levels. These recommendations, however, are more applicable to illustrations for posters or slides than for most published works.

Cleveland and McGill (28) provide experimental evidence that specific graph types are interpreted more accurately than are certain other types. In particular, they recommend dot or bar charts in place of pie charts, and dot or bar charts with grouping in place of stacked bars. Dot charts use dots to represent a particular number of individuals or data elements. Component (ie, stacked) bar graphs merit special attention because they are widely used to depict the components of a whole and are easy to create with graphics software. A major problem with these graphs is that they require estimation of length along nonaligned scales.

Cleveland and McGill (28) further recommend the direct display of the differences between two curves in place of the curves themselves. Messages conveyed by curve-difference graphs are greatly different from those conveyed by graphs that depict the two curves separately. If the object is to show that one treatment consistently produces better results than another, a graph showing the two curves is more appropriate to use. If the difference between values at various time points is important, curve-difference graphs or a table of differences would be superior.

Determine whether the difference between the curves warrants emphasis. Some readers who compare graphs in which the curves are close together suspect an error because of the great difficulty of visually perceiving absolute differences between two adjacent curves.

OTHER FORMS OF ILLUSTRATIONS

Histograms

Histograms display frequency distributions; the areas of the rectangles in the histogram represent the frequency of the data. Accurate scaling of the horizontal axis must be maintained. Thus, if intervals are unequal (eg, they represent different time periods), the width of the rectangle should reflect this inequality. As shown earlier in Figure 30.1, graphics programs allow researchers to choose any one of many graph variations, not all of which are acceptable. A better alternative might be to use horizontal bar graphs (Figure 30.1e) so that complete labels can be used rather than abbreviations or other, sometimes awkward strategies.

TABLE 30.3   Elementary Tasks in Graphical Perception in Decreasing Order of Accuracy

Elementary Estimation Task	Examples
1. Position along a common scale	Height or length of a bar that is part of a bar graph
2. Position along nonaligned scales	Heights of segments in identical closed rectangles
3. Length, direction, angle	Comparison of line lengths without any point of reference; relative sizes of segments in a pie chart
4. Area	Difference in size of two charts
5. Volume, curvature	Difference in volume of two or more spheres
6. Shading, color saturation	Differences in shading on distribution maps

Data are from reference 28.

Distribution Maps

Distribution maps focus on the location of data and can be useful in depicting differences in rates, ratios, total amounts, or percentages by area. For example, a map of the United States in which states are grouped by census regions can be used to depict differences in breastfeeding rates in different parts of the country. A state map can be used to identify counties with an unusually high or low prevalence of obesity, and a city map can be used to identify census tracts where members of an ethnic minority reside in large numbers. Shades from light to dark are often used to depict numerical values from low to high. This practice has some drawbacks: regardless of the numerical value, large areas tend to appear more important, and differences in the shades of gray may be overestimated, implying larger differences in the numerical values (13). If such maps are used, seven intervals for the data should be the maximum number.

Cleveland and McGill (28) suggest the use of framed rectangle (ie, blocked rectangle) charts as replacements for distribution maps in which shading denotes quantitative information. Framed rectangles show the level of a variable within a particular population group or region. They can be overlaid on a map to show how a variable varies geographically.

Photographs

Photographs bring the element of reality to the reader. A photograph showing clinical signs of a rarely seen nutrient deficiency reinforces the author's statement that a specific treatment can lead to serious nutrition problems and thus the importance of nutrition intervention. *Illustrating Science: Standards for Publication* (13) and *A Guide to Medical Photography* (30) contains detailed information on photography and points to consider in the reproduction of photographs. Staged photographs need to be used with care to avoid being misleading. Authors should ensure that the correct message is conveyed by a photograph. Differing cultural perceptions need to be considered.

Images of gel electrophoresis are an example of a specialized use of photography entering the nutrition literature. Genetic researchers use these techniques to investigate the response of different tissues to a stimulus. If a gene is present or activated, a dark band is present at a particular point on the gel. Photographs of these gels are used to show results of an experiment.

Algorithms and Flowcharts

Increasing numbers of algorithms and flowcharts are appearing in the dietetics literature. Algorithms are used for clarifying complex decision-making processes; algorithms list each step in a process, indicating points where various actions occur. Flowcharts are graphic representations of algorithms and make it easier for the reader to visualize steps in the process. The major tasks involved in the process are placed within carefully selected shapes and arranged logically. The shapes used are informative for those familiar with standard conventions, but knowledge of these conventions is not required for understanding the diagram. Drawings used as part of a flowchart should be easily recognizable. Decision points may be highlighted by question marks or branching of the flowchart to show the impact of various decisions. Because the difference in time required by the two data collection methods was one of the reasons for the research, this information is included in the diagram in concise form.

The same symbol should not be used to represent two different variables. For example, if N is used in the legend to denote the number of an activity node, a different symbol, such as T, should be used to denote the time required for the activity. Different codes should be used to denote times at various steps so that the reader realizes that each time is different.

CONCLUSION

Researchers preparing research illustrations should select the proper type of illustrations to serve specific functions, identify the messages to be conveyed, and develop the illustrations as a compatible set. They should pay particular attention to conveying important messages with clarity, simplicity, consistency, and accuracy. Once the illustrations are prepared, the investigator should examine the visual effect of those illustrations, both individually and as a set, and make adjustments as needed. Peer review of illustrations can be extremely helpful in identifying potential areas for misinterpretation and to determine whether key points are accurately conveyed.

REFERENCES

1. Willows DM, Houghton HA. *The Psychology of Illustration: Basic Research.* Vol 1. New York, NY: Springer-Verlag; 1987.

2. Goldsmith E. *Research into Illustration: An Approach and a Review.* Cambridge, UK: Cambridge University Press; 1984.

3. Duchastel PC. Research on illustrations in text: issues and perspectives. *Educ Commun Technol J.* 1980;28: 283–287.

4. Levie WH, Lentz R. Effects of text illustrations: a review of research. *Educ Commun Technol J.* 1982;30: 195–232.

5. Bailar JC III, Mosteller F. Guidelines for statistical reporting in articles for medical journals: amplifications and explanations. *Ann Intern Med.* 1988;108: 266–273.

6. Jackson K, Sheldon L. Poster presentation: how to tell a story. *Paediatr Nurs.* 1988;10:36–37.

7. Warmuth JF. Perspectives on research. *J Nurs Staff Dev.* 1988;4:192–193.

8. Ryan NM. Developing and presenting a research poster. *Appl Nurs Res.* 1989;2:52–55.

9. Kroenke K. The 10-minute talk. *Am J Med.* 1987;83: 329–330.

10. Garson A Jr, Gutgesell HP, Pinsky WW, McNamara DG. The 10-minute talk: organizations, slides, writing, and delivery. *Am Heart J.* 1986;111: 193–203.

11. Johnson V. Picture-perfect presentations. *Training Develop J.* May 1989;45–47.

12. Fiedler KM, Raguso A, Morgan G, Renker L. A retrospective study of graduates of a coordinated internship/master's degree program. *J Am Diet Assoc.* 1990;90:591–596.

13. Scientific Illustration Committee of the Council of Biology Editors. *Illustrating Science: Standards for Publication.* Bethesda, Md: Council of Biology Editors; 1988.

14. *The Chicago Manual of Style.* 15th ed. Chicago, Ill: University of Chicago Press; 2003.

15. Day RA. *How to Write and Publish a Scientific Paper.* 6th ed. Westport, Conn: Greenwood Press; 2006.

16. Colton T. *Statistics in Medicine.* Boston, Mass: Little, Brown and Co; 1974.

17. Ehrenberg AC. The problem of numeracy. *Am Statistician.* 1981;35:67–71.

18. Clark N. Tables and graphs as a form of exposition. *Scholarly Publishing.* 1987;19:24–42.

19. Lang TA, Secic M. *How to Report Statistics in Medicine: Annotated Guidelines for Authors, Editors, and Reviewers.* 2nd ed. Philadelphia, Pa: American College of Physicians; 2006.

20. Burns PE, McCall L, Wirsching R. Physical compatibility of enteral formulas with various common medications. *J Am Diet Assoc.* 1988;88:1094–1096.

21. Fuhrmann S, MacEachren A, DeBerry M, Bosley J, Taulor RL, Gahegan M, Downs R. MapStats for kids: making geographic statistical facts available to children. *J Geography.* 2005:104:233–241.

22. Hartley J. Planning the typographical structure of instructional text. *Educ Psychol.* 1986;21:315–332.

23. Tufte ER. *The Visual Display of Quantitative Information.* 2nd ed. Cheshire, Conn: Graphics Press; 2001.

24. Williamson DF, Parker RA, Kendrick JS. The box plot: a simple visual method to interpret data. *Ann Intern Med.* 1989;110:916–921.

25. Hebert JR, Waternaux C. Graphical displays of growth data. *Am J Clin Nutr.* 1983;38:145–147.

26. Worthington-Roberts BS, Breskin MW, Monsen ER. Iron status of premenopausal women in a university community and its relationship to habitual dietary sources of protein. *Am J Clin Nutr.* 1988;47: 275–279.

27. Stevens J, Cai J, Juhaeri, Thun MJ, Wood JL. Evaluation of WHO and NHANES II standards for overweight using mortality rates. *J Am Diet Assoc.* 2000; 100:825–827.

28. Cleveland WS, McGill R. Graphical perception: theory, experimentation, and application to the development of graphical methods. *J Am Stat Assoc.* 1984;79:531–554.

29. Marcus A. Computer-assisted chart making from the graphic designer's perspective. *Comput Graphics.* 1980;14:247–253.

30. Hansell P, ed. *A Guide to Medical Photography.* Baltimore, Md: University Park Press; 1979.

31

Research Publications: The Perspectives of the Writer, Reviewer, and Reader

Jeffrey E. Harris, DrPH, MPH, RD

The writer, the reviewer, and the reader have different perspectives as they approach research publications. The writer wishes to publish his or her findings to advance knowledge in the scientific community. The reviewer volunteers time to help ensure the quality and clarity of research in the literature in as timely a fashion as possible. The reader wants to familiarize himself or herself with areas of research in order to engage in evidence-based practice.

The registered dietitian (RD) has the opportunity to assume the roles of writer, reviewer, and reader of research publications. Meaningful research that is original, designed to answer specific research questions, current, well organized, meticulously conducted, and effectively communicated characterizes the ideal within the perspectives of all three roles. Guidelines have been developed that assist the writer, the reviewer, and the reader in the implementation, interpretation, and communication of research. Recently, a Publishing Nutrition Research series of articles has been published in the *Journal of the American Dietetic Association* to provide guidance in research design and data analysis to assist with manuscript preparation and evaluation (1–5). World Wide Web–based literature archives and databases and online publishing provide writers with enhanced access, reduced costs, flexible publication formats, and faster publication of articles. Also, there is much easier access to journal articles and systematic reviews to study various subjects. Literature searches are easy to conduct. These developments, however, have raised some issues related to intellectual property, the peer review process,

and the dissemination of research findings to populations without access to current technology (eg, most of the developing world) (6–9). This chapter addresses the three different roles an RD can play in the area of research.

THE WRITER'S PERSPECTIVE

The writer is responsible for scrupulous behavior in the design and completion of research studies, intellectual honesty, and responsible coauthorship (10). The writer, as scientist, has an idea that emerges from an area of interest, from professional experience, or from the literature. He or she develops this idea into a research protocol and fosters it through the stages of implementation, data collection, and data interpretation. Much of this book addresses these issues. The author has an ethical obligation to society to design research that furthers the advancement of the science and submit research protocols and results for peer review. Intellectual honesty, a responsibility of manuscript authors, is essential for the continued professional and public trust of scientific research (10). Scientific dishonesty was defined in 1830 (11) as "trimming," "cooking," or "forging" data, and that definition still applies to published literature today. Chapter 3 discusses ethical issues more thoroughly. The following three suggestions can lead to rational inquiry and intellectual honesty: (a) write only what you mean, and mean what you write; (b) provide all the evidence (including negative findings) honestly obtained, and reason logically from the evidence; and (c) be aware of, and discuss, all substantive counterclaims (based on evidence) to your claim (based on evidence) (10). In addition, do not overstate conclusions, express a biased opinion because of a source of financial support, exclude published credit to ghost-writers, or give published credit to those who contributed very little to a manuscript.

Consultation with a statistician during the design phase and when results are analyzed is essential to prevent the collection of potentially worthless data that do not fit into an appropriate design for statistical analysis (12,13). It may be necessary to establish a network within one's institution and work with identified people who have statistical expertise. It is important to identify a statistician who can assist in the specific domain of the researcher, whether it be foodservice management, clinical nutrition, dietetics education, or community nutrition. Chapters 2, 27, and 28 of this book review methods for design, data analysis, and presentation of research methods in nutrition and dietetics, as well as provide a statistics review and update for the researcher. As previously mentioned, the *Journal of the American Dietetic Association* Publishing Nutrition Research series can be of great assistance when you are in need of statistics guidance (1–5).

Authors should be familiar with the 1997 (printed) and 2006 (on-line, updated) editions of the *Uniform Requirements for Manuscripts Submitted to Biomedical Journals* (14,15). This text, created by the International Committee of Medical Journal Editors (ICMJE), describes the format in which editors agree to receive articles and includes guidelines for presenting statistical aspects of scientific research in ways that are clear and helpful to readers (15). The American Dietetic Association (ADA) also has its own guidelines for the preparation of manuscripts that were substantially revised and published in 2006 (16).

The writer, as communicator, needs to be logical, clear, and accurate in describing the research. He or she should read the literature and learn which journals would be most appropriate for publication of a specific manuscript. Tailoring the format of the manuscript to suit the chosen journal and following that journal's guidelines for authors can expedite the reviewing process (14–20). For instance, the *Journal of the American Dietetic Association* has a format that is different from that of the *American Journal of Clinical Nutrition* or the *Journal of Foodservice Management and Education*.

Submitting a manuscript for peer review can be an invaluable educational experience for the author. Authors are entitled to expect a consistent response from the editor and prompt and courteous treatment of their articles. They should feel free to question why a paper has been turned down. Frequently, authors complain that the months of time spent in reviewing and fine-tuning a paper delays the transmission of knowledge. The time spent refining a manuscript, however, is well spent and relatively minor when compared with the time spent completing the research and writing (21). A review can be facilitated by the author's inclusion of page and line numbers throughout the manuscript and specifically following author guidelines.

An author can best interpret and respond to reviewers' and editors' comments by putting emotions aside. It is important to take constructive criticism not as rejection, but as an opportunity to learn. Adherence to the following suggestions can facilitate communication between the author and the editor about a particular manuscript, as well as future manuscripts (22):

- Consider and respond to all comments and suggestions made by both the editor and the reviewers.
- Do not resubmit a manuscript to the same journal if it is refused for publication; instead, consider the reviewers' and editor's comments and submit to another journal.
- Do not call the editor directly, unless invited to do so.
- Do not approach the editor personally at the annual meeting or elsewhere to discuss a particular manuscript.
- Use restraint in the last paragraph of the manuscript; do not make naive policy recommendations or generic calls for more research. Also, do not overstate conclusions, such as making cause-effect deductions from a research design that does not warrant such deductions.

Irresponsible authorship and wasteful publication in scientific publishing is considered offensive and may be more damaging than fraud or plagiarism (23). Irresponsible authorship is identified as the inclusion, as authors, of persons who made little or no contribution to the work reported or the omission of persons who made major contributions. The responsible writer, as collaborator, acknowledges the complexity of modern dietetics research, which may require a variety of skills and techniques available only from the joint efforts of several people. Principles that can be used for justification for multiple authorship are included in the *Uniform Requirements for Manuscripts Submitted to Biomedical Journals* (see Box 31.1) (14,15,24).

BOX 31.1   Authorship Guidelines

- All persons designated as authors should qualify for authorship. Each author should have participated sufficiently in the work to take public responsibility for the content.
- Authorship credit should be based on only substantial contributions to (a) conception and design, or analysis and interpretation of the data; (b) drafting the article or revising it critically for important intellectual content; and (c) final approval of the version to be published. Conditions a, b, and c must all be met. Participation solely in the acquisition of funding or the collection of data does not justify authorship. General supervision of the research group is not sufficient for authorship. Any part of an article critical to its main conclusions must be the responsibility of at least one author.
- Editors may ask authors to describe what each contributed; this information may be published.
- Increasingly, multimember trials are attributed to a corporate author. For example, this type of author citation is used in articles based on the Women's Health Initiative Randomized Controlled Dietary Modification Trial (24). All group members who are named as authors, either in the authorship position below the title or in a footnote, should fully meet the above criteria for authorship. Group members who do not meet these criteria should be listed, with their permission, in the acknowledgments or in an appendix.
- The order of authorship should be a joint decision of the coauthors. Because orders are assigned in different ways, the meaning of a particular order cannot be inferred accurately unless it is stated by the authors. Authors may wish to explain the order of authorship in a footnote. In deciding on the order, authors should be aware that many journals limit the number of authors listed in the table of contents, and that the US National Library of Medicine (NLM) lists in MEDLINE only the first 24 authors plus the last author when there are more than 25 authors.

Source: Adapted from International Committee of Medical Journal Editors. Uniform Requirements for Manuscripts Submitted to Biomedical Journals (updated February 2006). Available at: http://www.icmje.org. Accessed June 22, 2006.

Abuse with regard to authorship has in part been attributed to the system of academic promotion and reward (25). Many peer-reviewed journals provide clear guidelines for authorship. A summary of policies of several medical journals regarding author criteria and responsibilities indicates that issues related to the ordering of authors and alternative forms of recognition are not addressed by the current guidelines of the ICMJE (26). A different system has recently been proposed that would require that all participants be named as contributors with the intent "to eliminate the artificial distinction between authors and acknowledge and enhance the integrity of publication" (27). Compared with the ICMJE's suggested guidelines for author acknowledgment in manuscript submission (14,15), the alternative system provides more complex, detailed, and accurate descriptions of contributors that better define the efforts of the individuals involved in the work and publication (27). This system substitutes the word *contributor* for *author*. It also designates the role of *guarantor* to contributors who are responsible for the integrity of the entire work. Furthermore, this system helps the reader by identifying for

each contributor the following job descriptions with regard to the work and publication:

- Design of the review, the literature search, the data extraction, the data analysis, the production of the first draft, the revision of subsequent drafts, and the coordination of communication among all investigators
- Literature search, retrieval of articles, creation of data extraction forms, data extraction, data analysis, comments on first draft, creation of first draft of tables, and comments on subsequent drafts
- Generation of the idea for a review on this topic, design of the review, and financial support comments on drafts

Also, contributors are listed in order of percentage of contribution to the entire project.

A scale to determine the order of contributors in a work that involves multiple investigators and contributors has been described (28). Agreements about contributor order at the beginning of collaboration may change by the time the work is ready for publication, based on the actual contributions of collaborators rather than intended activities (29).

Authors should avoid wasteful publication, which includes reporting the results of a single study in two or more papers (or, as Huth puts it, "salami science") and republishing the same material in successive papers that differ only in format and how the content is discussed (23). Wasteful publication also includes blending data from one study with additional data that are insufficient to stand on their own to create another paper, or "meat extending" (23).

The author is required to sign a copyright form stating that the article being submitted is exclusive and has not been published elsewhere. This procedure is designed to prevent the problem of repetitive publication (23).

Electronic databases such as MEDLINE have made literature review for authors easier and far less time-consuming. With the many sources a literature search can generate, the author is responsible for finding, assessing the quality of, and referencing the primary source of the information upon which the submitted work is based.

Many journals currently make their publications available online to increase the ease and speed of access to the most up-to-date information from scientists. The *Journal of the American Dietetic Association* offers ADA members access to current and past journal articles through its Web site. Some databases such as MEDLINE direct readers to journal Web sites where full-text articles can be accessed either for a price or for free. Some journals post manuscripts on their Web sites as they are being reviewed so that scientists get fast access to the most current information and can post comments about the research. If manuscripts are rejected by the journal for publication, they can be withdrawn from the journal's Web site.

Many journals have online systems for submission and review of manuscripts. For instance, the *Journal of the American Dietetic Association* has an on-line editorial manager that the author, reviewers, and the editor use to process manuscripts (30). Anyone interested in publishing in the *Journal of the American Dietetic Association* should become familiar with this Web site.

The advancement of technology during the past decade has created controversy around the issue of copyright control between authors and publishers involved in scholarly communication. Academic authors historically have viewed their work as having "barter value" only—value in achieving tenure, obtaining time and money for research, and building and maintaining a reputation (9). Four areas where academic authors are beginning to seek

copyright control over scholarly communication have been identified. The first area is electronic prepublication, which allows anyone to see preprinted work and work that has not yet been peer-reviewed. The second area is emerging knowledge environments in which the literature of an entire discipline or subdiscipline is brought together digitally for convenience. Authors in these environments are interested in securing the greatest possible flexibility in publishing. The third area in which authors seek more copyright control is personal or laboratory Web sites, where authors can post original writings for teaching purposes. The final area is distance education, which requires printed material and streaming video (ie, transmission to a personal computer via the Internet of audio or video content that is seen and/or heard as the content is received) in lieu of the traditional verbal classroom lecture. Advancements in technology and the changing marketplace for education will likely increase the need for authors to negotiate copyright agreements that will allow the widest possible dissemination of their work and ensure that authors, rather than the publishers, have control over, and barrier-free access to, the accumulating body of scholarship on which future teaching and research will build (9).

There is a wealth of resources that address the issue of copyright. Many are electronically available to writers interested in learning about authors' intellectual property rights (9,31–35).

Three current controversial issues are the publishing of qualitative research, freedom of access to full-text journal articles, and publishing research by dietetics practitioners. Qualitative research has often been considered by the research community to be inferior to quantitative research. Scientists have felt discouraged in their attempts to publish qualitative research. There is a current movement to recognize qualitative research as being useful because it addresses research questions that cannot be explored using quantitative research (36,37).

Some scientists believe that full-text publications should be free of charge online. Some researchers avoid publishing in journals that charge exorbitant prices for access to full-text articles. Many argue that it is the obligation of the research community to make the most current information available to all people. This can be a costly endeavor for journals. Because of cost issues, many "open-access" journals follow a different business model in that they charge authors a fee to publish their manuscripts and therefore can offer free on-line access to full-text articles (38). Open access has its challenges and critics, and the research community is far from agreement regarding on-line access to journal articles.

The number of practicing RDs far exceeds the number of articles published by dietitians (39). The information practitioners could provide could be very valuable when we understand that evidence-based practice has as a foundation the marriage between the best available scientific facts and experience in real-life contexts. Because of lack of time and resources, practitioners are discouraged from conducting applied research (40,41). Ways to encourage research by practitioners must be explored. A recent suggestion is that practitioners collaborate by forming practice-based research networks (PBRNs) (42). Combining resources and efforts may facilitate a greater volume of research activities.

THE REVIEWER'S PERSPECTIVE

Peer review is defined as the critical, judicious evaluation of a manuscript performed by one's equals (43). Peer review plays a critical role in determining the value of a manuscript for publication. Approximately three-quarters of the major scientific journals use some sort of peer review (21). A historical perspective of peer review and guidelines for the reviewer presented by Godlee and Jefferson (21), both affiliated with the *British Medical Journal,* is of interest to authors and critical readers, as well as reviewers. In their guidelines for the reviewer, Godlee and Jefferson emphasize that the unpublished manuscript is a privileged document and should be protected from any form of exploitation. Reviewers are expected not to cite a manuscript or refer to the work it describes before the manuscript has been published, as well as to refrain from using the information contained in an unpublished manuscript for the advancement of their own research. This has become a complicated issue with the posting of manuscripts on journal Web sites before they have been accepted for publication. The reviewer, as confidant, must not plagiarize or use in any form the work that is being reviewed during the lengthy editorial process (44). Therefore, the reviewer, as impartial referee, may be faced with important ethical questions, especially because the author and reviewer often are competitors. A reviewer with an expertise in pediatric obesity may be tempted to use information in a manuscript to further her research agenda, or to reject the manuscript if it competes or predates her findings.

The peer review is a positive, usually constructive critical process that allows the author to enhance the publication. In comments to the author, the reviewer should present criticism dispassionately and avoid abrasive remarks (21). The reviewer assesses organization, originality, scientific reliability, clinical importance, clarity,

correct and current referencing, and suitability for publication. The Guidelines for Manuscript Review used by reviewers for the *Journal of the American Dietetic Association* can be found at the journal's editorial manager Web site (30). In addition, the Web site for the World Association of Medical Editors can be a valuable resource for guidelines for peer review (45).

At the end of the process, the reviewer makes a recommendation to accept the paper for publication, accept it for publication after modification, or reject it for publication in a particular journal. The reviewer may recommend that the manuscript be submitted to another journal and may cite a particular journal (44). Specific statements about the acceptability of a paper are directed to the editor in a confidential cover letter or on a form provided for that purpose. The editor gratefully receives a reviewer's recommendations. However, editorial decisions are usually based on evaluations derived from several sources, and a reviewer therefore should not expect the editor to honor every recommendation (46). Keep in mind the subjectivity of peer review due to the lack of formal training of reviewers. Very few journals offer their reviewers formal training in the task of manuscript review. At times reviews can lack ideal objectivity and a systematic application of guidelines for review. Short-term training workshops have been minimally effective in increasing review quality by reviewers over the long term (47,48).

The peer review not only influences the content of dietetics literature but also directly affects dietetics education in the classroom and in the workplace. The process influences the use or rejection of various dietetics-related interventions, educational models, preventive activities, behavior change strategies, or processes (49). Peer review also benefits the readership by reducing the number of gross errors that appear in the literature, enforces some set of standards for practice, exerts a mechanism for quality control, and stimulates efforts to produce better work and better writing. Potential risks of peer review include delay in transmission of helpful information, as well as the exclusion of new ideas or approaches that conflict with orthodoxy; both of these practices can retard progress (49).

Even though the current referee system may fail from time to time, it represents today's single greatest protection of scientific integrity and excellence (44). If the reviewer accepts the role of teacher by giving constructive criticism and remains open to feedback from the investigator, as in the case of a rebuttal, both investigator and reviewer are provided an educational experience. This effective communication within the editorial review process makes a good paper better and an excellent paper superb (44). Nearly 50% of rejected manuscripts that had the benefit of additional peer review eventually were accepted for publication (46).

The current peer review process has been challenged by some as an area "ripe for systematic research and review" (49). In an interesting study, reviewer performance was evaluated using a preconceived manuscript into which purposeful errors were placed; the study showed that reviewers failed to identify two-thirds of the major errors (50). An International Congress on Peer Review in Biomedical Publications, sponsored by the American Medical Association, emphasized responsibility as it applies to authors and editors and the improvement of quality control over the entire peer review process, the intent being to improve the process (51).

Electronic publication does allow a path for the peer review process to continue. However, concern has been expressed that immediate unreviewed publication, even if only temporary while the peer review process is ongoing, "is risky and might well fill the clinical databases with misleading and inadequately evaluated information." Furthermore, "the few weeks saved between acceptance and print would not justify the confusion and misunderstanding that would attend the immediate electronic posting and subsequent publicizing of clinical studies" (52).

Traditionally, reviewers would conduct a blind review. In a blind review, the reviewer and author are unaware of each other's identity. Recently, some journals, such as the *British Medical Journal,* have gone to what is called "open peer review" or "unblinded review." In this type of review, reviewers and authors are not blind to one another, and they can discuss questions raised by the review of the manuscript. Some journals provide open posting of the manuscript and reviewer comments on their Web sites and allow community comment. The hope is that this process will lead to the publishing of high-quality manuscripts. *Nature* recently attempted to adopt an open peer review process but has since discontinued it. Open peer review is controversial and being debated in the peer review community. An editorial in the *British Medical Journal* published in 1999 effectively framed the debate (53). Since that time, the debated has evolved through postings on science-related blogs.

THE READER'S PERSPECTIVE

People read reports of research in the literature to keep abreast of current findings in their profession and areas of specialty and improve their job performance and practice.

Evidence-based practice is now emphasized in the field of dietetics and its subdisciplines (see Chapter 12). Evidence-based practice is a model of decision making that uses a systematic process to integrate the best research evidence with actual practice and patient or consumer values to optimize outcomes (54). A good example of the importance of evidence-based practice is its integration in the ADA-accepted nutrition care process model in clinical dietetics (55). Also, the ADA is working to provide resources to help RDs engage in evidence-based practice (56). Therefore, RDs must be effective miners of research evidence from the existing scientific literature so that they can engage in effective practice. With so many journals, it is hard to keep track of all findings and developments in dietetics. A recent study described the difficulty RDs have with staying current with scientific evidence and critically evaluating journal articles (54). Current emphasis on compiling systematic reviews is helping practitioners stay abreast of specific research evidence.

The reader, as student and critic, looks for scholarly articles that contribute to the scientific knowledge base, are clearly communicated, can be applied, and promote individual professional development. University-gained knowledge in dietetics is substantially outdated after a few years; RDs must review and update their knowledge regularly through journal publications.

Students generally receive little exposure to any organized method for reading articles in the literature. Critical evaluation of journal articles, however, can be taught to dietetics students by presenting methodological criteria for determining the validity and usefulness of published data. The critical evaluation of dietetics-related literature can be incorporated into a dietetics research course and throughout advanced dietetics courses. Students, as future dietetics professionals, need to be competent in reading scientific journals and understand basic statistics. As previously mentioned, the Publishing Nutrition Research series of articles on research design and statistical methods were published in the *Journal of the American Dietetic Association* to help readers of the journal better understand and interpret statistics (1–5). In addition, Greenhalgh has published the "how to read a paper" series on interpreting statistics and reading scientific papers in the *British Medical Journal* (57). The reader who is trained to be more critical and skeptical of the printed word recognizes the limitations of individual papers, as well as the limitations of the scientific method as applied to a given discipline (49).

Strategies mentioned for keeping current with the literature included forming a journal club at work and allowing professional colleagues and students to share research articles. Another strategy was to read only articles specific to one's interest or area of expertise.

The following steps serve as a guide to readers for the critical selection of articles from the printed literature.

- Look at the title, and determine whether the article is of interest or use to you. If not, go on to the next article.
- Review the list of authors and/or the institution where the research was completed. If the authors are well-known authorities in the subject area and have a good track record of careful and thoughtful work, read on.
- Determine the intent of the article as a practice-oriented piece, a review article, an original research article, or a research or professional brief. If it piques your interest and meets your needs, read on.
- For a practice-oriented piece, a review article, or an original research article, read the abstract. Then decide whether the brief descriptions of the purpose, methods, and sample seem reasonable and the results and conclusions seem valid and useful. If further reading would be of value to you, read on.
- For a practice-oriented or review article, read the text and check it for clarity. Check also the references for appropriateness and sufficiency in number and scope.
- For a research article, read the Materials and Methods section, and critically review it for scientific accuracy, research design, sample selection, and suitability of applied statistical tests.
- For a research article, read the Results and Discussion sections, and critically review them for clarity and appropriateness in interpretation. Check the references for appropriate incorporation into the discussion.
- For all types of articles, read the sections on conclusions, implications, and recommendations, and critically review them for relevant application into practice.

Refer to Chapter 12 for information on evaluating the scientific quality of a journal article.

Once a reader knows how to choose and evaluate articles, he or she must know how to access them. At present, many dietetics-related journals have a Web site from which readers can obtain limited parts of the printed journal's content shortly before, or on the date of, publication. Full-text versions, however, often require a subscription. As mentioned previously, some journals allow

free access to full-text articles. PubMed does not require a subscription (7). Some on-line journals allow readers to review the archives of all papers published by the journal on a particular topic and inform the journal of select topics about which they want to be kept routinely updated. Readers are then alerted by the on-line journal when articles are published that match their interests—an important time-saving service. Authors will automatically receive editorial responses to their work by e-mail (8). The future of on-line articles will also include the publication of abridged forms as hyperpapers (electronic texts with "clickable" [hyperlinked] phrases that take the reader to areas of interest within the paper) (8). This approach is likely to be instituted for all original papers in the *British Medical Journal.*

The Internet makes information readily available worldwide. For the foreseeable future, however, clinicians in developing areas of the world will continue to rely on printed media. Professional development infrastructures in developing countries should expand to include the delivery of Internet resources to support medical education and clinical practice decisions (58).

Often professionals put too much faith in the results of a single publication. Every individual research study has weaknesses and limitations that reduce the validity and reliability of the results. Conclusions from scientific evidence are best made from multiple studies. In the past, writers would compile review articles in an attempt to summarize the research findings of several studies. However, these reviews did not use standardized criteria for including and evaluating articles and making conclusions. Currently, certain groups, such as the Cochrane Collaboration and the ADA, are conducting systematic reviews on a variety of topics using standard procedures and criteria for analyzing evidence (59). Various groups within the Cochrane Collaboration use a consistent system of evidence analysis to review existing studies on various health care–related topics. These systematic reviews are published in the Cochrane Library and posted at the Cochrane Web site. ADA's Evidence Analysis Library published systematic reviews and evidence-based guidelines for practice on its Web site (60). For more on this topic, refer to Chapter 12.

Research shows that RDs in general are struggling to keep up with the scientific literature and many are unfamiliar with systematic reviews (54). A recent study highlighted the barriers to actively reviewing the literature (54). It is vital that dietetics education programs better prepare future RDs to analyze evidence. In addition, practicing RDs need continuing education to help them more efficiently and effectively stay current.

CONCLUSION

RDs have the opportunity to be viewed as the expert resources for nutrition knowledge and the primary communicators of that knowledge to their scientific and administrative colleagues, as well as to the lay public. The tools needed to fulfill these challenging roles lie in the development of a critical readership, a responsible authorship, and an invested group of peer reviewers. Critical readers will become critical reviewers of noteworthy information. Responsible authors will continue to be stimulated to research worthwhile ideas and effectively communicate the findings. Peer reviewers, through their efforts and expertise, guarantee high-quality, valid published knowledge. Journals are, and will continue to be, the most current source of nutrition knowledge; therefore, personal commitment to develop and maintain skills in all aspects of the periodical arena is necessary for RDs to become the readers, writers, and reviewers that they are called on to be.

REFERENCES

1. Boushey C, Harris J, Bruemmer B, Archer SL, Van Horn L. Publishing nutrition research: a review of study design, statistical analyses, and other key elements of manuscript preparation, part 1. *J Am Diet Assoc.* 2006;106:89–96.
2. Boushey C, Harris J, Bruemmer B, Archer SL. Publishing nutrition research: a review of sample size selection and parametric statistics, part 2. *J Am Diet Assoc* (in press).
3. Harris J, Boushey C, Bruemmer B, Archer SL. Publishing nutrition research: a review of nonparametric statistics, part 3. *J Am Diet Assoc* (in press).
4. Bruemmer B, Boushey C, Harris J, Archer SL. Publishing nutrition research: a review of epidemiologic methods, part 4. *J Am Diet Assoc* (in press).
5. Archer SL, Boushey C, Harris J, Bruemmer B. Publishing nutrition research: a review of measurement and diagnostic testing, part 5. *J Am Diet Assoc* (in press).
6. McConnell J, Horton R. Lancet electronic research archive in international health and eprint server. *Lancet.* 1999;354:2–3.
7. Biomedical research publishing: radical changes ahead. *Bull World Health Organ.* 1999;77:610–611.
8. Schroter S, Barratt H, Smith J. Authors' perceptions of electronic publishing: two cross sectional surveys. *BMJ.* 2004;328:1350–1353.
9. Gurry F. The growing complexity of international policy in intellectual property. *Sci Eng Ethics.* 2005;11:13–20.
10. Schiedermayer DL, Siegler M. Believing what you read: responsibilities of medical authors and editors. *Arch Intern Med.* 1936;146:2043–2044.
11. Babbage C. *Reflections on the Decline of Science in England and on Some of Its Causes.* London, UK: Gregg International; 1969.
12. Bailar JC, Mosteller E. Guidelines for statistical reporting in articles for medical journals. *Ann Intern Med.* 1988;108:266–273.
13. Gardner MJ, Machin D, Campbell MJ. Use of check lists in assessing the statistical content of medical studies. *BMJ.* 1986;292:810–812.
14. International Committee of Medical Journal Editors. Uniform requirements for manuscripts submitted to biomedical journals. *Ann Intern Med.* 1997;126: 36–46.
15. International Committee of Medical Journal Editors. Uniform Requirements for Manuscripts Submitted to Biomedical Journals (updated February 2006). Available at: http://www.icmje.org. Accessed June 22, 2006.
16. *Journal of the American Dietetic Association* guidelines for authors. *J Am Diet Assoc.* 2006;106: 140–147.
17. Stein K. Journal adopts use of conventional and SI units. *J Am Diet Assoc.* 2005;105:1186–1187.
18. Chernoff R, ed. *Communicating as Professionals.* 2nd ed. Chicago, Ill: American Dietetic Association; 1994.
19. Day RA, Gastel B. *How to Write and Publish a Scientific Paper.* 6th ed. Phoenix, Ariz: Oryx Press; 2006.
20. Huth EJ. *Scientific Style and Format: The CBE Manual for Authors, Editors, and Publishers.* 6th ed. New York, NY: Cambridge University Press; 1994.
21. Godlee F, Jefferson T. *Peer Review in the Health Sciences.* London, UK: BMJ Publishing Group; 2003.
22. Samet JM. Dear author—advice from a retiring editor. *Am J Epidemiol.* 1999;150:433.
23. Huth EL. Irresponsible authorship and wasteful publication. *Ann Intern Med.* 1986;104:257–259.
24. Prentice RL, Caan B, Chlebowski RT, et al. Low-fat dietary pattern and risk of invasive breast cancer: the Women's Health Initiative randomized controlled dietary modification trial. *JAMA.* 2006; 295:629–642.

25. Marusic A, Marusic M. Authorship criteria and academic reward. *Lancet.* 1999;353:1713–1714.

26. Gaeta TJ. Authorship: "law" and order. *Acad Emerg Med.* 1999;6:297–301.

27. Rennie D, Yank V, Emanuel L. When authorship fails: a proposal to make contributors accountable. *JAMA.* 1997;278:579–585.

28. Ahmed SM, Maurana CA, Engle JA, Uddin DE, Glaus KD. A method for assigning authorship in multiauthored publications. *Fam Med.* 1997;29: 42–44.

29. Baughman AL. Invited commentary: what can we infer from author order in epidemiology? *Am J Epidemiol.* 1999;150:663.

30. American Dietetic Association Editorial Manager Web site. Available at: http://www. editorialmanager.com/adaj. Accessed June 5, 2006.

31. Bailey CW Jr. Legal issues: intellectual property rights. In: *Scholarly Electronic Publishing Bibliography.* Houston, Tex: University of Houston Libraries; 1996–2001. Available at: http://info.lib.uh.edu/sepb/1copyr.htm. Accessed January 21, 2003.

32. Rozenberg P. Developing a Standard for Legal Citation of Electronic Information. Available at: http://www.murdoch.edu.au/ elaw/ issues/v4n4/rozen44.html. Accessed January 21, 2003.

33. EFF "Intellectual Property Online: Patent, Trademark, Copyright" Archive. Available at: http://www.eff.org/ pub/Intellectual_property/#files. Accessed January 21, 2003.

34. The Center for Advanced Research and Study on Intellectual Property (CASRIP) of the University of Washington School of Law. Available at: http://www.law.washington.edu/casrip. Accessed June 21, 2006.

35. US Copyright Office, Library of Congress. Available at: http://lcweb.loc.gov/copyright. Accessed June 20, 2006.

36. Draper AK. The principles and application of qualitative research. *Proc Nutr Soc.* 2004;63:641–646.

37. Abusabha R, Woelfel ML. Qualitative vs quantitative methods: two opposite approaches that make a perfect match. *J Am Diet Assoc.* 2003;103: 566–569.

38. Brown D. Open-access journals offer a new way of publishing. *J Am Diet Assoc.* 2004;104:1060–1062.

39. Slawson DL, Clemens LH, Bol L. Research and the clinical dietitian: perceptions of the research process and preferred routes to obtaining research skills. *J Am Diet Assoc.* 2000;100:1144–1148.

40. Gardner JK, Rall LC, Peterson CA. Lack of multi-disciplinary collaboration is a barrier to outcomes research. *J Am Diet Assoc.* 2002;102:65–71.

41. Byham-Gray LD, Gilbride JA, Dixon LB, Stage FK. Predictors for research involvement among registered dietitians. *J Am Diet Assoc.* 2006;106: 2008–2015.

42. Trostler N, Myers EF. Blending practice and research: practice-based research networks an opportunity for dietetics professionals. *J Am Diet Assoc.* 2003;103:626–632.

43. Sylvia LM, Herbel JL. Manuscript peer review: a guide for health care professionals. *Pharmacotherapy.* 2001;21:395–404.

44. Soffer A. Proponent view. *Chest.* 1987;91:255.

45. World Association of Medical Editors Web site. Available at: http://www.wame.org. Accessed June 22, 2006.

46. Robin ED, Burke CM. Peer review in medical journals. *Chest.* 1987;91:252–257.

47. Schroter S, Black N, Evans S, Carpenter J, Godlee F, Smith R. Effects of training on quality of peer review: randomized controlled trial. *BMJ.* 2004; 328:673.

48. Calaham ML, Schriger DL. Effect of structured workshop training on subsequent performance of journal peer reviewers. *Ann Emerg Med.* 2002;40: 323–328.

49. Jefferson T, Alderson P, Wager E, Davidoff F. Effects of editorial peer review: a systematic review. *JAMA.* 2002;287:2784–2786.

50. Baxt WG, Waeckerle JF, Berlin JA, Callaham ML. Who reviews the reviewers? Feasibility of using a fictitious manuscript to evaluate peer reviewer performance. *Ann Emerg Med.* 1998;32: 310–317.

51. Rennie D. Guarding the guardians: a conference on editorial peer review. *JAMA.* 1986;256:2391–2392.

52. Relman AS. The NIH "E-Biomed" proposal—a potential threat to the evaluation and orderly dissemination of new clinical studies. *N Engl J Med.* 1999; 340:1828–1829.

53. Smith R. Editorial: a beginning that should lead to complete transparency. *BMJ.* 1999;318:4–5.

54. Byham-Gray LD, Gilbride JA, Dixon B, Stage FK. Evidence-based practice: what are dietitians' perceptions, attitudes, and knowledge? *J Am Diet Assoc.* 2005;105:1574–1581.

55. Lacey K, Pritchett E. Nutrition care process and model: ADA adopts road map to quality care and outcomes management. *J Am Diet Assoc.* 2003;103:1061–1072.

56. Laramee SH. Evidence-based practice: a core competency for dietetics. *J Am Diet Assoc.* 2005; 105:333.

57. Greenhalgh T. How to read a paper: statistics for the nonstatistician. I: Different types of data need different statistical tests. *BMJ.* 1997;315:364–366.

58. Godlee F, Pakenham-Walsh L, Ncayiyana D, Cohen B, Packer A. Can we achieve health information for all by 2015? *Lancet.* 2004;364:295–300.

59. The Cochrane Library. The Cochrane Collaboration Web site. Available at: http://www.cochrane.org. Accessed June 22, 2006.

60. American Dietetic Association Evidence Library Web site. Available at: http://www. adaevidencelibrary.com. Accessed June 22, 2006.

CODA

—⧕—

Applications of Research to Practice

32

Bridging Research into Practice

Judith A. Gilbride, PhD, RD, FADA, and Laura Byham-Gray, PhD, RD

The profession of dietetics requires a broad theoretical and applied research base because it is the integration of several disciplines. Since the beginning of the profession, research and its applications have been valued and sought after. In fact, research has been described as the "body" and the "backbone" for the dietetics profession (1); it has been suggested that "stronger links [be] built between research and practice to strengthen [the dietetics] profession [since] research is driven by practice, and practice is supported by research" (2). Unfortunately, registered dietitian (RD) involvement has not changed substantially in the past 20 years, despite an increased focus in the dietetics curriculum and widely publicized research initiatives by the American Dietetic Association (ADA) (3). This chapter explores some ways to bridge the gap between research theory and practice. This chapter—and indeed, this book—has been designed to provide background and technical information that will further the effort to increase the investigative opportunities for RDs.

EMERGENCE OF RESEARCH IN DIETETICS PRACTICE

The discovery of new knowledge is the foundation and framework of our profession (1–5). Research helps RDs develop professionally and allows them to integrate findings into their work. Nutrition professionals who work with the public must keep up to date on nutrition science and be able to interpret scientific research accurately and thoroughly and

correct misinformation (5). In all practice settings, the generation of scientific data supports accurate practice and gives credibility to what practitioners say (1,5).

A research perspective is useful in monitoring ongoing activities in all areas of dietetics and provides evidence that serves as a basis for changing policies, protocols, or procedures to improve the general health of clients. Well-designed studies can also provide data to improve food and nutrition services, to ensure quality, to evaluate systems, to determine effectiveness of medical nutrition therapy, and to substantiate cost savings from dietetics interventions (6). Monsen stated that "research advances practice and allows effective decision-making. In turn, questions arising from practice provide a practical focus for research" (6, p. 459).

The proliferation of nutrition articles in the health and medical journals and the explosion of information on the Internet make targeted reading of research critical for today's busy practitioners. Although evidence analysis summaries and abstracts help in making decisions at the bedside, reflection is important to consider the body of evidence that exists and to determine gaps in our knowledge that affect practice. RDs who want to improve their analytic skills and better understand statistical tests and interpretation of significance (both clinical and statistical) should adopt a disciplined approach to reading the literature.

According to Gehlbach, "the ultimate interpretation and decision about the value of an article rests with the reader" (7). Acquiring the ability to judge the value, methods, and clinical and practical usefulness of research studies can ultimately enhance the care of patients and clients.

What do the studies really say? Are the results relevant to my patients? Here are some suggestions to consider:

- Avoid the abstract, introduction, and discussion unless you are simply scanning the literature or gaining an overall perspective.
- Concentrate on the design and methods section first and determine how the study was planned and executed.
- Analyze what the statistical significance means as well as the clinical (ie, impact on patient care) and practical (ie, relevance to altering practice) implications. Gain confidence in interpreting tables and graphs because they usually summarize the main findings of the study.
- Reflect on the soundness and reliability of the methods and the strengths and weaknesses of the study before you analyze other references from the bibliography and design your own project (7).

Although many questions can be answered from research, job demands, limited resources, and time constraints may hamper investigators' efforts to solve practice problems (8). Practitioners are often so busy concentrating on meeting their routine responsibilities that they have little time to begin a research project or even become involved in an ongoing study. Sometimes practitioners, in their eagerness to solve clinical problems, attempt to incorporate findings that have not been studied and tested adequately (5). Collaborating with faculty in academic settings and finding research mentors have been identified as helpful ways clinical dietitians can increase their participation in research (9,10).

A survey for the ADA Research Committee identified research activities of ADA members and examined trends in research funding, gaps, and priorities. According to the 545 responses of ADA members, dietetics research encompassed nutrition intervention of specific disorders and nutrition support, dietetics education, medical nutrition therapy, outcomes research, and a variety of other miscellaneous areas. Other activities were identified as nutrition research, behavioral and social science research, management research, basic science research, food science research, and general research methods (11).

Dietetics research, based on the understanding of food composition, nutrition, metabolism, and management principles, is used to demonstrate the application of knowledge in the field to help people choose a healthy diet and lifestyle. The ADA set a goal in 1993 to increase member involvement in dietetics research in four practice areas:

disease prevention and health promotion, acute and long-term care, food service, and consumer education (12). Research topics and priorities were established by the ADA Research Agenda (12,13) and are reexamined periodically by the association. The ADA research priorities, recently approved by the ADA Board of Directors (14), are presented in Box 32.1.

BOX 32.1   American Dietetic Association Research Priorities

Core Research Priorities
- Nutrition and lifestyle change interventions to prevent or treat obesity and chronic diseases
- Safe, secure, and sustainable food supply
- Nutrients and systems biology (eg, nutrigenetics and nutrigenomics)

Dietetics-Specific Research Priorities
- Nutrition care process and health outcome measures
- Delivery and reimbursement of dietetics services
- Dietetics education and retention

Source: Data are from reference 14.

ADA's emphasis on research in dietetics has led to the generation of the ADA's online Evidence Analysis Library (EAL) (http://www.adaevidencelibrary.com) and the formation of a dietetics practice-based research network (DPBRN). This new collaborative model has emerged to involve more practicing clinical RDs in the research process, whose purpose is to "conduct, support, promote, and advocate research in practice-based settings" (15). The DPBRN exemplifies how practitioners can become involved in research and add to the body of dietetics literature while being mentored (16).

Practice-based studies can document dietetics and assess the effectiveness of nutrition procedures and treatment (17–22). Once effectiveness is determined, it is possible to evaluate the costs of intervention procedures and measure those costs against the efficacy of outcomes. Outcome evaluation will keep dietetics competitive as a profession (21,23). The need for more nutrition science has also been addressed by the National Institutes of Health (NIH) through increased support of randomized controlled nutrition trials, often with required input from RDs. In this era of shrinking financial resources in health care, the evaluation of the provisions of dietetics care and intervention can demonstrate the value of nutrition services in competing for limited funds (24).

Scholarly activities begin with a strong foundation in research. The ADA Standards of Education support the development of research skills by dietetics students (25), including a basic knowledge of research methods, needs assessments, and outcomes research and in-depth knowledge of the scientific method and quality improvement methods. Educators have initiated novel approaches to applied research skills, heeding the call to increase research content in curriculums (9,10,26). The criteria for evaluating dietetics education programs rely on the ability of graduates to interpret current research and basic statistics (10,27).

APPLICATION OF RESEARCH TO PRACTICE

Research studies do not always have immediate, practical application; sometimes they build on what was learned in previous studies. The application of sound research principles can confirm impressions or observations about patient care. Research is a systematic process of deductive-inductive reasoning designed to provide answers to questions and to help researchers develop theories (28). Such answers may be abstract and general in qualitative studies; they may be concrete and specific in clinical trials. In both descriptive and analytic research, the investigator uncovers facts and then formulates a generalization based on the exploration, description, and explanation of those facts (29).

Applying research to practice is the central element of evidence-based medicine (EBM). EBM, now more broadly termed as evidence-based practice (EBP), is a model of clinical decision making that uses a "systematic process to integrate the best [research] evidence with clinical expertise and patient values to answer a question about one patient's plan of care in order to optimize outcomes" (30). This model incorporates a five-step process for making appropriate patient care decisions, inclusive of writing an answerable clinical question, effectively searching the literature, critically appraising the literature, applying research findings to practice, and evaluating patient and practitioner outcomes. Such methodologies allow the RD to link the best research evidence to clinical decisions and practice. Investigations by Byham-Gray and others (3,31) indicated that EBP is the bridge across the theory-practice gap in dietetics—in other words, the higher the knowledge of EBP among RDs, the greater their level of research involvement.

Linking Research and Practice

The application of research techniques to practice focuses on everyday operations and problem solving (31). Data collection and data interpretation can provide insight and direction for doing collaborative projects with colleagues and health care professionals (32). The cycle of practice-based research begins with questions generated by practice; a workable research question is clarified through an extensive literature search, and the research methods are refined (6, p. 463). Through the design and implementation of the research project, researchers seek to answer unresolved problems in practice. Conducting the project produces new facts that necessitate careful analysis. However, integrating that new information into practice requires determining its practical relevance to current procedures. The final steps are disseminating findings to colleagues and other practitioners and applying the new knowledge to improve practice. Thus, the cycle is completed and starts again as other practice questions are raised and solutions to new, perplexing problems are sought.

The Cycle of Research in Practice

A nutrition intervention study can illustrate the cycle of research. The following discussion illustrates these interactions through the study titled "Medical Nutrition Therapy Lowers Serum Cholesterol and Saves Medication Costs in Men with Hypercholesterolemia" (32).

The Problem

Does medical nutrition therapy (MNT) for patients with hypercholesterolemia lead to a decrease in serum cholesterol and save medication costs?

Clarifying the Question

The investigators developed a protocol in the dietary intervention phase of a clinical trial using an experimental lipid-lowering medication. The dietary protocol required at least two (and a maximum of four) intervention visits with an RD to determine the following:

- Did the MNT sessions lead to a reduction in serum cholesterol level and low-density lipoprotein cholesterol (LDL-C)?
- How many MNT sessions improved LDL-C and outcome?
- Is the cost of treating hypercholesterolemia patients with MNT from an RD substantially less than with lipid-lowering drug therapy?

Conducting the Study

Ninety-five male outpatients with hypercholesterolemia took part in a nutrition intervention program prior to treatment with a lipid-lowering medication. The participants took part in a 6-week to 8-week program using the National Cholesterol Education Program (NCEP) Step I diet. Patients' records were reviewed retrospectively to determine plasma lipid levels at the beginning and end of the program and the number and length of sessions with an RD. Participants returned at weeks 6, 7, and 8 for blood lipid evaluations to qualify for the lipid-lowering drug therapy using NCEP criteria. Initial and final evaluations for total cholesterol, LDL-C, high-density lipoprotein cholesterol (HDL-C), triglycerides, and weight were recorded. Height, number of RD visits, and estimated RD intervention time (in minutes) were also noted. Costs for the intervention and medication costs were also calculated and compared. Later, a sensitivity analysis was done to calculate cost-effectiveness ratios for MNT. Provision of MNT varied for differing RD consultation charges.

Intervention

The MNT protocol was administered by an RD in at least two 60-minute and two 30-minute sessions. A 4-day food record was reviewed at each visit, and appropriate recommendations were made based on the NCEP guidelines.

Interpreting and Determining Relevance to Practice

Findings indicated a marginal difference between the number of visits and change in LDL-C. By estimating cost savings by avoiding medications, researchers concluded that three or four sessions with a RD over 7 weeks were associated with a reduction in serum cholesterol and cost savings. Continuation and expansion of an outpatient intervention program is indicated by these findings to help patients reduce cholesterol levels. A case for sufficient counseling sessions by an RD could be supported by data generated by this study.

Dissemination of Findings and Application to Practice

The findings were shared with the intervention team and administrators in the lipid clinic. As research results are incorporated into clinical practice, more questions arise that warrant additional study. In this case, the investigators raised two questions:

- Are individuals who do not respond to MNT in need of more intense intervention, or are they resistant to diet?

- What are the optimal number and frequency of intervention visits to RDs to maintain normal lipid levels?

Thus, new research questions are devised and the practice-research-practice cycle continues.

Related or Follow-up Studies

Several studies have been conducted with patients who receive MNT as part of the intervention for lipid disorders. Some studies have evaluated diet alone, and others have considered diet, exercise, and medication for treating patients with hypercholesterolemia (33). The researchers made recommendations for doing a cost-effectiveness analysis in a clinical setting, including a well-controlled pilot study and detailed documentation for doing a prospective economic analysis. Follow-up studies were conducted to examine the long-term outcomes for these patient populations (34).

READING RESEARCH LITERATURE

RDs should look for ways to integrate research findings into practice and carefully weigh the scientific evidence. When reading and examining reports, RDs should ask themselves the following questions: "Are there practical applications for these investigative findings?" "What is the impact of this study on patients or the setting?" "Can I apply this information to my setting?" Such questions are the foundation of EBP (29).

Knowledge of research methods is required to understand scientific articles (35). Critical analysis is useful when reading investigative reports and articles to determine whether the purpose and need of the study are supported, the methods are appropriate, the conclusions indicate accurate interpretation of the data, and the references are well chosen and up-to-date. Some research studies may contain limitations or gaps in knowledge. Practitioners should evaluate the quality of each report and determine whether the study has weaknesses that limit its application to a particular health care setting. After a literature search involving a myriad of information sources, the clear clinical question can be further refined to include the patient or problem; the intervention (ie, cause, prognostic factors, and treatment); the comparison intervention, if appropriate; and the outcomes to be measured. The ADA uses a Quality Criteria Worksheet, available as part of the EAL, that can assist the practitioner with the appropriate questions for guiding the critical appraisal in relation to analyzing the study's relevance and validity to practice (36). (See Chapter 12.)

To develop a framework for investigating nutrition intervention, grounded research theory—an inductive approach to understanding a phenomenon built on actual data—can be employed to collect data about the patient population, the institution, and the community. (See Chapter 6.) This information is vital in planning and testing the most efficient and effective delivery of nutrition services. An instrument can be developed to collect pertinent information, or one that incorporates the nutrition care process can be adapted to a specific setting. Questions such as the following can be asked:

- What is the population serviced by this institution or agency (eg, numbers, age, gender, or economic status)?
- What are their nutrition needs (eg, diagnosis, health status, or mobility)?
- What resources are available to help deliver nutrition services (eg, infrastructure, time, funds, personnel, or other health care professionals)?

In the past two decades, the number of randomized clinical trials that include nutrition has increased. Research sponsored by the NIH and pharmaceutical companies has prompted RDs to assume the roles of study managers and coordinators (37), investigators in clinical research centers (38), and employees in independent research organizations (39). RDs who are entering these positions or embarking on research in clinical settings can benefit by perusing the ADA's EAL or other systematic databases; these resources help the investigator review the published research to determine the clinical relevance of treatment protocols before changing or testing them (13). Data should be carefully scrutinized to determine the validity of the study, the controls, and the relevance to clinical and patient outcomes for one's individual setting.

Research to Measure Practice

Documentation and measurement of practice standards can provide evidence of the effectiveness of nutrition care. Standards of practice and evidence-based guidelines (40,41) are intended to help RDs make decisions on how various nutrition-related conditions are most effectively prevented and treated. If effectiveness is not demonstrated, the findings can provide a framework for further study that changes practice and produces more positive outcomes.

EXAMPLE TO MEASURE PRACTICE. A descriptive study examined changes in health and lifestyle factors in persons with type 2 diabetes during a 6-month period with counseling from RDs. The sample consisted of 244 adults with type 2 diabetes from 31 sites who were referred for nutrition counseling by physicians. Traditional diet counseling, glycemic control, coronary heart disease risk, self-management behaviors, and quality of life were measured with participants at baseline, at 3 months, and at 6 months. Using analysis of variance and other statistical tests, researchers found that these variables plus weight and body mass index (BMI) improved substantially between baseline and 3 months and baseline and 6 months for the participants. These findings suggested that ongoing intervention and nutrition counseling are needed to support continuous clinical improvements. This study indicates the value of outcome measures in documenting the effectiveness of MNT among adults in a variety of health care settings (42).

Research to Change Practice

Research is useful to monitor activities or procedures, solve problems, and change practice by finding a better way to deliver nutrition services.

EXAMPLE TO CHANGE PRACTICE. A clinical study investigated whether body fat percentages estimated from BMI could accurately assess nutritional status in individuals with cystic fibrosis. Thirty-five patients agreed to participate in a comparison of four methods of estimating the percentage of body fat: the reference standard of whole-body bioimpedance, BMI, skinfold thickness, and leg-to-leg bioimpedance. A food frequency questionnaire and a physical activity questionnaire were also used to rank participants according to energy, fat, fatty acid, and cholesterol intakes. Using descriptive statistics and correlation coefficients to compare methods of body composition, the investigators found BMI to be a good indicator of nutritional status compared with whole-body bioimpedance. They concluded that RDs can use BMI as a reliable, easy-to-use indicator to assess nutritional status of adults with cystic fibrosis (43).

Research to Document Effectiveness

More and more research studies and projects exemplify the documentation of patient and cost outcomes when MNT is provided by RDs. The advent of EBP has made a difference in assessing the effectiveness of RDs who deliver MNT to individuals with chronic diseases (38). Early intervention and monitoring of patients can help reduce the incidence of diabetes, cardiovascular disease, and cancer (38,44,45). Besides EBP, the adoption of the nutrition care process in dietetics helps to solidify a strong foundation for research in the profession. Use of the nutrition care process encourages RDs and dietetics students to increase the body of dietetics research through the measurement of outcomes (46).

EXAMPLE OF EFFECTIVENESS IN PRACTICE.
The systematic collection of a body of scientific evidence can be used to incorporate new approaches into dietetics practice. A systematic review was done by an ADA Evidence Analysis Working Group to answer the question, Which predictive equation works best to estimate the metabolic rate of adults, and how accurate is it? Four predictive equations—Mifflin-St Jeor, Harris-Benedict, Owen, and World Health Organization/Food and Agriculture Organization—for measuring resting metabolic rates (RMR) in healthy nonobese and obese adults were compared. The Mifflin-St Jeor equation was the most likely equation to estimate RMR to within 10% of measurement. The working group advised practitioners to use clinical judgment when selecting any method to assess individuals or when generalizing to ethnic and age groups underrepresented in the research on this topic. The working group recommended that indirect calorimetry can be an important technique when predictive equations fail an individual in a clinical meaningful way (47).

EXAMPLE OF EFFECTIVENESS IN PRACTICE.
Researchers investigated whether, within a low-income population serviced by the Special Supplemental Nutrition Program for Women, Infants, and Children (WIC), breastfeeding was associated with a reduction in Medicaid expenses during the first 6 months of life (48). The study participants included 470 formula-fed infants and 406 exclusively breastfed infants who were tracked prospectively for 6 months to determine WIC costs and Medicaid expenditures. Using economic analyses, the comparison showed that breastfeeding of infants saved an average of $478 in WIC costs and Medicaid expenditures, or $161 after considering the manufacturer's rebate. The researchers concluded that the promotion of breastfeeding in WIC supplemental nutrition programs was cost-effective.

USING RESEARCH REPORTS TO HELP SOLVE PROBLEMS

The earlier discussion of the practice-based research model drew on the study of Sikund, Kashyap, and Yang (32) to illustrate implications of the model. An examination of the other steps to developing a research project helps to clarify further the process of incorporating research into practice.

Planning the Project

When confronting a practice problem, researchers may find that some steps serve to facilitate planning the project and moving it along. These steps include appointing a committee or work group, defining the problem and subproblems, making assignments to committee members, setting a time frame, and organizing ongoing meetings to discuss progress, refocus if necessary, and keep the project progressing toward completion. A subproblem, often used in academic settings to develop the skills of beginning researchers, breaks the problem statement down into small units according to each hypothesis or type of analysis.

EXAMPLE.   Collaborative teamwork is illustrated in the development of a research project by RDs at the Cleveland Clinic. They had made a commitment to outcomes research by putting it in the departmental strategic plan. A team of 11 inpatient RDs worked jointly to examine the effect of their training on patients and patients' families and to identify potential areas for improvement (49).

The problem was to examine the outcomes of patients who received home enteral feeding training. The first step was to establish a committee of RDs to determine the research design, methods of data collection, and responsibilities. The committee met and defined their research objective—to "examine the outcomes of patients who received home enteral nutrition training by dietitians." The first phase included a literature search by committee members to learn what had been reported and to refine the project design.

RDs were trained on how to collect and document patient outcomes to ensure that consistent and accurate data were obtained. The follow-up telephone survey was drafted so that the same information was collected on all patients and their caregivers. The project was completed in 1 year, with meetings held at intervals during that time. When the project was completed, the team disseminated the results to their colleagues at a meeting and to other health providers in their institution through an agreed-upon outcomes report format and gave presentations to the nurses and physicians. Braga and colleagues (50) have done a related study that documents improved outcomes.

Defining the Problem

The research project begins with a clearly written and definitive practice question that is specific to what will be measured. Using the EBP framework, the practice question may contain four critical components: statement of the patient or problem of interest (P), the intervention (I), the comparison with a control group (C), and the measured outcomes (O). The following is an example of a practice-based question related to nutrition and chronic kidney disease (CKD): Does a modular supplement (I) increase serum albumin levels (O) higher than a nutritionally complete product (C) does in patients on maintenance dialysis (P)? (24). Research begins with a problem or question, that is, what one wants to know about one's practice that would be useful. The question should be clearly defined at the outset and should have an answer that is measurable. After putting the question in writing, the practitioner should work on refining and clarifying it. With further thought, the question usually expands and evolves into a broader statement; however, an effort should be made to tighten and focus the problem and allow measurement of very specific variables. Coulston (51, p. 30) summarized three prototypical formats for research questions in clinical dietetics practice:

- What is the nutritional status of patients with, or at risk of developing, specific diseases?
- What are the nutrient requirements of patients with specific diseases, and how do these requirements differ from the requirements of the healthy population?
- What is the efficacy of nutrition intervention: in the prevention of disease, as adjunctive therapy, as primary treatment for specific diseases?

The Literature Search

Literature related to the selected problem provides the foundation for the planned study. A review of the literature provides ideas for methodology and shows how other researchers have handled similar questions. For RDs embarking on new ventures, scientific databases and systematic reviews have greatly expanded access to current investigations and researchers worldwide. Searching evidence-based resources is an efficient way to survey the literature in order to locate the strongest research evidence; examples of resources include EAL, the National Guidelines Clearinghouse, American College of Physicians Journal Club, Evidence-Based Medicine Reviews, Cochrane Database of Systematic Reviews, and Database of Abstracts of Reviews of Effectiveness (DARE) (30).

In reviewing the literature, researchers may find it advantageous to begin with the EAL to determine what questions have been asked and to discern the gaps in the research related to dietetics practice. Such reviews may pose additional questions that help researchers clarify the problem and develop the study (eg, Can this information help solve the problem?). A literature review sometimes provides the information that answers the question without further study. This is an efficient use of existing research.

Another useful question is whether there is a theoretical model that can be used to study the problem. Some studies may provide such a model and eliminate some steps in the research process. Researchers should determine whether the information in the literature can be modified or adapted for the case in question. Other models, findings, methodologies, or instruments may be discovered through the literature review and discussion with peers—especially peers with research experience—that would be appropriate for the study under consideration. Collaborative partnerships have been devised for joining professionals in educational institutions, research centers, and practice settings to conduct projects that benefit the community served (38,42–45).

Implementing the Plan

After developing the question and conducting the literature search, researchers select a design for the study. Preparation of a proposal or research protocol is necessary to delineate clearly the procedures and processes for data collection. A pilot study is useful to test for any problems in the methodology and provide an opportunity to make adaptations prior to undertaking the larger investigation.

Analysis of Results

The procedures for analysis of data should be planned at the beginning of the study, not after the data are collected. In conducting research in the practice setting, researchers may find that resources for collection, analysis, and interpretation of data are limited. Researchers may need to simplify the process to complete the project with the resources available in the health care setting. Assistance can often be obtained from a statistician or an academician interested in practice-based research. Researchers need to be careful of certain pitfalls in interpreting data: inaccurate observations, poor reasoning, overgeneralization, selection bias, and selective observations (7,28).

BARRIERS TO QUALITY RESEARCH

Despite the concerted effort to enhance and increase research involvement, RDs still have limited activity in the research process (3,52). Some of the factors that affect dietitians' research involvement are related to their level of education, research knowledge and skills, areas of practice, and perceptions, attitudes, and knowledge of EBP. Nonetheless, there are a number of barriers to conducting research, and they are well documented in the literature (3,31). Approaches to overcome some of the barriers to research involvement are outlined here.

OVERCOMING BARRIERS TO RESEARCH IN THE PRACTICE SETTING

Getting started with research in the practice setting is the first giant step. Reading the research literature and one's own curiosity help generate ideas. Identifying possible questions to address is a good starting point. Assessment of the needs of the population and the resources available to implement investigations are crucial to productive planning. Creativity and imagination are useful tools to assist with conducting research and managing the barriers that may impede implementation of practice-based research projects. These barriers include time, staffing, money, permissions, and knowledge.

Time Constraints

Time must be found to conduct practice-based research. Unfortunately, sufficient time for research generally needs to be carved out of an already full schedule. An evaluation of existing responsibilities to determine whether some can be simplified, delegated, or eliminated may open up some blocks of time. Consulting evidence-based resources, in which the content is already critically appraised, may assist the practitioner in staying abreast of emerging research findings—an especially helpful technique when time is limited. Reading articles on time management may help with this task. Incorporating professional reading time or journal clubs into daily activities is positive time management. It not only helps keep the practitioner current about professional development but also helps generate research ideas. However, a willingness to devote some personal time to the early development of a research investigation is usually necessary.

Staffing Constraints

Staff members may not be available or interested in assisting the principal investigator when she or he is planning a research project. Enlisting other staff members to collaborate in at least part of the project is crucial. It may be easier to motivate staff members if the investigation has the potential to make their jobs easier or more efficient. Other health care personnel within an institution may be interested in the project, and volunteers or students sometimes may be eager to participate.

Money Constraints

A practitioner must recognize that funds generally are not allocated for his or her first efforts at research. Selecting data that are readily available is desirable. Some pertinent questions to ask include the following: Can any established laboratory values be used as end points? Are data analysis systems in place in the institution? Working through a pilot study can be an excellent way to learn how to use an existing data analysis program. When planning the project, researchers should be careful not to exceed available resources. If the investigator must input data manually, the study design should be consistent with this limitation. Even though new investigator funds are limited, occasionally institutions or dietetics-related groups contribute funds for projects that can advance practice or improve systems of care.

Need for Permission and Cooperation

Implementing any research necessitates permission from supervisors or superiors. Reorganization of duties or staffing must be authorized. Cooperation and permission are needed to make use of facilities such as computer time. Permission from physicians, patients, and internal review boards is necessary for human subject research. To protect patient privacy, Health Insurance Portability and Accountability Act regulations must be adhered to. The practitioner must go through the appropriate channels to organize the project, or the barriers could lead to frustration. Explaining the potential benefits of the study or the potential for higher productivity will often encourage cooperation from the institutional or agency administration.

Knowledge Constraints

Learning how to conduct research is essential for success. Taking a course or courses is a good way to learn. However, reading research literature and talking with researchers is also very helpful. Many people are afraid to initiate investigations, but involvement usually builds confidence. Published and tested protocols and validated practice guidelines are useful for developing a research project. Researchers often share their experiences in developing and conducting research projects in the hope that by revealing potential problems, they can help other practitioners to avoid some of the pitfalls and to develop and implement successful designs. The DPBRN is one avenue for reaching out to other investigators for practical advice and encouragement; one could also consult with dietetics research faculty members from local universities.

SUGGESTIONS FOR FUTURE RESEARCH

A vast array of topics (5,13,14) could be studied by practitioners to improve practice and open up new vistas for the profession. The following research topics might be addressed to expand the body of research literature in dietetics:

- Documentation of clinical practice and assessment of the effectiveness of MNT in selected nutrition-related diseases
- Investigation of the team approach to determine what aspect of care provided by RDs contributed to improved patient or client outcomes
- Comparison of different prevention and treatment models of nutrition intervention and the outcomes for clients over time

- Evaluation of the achievement of quality improvement methods of foodservice systems in various settings
- Participation in joint projects across institutions as a contributor to the DPBRN

CONCLUSION

By incorporating research, investigators can uncover endless opportunities to refine and change dietetics practice. Important to making research a part of an RD's responsibilities are good analytic skills and a commitment to building the evidence base for ethical and scientific dietetics practice. RDs should contribute to the advancement of the profession by reading critically, designing and executing studies carefully, and disseminating findings broadly.

REFERENCES

1. Smitherman AL, Wyse BW. The backbone of our profession. *J Am Diet Assoc.* 1987;87:1394–1396.
2. Monsen ER. New practices and research in dietetics: the 1988 journal. *J Am Diet Assoc.* 1988;88:15.
3. Byham-Gray LD, Gilbride JA, Dixon LB, Stage FK. Predictors for research involvement among dietitians. *J Am Diet Assoc.* 2006;106:2008–2015.
4. Sims LS, Simko MD. Applying research methods in nutrition and dietetics: embodiment of the profession's backbone. *J Am Diet Assoc.* 1988;88:1045–1046.
5. Dwyer JT. Scientific underpinnings for the profession: dietitians in research. *Challenging the Future of Dietetics Education and Credentialing Proceedings.* Chicago, Ill: American Dietetic Association; 1993.
6. Monsen ER, ed. *Research: Successful Approaches.* 2nd ed. Chicago, Ill: American Dietetic Association; 2003.
7. Gehlbach SH. *Interpreting the Medical Literature.* 5th ed. New York, NY: McGraw-Hill; 2006.
8. Slawson DL, Clemens LH, Bol L. Research and the clinical dietitian: perceptions of the research process and preferred routes to obtaining research skills. *J Am Diet Assoc.* 2000;100:1144–1148.
9. Shatz PE, Bush-Zurn TJ, Ceresa C, Freeman KC. California's professional mentoring program: how to develop a statewide mentoring program. *J Am Diet Assoc.* 2003;103:73–76.

10. Hays JE, Peterson CA. Use of an outcomes research collaborative training curriculum to enhance entry-level dietitians' and established professionals' self-reported understanding of research. *J Am Diet Assoc.* 2003;103:77–84.

11. Myers EF, Beyer PL, Geiger CJ. Research activities and perspectives of research members of the American Dietetic Association. *J Am Diet Assoc.* 203;103:1235–1243.

12. *The Research Agenda for Dietetics: Conference Proceedings.* Chicago, Ill: American Dietetic Association; 1993.

13. Castellanos VH, Myers EF, Shanklin CW. The ADA's research priorities contribute to a bright future for dietetics professionals. *J Am Diet Assoc.* 2004;104:678–681.

14. American Dietetic Association. *Priorities for Research: Agenda to Support the Future of Dietetics* (April 17, 2007, draft). Distributed in American Dietetic Association Board of Directors meeting packet, May 5–6, 2007.

15. Trostler N, Myers EF. Blending practice and research: practice-based research networks, an opportunity for dietetics professionals. *J Am Diet Assoc.* 2003;103:626–632.

16. Jewell MB. *Level of Participation in the Dietetics Practice-Based Research Network among Members of the American Dietetic Association.* Master's thesis. Newark, NJ: University of Medicine and Dentistry of New Jersey; 2006.

17. Brody RA, Touger-Decker E, VonHagen S, Maillet JO. Role of registered dietitians in dysphagia screening. *J Am Diet Assoc.* 2000;100:1029–1037.

18. Barr SI, McCarron DA, Heaney RB, Dawson-Hughes B, Berga SL, Stern JS, Oparil S. Effects of increased consumption of fluid milk on energy and nutrient intake, body weight, and cardiovascular risk factors in healthy older adults. *J Am Diet Assoc.* 2000;100:810–817.

19. Jonnalagadda SS. Effectiveness of medical nutrition therapy: importance of documenting and monitoring nutrition outcomes. *J Am Diet Assoc.* 2004;104:1788–1792.

20. Pavlovich WD, Waters H, Weller W, Bass EB. Systematic review of literature on cost-effectiveness of nutrition services. *J Am Diet Assoc.* 2004;104:226–232.

21. August DA. Nutrition support research: it is our obligation to do better! *JPEN J Parenter Enteral Nutr.* 2004;28:201–209.

22. Trostler N, Myers EF. Mainstreaming international outcomes research in dietetics. *J Am Diet Assoc.* 2004;104:279–281.

23. Kaye GL. *Outcomes Management: Linking Research to Practice.* Columbus, Ohio: Ross Products Division, Abbott Laboratories; 1996.

24. Byham-Gray LD. Outcomes research in nutrition and chronic kidney disease: perspectives, issues in practice, and processes for improvement. *Adv Chron Kidney Dis.* 2005;12:96–106.

25. *Accreditation/Approval Manual for Dietetics Education Programs.* 5th ed. Chicago, Ill: American Dietetic Association; 2002.

26. Rebovich EJ, Wodarski LA, Hurley RS, Rasor-Greenhalgh S, Stombaugh I. A university-community model for the integration of nutrition research, practice, and education. *J Am Diet Assoc.* 1994;94:179–182.

27. Vaughan L. Research and the dietetics profession: initiating undergraduate students into the culture of research. *J Am Diet Assoc.* 2003;103:815–816.

28. Batavia M. *Clinical Research for Health Professionals.* Boston, Mass: Butterworth Heinemann; 2001.

29. Strauss SE, Richardson WS, Glasziou P, Haynes RB. *Evidence-Based Medicine: How to Practice and Teach EBM.* 3rd ed. New York, NY: Elsevier/Churchill Livingstone; 2005.

30. Byham-Gray LD, Gilbride JA, Dixon LB, Stage FK. Evidence-based practice: what are dietitians' perceptions, attitudes, and knowledge? *J Am Diet Assoc.* 2005;105:1574–1581.

31. Wylie-Rosett J, Wheeler M, Krueger K, Halford B. Opportunities for research-oriented dietitians. *J Am Diet Assoc.* 1990;90:1531–1534.

32. Sikund G, Kashyap ML, Yang I. Medical nutrition therapy lowers serum cholesterol and saves medication costs in men with hypercholesterolemia. *J Am Diet Assoc.* 1998;98:889–894.

33. Naglak MC, Mitchell DC, Shannon BM, Pearson TA, Harkness WL, Kris-Etherton PM. Nutrient adequacy of diets of adults with hypercholesterolemia after a cholesterol-lowering intervention: long-term assessment. *J Am Diet Assoc.* 2000;100:1385–1388.

34. Sikund G, Kashyap ML, Wong ND, Hsu JL. Dietitian intervention improves lipid values and saves medication costs in men with combined hyperlipidemia and a history of niacin noncompliance. *J Am Diet Assoc.* 2000;100:218–224.

35. Glore S. Show me the science. *J Am Diet Assoc.* 2001;101:186.

36. American Dietetic Association Evidence Analysis Library. Available at: http://www.adaevidencelibrary.com. Accessed August 1, 2006.

37. Schmidt L. A new career for dietitians: study coordinators. *J Am Diet Assoc.* 1993;93:749–751.

38. Delahanty LM, Nathan DM. Research navigating the course of clinical practice in diabetes. *J Am Diet Assoc.* 2004;104:1846–1852.

39. Peterson DA, Albers JE, Mertz JR, McCoy RA. Broadening career opportunities in dietetics: employment in independent research. *J Am Diet Assoc.* 1999;99:799–801.

40. Kieselhorst KJ, Skates J, Pritchett E. American Dietetic Association: standards of practice in nutrition care and updated standards of professional performance. *J Am Diet Assoc.* 2005;105:641–645.

41. Blumberg-Kason S, Lipscomb R. Evidence-based nutrition practice guidelines: a valuable resource in the Evidence Analysis Library. *J Am Diet Assoc.* 2006;106:1935–1936.

42. Lemon CC, Lacey K, Lohse B, Hubacher DO, Klawitter B, Palta M. Outcomes monitoring of health, behavior and quality of life after nutrition intervention in adults with type 2 diabetes. *J Am Diet Assoc.* 2004;104:1805–1815.

43. Hollander FM, De Roos NM, De Vries JHM, Van Berkhout FT. Assessment of nutritional status in adult patients with cystic fibrosis: whole-body bioimpedance vs body mass index, skinfolds and leg-to-leg bioimpedance. *J Am Diet Assoc.* 2005;105:549–556.

44. Nasser R, Cook SL, Dorsch KD, Haennel RG. Comparison of two nutrition education approaches to reduce fat intake and serum lipids reveals registered dietitians are effective at disseminating information regardless of the educational approach. *J Am Diet Assoc.* 2006;106:850–859.

45. Fagciglia GA, Whittle KM, Levin LS, Steward LD. A clinical-based intervention improves diet in patients with head and neck cancer at risk for second primary cancer. *J Am Diet Assoc.* 2005;105:1609–1612.

46. Byham-Gray LD. Research: a review of the "body" and the "backbone" of the dietetics profession. *Top Clin Nutr.* 2005;20:2–15.

47. Frankenfeld D, Roth-Yousey L, Compher C, for the Evidence Analysis Working Group. Comparison of predictive equations for resting metabolic rate in healthy nonobese and obese adults: a systematic review. *J Am Diet Assoc.* 2005;105:775–789.

48. Montgomery DL, Splett P. Economic benefit of breast-feeding infants enrolled in WIC. *J Am Diet Assoc.* 1997;97:379–385.

49. Carr-Davis E, Polisena C, Austhof S, Blakely-Adams C, Cook K, DelRoso L, Morris MP, Mueller C, Reardon L, Schupp K, Verdi P, Willis-Hall T. The effectiveness of instruction of home enteral nutrition. *J Am Diet Assoc.* 1997;97:S30.

50. Braga JM, Hunt A, Poppe J, Molaison E. Implementation of dietitian recommendations for enteral feeding results in improved outcomes. *J Am Diet Assoc.* 2006;106:281–284.

51. Coulston AM. Make a career of clinical nutrition research. *Top Clin Nutr.* 1995;10:29–33.

52. Genovese S. *Research Involvement among Members of the New Jersey Dietetic Association.* Master's thesis. Newark, NJ: University of Medicine and Dentistry of New Jersey; 2006.

Index

Page numbers with *b* indicate boxes; page numbers with *f,* figures; and page numbers with *t,* tables.

453